GENERAL SURGICAL OPERATIONS

AF669491

GENERAL SURGICAL OPERATIONS

SECOND EDITION

Editor

Dhiraj Choudhury

MS (Cal) FRCS (Eng and Edin)

Consultant

Department of Surgery

Peerless Hospital and Ruby General Hospital

Kolkata, West Bengal, India

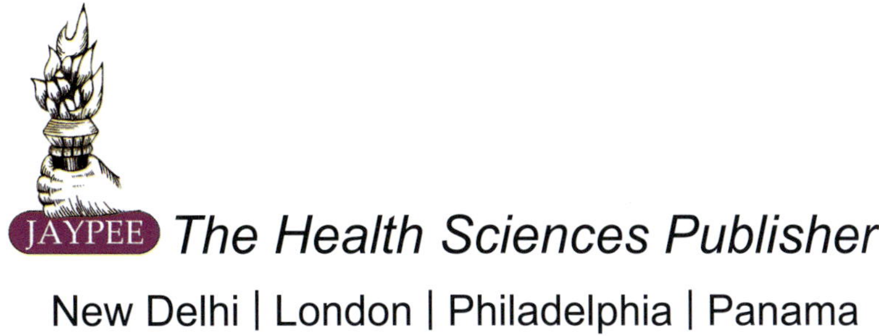

The Health Sciences Publisher

New Delhi | London | Philadelphia | Panama

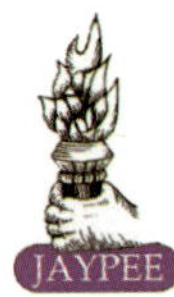

Jaypee Brothers Medical Publishers (P) Ltd.

Headquarters
Jaypee Brothers Medical Publishers (P) Ltd.
4838/24, Ansari Road, Daryaganj
New Delhi 110 002, India
Phone: +91-11-43574357
Fax: +91-11-43574314
E-mail: jaypee@jaypeebrothers.com

Overseas Offices

J.P. Medical Ltd.
83, Victoria Street, London, SW1H 0HW (UK)
Phone: +44-20 3170 8910
Fax: +44(0) 20 3008 6180
e-mail: info@jpmedpub.com

Jaypee-Highlights Medical Publishers Inc.
City of Knowledge, Building 235, 2nd Floor
Clayton, Panama City, Panama
Phone: +1 507-301-0496
Fax: +1 507-301-0499
E-mail: cservice@jphmedical.com

Jaypee Medical Inc.
325, Chestnut Street
Suite 412, Philadelphia, PA 19106, USA
Phone: +1 267-519-9789
E-mail: support@jpmedus.com

Jaypee Brothers Medical Publishers (P) Ltd.
17/1-B, Babar Road, Block-B
Shaymali, Mohammadpur
Dhaka-1207, Bangladesh
Mobile: +08801912003485
E-mail: jaypeedhaka@gmail.com

Jaypee Brothers Medical Publishers (P) Ltd.
Bhotahity, Kathmandu, Nepal
Phone: +977-9741283608
E-mail: kathmandu@jaypeebrothers.com

Website: www.jaypeebrothers.com
Website: www.jaypeedigital.com

© 2017, Jaypee Brothers Medical Publishers

The views and opinions expressed in this book are solely those of the original contributor(s)/author(s) and do not necessarily represent those of editor(s) of the book.

All rights reserved. No part of this publication may be reproduced, stored or transmitted in any form or by any means, electronic, mechanical, photocopying, recording or otherwise, without the prior permission in writing of the publishers.

All brand names and product names used in this book are trade names, service marks, trademarks or registered trademarks of their respective owners. The publisher is not associated with any product or vendor mentioned in this book.

Medical knowledge and practice change constantly. This book is designed to provide accurate, authoritative information about the subject matter in question. However, readers are advised to check the most current information available on procedures included and check information from the manufacturer of each product to be administered, to verify the recommended dose, formula, method and duration of administration, adverse effects and contraindications. It is the responsibility of the practitioner to take all appropriate safety precautions. Neither the publisher nor the author(s)/editor(s) assume any liability for any injury and/or damage to persons or property arising from or related to use of material in this book.

This book is sold on the understanding that the publisher is not engaged in providing professional medical services. If such advice or services are required, the services of a competent medical professional should be sought.

Every effort has been made where necessary to contact holders of copyright to obtain permission to reproduce copyright material. If any have been inadvertently overlooked, the publisher will be pleased to make the necessary arrangements at the first opportunity.

Inquiries for bulk sales may be solicited at: jaypee@jaypeebrothers.com

General Surgical Operations

First Edition: 2008

Second Edition: **2017**

ISBN: 978-93-5152-520-2

Printed at Sanat Printers

Dedicated to

My Parents

Contributors

Abhijit Chatterjee FRCS
Consultant
Department of Urology
Peerless Hospital
Kolkata, West Bengal, India

Abir Banerjee MS FRCS
Consultant
Department of Surgery
Peerless Hospital
Kolkata, West Bengal, India

AK D'Cruz MS DNB
Chief
Department of Head and Neck Surgery
Tata Memorial Hospital
Mumbai, Maharashtra, India

Alexander H Mirnezami BSc (Hons) BM PCME Phd FRCS Cancer Research UK
Clinician Scientist and Honorary Consultant
Department of Colorectal Surgery
University of Southampton
School of Medicine
Southampton, United Kingdom

C Palanivelu MS MCh MNAMS FACS FRCS (Ed)
Professor
Department of Laparoscopic Surgery
Gastroenterology Medical Centre and Hospital
Coimbatore, Tamil Nadu, India

CS Pramesh MS
Assistant Professor
Department of Thoracic Surgery
Tata Memorial Hospital
Mumbai, Maharashtra, India

Debasish Banerjee MS FRCS Fellowship in Liver Transplantation (UK)
Consultant
Department of Gastrointestinal and Transplant Surgery
Peerless Hospital
Kolkata, West Bengal, India

Dhiraj Choudhury MS (Cal) FRCS (Eng and Edin)
Consultant
Department of Surgery
Peerless Hospital and Ruby General Hospital
Kolkata, West Bengal, India

Dipak Kr Ghosh MS FRCS
Consultant
Department of Surgery
AMRI Hospital
Kolkata, West Bengal, India

Dipankar Sen Gupta MS FRCS
Consultant Surgeon
Department of Gastroenterology
Peerless Hospital
Kolkata, West Bengal, India

Gautam Mukhopadhya MS
Consultant
Department of Head and Neck Surgery
Ruby General Hospital
Kolkata, West Bengal, India

Kalyan Kar MS FRCS
Consultant
Department of Surgery
Ruby General Hospital
Kolkata, West Bengal, India

Kaushik Sen MS
Registrar
National Neuroscience Center
Kolkata, West Bengal, India

Krishnendu Mukherjee MS (Cal) FRCS (Eng) FRCS (Ed)
Consultant (General/Vascular Surgeon)
Belle Vue Clinic
AMRI Hospital
Kolkata, West Bengal, India

Marc D Bullock BM Bch MA (Oxon) MRCS
Clinical Research Fellow and Specialist Registrar
Department of Surgery
University of Southampton
School of Medicine
Southampton, United Kingdom

Niraj Khetan FRCS
Consultant
Department of Surgery
Wrexham Maelor Hospital
Wrexham, United Kingdom

Om Tantia MS
Consultant
Department of Endosurgery
Institute of Laparoscopic Study
Kolkata, West Bengal, India

Parul Shukla MS FRCS
Chief
Department of Gastrointestinal Surgery
Tata Memorial Hospital
Mumbai, Maharashtra, India

Peter J Billings FRCS
Consultant
Department of Surgery
Wrexham Maelor Hospital
Wrexham, United Kingdom

RA Badwe MS
Chief
Department of Surgery
Tata Memorial Hospital
Mumbai, Maharashtra, India

Rahul Dey MS
Consultant Neurosurgeon
National Neuroscience Center
Kolkata, West Bengal, India

Rajesh Mistry MS
Consultant and Head
Department of Thoracic Surgery
Tata Memorial Hospital
Mumbai, Maharashtra, India

RS Rao MS FRCS
Ex-Director and Chief
Department of Surgery
Tata Memorial Hospital
Mumbai, Maharashtra, India

Samik Kumar Bandyopadhyay
MS FICS (USA)
Fellow
Department of Minimally Invasive Surgery
Institute of Laparoscopic Study
Kolkata, West Bengal, India

Satish Rao MS
Consultant
Department of Oncology
Bhatia and Shushrusha Hospital
Mumbai, Maharashtra, India

Saugata Deb MS FRCS
Consultant
Department of Surgery
Ruby General Hospital
Kolkata, West Bengal, India

Subhayan Bera MS FRCS
Consultant
Department of Surgery
Peerless Hospital and BK Roy Research Center
Kolkata, West Bengal, India

Sunanda Roy Mahapatra FRCS
Associate Specialist
Department of General and Colorectal Surgery
Countess of Chester NHS Foundation Trust
Chester, United Kingdom

Vani Parmar MS
Registrar
Tata Memorial Hospital
Mumbai, Maharashtra, India

X Escofet FRCS
Consultant
Department of Surgery
Wrexham Maelor Hospital
Wrexham, United Kingdom

Preface to the Second Edition

I had been overwhelmed by the wide acceptance of the first edition of the book *General Surgical Operations* by medical fraternity all over the world. The feedback that I received prompted me to revise and update it for the second edition by paying special attention to the deficiencies. So, this present edition has been prepared to include a wide range of procedures, which are essential in modern surgical practices. Both conventional and laparoscopic procedures have been given due weightage. This book has been enriched by the outstanding authors from different parts of the world.

This edition has been divided into 19 sections containing 101 chapters. Many new chapters have been added such as Surgery for Liver, Surgery for Portal Hypertension, Principles of Day-case Surgery, Management of Rectal Cancer, Surgery of Adrenals, Parathyroidectomy, and Bariatric Surgery—in view of their growing importance and demand in the current surgical practices. The chapter Management of Rectal Cancer has been updated by the authors, who are devoted to colorectal surgery; and, the chapters under the section Vascular Surgery have been rewritten by the promising surgeons expert in vascular surgery. This edition, like the previous one, presents step-by-step description of the common surgical operations intended for the medical students, postgraduate trainees and practicing surgeons.

Dhiraj Choudhury

Preface to the First Edition

There has been a long-felt need for a compilation of the stepwise procedures of operative surgery for general surgeons and postgraduate trainees. The idea was first suggested to me by Shri Jitendar P Vij (Group Chairman), M/s Jaypee Brothers Medical Publishers (P) Ltd, New Delhi, India, at a meeting in Kolkata. I immediately accepted the offer. The task of mobilizing multiple authors from India and abroad representing various aspects of general surgery was an uphill task. I am glad and relieved that the book has now seen the light of the day.

This compilation is intended to provide concise and step-by-step account of various surgical procedures, supported by diagrams and photographs, essential to general surgeons in their day-to-day practice. It should also be a valuable guide to postgraduate trainees in the field of surgery. This book has a total of 87 chapters covering both conventional and laparoscopic methods used in general surgery. We have tried to describe the various operations in detail so that the surgeon and his team can finish their task by following the steps as necessary.

I have included one chapter on neurosurgery titled Burr Hole Procedures, which a general surgeon is also required to perform occasionally.

Dhiraj Choudhury

Acknowledgments

I am grateful to each of the contributors for the brilliant job done in preparing the comprehensive chapters in spite of their busy schedules. I am also indebted to my colleagues for their suggestions, support and supply of the photographs.

I must thank my wife Gouri Choudhury; sons Dr Prithwiraj Choudhury and Dr Gourab Choudhury; and my grandson Uraan Choudhury, for their encouragement, support and sacrifice of time during preparation of this edition.

Last but not least, my deep appreciation is for Shri Jitendar P Vij (Group Chairman), Mr Ankit Vij (Group President), Mr Tarun Duneja (Director-Publishing), Ms Samina Khan (Executive Assistant to Director-Publishing), Mr KK Raman (Production Manager), Mr Sabyasachi Hazra (Commissioning Editor), Mr Ashutosh Srivastava (Assistant Editor), Mr Himanshu Sharma (Proofreader), Mr Vinod Sharma (Typesetter), Mr Pawan Kumar (Graphic Designer), and the other staff of M/s Jaypee Brothers Medical Publishers (P) Ltd. New Delhi, India, for their help and support.

Contents

SECTION

1

General Principles

CHAPTER

1

Decision Making in Surgery

Dhiraj Choudhury

A successful operative strategy begins with decision making: how to operate; when to operate; when not to operate. The decision should be evidence-based supported by clinical diagnosis, investigations and previous experience. Patients are often referred to surgeon with a provisional diagnosis and results of investigations for operation. Sometimes a decision for further investigations or consideration of an alternative therapeutic option may lead to postponement of operation. It is important on the part of the surgeon to explain the nature of illness, decision to proceed with operation or postpone operation, the benefits of surgery and risk involved, to the patient.

Once surgery is decided, a number of considerations must be addressed.

TIMING

If surgery is the treatment of choice, the question is when to proceed? *Elective operations* are planned routine operations decided from outpatient department. For daycare surgery patients are prepared from clinics, e.g. operations for groin hernias, varicose veins, biopsy, excision of superficial lumps. For operations involving body cavities or patients having medical problems, they have to be admitted 2–3 days prior to surgery.

Emergency operations mean immediate surgery where resuscitation and operation are carried simultaneously. Very few patients seen in emergency require operation within minutes of admission. Penetrating wounds of heart and neck require emergency operation.

Urgent operations are undertaken as soon as possible after resuscitation, e.g. operation for perforated peptic ulcer and acute intestinal obstruction.

PROCEDURE

Procedures standardized to give best results in majority of circumstances, should be followed.

APPROACH

Once the procedure has been decided, the next important decision is selection of type of approach. In the present time, the choice lies between conventional open method or minimally invasive method. The decision should be based on training and experience of the surgeon, availability of facilities and choice of the patient.

CHAPTER

2

Preparations for Operation

Dhiraj Choudhury

PREOPERATIVE PREPARATION OF THE PATIENT

Ideally preoperative preparations should begin as soon as a patient is advised operation following a diagnosis and patient agrees. Assessment of fitness for anesthesia and operation should be given top priority.

Assessment of Fitness

The aim of preoperative assessment of fitness is to improve outcome of operation. It can be carried out in surgical clinics, and in ward, if the patient is admitted before surgery. For daycare surgery, it should be completed in surgical clinics because the patient is admitted on the day of operation. The assessment of the fitness is based on history taking, clinical examinations and appropriate investigations. Patient should be examined both by surgical team and anesthetist. Apart from evaluation of the condition for which operation has been advised, a systemic examination should include cardiovascular system, respiratory system, gastrointestinal system, genitourinary and metabolic system.

Routine preoperative tests should include:

- Full blood count
- Blood sugar
- Renal function
- Clotting profile
- Urine analysis
- Plain X-ray chest
- ECG
- Preoperative serology
- Hepatitis B, HIV.

Grading of patients according to American Association of Anesthesiology (ASA):

- *ASA1*: Normal healthy patient
- *ASA2*: Patient with mild systemic disease
- *ASA3*: Patient with severe systemic disease definite functional limitation
- *ASA4*: Patient with severe systemic disease constant threat to life
- *ASA5*: Moribund patient
- *ASA6*: Brain dead, awaiting organ donation

Routine Preoperative Directions

- *Consent:* Written consent should be obtained containing simple description of the operation, the risk and side-effects accompanying the operation and outcome.
- *Fasting*
  All patients are fasted for general anesthesia as follows:
  - 6 hours for solid food
  - 4 hours for breast milk
  - 2 hours for clear fluid
- *Shaving:* Shaving the operation site before surgery increases the risk of surgical site infection. Ideally it should be done immediately before operation.
- *Marking operation site:* This is important in case of hernia and amputation.
- *Bowel preparations:* For colorectal surgery, patient is put on nonresidual diet for 2–3 days. Complete mechanical bowel wash is given in the morning with peglac.
- *Medication:* Prescribe prophylactic antibiotics, DVT prophylaxis in appropriate cases. Issue special instructions regarding medications like insulin, steroids.

Special Preparations

High-risk Patients

The medical problems most commonly associated with increased surgical morbidity and mortality which require special care are discussed below:

- *Ischemic heart disease*: No elective operation should be done within six months of an attack of acute myocardial infarction.
- Congestive cardiac failure should be adequately controlled before elective operation.
- Cardiac arrhythmias should be treated before surgery.
- Chronic obstructive pulmonary disease (COPD) should be treated by chest physiotherapy, prophylactic antibiotic and bronchodilator before surgery.
- *Diabetes mellitus*: For elective operation blood sugar should be adequately controlled by insulin, diet or oral hypoglycemic before surgery.
- Anemia should be corrected by blood transfusion.
- Obstructive jaundice requires preparation like rehydration, vitamin K injection and infusion of 20% mannitol.

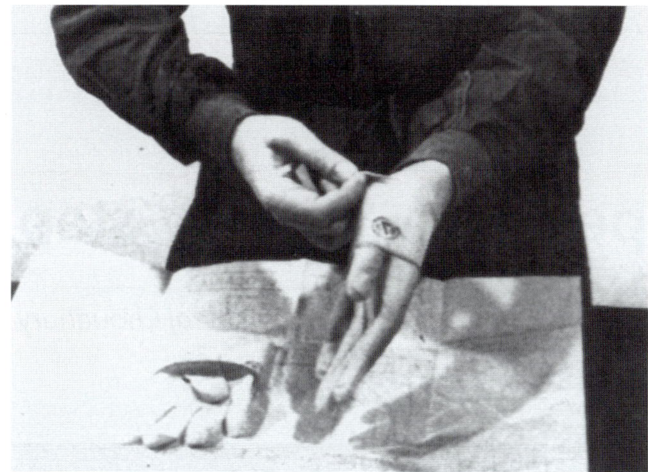

Fig. 2.1 Putting left gloves

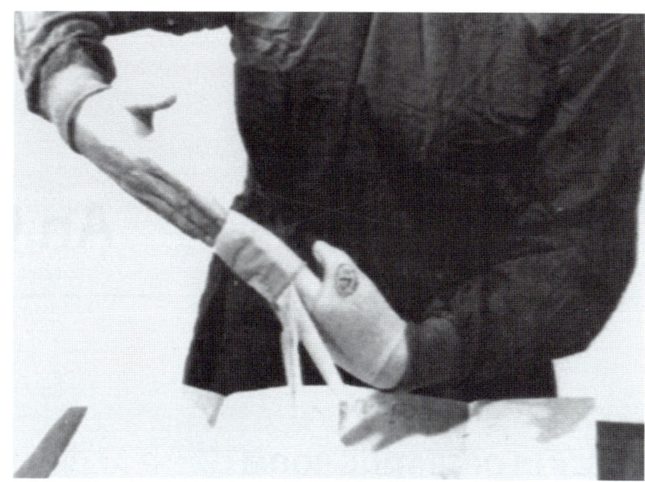

Fig. 2.2 Putting right gloves

PREOPERATIVE PREPARATIONS OF SURGICAL TEAM: SCRUB-UP TECHNIQUE

Entry to Operation Theater

Only members of surgical team and operation theater (OT) staff should be allowed to enter theater from changing room after putting OT dresses, mask, cap and shoes.

Scrubbing

Scrubbing is washing of hands and arms of the surgical team before putting gown and gloves. The aim is to minimize microbial loads on the parts of surgical team members. One should not scrub if he or she has an open wound or infection. All jewellery on hands should be removed before washing. Clean dirt from under nails. The hands are washed systematically with 7.5% povidone-iodine or chlorhexidine. The hands should be dried with sterile towels.

Gowning

The sterile gown is grasped firmly at the neckline and allowed to unfold completely. The arms are introduced in armholes simultaneously. The theater nurse should secure the gown at the neck and the waist.

Gloving

The importance of surgical gloves has been reemphasized in view of hepatitis B and HIV infection. It has been recommended that surgical gloves should not be reused because 50% of them develop perforations not detectable at the time of use. Double gloving is also advised in high-risk cases.

Technique of Putting Gloves

The hands should be well-dried and powdered. Select gloves of correct size. The turned up cuff of the left hand glove is held in the right hand and the glove is slipped on to the left hand (Fig. 2.1).

Now, the fingers of the gloved left hand is slipped into the turned down cuff of the right hand glove and the glove is slipped on the right taking care not to touch the bare right hand with gloved left hand (Fig. 2.2).

Finally, the cuff of the gloves are slipped over the sleeves of the gown without allowing gloved hand to come in contact with bare skin.

CHAPTER

3

An Operation: Step-by-step

Dhiraj Choudhury

CHECK IN OPERATING ROOM

Before induction of anesthesia, the patient should be checked up by surgical, anesthesia and nursing team. The check list should include: Patient's identification, diagnosis, procedure proposed, consent and investigations.

ANESTHESIA

Some forms of anesthesia is required for almost every surgical procedure to prevent pain, minimize stress and help surgical method. The choice of anesthesia may be general with endotracheal intubation, spinal or epidural or local. The choice is made by joint consultation between anesthetist, surgeon and the patient.

PATIENT POSITION

The patient may be placed in any of the following positions:

Supine Position

This is used for operations on face, neck and abdomen (Fig. 3.1).

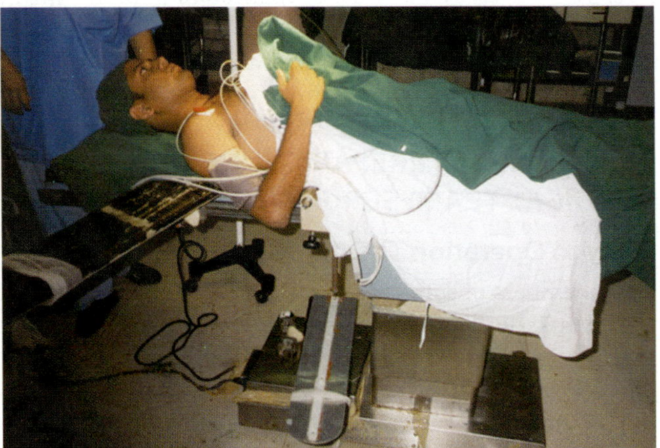

Fig. 3.1 Patient in supine position

Lateral Position

It allows position of extension on right or left side with uppermost arm raised above and in front of head. The center of the table may be angled to improve access. This position is used during operations on kidney, ureter and chest.

Lithotomy Position

This is a supine position with hips and knees flexed and ankles supported with stirrups. This is used during operations on perineum, perianal region and external genetalia.

Trendelenburg's Position (Fig. 3.2)

This is supine position with patient tilted 30° head down. This is used for intrapelvic operations to allow displacement of intestine away from pelvic cavity.

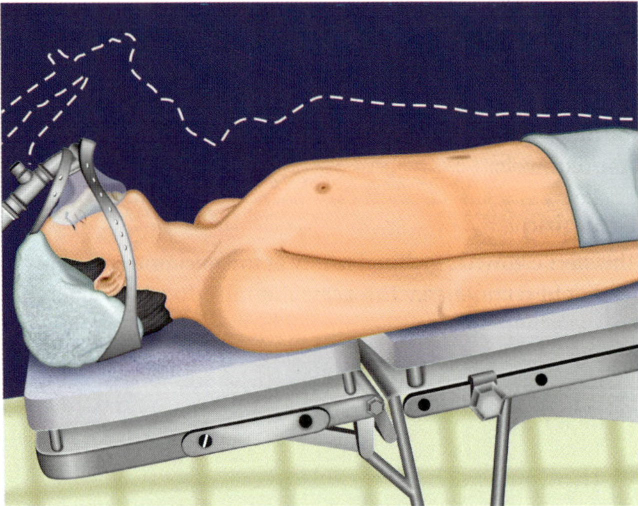

Fig. 3.2 Trendelenburg's position

Lloyd–Davies Position

This is Trendelenburg's position in which legs are widely abducted and hips and knees slightly flexed. This is used for abdominoperineal resection (APR) of rectum for cancer.

Prone Position

This position is required for operation on the back.

Prone Jack-knife Position

Nearly all anal operations can be done in this position.

The patient should be held securely on the operation table and all pressure points should be adequately protected. The diathermy plate should be well-positioned and secured.

SKIN PREPARATIONS

'Prep' and 'Drape'

The prep area should include the operative site and a considerable surrounding area in order to minimize migration of organisms from unclean area. In general, 2% povidone-iodine is applied with a swab on a sponge holding forceps over the prep area. Start application from the line of incision working outwards in continually expanding circles.

Surgical draping consists of covering the area immediately surrounding the operative site with sterile barrier materials (drape). The purpose of surgical draping is to create and maintain a protective zone called sterile field. Drapes can be both disposable or reusable. Draping should allow free access to the whole surgical incision and allow further extension if necessary. The edge of the drape nearest to incision should be struck down on to skin with clips. The diathermy and suction tubes should be firmly attached to drapes.

Position of Surgeon

Usually a right-handed surgeon stands on right side of the patient. During laparoscopic surgery, surgeon stands on left side of the patient.

OPERATIVE TECHNIQUE

Incision

For an open surgery, the ideal incision should:

- Allow ready and direct access to the site of operation
- Be of adequate length
- Allow any change in surgical procedure
- Leave the part as strong as before
- Be parallel to important blood vessels and nerves
- Offer cosmetically acceptable scar.

For best result, place the skin incision along skin crease or Langer's line.

For laparoscopic surgery, skin incisions for insertion of laparoscope and other instruments have been standardized to suit the procedure.

Method of Making an Incision

Hold the scalpel handle in the palm of the hand and rest your index finger along the back of the handle towards the blade (dinner knife position). The blade is pressed into the skin at right angles to required depth and then drawn along parallel to surface. Keep the skin under tension by using thumb and forefinger (Fig. 3.3).

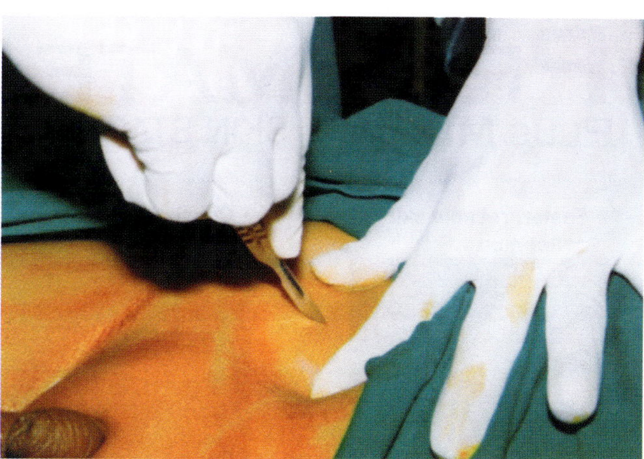

Fig. 3.3 Method of making skin incision

EXPOSURE/DISSECTION

An adequate exposure is essential for safe operations. The subcutaneous fat can be incised with scalpel producing a clean edge or with diathermy knife. Muscles can be divided or split along the fibers. Exposure in the deeper plane requires adequate retraction of wound edges. This can be done by assistants applying retractors or by applying self-retaining retractors.

Dissection in the deepest plane can be blunt dissection with gauze (peanut) or finger, or sharp with knife and scissors. For sharp dissection, anatomy should be well-known.

Hemostasis: It will be described in Chapter 4.

PROCEDURES

The common surgical procedures are:

- Otomy, surgical incision into an organ or cavity, e.g. laparotomy
- Ostomy, surgically created connections between two viscus, e.g. gastrojejunostomy
- Ectomy, removal of a part or all of an organ, e.g. appendicectomy
- Orrhaphy, a repair operation, e.g. herniorraphy
- Pexy, an operation to secure an organ, e.g. orchidopexy
- Plasty, an operation to alter structure or function of an organ, e.g. pyloroplasty.

CLOSURE

Before closure of any surgical wounds (particularly laparotomy, thoracotomy):

- Ensure adequate hemostasis
- Count instruments, mops and gauzes
- Insert a drain when indicated, and check its position.

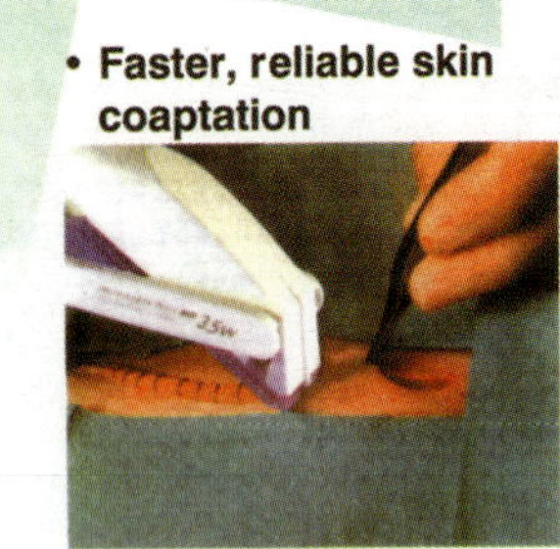

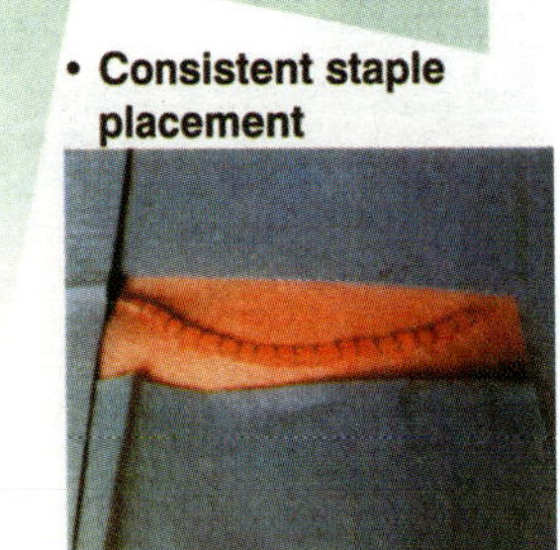

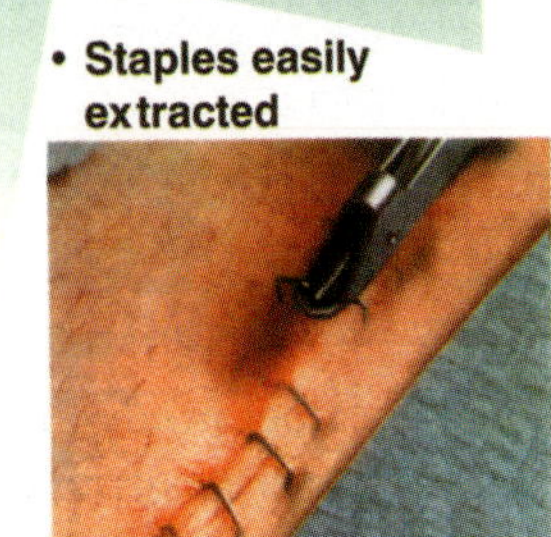

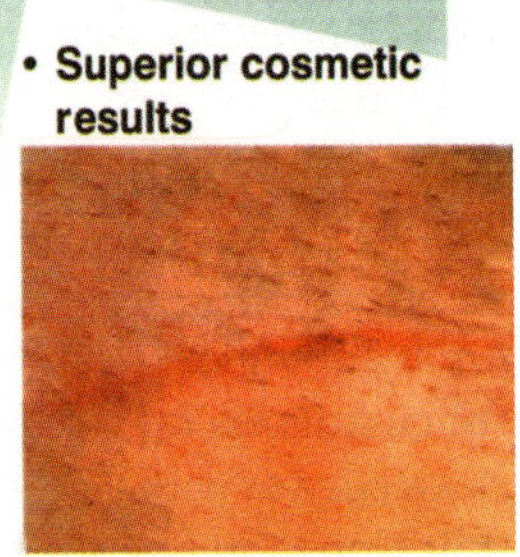

Fig. 3.4 Proximate plus MD skin stapler

Methods of Closure of Skin Wounds

- *By suturing:* With nonabsorbable (silk, ethilon) or absorbable (vicryl) suture materials. This is the traditional method, which will be described in details in Chapter 5.
- *By application of clips:* Mitchel's clips are being used for many years for skin closure, particularly after thyroidectomy. It is simple and cosmetically acceptable.

  Method: The skin margins may be apposed by putting subcuticular sutures before applying clips. The wound edges are held by forceps beyond the point of application of clips and the clips are applied with pressure by Mitchel's clip applicator.
- *By application of staples:* Skin staples are now available (Proximate plus MD skin stapler) for skin closure. It is a faster and reliable skin coaptation. Staples are easily applied and extracted and have superior cosmetic result (Fig. 3.4).
- *Sutureless closure*:
  Micropores, adhesive tapes: Steristrip, ethistrip and more recently microporous films (op-site) have been introduced to be laid across the wound to offer cosmetically better scar. A subdermal or intradermal stitch will reduce destructive forces at the line of incision.

  Tissue adhesive (Glue): Medical tissue adhesive has been produced as a sterile solution of n-butyl-2 cyanoacrylate (e.g. Nectacryl). When applied to cut margins of skin, it rapidly polymerizes into a firm adhesive bond. This should not be used in infected wounds, vascular wounds.

CHAPTER

4

Methods of Hemostasis in Surgery

Dhiraj Choudhury

Bleeding is an unavoidable part of surgery. Minimizing blood loss is an important aspect of surgery which requires adequate steps preoperatively, intraoperatively and postoperatively.

PREOPERATIVE

Identify patients having bleeding diathesis which may be congenital, e.g. hemophilia or acquired, e.g. obstructive jaundice or drug-induced coagulopathy. Adequate steps should be taken to prepare such patients, starting preoperatively.

INTRAOPERATIVE

The *three main techniques* used during operation to stop bleeding are:

- Compression
- Ligation or clipping
- Thermal coagulation.

COMPRESSION

Pneumatic tourniquet, Esmarks bandage is used during surgery of limbs to achieve bloodless field during operation. They should not be used in ischemic conditions.

Direct pressure is a useful means of controlling bleeding until platelet aggregation, reactive vasoconstriction and blood coagulation takes over. Packing bleeding cavity or surface is an useful method to stop bleeding, five minutes of compression can achieve hemostasis.

LIGATION OR CLIPPING

Cut end of blood vessel may be closed with metal or synthetic clips carried on special forceps. This is particularly useful during minimally invasive surgery.

Ligation is obligatory when large vessels are divided (larger than 1 mm caliber). The mouth of the divided vessels is picked up with hemostatic forceps and tied with ligature either absorbable (catgut) or nonabsorbable (silk). This is the commonest method of hemostasis during open surgery.

Ligation in continuity: A free window is created around the vessel through which tips of a hemostat can be introduced. The assistant passes the ligature below the tip of the instrument sitting under the vessel. The ligature can be easily grasped and passed beneath the vessel as the assistant releases the hemostat. The ligature is then tied.

Pedicle ligation: For ligation of a pedicle, it is necessary to dissect it free of surrounding tissues. Two hemostats are placed on pedicle with curves of the jaws facing each other. The pedicles are then divided and both ends of the pedicle are ligated individually.

Pedicle transfixation: If a pedicle contains a significant vessel it is desirable to transfix the pedicle. The vessel is divided after applying two hemostats. Using monofilament suture, a curved needle is passed through the center of one pedicle. The suture is tied first with backhand throws around one side of the pedicle. The free ends of the suture are then passed beneath the hemostat to other side of the pedicle. After the next throw is created and tightened down, the hemostat is removed.

FLUID INFILTRATION

Bleeding can be minimized by infiltrating subcutaneous tissues with 0.9% saline containing 1 in 200,000 adrenaline. This technique is preferred in case of thyroidectomy and perianal operations.

THERMAL COAGULATION/DIATHERMY

Diathermy achieves hemostasis by local intravascular coagulation caused by heat generated by high frequency electric current. It is a rapid valuable means of hemostasis but should not be used for vessels having diameter more than 2–3 mm.

There are two basic forms of diathermy, monopolar diathermy and bipolar diathermy, of which monopolar diathermy is the most commonly used form.

In monopolar diathermy, an alternating current is produced by suitable generator and passed to patient through an active electrode. The current then passes through the tissues and returns via a very large surface plate back to earth pole of the generator (Fig. 4.1).

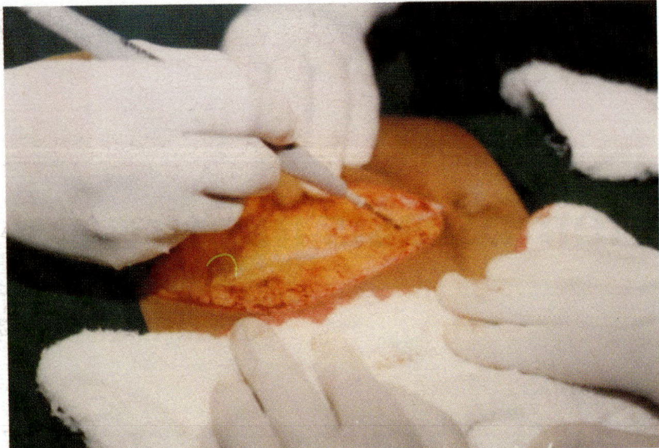

Fig. 4.1 Cutting diathermy

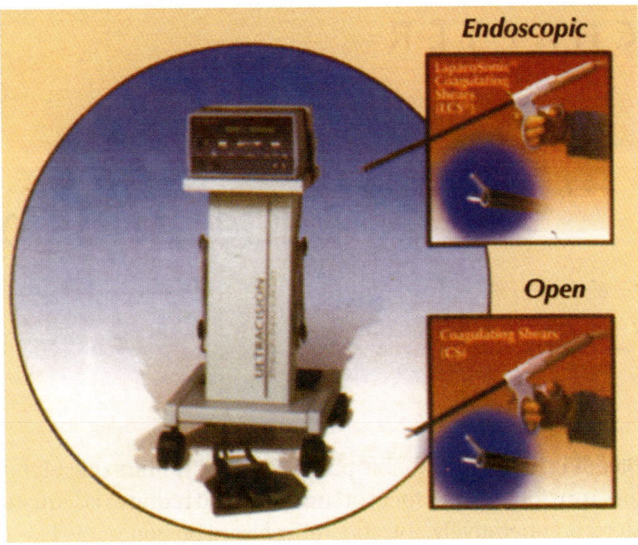

Fig. 4.2 The harmonic scalpel system

In bipolar diathermy the two active electrodes are usually represented by the limbs of a pair of diathermy forceps. This form of diathermy is used when it is essential that the surrounding tissue should be free from either the risk of being burned or having current passed through it. It is safe for patients having pacemaker.

Diathermy can be used for three purposes:

1. *Coagulation*: Sealing of blood vessels
2. *Cutting*: To divide tissues during bloodless surgery
3. *Fulguration*: Destructive coagulation of tissues with charring.

ULTRASOUND

Surgical aspirator: There are various ways in which liver parenchyma may be dissected with minimum blood loss. Cavitron ultrasonic aspirator (CUSA) works by converting electromagnetic energy to mechanical movements.

Harmonic shear (Harmonic scalpel): These are new tools with vibrating blades that oscillate at 50,000 cycles per second, producing heat by friction and resulting in a coagulation process that can seal structures such as small vessels or ducts (Fig. 4.2). Harmonic shears can be used on most of unnamed vessels up to a diameter of 5 mm, above which it is safer to apply clips or ligatures. Advantages of harmonic scalpel are: precise cutting with minimum lateral thermal damage and bleeding, avoidance of electric current, and minimal desiccation of tissues.

LASER

Light amplification by stimulated emission of radiation use photons to excite the chromophore molecules within target tissues generating kinetic energy that is released as heat causing protein denaturation and coagulation necrosis. The neodymium: Yttrium aluminum garnet (Nd: YAG) laser is currently favored to control gastrointestinal hemorrhage from stomach, esophagus, duodenum and for palliative resection of advanced cancer.

Photodynamic Therapy

It works on administration of a target specific photosensitizer that is eventually concentrated in target tissue. This is used to treat different type advanced cancers with minimum blood loss.

LOCAL HEMOSTATS

The general surgeon performs numerous procedures in which a topical absorbable hemostat such as surgicel is an adjunct to control bleeding. The operations include:

- Cholecystectomy
- Repair of trauma to spleen or liver
- Partial hepatectomy
- Herniorrhaphy.

Procedures

Spongostan surgical have particular utility in these procedures all of which involve capillary or small vessel bleeding that is difficult to control by conventional measure.

Removal of the gallbladder leaves an oozing bed. Most often there is generalized persistent ooze that creates a film by blood over the area. Pressure alone cannot control it with any rapidity. Spongostan surgical is placed over the oozing gallbladder bed and pressure is applied for 2–3 minutes. Recently, 1% feracrylum uniheal solution by Themis medicare (Uniheal) has been introduced as a local hemostatic and antiseptic agent. The hemostatic effect is based on formation of Feracrylum-albumin complex.

Fibrin tissue glue works on the conversion of fibrinogen by thrombin to fibrin with crosslinking by factor XIII. The fibrinous network has been used for hemostasis in liver and spleen. Fibrin glue has also been used to control gastrointestinal hemorrhage by endoscopic injection.

CHAPTER

5

Sutures, Ligatures and Knots in Surgery

Dhiraj Choudhury

SUTURE AND LIGATURE MATERIALS

An ideal suture material should:

- Possess good tensile strength
- Cause minimum tissue reaction
- Be easy in handling and application of knot
- Be easily sterilized.

TYPES

Absorbable

- Plain catgut natural monofilament, durability 7–10 days
- Chromic catgut natural monofilament, durability 21–28 days
- Polyglactin synthetic braided (vicryl), durability 60–90 days
- Polyglactin acid synthetic braided (dexon) durability 60–90 days
- Polydioxanone (PDS) synthetic monofilament, durability 180 days
- Polyglecaprone (Filapron) synthetic monofilament durability 90–120 days.

Nonabsorbable

- Silk natural braided
- Linen natural braided
- Nylon synthetic usually monofilament (Ethilon)
- Polypropylene synthetic monofilament (Prolene)
- Stainless steel wire synthetic monofilament or braided.

Advantages of Synthetic Polymeric Suture Materials

- Inflammatory reaction is less
- Strength is predictable
- Absorption is more complete
- Can be monofilament or braided.

SURGICAL KNOTS

A knot is an intertwining of threads for the purpose of joining them. Tying knot is one of the most fundamental techniques of surgery. A single throw (half hitch) forms the basis of most knots used in surgery.

Principles of Knot Tying

- The knot must be firm and secured
- The knot must be as small as possible to minimize foreign materials
- The suture should not be sawed while tying knot
- The suture should not be grasped with artery forceps except when tying a knot
- Use first throw for position and second throw for tension.

Types of Knots

Granny Knot

After applying a single throw, apply a second throw of the same type. This is an unsafe knot (Fig. 5.1A).

Reef Knot

After tying a single throw, apply a second throw of different type. This is simple but reliable (Fig. 5.1B).

Triple-throw Knot

After applying a reef knot, produce a third knot. This is very reliable.

Surgeon's Knot

Apply a double-throw on first loop, to be followed by two single throws. The double throw helps to prevent slacking while second throw is made. It is suitable for large pedicle (Fig. 5.1C).

Aberdeen Knot (Figs 5.1 D to I)

It is applied for tying continuous suture during abdominal closure. A loop is held before the last stitch is applied. After the stitch is completed, a loop of free thread is pulled through the first loop, a further loop is pulled through second and so on, each loop being pulled tight in turn. The tie is secured by passing the free end through the last loop, pulling it tight and cutting it off, leaving a generous free end.

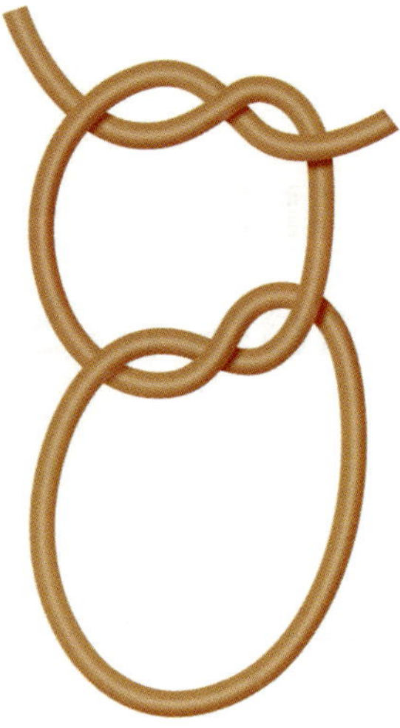

Fig. 5.1A Granny knot

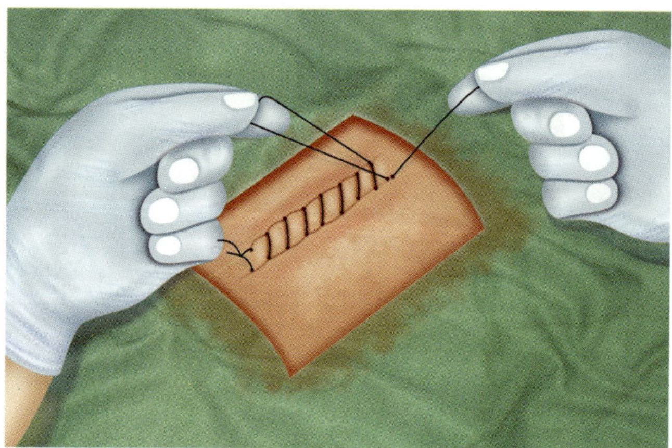

Fig. 5.1D Aberdeen knot a loop is held before last stich

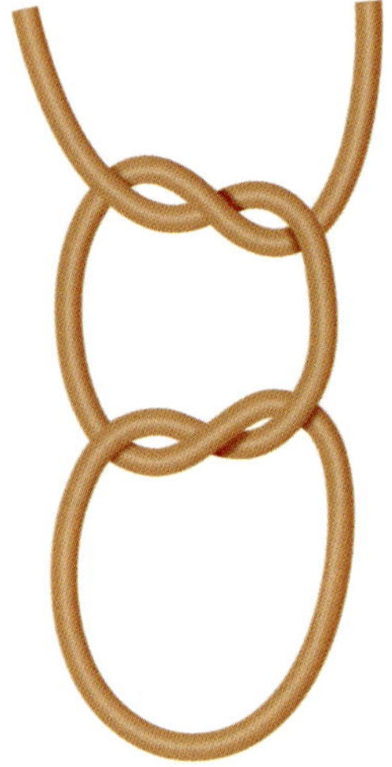

Fig. 5.1B Reef knot

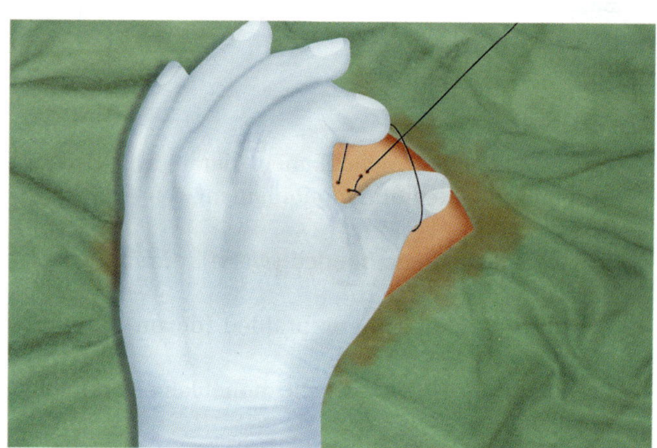

Fig. 5.1E Aberdeen knot continued by pulling a loop of free thread through first loop

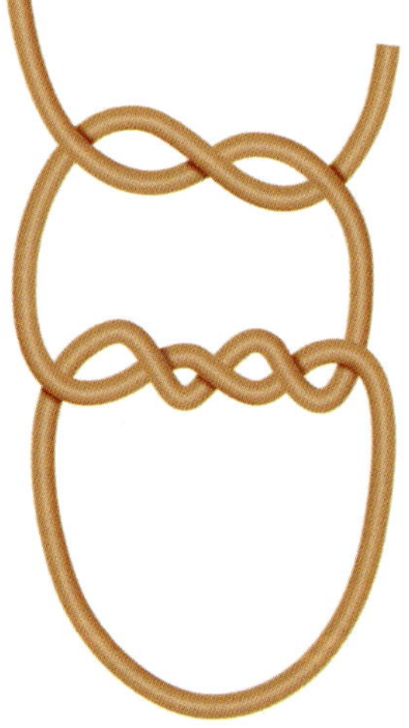

Fig. 5.1C Surgeon's knot

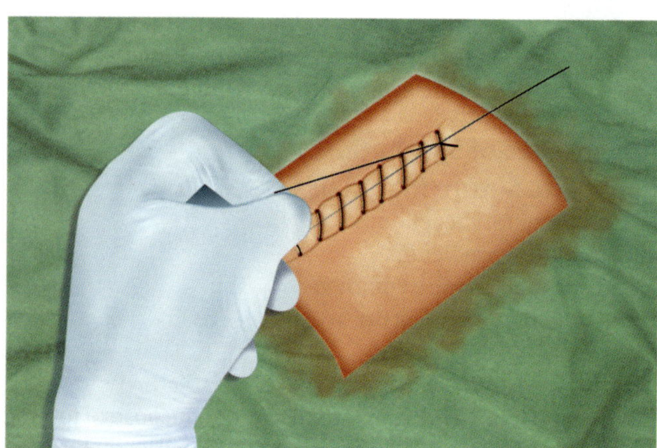

Fig. 5.1F Aberdeen knot continued as in Figure 5.1E

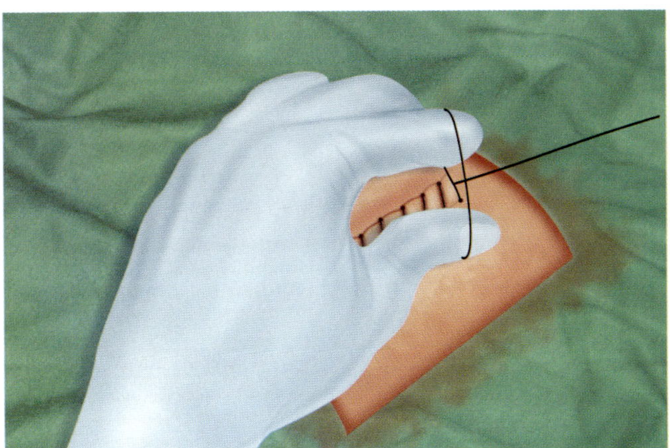

Fig. 5.1G Aberdeen knot continued as in Figure 5.1F

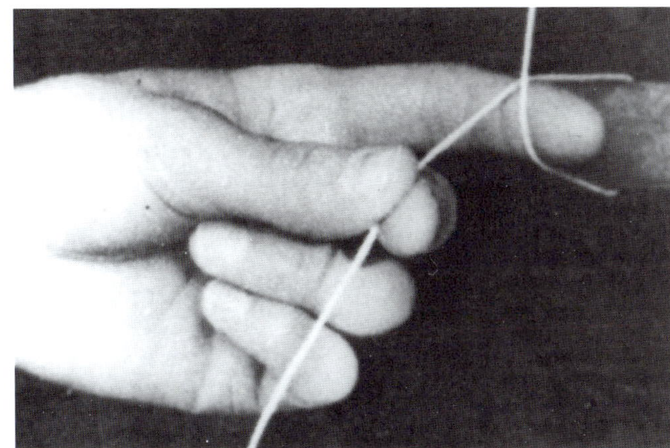

Fig. 5.2A Tying reef knot with left hand

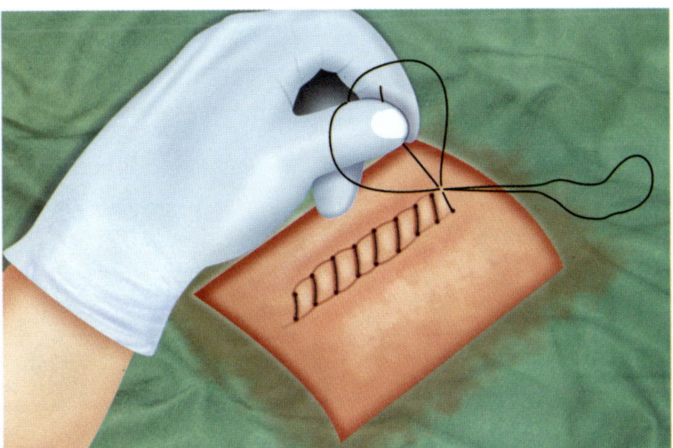

Fig. 5.1H Aberdeen knot continued as in Figure 5.1G

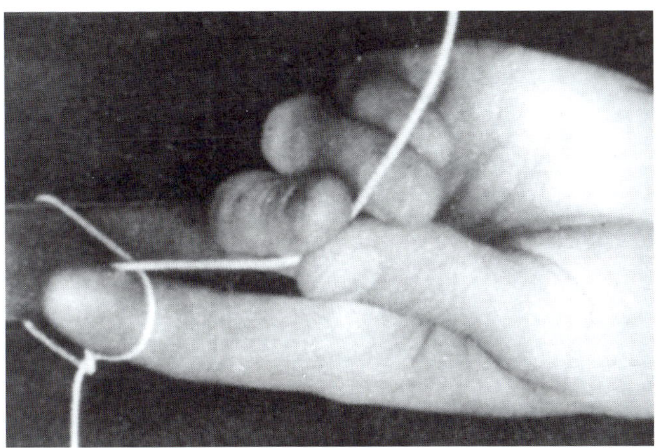

Fig. 5.2B Formation of a loop of short thread

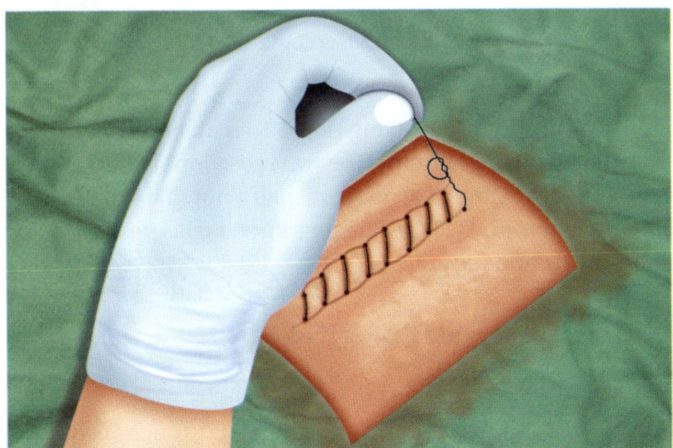

Fig. 5.1I Aberdeen knot completed

Methods of Tying Knots

By Both Hands

This is safest and surest method and should be used while tying knot around vessels in a deep or poorly accessible sites. The three-point technique is important when tying a blood vessel. The surgeon's hand holding two ends of the ligature and the vessel to be ligated should be in a straight line. The type of knot to be applied should be decided on the basis of ligature material used.

By One Hand

Method of tying reef knot with left hand: Hold the short end of the thread between thumb and middle finger of the left hand. A crossing of thread is formed over the left index finger (Fig. 5.2A).

A loop of short thread is drawn under the crossing with left index finger (Fig. 5.2B).

The short end of the thread is now released, drawn under the crossing and recaptured between index and middle finger of the hand to form a single throw/hitch (Fig. 5.2C).

Tighten the hitch by carrying short end towards body and long end away from it. Now hold the short end between thumb and index finger, and lay the thread over middle and ring finger (Fig. 5.2D).

Bring the long end of the thread over palmer aspect of these fingers at the level of distal interphalangeal joints.

Straighten the middle finger in front of the loose thread, so that it passes between middle and ring fingers (Fig. 5.2E).

Slide the fingers out of the loop and you will have second throw (Fig. 5.2F).

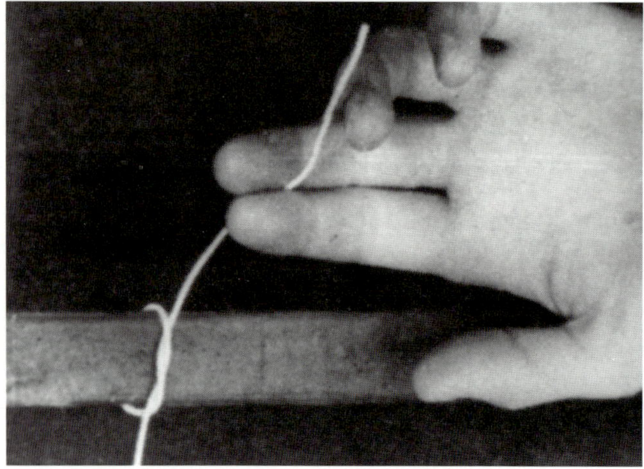

Fig. 5.2C Formation of single throw

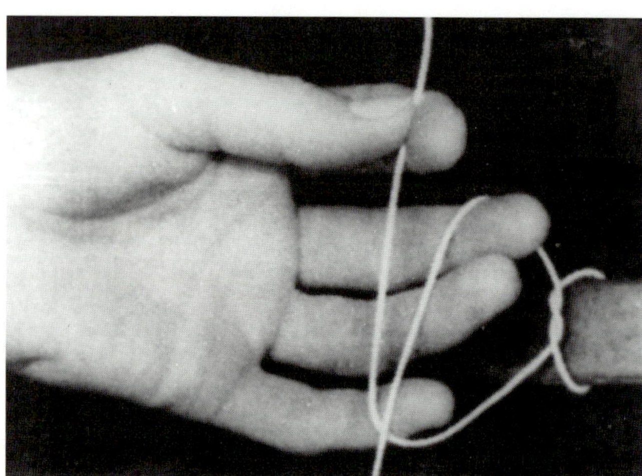

Fig. 5.2D First step in formation of second throw

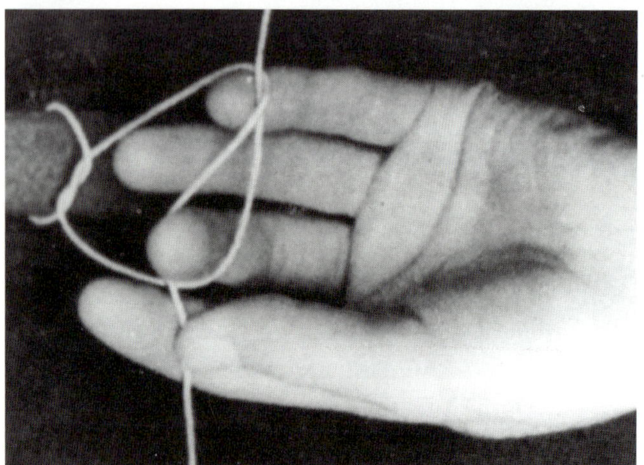

Fig. 5.2E Second step in formation of second row

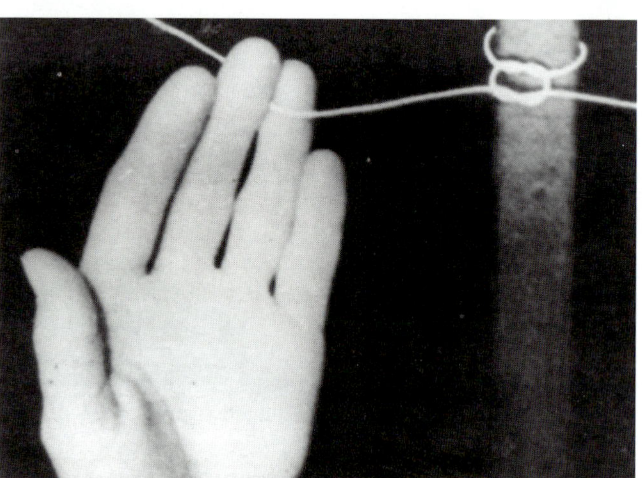

Fig. 5.2F Completion of second throw

By Instrument

Loop the long end of the suture material around the instrument, the instrument being placed over the thread. Grasp the short end at its free end within the jaws of the instrument and pull it through the loop and complete the first hitch. Now form a similar loop around the instrument again placing the instrument over the distal thread, draw it towards the operator and grasp the free end of the short end again, pulling it through to complete classical reef knot. For security, three throws should be used.

Laparoscopic knot-tying

There are two options: Intracorporeal and extracorporeal knot-tying. A general principle of intracorporeal knot-tying is that the needle should 'smile' at the surgeon and the tip of the needle should be at the loose end of the thread, when the loose end is on the right side of the surgeon. This will allow rotation of the needle holder held with the right hand around the left grasper, and the tip of the left grasper will then grab the loose end at the right side and bring it inside the loop.

Extracorporeal knot-tying (Fig. 5.3) is achieved by using a long thread (at least 90 cm). The two most popular techniques are: (1) The creation of an external half-knot that is pushed by a knot-pusher, and (2) the Roeder's knot, that is pushed inside using an atraumatic grasper.

METHODS OF SUTURING SKIN

Closure of Wounds

Suturing should be undertaken using a no-touch technique whenever possible to reduce risk of needle injury.

- Wound edges should be everted
- Wound edges should be slightly gaping
- The knot should be placed to one side of the wound edge
- Knot must be secure.

Types of Skin Closure

Simple Interrupted Suturing

This is gold standard for closure of skin wounds. Apply the stitch 1 mm from the margin and 1 mm from the each other.

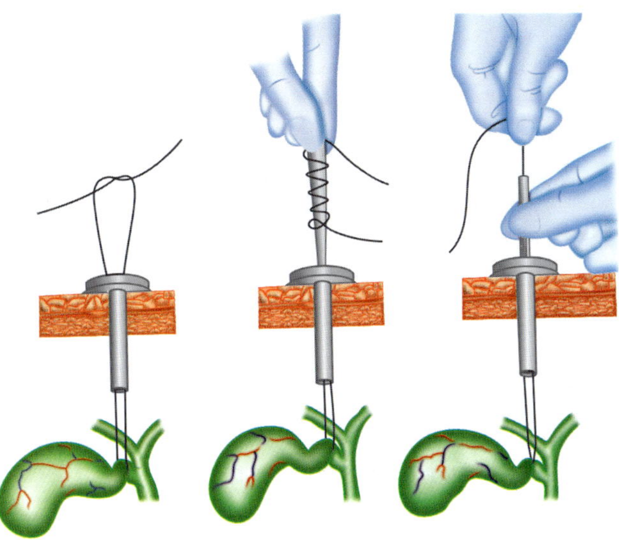

Fig. 5.3 Roeder's knot

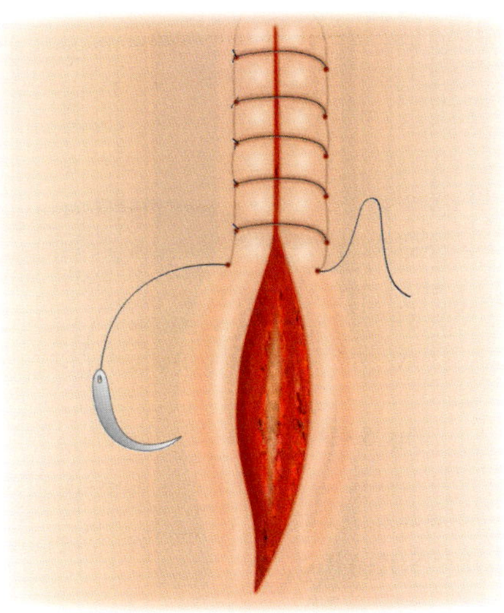

Fig. 5.4A Simple interrupted suturing

The needle is passed through skin and small amount of subcutaneous tissue perpendicular to the surface add the suture is completed with mirror image. The knot is preferably placed to one side. The stitches have advantage that failure of one stitch does not prejudice other. A potential disadvantage is the number of knots which are weak points (Fig. 5.4A).

Simple Continuous Suturing

This is a rapid and efficient method of closure, commonly applied in case of peritoneum and sheath. It is also hemostatic. But it may cause overlapping of edges and failure of wound closure if one stitch is dissolved early or if it breaks. Hence, it is contraindicated in contaminated wounds (Fig. 5.4B).

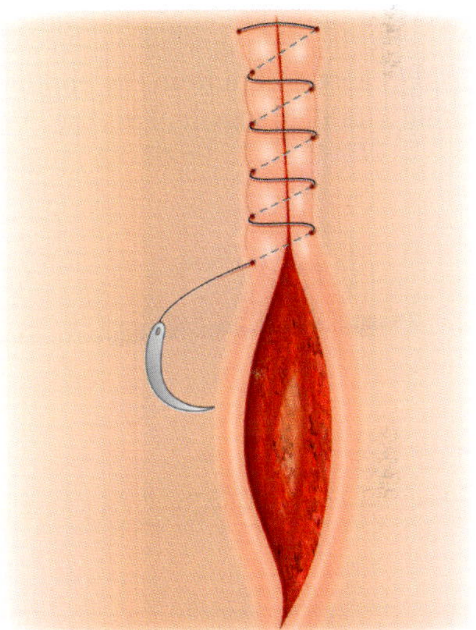

Fig. 5.4B Continuous suturing

Continuous Locked Suturing

This is a type of continuous suturing where needle is passed through a loop at each stitch. This allows hemostasis and apposition.

Mattress Suturing

This is a double stitch, which aims to close the deep part of the wound, to obliterate dead space and slightly invert the edges. It may be horizontal or vertical (Fig. 5.4C).

Method: Starting from one margin, the needle passes through other edge, and is then returned to the starting side through separate bite. It is most useful where skin is loose or hemostasis is required.

If the entry and exit holes lie parallel to the edges, these are called horizontal mattress stitches. If the entry and exit holes are perpendicular to the edges, these are vertical mattress stitches. In each variety, there is a bridge of suture on the upper surface which draws in the surface away from the edge so that edge itself is everted.

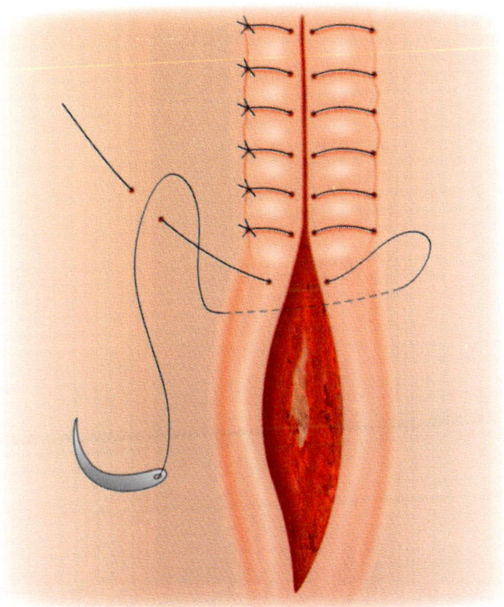

Fig. 5.4C Mattress suturing

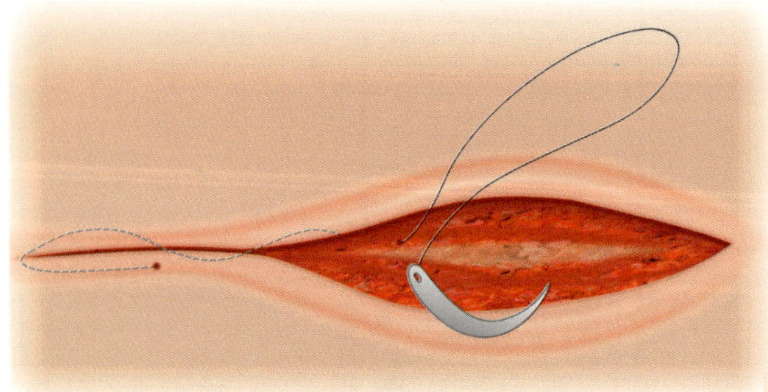

Fig. 5.4D Subcuticular suturing

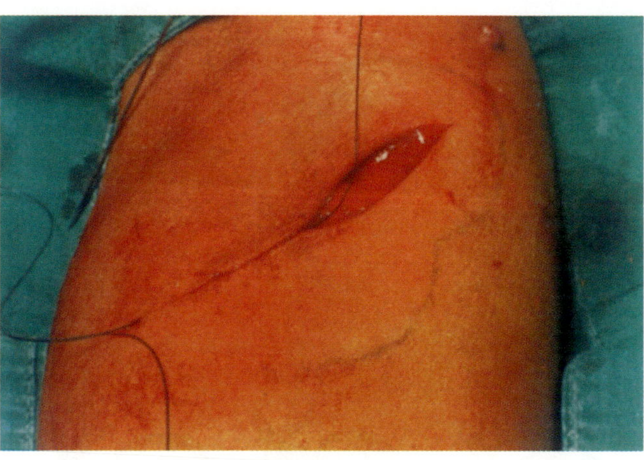

Fig. 5.4E Subcuticular stitch

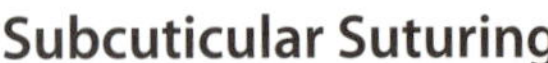

Subcuticular Suturing

It is less prone to infection, easier to remove and is cosmetically better. The suture material may be absorbable (Chromic catgut) or nonabsorbable (3/0 ethilon) (Fig. 5.4D).

Enter the skin about 1 cm from the end of the incision using preferably a straight needle. Pass the needle through subcuticular layer and dermis along the wound in regular step-wise fashion. Regular progression ensures good apposition of the wound margins when the stitch is pulled straight (Fig. 5.4E).

Methods of closure of skin wounds have been also mentioned in Chapter 3.

CHAPTER

6

Role of Surgical Drains

Dhiraj Choudhury

A drain is a channel along which fluids (blood, bile, pus, serum) can reach the surface while allowing normal healing of the main wound.

INDICATIONS

- To remove collection of blood or bile from the field of operation, e.g. corrugated drain in pouch of Morrison following cholecystectomy
- To drain contents of a hollow organ or tube, e.g. T-tube drain following exploration of CBD
- To facilitate drainage of pus from an abscess and allow shrinkage of cavity
- To allow irrigation of serous lined cavities, e.g. peritoneal cavity.
- To provide drainage of abnormal channel
- To provide early warning of complications such as anastomotic leak or bleeding.

Disadvantages claimed by opponents of surgical drain are:

- Increase of infection by acting as a route for bacterial entry
- Damage by mechanical pressure and use of suction
- Delay in wound healing.

TYPES OF DRAINS

Figure 6.1 shows type of open and closed drains.

Drains may be *active* or *passive*. Active drainage works by suction forces provided by vacuumed container. Passive drains function by different pressure between body and exterior and are dependent on gravity or capillary action to drain fluids.

Drains may be *open* or *closed*. Open drains are used to establish a tract from a body cavity into skin surface, e.g. corrugated rubber or silastic sheet. These can effectively drain pus, blood, serum from body cavity. Closed tube system drain directly into a container with or without suction.

Open Drains

These establish a tract from a body cavity to the skin surface and can effectively drain pus, serum or blood.

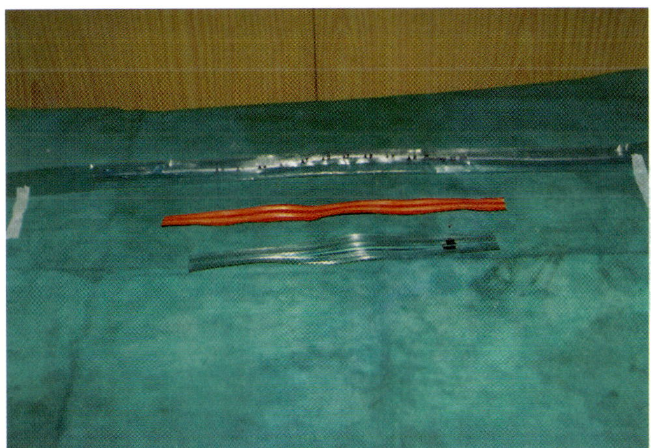

Fig. 6.1 Types of drains

Corrugated Rubber or Silastic Sheet

These are made of radiopaque sheet of rubber or silastic material. They are traditional methods of drainage. They drain by capillary action or gravity into dressings or stoma bags. Their efficiency depends on position of the patient, site and amount of collection (Fig. 6.2).

Advantage: These are economical.

Disadvantage: They do not permit irrigation of cavity. They require relatively large stab wound.

Closed Drains

Rubber Tube Drain

They are used to drain bile from CBD or fluids from peritoneal cavity. They are mildly reactive to tissues. One disadvantage of rubber tube drain is that it can become blocked with clotted serum. These drain into bags by low-pressure suction working on the Siphon principle.

Silicon Tube Drain

They are less reactive but can be easily blocked by clotted serum.

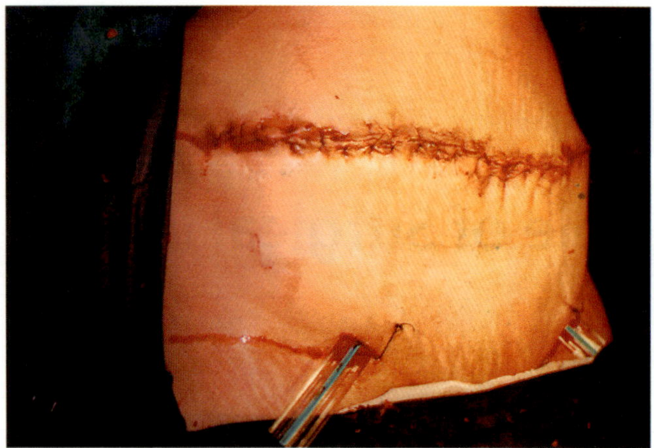

Fig. 6.2 Corrugated silastic drain

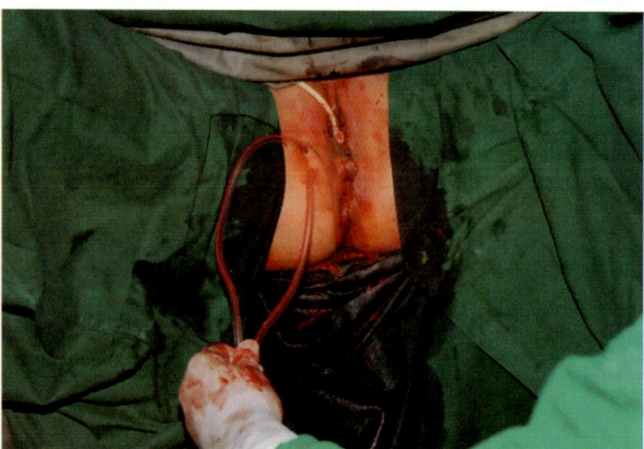

Fig. 6.3 Closed suction drain

Penrose Drain

It is a soft latex tube drain of various diameter.

Closed Suction Drain

These may be either reusable or disposable system of active drains. These consist of one or two multiperforated silicone or polyethylene catheters attached to a sterile plastic container. It is a closed system. The container is the source of continuous suction. The catheters are brought through separate stab wounds. The bulbs can be re-expanded. They are commonly used in clean wounds, e.g. neck dissection or axillary clearance (Fig. 6.3) abdominoperineal resection of rectum.

Sump Drain

These contain an air inlet lumen which prevents blockage by soft tissue. Sump drains are large caliber multilumen tubes which provides continuous irrigation and aspiration. They are generally used for drainage of intra-abdominal spaces that might benefit from continuous irrigation, e.g. pancreatic abscess.

Percutaneous Drainage

These are thin walled plastic tubes which are inserted percutaneously under guidance of ultrasound or CT scan.

Fixation of Drains

A drain should be fixed to skin wound by silk suture so that it does not get displaced.

Removal of Drains

A drain should be removed as soon as it stops draining substantial amount.

CHAPTER

7

Techniques of Achieving Skin Cover

Dhiraj Choudhury

DIRECT CLOSURE BY SUTURING

This is the method of choice in case of surgical incisions, clean lacerations—which has been described in Chapter 5.

SKIN GRAFTING

A skin graft is a piece of skin taken from a donor site and moved to a recipient site.

Indications

- Considerable loss of skin due to trauma
- Full thickness burns
- Chronic ulcers like varicose ulcer
- Radical excision of malignant tumors.

Types

Free Skin Graft

A free skin graft is the transfer of a segment of skin, which has been totally separated from its blood supply. They have to be revascularized from recipient site.

Partial Thickness/Split Graft/Thiersch Graft

This consists of epidermis and dermis. This procedure will be described in details, because general surgeons are often required to perform this simple method of obtaining skin cover of wounds. A disadvantage of split skin graft is their tendency to contract.

Indications:

- Granulating wounds
- Large denuded areas.

Instrument: Hand dermatomes like Humby's knife, Waston knife are commonly used as they are cheap and readily available. Electric dermatomes are especially useful for difficult donor sites (such as abdomen and scalp) (Fig. 7.1).

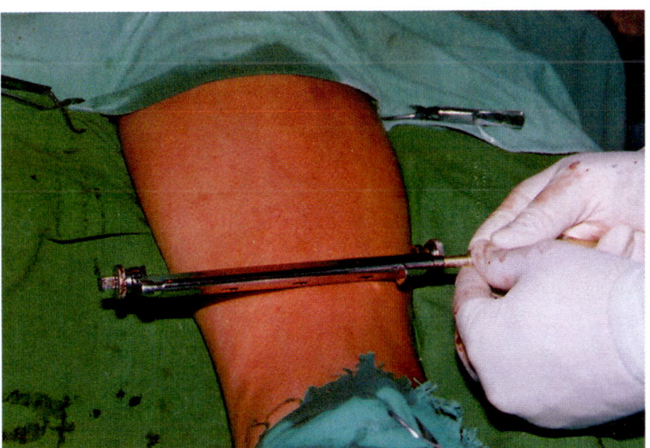

Fig. 7.1 Donor area and hand dermatome

OPERATIVE PROCEDURE

Anesthesia

Local

Local anesthesia with 0.5% lignocaine may be used for:

- Small graft
- Elderly people.

General

General anesthesia is usually necessary for:

- Children
- Large graft.

Preparation of Donor Site

The most commonly used donor sites are thigh and upper inner aspect of arm. The donor site is painted with Sevlon.

Graft Cutting

The donor site and under surface of knife are well-lubricated with liquid paraffin. The site to be cut is rendered tense in two

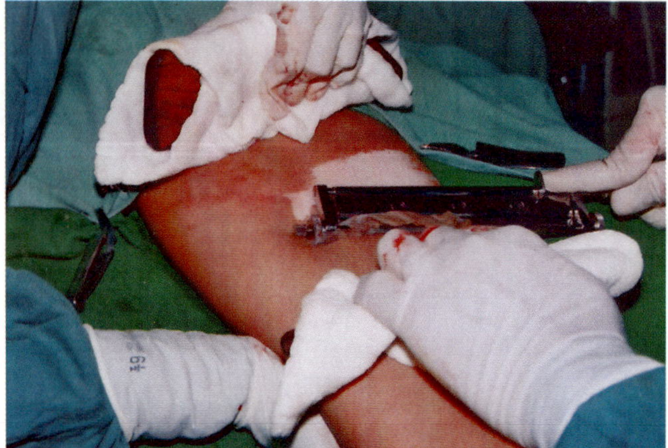
Fig. 7.2 Graft cutting

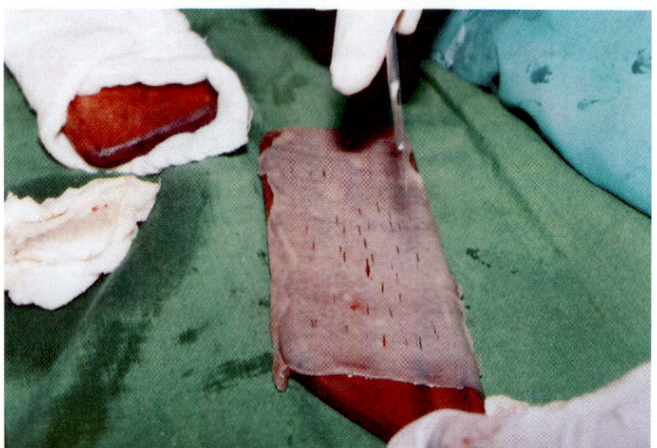
Fig. 7.3 Graft treatment

dimensions with wooden boards, covered with mop-held by the assistant at upper end and surgeon's nondominant hand at lower end (Fig. 7.2).

The knife is held firmly with blade angled at 5° to 10° to skin. The grafts are cut with a bold sawing motion. The knife should be advanced with minimal side-to-side swing.

Graft Treatment

The graft after being taken, is placed on a wooden board and multiple punctures are made with tip of knife (Fig. 7.3).

Graft Application

The recipient site is prepared by scraping granulation tissues. Now apply the graft (Fig. 7.4).

Graft Fixation

Grafts are anchored at edges with sutures, staples or glue. Graft can be fixed in position by sutures. Shearing can be prevented by a firm tie-over bolster dressing or quilting the graft into place. Pressure dressing is vital to prevent collection of serous exudates or pus between graft and its bed. Apply firm pressure dressing, which is evenly distributed over the graft (Fig. 7.5). Careful dressing is applied to avoid infection, hematoma or seroma and shearing.

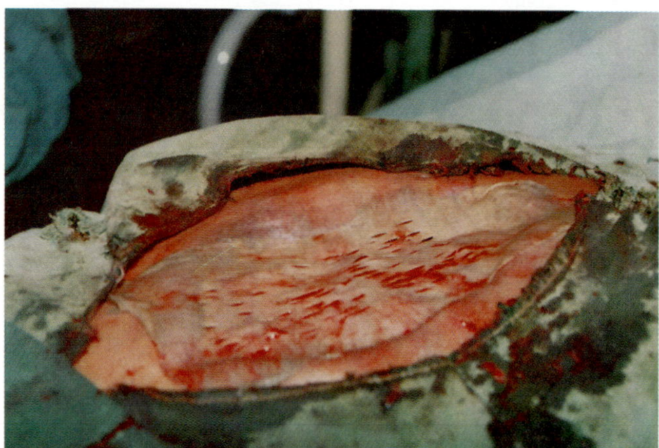
Fig. 7.4 Graft application

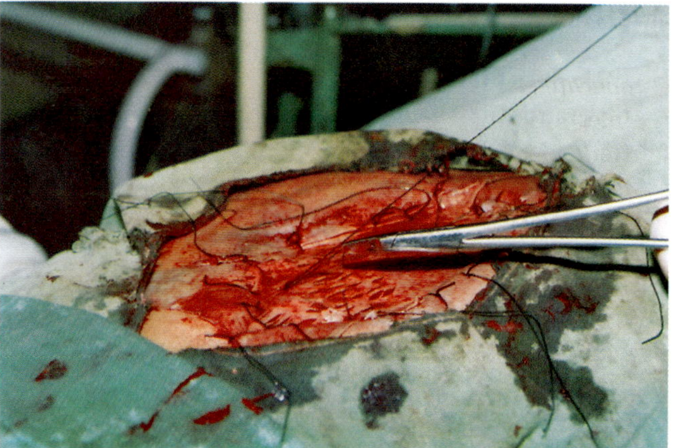
Fig. 7.5 Graft fixation

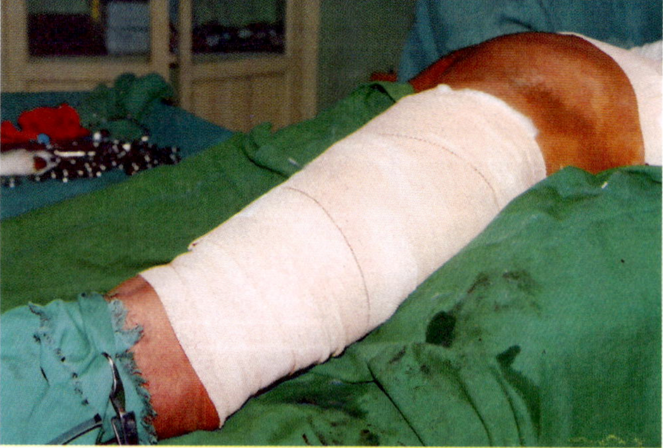
Fig. 7.6 Dressing on donor site

Dressing of Donor Site

The donor site is dressed with gauze and wools, which are kept in position by elastic crepe bandage (Fig. 7.6).

Full-thickness (Wolfe) Graft

This consists of full skin thickness with no subcutaneous fat. It is indicated for replacement of small area on the face and hand where blood supply is excellent, where contracture will be disastrous and where excellent result is required.

Donor site: Postauricular sulcus is the best match for face.

Graft fixation: The graft is sutured to recipient site avoiding any tension and carefully dressed.

Disadvantage: It is not easy to take.

Pinch Grafts

These are cone-shaped pieces of full-thickness grafts which have better survival in presence of sepsis.

Complications

- Infection
- Hematoma
- Failure
- Flap necrosis
- Contraction
- Scarring.

FLAPS

The flap consisting of skin and subcutaneous tissue is transferred from one site of an individual to another site of the same individual, while maintaining is vascular supply. A flap is a block of tissue that brings its own blood supply with it.

Indications

- Where the defect has inadequate blood supply to support a graft
- To cover exposed bone, cartilage, joint and tendon.

Types

Flaps can be classified on the basis of their blood supply or movements, e.g. advancement or free flaps (the latter involving vascular or microvascular anastomosis), or *tissue content*, either single (cutaneous, fascial or bone) or composite (myocutaneous or fasciocutaneous).

Advantages: They can cover many defects (cartilage, bone or bare tendon) and healing time is faster than grafts.

Disadvantages: Include the level of expertise required. The donor site may be left with cosmetic or functional defect.

Random Pattern Flaps

In random pattern flaps, there is no specific blood vessel in the pedicle, the flap being nourished by dermal plexus.

Axial Flaps

Groin flap, deltopectoral flap are supplied by specific blood vessel and the artery is included in base of the flap.

Myocutaneous Flaps

The principle of a myocutaneous flap is that the skin overlying a muscle will survive provided the pedicle to the muscle which is usually a dominant vessel at one end, is not divided, e.g. latissimus dorsi flap.

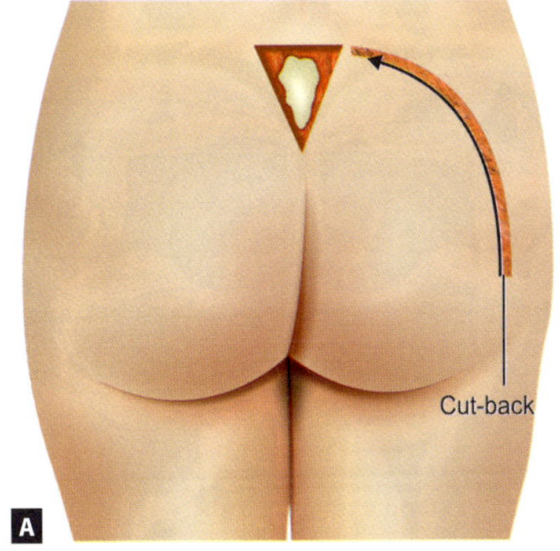

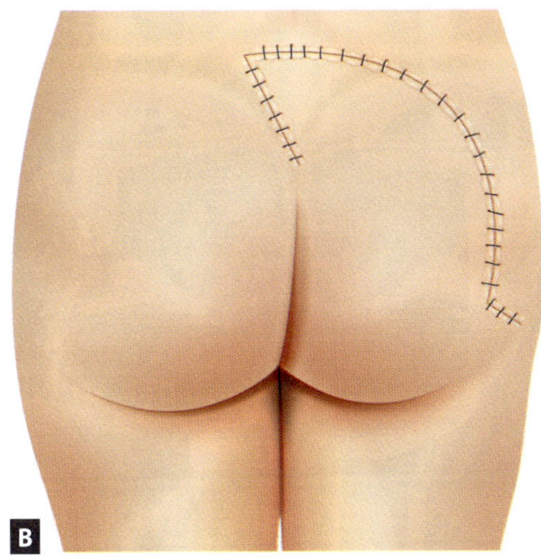

Figs 7.7A and B Rotation flaps

The simplest type of tube pedicle grafts is carried in 3 stages; In first stage, the flap is cut but left attached at both ends converted into a tube. In second stage, after six weeks, one end is freed and implanted into recipient area. At third stage, the transplanted skin is severed from the pedicle.

Rotation Flaps (Figs 7.7A and B)

The rotation flap closes defects by mobilizing the surrounding tissue in a rotational manner. A back cut or a triangle excision are useful methods (Fig. 7.7A). The defect may be closed primarily (Fig. 7.7B) or by thin grafting. Double rotation flap with split thickness skin grafts at donor area is frequently used in scalp. In cheek area, V-Y-advancement transposition flap, rhomboid flap may be used.

TISSUE EXPANSION

Recently tissue expanders are being increasingly used to repair local defects. It relies on the tissues' ability to stretch and proliferate under continuous moderate tension.

CHAPTER

8 Principles of Minimal Access Surgery/ Minimally Invasive Surgery

Dhiraj Choudhury

The term minimal access surgery or "minimally invasive surgery" (alternative terminology coined by Wickham and Fitzpatrick) indicates surgical innovation which aims to achieve surgical therapeutic goal with minimal physical and psychological trauma with the help of modern technology.

NATURE OF MINIMAL ACCESS/ MINIMALLY INVASIVE SURGERY

The hallmark of such procedure is the reduction of the trauma of access without compromise. Surgical operations are conducted by remote surgical manipulations carried out within closed confines of body cavities or lumen of hollow organs under visual control via telescopes which incorporate the Hopkins rod lens system linked to charge couple device (CCD) cameras such that the surgeon can operate across the television screen.

SCOPE OF MINIMAL ACCESS/INVASIVE SURGERY

This involves several procedures like:

- *Laparoscopic surgery*: This is the most important development in the field of minimally invasive surgery
- Thoracoscopic surgery
- Endoluminal surgery
- Perivisceral endoscopic surgery
- Arthroscopic surgery
- Combined surgery.

ADVANTAGES

- Improved visualization of anatomy
- Avoidance of large painful access wounds by smaller incision
- Less postoperative pain
- Least psychological
- Shorter hospital stay
- Decreased contact with pathogens like HIV, hepatitis
- Earlier return to normal activities
- Cosmetically acceptable
- Diminished cost of treatment debatable
- Decreased perioperative complication rate
- Decreased wound-lelated complications.

DISADVANTAGES/RISKS

- Lack of tactile feedback from tissues
- Depth perception is diminished
- Hemostasis is difficult
- Suturing is difficult
- Requires training in handling instruments
- Iatrogenic injuries are relatively more
- Role in treatment of malignant lesions is debatable
- Laparoscopy is resource-intensive.

FUNDAMENTALS OF LAPARO (INSIDE) SCOPIC (TO SEE) SURGERY

'Lapara' is derived from Greek word (*Lapar*) meaning Flank. 'Scope' is coined from Greek word (*Skopein*) meaning to view or examine.

Indications

Diagnostic

Most useful tools in:

- Undiagnosed abdominal pains
- Acute abdomen
- Blunt injury abdomen
- *Tumors*: For diagnostic, biopsy, staging.

Therapeutic

- Lap cholecystectomy has achieved gold standard
- Lap appendicectomy
- Lap fundoplication
- Lap surgery for peptic ulcer
- Lap repair of hernia.

Contraindications

Absolute

- Unfit for general anesthesia
- Generalized peritonitis

- Intestinal obstruction
- Clotting abnormalities
- Cirrhosis of liver.

Relative

- Gross obesity
- Pregnancy first and third trimester
- Multiple adhesions.

Operation Room Setup

- OT should be adequate in size ideally 20 × 20
- God earthing with enough power supply lines with stabilizers
- Alternative power supplies.

Equipment

- CD cameras
- Video monitors
- Carbon dioxide insufflator
- Light source (Halogen/Xenon)
- VCR
- Cautery
- Suction irrigation cannula
- Telescopic 0° (bright picture) or 30°
- Carbon dioxide cylinder.

Hand Instruments/Equipment

- *Creating and maintaining pneumoperitoneum*: Veress needle, insufflator
- *Access ports*: 5 mm, 10 mm and 12 mm

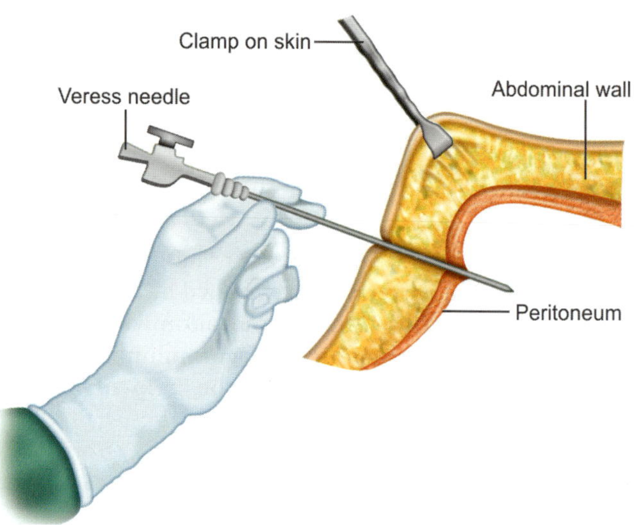

Fig. 8.1 Technique for inserting the Veress needle into the abdominal wall and the layers the needle passes through

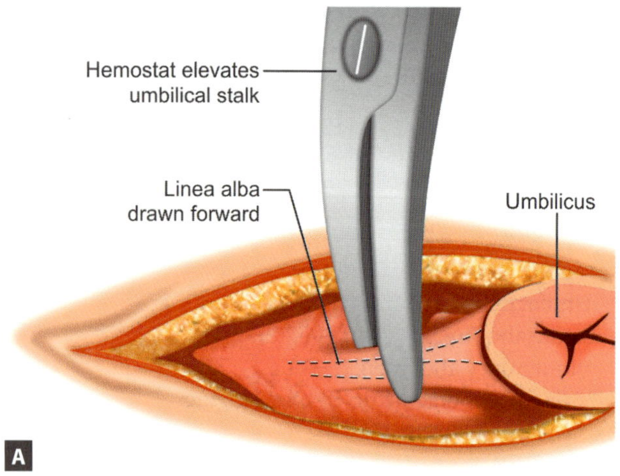

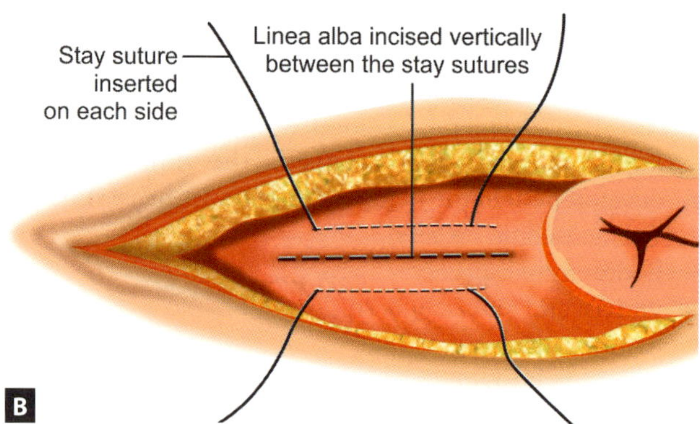

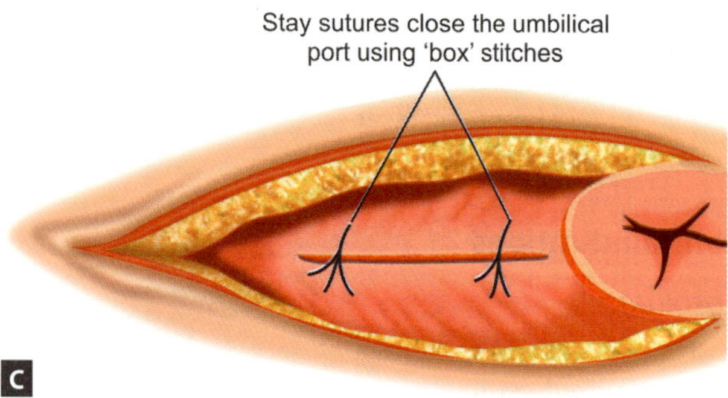

Figs 8.2A to C Insertion of a Hasson port just below the umbilicus. (A) Vertical incision made just below the umbilicus, dissected down to the linea alba; (B) Longitudinal absorbable stitches (Vicryl) have been inserted on each side of the midline; the vertical midline incision will be made between them through which the Hasson port will be inserted; (C) On completion and removal of the port, close the defect by tying the sutures across to produce a 'box' or 'mattress' stitch

- *Imaging equipments*: Telescope, light source, camera, monitor
- *Instruments*: Dissection, grasping and cutting
- Hemostasis, suturing and stapling retractors
- Bipolar applicator
- Clip applicator
- Suction irrigation cannula
- Knot pusher.

Operative Procedure

Anesthesia

General endotracheal.

OT Setup and Patient Position

- Patient is placed in a supine position
- Monitor placed on the right side head end of the patient on videocart
- All control panels within the reach of the anesthetist.

Operative Technique

Pneumoperitoneum: A working space is created in patients abdomen using CO_2 via either closed or open technique.

Closed technique: A Veress needle is placed most commonly at umbilicus through a small stab incision (Fig. 8.1). Two serial clicks are heard as the needle penetrates the fascia and peritoneum. Aspiration or gravity injection of sterile saline confirms the position. The abdominal cavity is insufflated via insufflator and pneumoperitoneum is produced.

Problems

- Return of blood or bilious fluid indicate necessity for needle reinsertion.
- Gas embolism.

Open technique: By direct cut-down through abdominal fascia, Hassan port can be placed under direct vision. Figures 8.2A to C show insertion of Hassan port and closure of the wound. See page 203 for picture of Hasson port.

Port placement: Location of ports have been standardized for most operations.

- Camera port should be behind and between surgeons to operative ports to maintain proper orientation.
- Working ports are placed laterally.

Actual technique: This will be described under individual procedure.

Operative Complications and its Avoiding

Attention is to be paid to detect intraoperative complications like hemorrhage, injury to duct and tackle them successfully.

Closure: The skin wounds can be closed with absorbable or nonabsorbable sutures.

CHAPTER

9

Principles of Day Case Surgery

Dhiraj Choudhury

It indicates types of surgery where the patient is discharged on the same day as admission. It is also called ambulatory surgery.

ADVANTAGES

- Early ambulation reduces the risk of thromboembolism.
- Reduces risk of cross-infection
- Reduces patient anxiety by avoiding overnight stay in hospital
- Quick return to normal activities
- Saves time and trouble for relatives visiting the patient
- Cost-effective.

CRITERIA FOR SELECTION

- Low risk of major complication following surgery
- Predictable recovery period
- Specialist postoperative therapy or treatment is not necessary
- Anesthesia not requiring invasive monitoring
- Postoperative analgesia does not need routine opiates.

BASIC NECESSITIES

- Preoperative assessment should include social, medical and surgical assessment
- Patient information system should be of high quality
- Day surgery ward
- Discharge protocol.

SELECTION OF CASES

- Age maximum 75 years and minimum above 3 years
- Patient has appropriate social support at home
- BMI below 35
- General fitness ASA grade 1–3
- No serious cardiac or respiratory disease
- Non-insulin diabetes only.

GENERAL SURGERY PROCEDURES

- Excision of lump
- Inguinal hernia
- Varicose vein operation
- Thyroidectomy
- Laparoscopic cholecystectomy.

UROLOGICAL PROCEDURES

- Cystoscopy
- Circumcision
- Orchidectomy
- Orchidopexy
- Hydrocele

DISCHARGE PROTOCOL

- Stable vital signs for at least one hour
- Adequate pain control
- Correct orientation of time, place and person
- Minimal nausea or vomiting
- Minimal bleeding on discharge
- Elderly male should pass urine
- Written or verbal instructions should be issued regarding postoperative management.

SECTION

2

Head and Neck

- **Burr Hole Procedures**
  Rahul Dey, Kaushik Sen
- **Excision of Cervical Lymph Nodes**
  Dhiraj Choudhury
- **Surgery for Parotid Tumors**
  Gautam Mukhopadhya
- **Simple Lithotomy for Submandibular Duct Stone**
  Dhiraj Choudhury
- **Excision of Submandibular Salivary Gland**
  Dhiraj Choudhury
- **Operations for Cancer of Face and Lip**
  Dhiraj Choudhury
- **Operations for Cancer of the Oral Tongue**
  RS Rao, Satish Rao
- **Neck Dissections**
  RS Rao, Satish Rao
- **Commando Operation**
  RS Rao, Satish Rao
- **Surgery for Thyroid Cancer**
  AK D' Cruz
- **Subtotal Thyroidectomy**
  Dhiraj Choudhury
- **Excision of Thyroglossal Cyst and Fistula**
  Dhiraj Choudhury
- **Parathyroidectomy**
  Dhiraj Choudhury
- **Excision of Branchial Cyst and Fistula**
  Dhiraj Choudhury
- **Tracheostomy**
  Dhiraj Choudhury

CHAPTER

10

Burr Hole Procedures

Rahul Dey, Kaushik Sen

INTRODUCTION

Burr holes are small round openings in the calvaria in order to gain access to the underlying brain and meninges. It is one of the basic neurosurgical procedures but also extensively used in general surgical setups, especially in context of situations like when a general surgeon encounters a patient with head injury. This is more pertinent in our country, where neurosurgical care is not readily available in distant setups and so any surgeon needs to have some knowledge of this procedure which can be life-saving in some patients.

HISTORY

Burr holes are known since ancient times. Peruvian mummies, some five thousands years old show marks of trephination in the skull. Similar trephines have been found in Indian, Sumatran and Mediterranean civilizations. People believed that 'evil spirits' would go away if the skulls were drilled. Hippocrates (460-370 BC) first described in writing, the use of trephine for contusions and depressed skull fracture. He also observed that it should never be done over the sutures due to risk of underlying dura. He also stressed the need of watering the skull to prevent overheating. As early as in 1000 AD, Albucasis, an Arabian physician, described the 'non-plunging trephine'. Lanfranchi of Milan (1306) described the classic guidelines for trephines in skull fracture. Ambroise Paré (1510-1590 AD) described the extensive use of trephines which was later modified to various designs by Giacopo Berengario da Carpi in his remarkable book *Tractatus* (1518 AD) Over the years, burr holes have become more refined, more precise, and simpler and it still remains the neurosurgeon's best diagnostic and therapeutic tool.

PROCEDURE

The instruments required to do burr holes are a perforator and a burr. A perforator is used first to penetrate the outer and inner tables of the skull and a burr of equal size is then used to enlarge the opening. (Fig. 10.1). Both can be assembled on to a handle for rotation called the Hudson's brace (Fig. 10.2). The end of perforation is determined when the perforator starts to wobble as it penetrates the inner table. The end of the burring is determined by the tendency of the burr to jam and a faint crackling noise, as the thin, innermost layer of bone, starts to disintegrate. When the skull is very thick, particularly in the midline anteriorly, it is necessary to undercut the burr hole with a small Kerrison's punch. In modern neurosurgical settings, the Hudson's brace has given way to power drills, either electrically or pneumatically operated (Fig. 10.3). They are more precise, quicker and easy to make. However, there are still some indications, for example while drilling over the venous sinuses, Hudson's brace is preferable as tactile feeling gives a better control over the instrument, thus minimizing injury to underlying structures. Similarly, in surgery for aneurysm, the Hudson's brace is preferable as the vibration of the power drills may cause early rupture of the aneurysm.

Sites of Placement

The site of the placement of burr holes on the cranial vault is so chosen that they overlie the maximum amount of underlying collection. In cases of planned operations, they

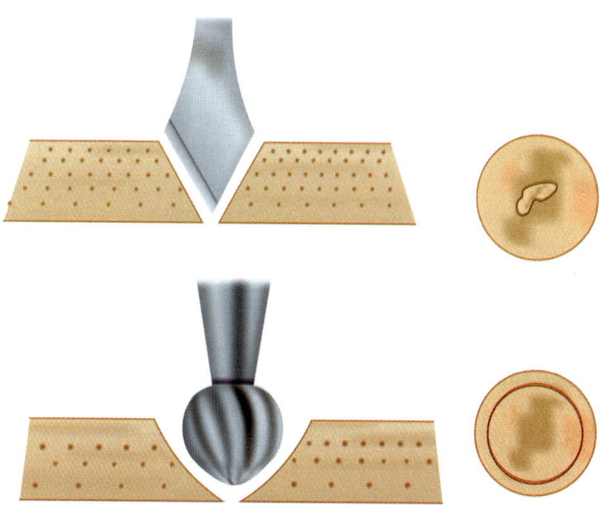

Fig. 10.1 Perforator and the burr

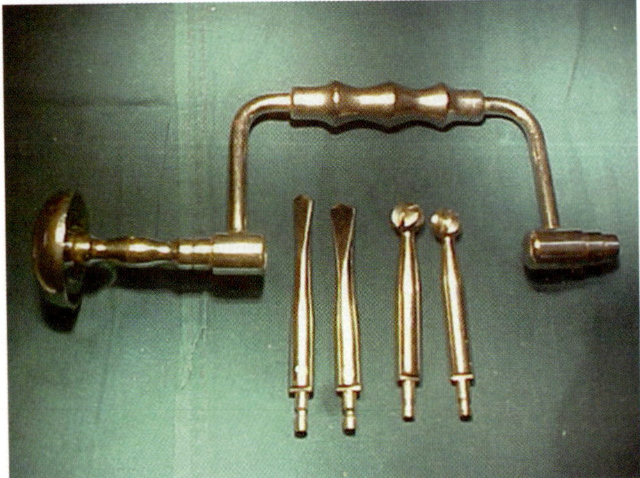

Fig. 10.2 Hudsons' brace

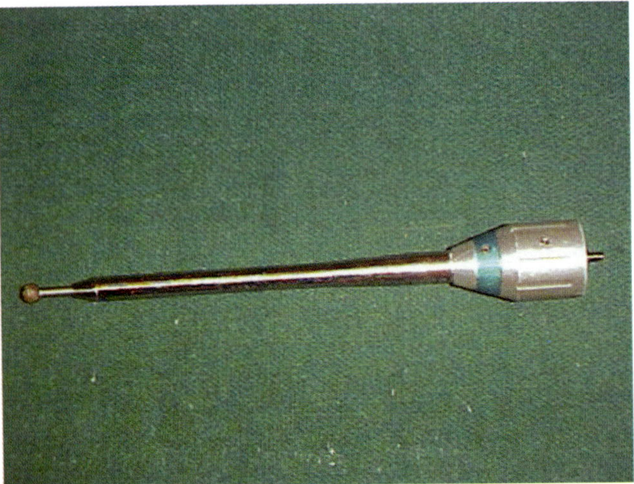

Fig. 10.3 Drill with burr

are placed along the line of proposed craniotomy flap, each 5–6 cm apart. However, if power drill is used, a single burr hole is sufficient to make room for the cutting craniotome. There are few principles in guiding the placement of burr holes.

- Normally, burr holes should not traverse air sinuses, like frontal air sinus or mastoid air cells.
- When access to the falx cerebri is required, it is required to put the burr holes on either side of the midline very close apart or on the midline, so that the underlying dura over the superior sagittal sinus is not torn.
- A burr hole if required close to the temporal crest, is usually cited below the crest, in order that the temporalis muscle may conceal it.

INDICATIONS AND PRESENT USAGE

Therapeutic Indications

- As part of a craniotomy bone flap opening
- Drainage of chronic subdural hematomas and hygromas
- Aspiration of brain abscess
- Stereotactic procedures of intracranial lesions
- CSF diversion procedures like external ventricular drainage or ventriculo-peritoneal shunt
- In neuroendoscopic procedures
- Functional neurosurgical procedures such as deep brain stimulation for Parkinson's disease and other movement disorders.

Diagnostic Indications

- Monitoring of intracranial pressure
- Ultrasound-based navigation during surgery
- Exploratory burr holes.

Craniotomy Flaps (Fig. 10.4)

In opening the skull as a flap, numerous burr holes are made in the margins of the proposed flap. They are then joined by cutting with a Gigli saw, so that the free bone flap comes out. Occasionally in the low temporal region, the bone flap is broken between two burr holes, called the osteoplastic flap. The 'key' burr hole is located on the sphenoid wing and is an important landmark as it separates the anterior and middle cranial fossa. If the flap crosses the midline, burr holes are needed to be placed either on or just adjacent to the venous sinus, so that the dura containing the sinus can be stripped off from the bone before cutting. In the posterior fossa, two adjacent burr holes are placed just below the transverse sinus called the 'spectacle' burr holes from which the craniectomy starts.

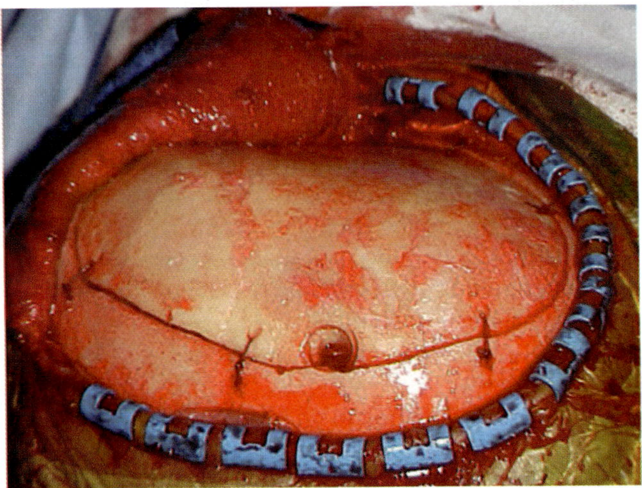

Fig. 10.4 Burr holes for craniotomy

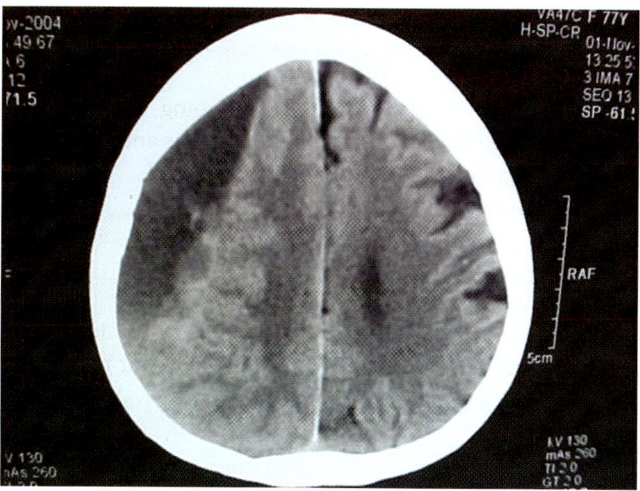

Fig. 10.5 Chronic subdural hematoma

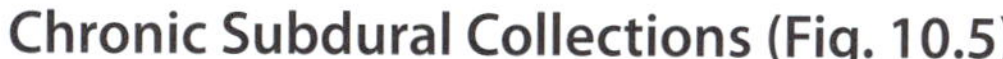

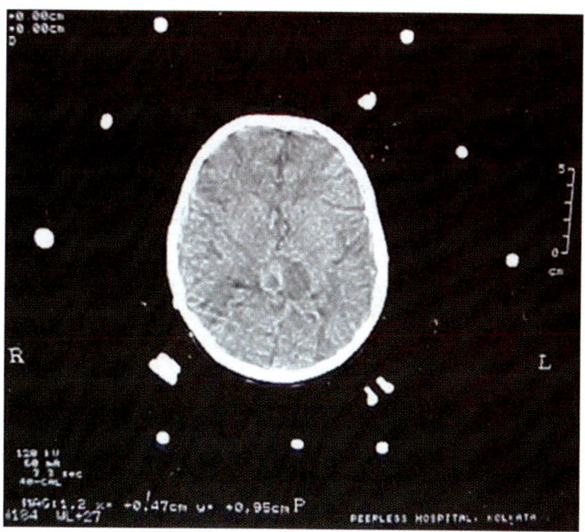

Fig. 10.6 Stereotactic localization

Chronic Subdural Collections (Fig. 10.5)

In the elderly, alcoholics and in those with coagulopathy, minor trauma may rupture the bridging veins leading to collection of blood in the subdural space. With time, the blood gets organized to liquid form and lie over the cerebral convexity within the subdural space. This liquid blood can easily be drained through a burr hole placed over the maximum depth of collection. This provides one of the gratifying responses to treatment of a very common neurosurgical problem.

Aspiration of Brain Abscess

Cerebral abscess is an intra-axial collection of pus mainly due to hematogenous spread of microorganisms. Since the patients are morbid due to infection, the safest procedure is to make a burr hole, aspirate the pus and follow-up with suitable antibiotic regime. The burr hole position is so chosen so that the path length to the abscess is minimized, avoiding traversing through the ventricles, and vital neural structures.

Stereotactic Procedures

This is an image-guided procedure where a lesion is localized geometrically with respect to the patient's skull after fixing a frame fixed on the head using three-dimensional coordinates. Then the burr hole is placed exactly over the target area and various procedures like biopsy, laser surgery, foreign body removal undertaken. This is useful when the lesion is small and deep (Fig. 10.6).

CSF Diversion Procedures

In treatment of hydrocephalus, ventricle is tapped and CSF is diverged either by a catheter connected to a drainage bag outside the body, or via a shunt connecting the ventricle with the peritoneal or pleural cavity. The burr hole is placed just in front of the coronal suture in case of external ventricular drainage (Kocher's point) and in the posterior parietal area (Keen's point) in case of shunt. An occipitoparietal burr hole (Frazier) is an important adjunct in posterior fossa surgeries for emergency ventricular access.

Neuroendoscopic and Functional Neurosurgical Procedures

Burr holes help to place the endoscope or electrode in procedures of third ventriculostomy for hydrocephalus, pallidal stimulation for movement disorders.

Monitoring of Intracranial Pressure

In following up a patient with raised intracranial pressure, burr holes are made to insert the various types of pressure gauges like intraventricular catheter, intraparenchymal monitor, subarachnoid screw, subdural bolt or epidural cup. This is a routine procedure in neurointensive units.

Ultrasound Navigation

Burr hole is placed and an ultrasound transducer is placed on it to locate a cystic lesion or the ventricle, thus plotting out the trajectory for biopsy or removal.

Exploratory Burr Holes

In days of pre-CT scan era, burr holes were used to be done on assumptive basis on the site and side of clinical localization of the intracranial lesion. Nowadays, they are infrequently indicated except in the following situations:

- Sudden onset rapid deterioration of neurological status of the patient like transtentorial herniation, where CT scanning and OT is logistically to be delayed.
- Some patient needed emergent surgery for multisystem injuries, where the condition is too poor to be transported to a scanner.

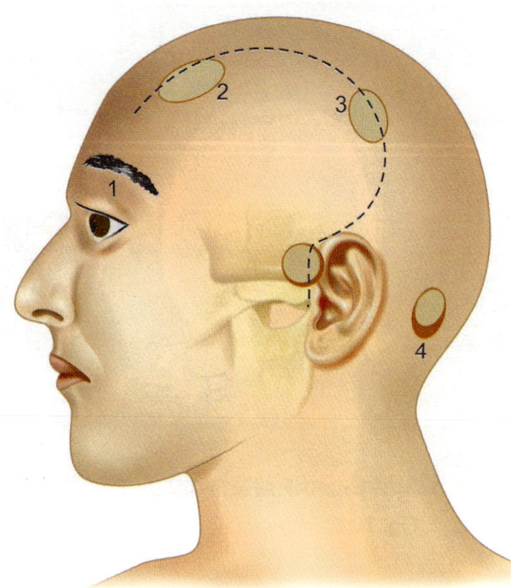

Fig. 10.7 Exploratory burr holes

Positions (Fig 10.7)

- First burr hole on the temporal region of the clinically suspecting side just superior to zygomatic arch. This provides access to middle cranial fossa, most of the thickness of a chronic subdural collection, as well as proximity to the middle meningeal artery
- If no epidural hematoma is found, the dura is opened, if it is tense and bluish
- If completely negative, usually perform temporal burr hole on the contralateral side
- If negative, ipsilateral frontal burr hole is done
- Subsequent burr holes are done in the parietal region and posterior fossa.

Choice of Initial Burr Hole

- Ipsilateral to blown pupil
- Ipsilateral to first dilated pupil
- Ipsilateral to obvious external trauma
- If no localization is possible, decompress the dominant hemisphere.

Rate of Positivity

There is 56% chance of an exploratory burr hole to give a diagnostic yield.

There is 86% chance of being on the correct side.

RISKS OF BURR HOLES

Uncontrolled trephination may lead to plunging of the perforator or burr causing dural, vascular and neural injury.

CLOSURE OF BURR HOLES

A burr hole is usually filled with bone dust that is collected during trephination to avoid unsightly deformities. Nowadays, artificial burr hole caps are available to seal them. A burr hole kept open helps to gauge the underlying intracranial pressure.

CONCLUSION

Burr holes are a neurosurgeon's window to the cranial cavity. However, may the science of noninvasive diagnosis and therapeutics progress, it will remain in the armamentarium of a neurosurgeon forever. Every young surgeon needs to acquire the skill of trephination that may be helpful to save an occasional patient's life if the need arises.

CHAPTER

11

Excision of Cervical Lymph Nodes

Dhiraj Choudhury

INDICATIONS

Excision biopsy of cervical lymph node is perhaps the best diagnostic method in establishing etiological diagnosis of cervical lymphadenopathy.

ANATOMY

The lymph node of the head and neck are arranged in superficial and deep chains. The superficial lymph nodes arranged in a circular way includes submental, submandibular, preauricular and suboccipital. The deep lymph nodes are situated deep to sternomastoid along the internal jugular veins and are divided into upper anterior, upper posterior, lower anterior and lower posterior groups. The two important groups are jugulo-omohyoid (lower anterior deep) and jugulodiagastric (upper anterior deep).

The supraclavicular lymph nodes are posteroinferior groups. A further group of deep cervical lymph nodes includes pre- and paratracheal lymph nodes (Fig. 11.1), also known as Delphic nodes.

PREOPERATIVE PREPARATIONS

Apart from routine blood tests, chest X-ray, preliminary laryngoscopy, esophagoscopy and bronchoscopy should be done if indicated.

OPERATIVE PROCEDURES

- *Anesthesia:* General anesthesia is preferred.
- *Position:* Supine with head tilted to opposite side.
- *Incision:* A crease incision is made according to position of the lymph node (Fig. 11.2).
- *Technique:* The incision is deepened through subcutaneous tissue and platysma. A plane is defined by dissection around the lymph node. In case of deep lymph node, the deep fascia is incised to define the anterior

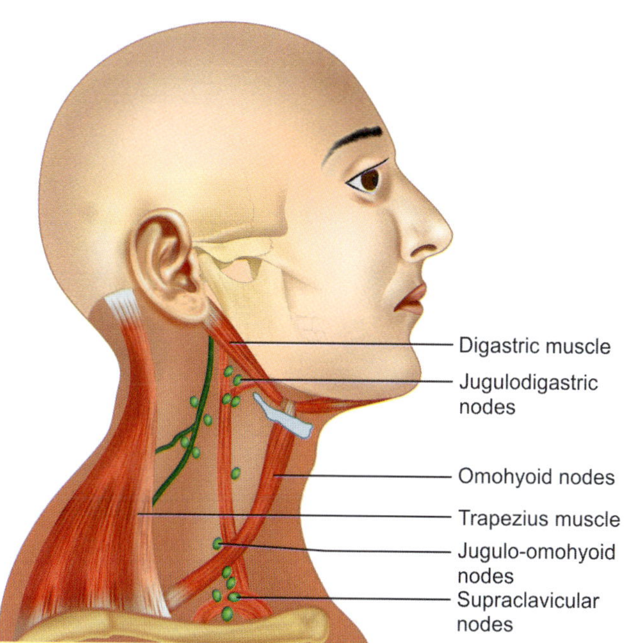

Fig. 11.1 Distribution of deep cervical lymph nodes

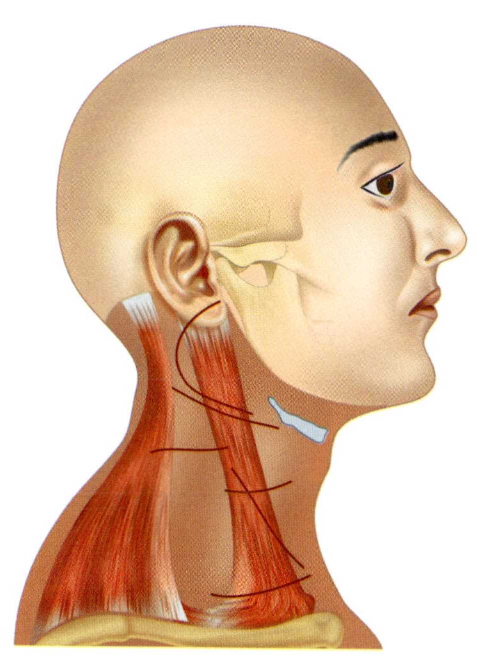

Fig. 11.2 Incisions for cervical lymph node biopsy

border of the sternomastoid. The lymph node is now held with Babcock's forceps gently and the feeding artery and draining vein is ligated and divided before removal of the node.

- *Closure:* Check hemostasis. Close the wound with interrupted nonabsorbable sutures.

POSTOPERATIVE CARE

Analgesic should be advised.

POSTOPERATIVE COMPLICATIONS

- Hemorrhage
- Sepsis.

CHAPTER

12

Surgery for Parotid Tumors

Gautam Mukhopadhya

SUPERFICIAL PAROTIDECTOMY

Indication

- Benign tumors of parotid
- Malignant tumors of parotid
- Uncommon situations like parotid calculi, chronic gland/duct fistula.

Preoperative Preparation

- Preoperative anesthetic checkup and control of medical problems like hypertension are mandatory
- Special consent along with explanation of the procedure to the patient and party are essential. Special reference need to be made regarding facial nerve neuropraxia/paralysis postoperatively
- In case of malignant tumor, implication of sacrificing part or all of the facial nerve should be discussed with patient
- Shaving anterior to ear and side of face is required.

Anesthesia

General anesthesia (GA) and hypotensive anesthesia may be necessary.

Position of Patient/Draping

After endotracheal intubation, the neck is extended and turned to the opposite side. The head end of the operating table is elevated if required. As in all head and neck surgeries, draping is done by three towel technique. After draping is complete, skin stitches are given all around to isolate the sterile area. The whole side of the face needs to be exposed. Bipolar diathermy and nerve stimulator are preferable. Sterile cotton plug is put in the ear.

Incision

Marking ink is used to mark the incision. The incision starts at the top of helix and proceeds inferiorly up to ear lobule and then is turned back up to 1 cm below the mastoid and then turns anteriorly to the tip of greater cornu hyoid following the skin crease. Figure 12.1 shows the standard S-shaped cervicofacial incision for parotidectomy.

Procedure

The incision is deepened and the skin flap is raised up to the anterior border of masseter. The tail of the gland is lifted of the sternomastoid muscle. The great auricular nerve is identified and divided close to the gland preserving its posterior branch which supplies the pinna. Preservation of most of the nerve may be useful if a facial nerve graft is required later on.

The sternomastoid muscle is retracted posteriorly and the posterior belly of digastric identified and followed up to the mastoid. The posterior border of the gland is now defined and retracted anteriorly. This allows identification of the point of tragal cartilage which along with the tip of mastoid, cartilaginous auditory canal and superior border of the posterior belly of digastric are the key landmarks to identify the main trunk of the facial nerve as it emerges from the stylomastoid foramen. The facial nerve lies 1 cm infero-medial to the point of tragal cartilage (Fig. 12.2).

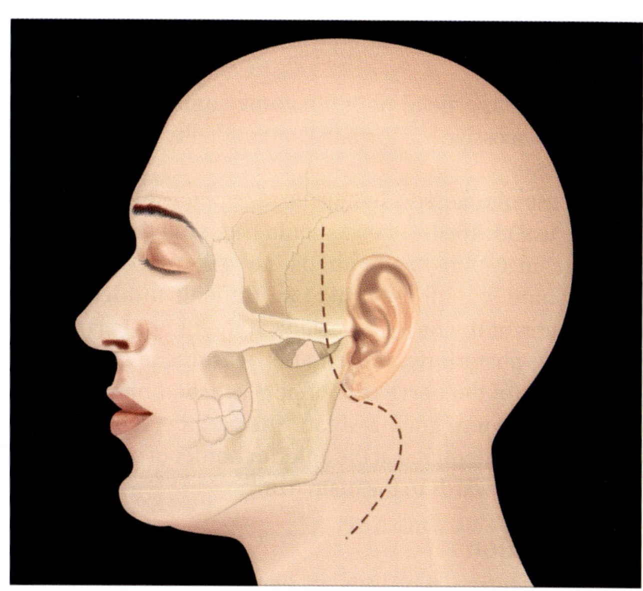

Fig. 12.1 Incision

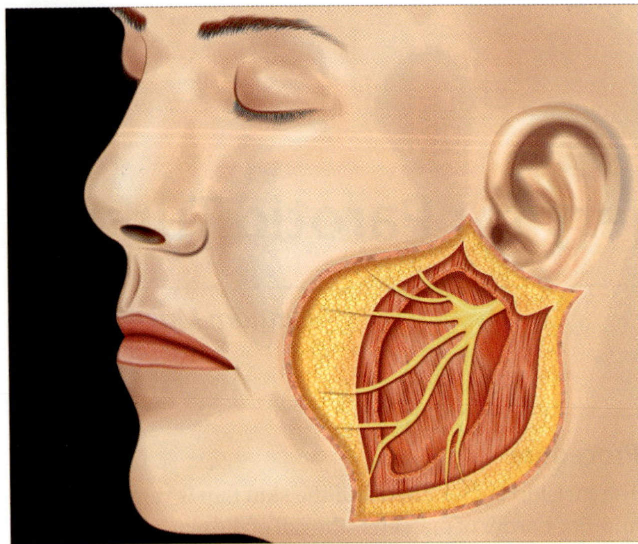

Fig. 12.2 Exposure of facial nerve

Once the main trunk of facial nerve is identified, it is followed forward. Usually, within 2 cm it divides into upper and lower division. The upper division is dissected first with mosquito artery forceps. Bleeding is controlled by bipolar diathermy, if available or sutured with 4/0 vicryl. The superior most branch crosses the midpoint of zygoma. The next division is very important as it supplies the eyelid. No attempt should be spared to save this vital branch of this facial nerve. The next is the buccal branch which lies close to the Stensen's duct and supplies the nose and upper lip. The branches of the lower division supplying the upper lip angle of the mouth and lower lip are now defined. The superficial lobe can now be dissected off and the specimen removed. Adequate hemostasis should be achieved prior to closure. The skin is closed with 4/0 prolene after suction drainage.

During superficial parotidectomy some problems may arise like excessive hemorrhage and difficulty in defining the facial nerve.

In case of excessive hemorrhage hypotensive anesthesia may be useful. The head end should be elevated as it reduces venous congestion. Rarely adrenaline soaks may be required.

In some situations, it may be difficult to identify the main trunk of the nerve especially, if the tumor is large and extending posteriorly. If even after reasonable attempt the main trunk of the nerve cannot be reached, it may be better to proceed in retrograde fashion. The peripheral branches of the nerve are identified at the anterior border of masseter and followed backwards to the main trunk.

Complications

- Facial nerve paralysis is usually uncommon after superficial parotidectomy. However, neuropraxia is common and recoverable with time. If the nerve is damaged accurate identification and primary suturing with 10/0 silk is advisable
- Postoperative hemorrhage is uncommon. However, if it occurs immediate drainage is essential
- Frey's syndrome may occur as a late complication. In this syndrome, when smell and taste are stimulated vasodilatation and sweating occurs. Fortunately, most resolve spontaneously.

EXCISION OF DEEP LOBE PAROTID TUMORS

Total Parotidectomy with Preservation of the Facial Nerve

Deep lobe parotid tumors are mostly benign. The surgical approach is similar to superficial parotidectomy. The superficial part of the gland is first dissected off, the branches of facial nerve identified and specimen removed. This exposes deep lobe tumors.

Delicate and meticulous dissection of the main trunk and peripheral branches are undertaken lifting the nerve off the tumor. Nerve hooks are used to lift the nerve and the tumor is mobilized by blunt and sharp dissection. The tumor can then be removed as one block saving the nerve.

Radial Parotidectomy

Radical parotidectomy with sacrifice of the facial nerve is required when there is clear histological evidence of high grade malignant tumor with extensive involvement of the facial nerve.

Radical parotidectomy involves removal of all parotid gland tissue and elective sacrifice of the facial nerve usually through the main trunk. The skin flap is reflected forward. The external carotid artery is identified at the lower pole of the gland and divided between ligatures. The trunk of the facial nerve is divided. The posterior aspect of the whole gland is now mobilized off the cartilaginous and bony external auditory meatus. The facial nerve branches are divided at the anterior border of the gland which is mobilized backwards off the masseter muscle. Now the gland is mobilized from below upwards. The superficial temporal and maxillary arteries are divided and doubly ligated. The whole gland with the facial nerve can now be removed.

Radical parotidectomy with block dissection: Patients suffering from proven malignancy of parotid gland and cytological evidence of node metastasis requires a formal block dissection in continuity radical parotidectomy. A modified Y incision may be applied for block dissection.

FOLLOW-UP/RESULTS OF TREATMENT

Although surgery is the mainstay of treatment, radiotherapy is useful in advanced cases especially in the adjuvant setting. Chemotherapy has no established role in malignant tumors of parotid.

Patient should follow-up every three monthly for the first two years, then six monthly for the next three years and thereafter once annually. The overall survival of malignant parotid tumors are approximately 60% at five years, 50% at ten years and 40% at twenty years. The clinical stage and tumor grade are the two most important prognostic indicators. For malignant parotid tumors, there is 95% survival for stage 1,70% for stage II and 25% for stage III at ten years. Postoperative radiotherapy has increased the survival status in advanced high grade malignant parotid tumors.

CHAPTER

13

Simple Lithotomy for Submandibular Duct Stone

Dhiraj Choudhury

INDICATION

Removal of a submandibular duct stone should be attempted only if the stone is confirmed radiologically lying within the duct and easily palpable well forward in the floor of the mouth. If the stone is located more posteriorly or the gland is chronically infected then excision of the submandibular gland is the procedure of choice.

OPERATIVE PROCEDURE

- *Position:* The patient lies in supine position.
- *Anesthesia:* The operation can be done under local or general anesthesia with endotracheal intubation and pharyngeal pack.
- *Exploration:* The mouth is kept wide open usually with a mouth gag. The tongue is drawn upwards and towards the opposite side with Alli's tissue forceps or tongue holding forceps. Localize the stone by palpation once the duct has been exposed (Fig. 13.1).
- *Technique:* Steady the duct by two stay sutures. Traction on the proximal one will prevent stone slipping proximally into the gland (Fig. 13.2).
- *Extraction of stone:* Make an incision with a 15 blade to open the duct directly over the stone. Remember the position of lingual nerve as it crosses the duct in the floor of the mouth to prevent its injury.

Once the lumen of the duct is opened, there is usually a gush of turbid saliva. Remove the stone with a scoop or dissecting forceps (Fig. 13.3).

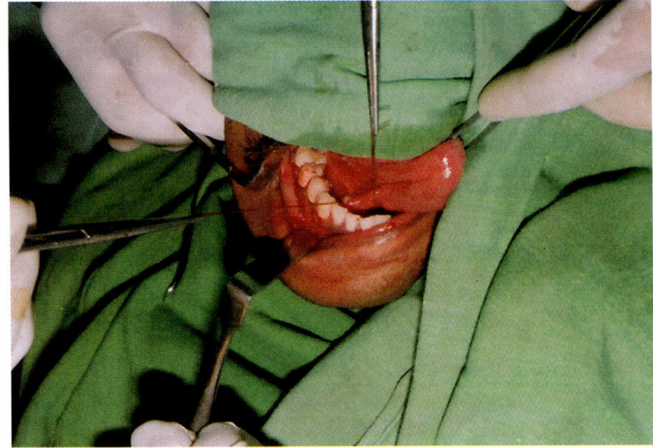

Fig. 13.2 Application of stay sutures

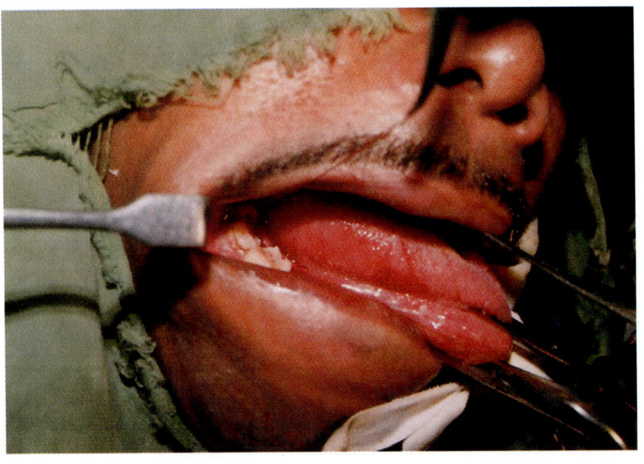

Fig. 13.1 Exposure of the duct

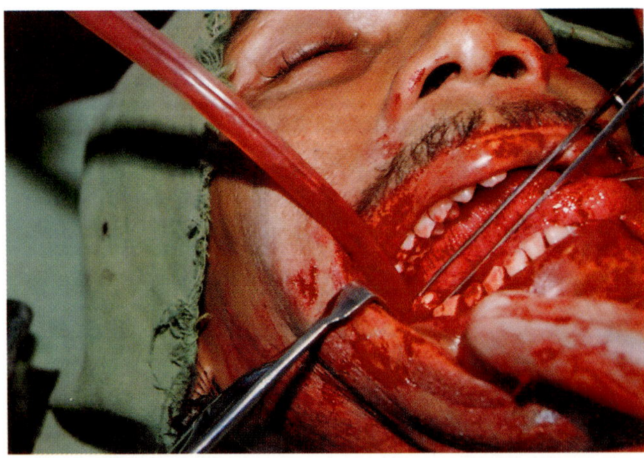

Fig. 13.3 Extraction of stone after making incision

- *Closure:* The duct is not sutured to prevent stenosis.
  Remove the stay sutures.
  Check hemostasis.

POSTOPERATIVE CARE

- Liquid is allowed orally as soon as the patient is allowed to swallow
- Mouth wash with betadine mouth wash solution
- Administer analgesic.

POSTOPERATIVE COMPLICATION

- Duct stenosis
- Damage to lingual nerve.

CHAPTER

14

Excision of Submandibular Salivary Gland

Dhiraj Choudhury

ANATOMY

The submandibular salivary gland lies in the submandibular fossa below the ramus of the mandible. It consists of a large superficial lobe and a small deep lobe which are continuous with each other around posterior border of the mylohyoid muscle (Fig. 14.1).

The superficial lobe is covered by platysma, deep fascia and fibrous capsule derived from deep fascia. It is crossed by cervical branch of facial nerve and facial vein. It is related to anterior belly of digastric anteriorly and posterior belly of digastric and stylohyoid posteriorly. Medially, it is related to mylohyoid, hyoglossus, lingual and hypoglossal nerve. Laterally, it lies on the medial surface of the mandible.

The facial artery is related to the posterior and superior aspect of the superficial lobe.

The deep part of the gland extends forward in the interval between the mylohyoid below and laterally and hyoglossus medially.

The submandibular duct emerges from the anterior end of the deep part of the gland. It passes forward along side of the tongue to open into the mouth on the summit of a papilla. It is crossed laterally by lingual nerve which loops around it.

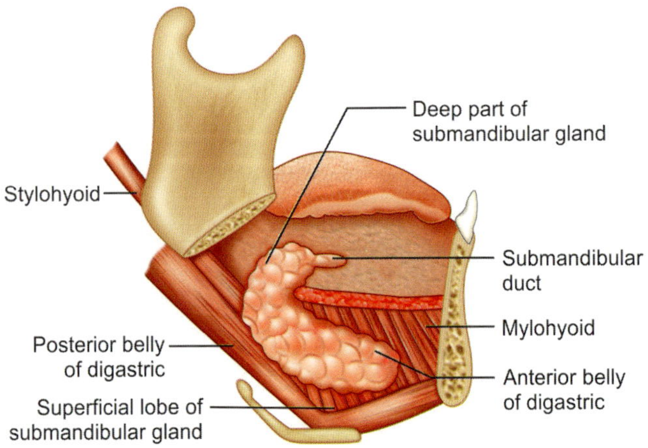

Fig. 14.1 Anatomy of submandibular gland

INDICATIONS

- Sialadenitis
- Tumors—adenoma or carcinoma
- As part of radical neck dissection.

PREOPERATIVE PREPARATION

- Plain X-ray of the floor of the mouth
- Fine needle aspiration cytology (FNAC) if there is clinical suspicion of neoplasm
- Explain the risk of injury to mandibular branch of facial nerve, lingual nerve and hypoglossal nerve before taking consent.

OPERATIVE PROCEDURE

Position

The patient lies in the supine position with a sandbag under the shoulder to extend neck and head turned to opposite side.

Anesthesia

General anesthesia with endotracheal intubation is used.

Draping

Apply a double head towel after painting the field of operation with povidone-iodine.

Incision

A 6 cm long crease incision is made 5 cm below and parallel to lower border of the mandible (Fig. 14.2) to avoid damage to marginal mandibular branch of the facial nerve.

Exposure

The incision is deepened through fat and platysma to deep fascia. Keeping the dissection as close as possible to the surface of the gland, dissect all around the superficial lobe rising superficial flap of tissues. The mandibular branch of the facial nerve will be safe if the dissection is kept close to the gland surface (Fig. 14.3).

Mobilization of Superficial Lobe (Fig. 14.4)

Free lower border of the gland and retract it upwards with tissue forceps. The tendon of the digastric muscle will be exposed which is retracted downward (Fig. 14.5).

Ligation of Facial Artery at Lower Border

Traction on the gland will reveal the tortuous facial artery which emerges from the deep to enter the posterior part of the gland. The artery is doubly ligated and then divided. The lower border of the gland is now free (Fig. 14.6).

Ligation of Facial Artery at Upper Border (Figs 14.7A and B)

Pull the gland inferiorly to free the upper attachment of the gland to lower border of the mandible. The facial artery and vein emerge from the upper border of the gland and should be divided and ligated guarding the mandibular of the facial nerve. The superficial lobe is free now.

A segment of the facial artery and vein will remain attached to the gland.

Mobilization of the Deep Lobe

Now identify the mylohyoid muscle which is overlapped by superficial lobe. The superficial lobe is retracted to ipsilateral side to expose the mylohyoid. Retract the mylohyoid muscle medially to expose the deep lobe. The lingual nerve and hypoglossal nerve are identified and preserved between deep lobe and hyoglossus muscle. Downward traction on the gland and careful dissection will expose the lingual nerve which is attached to the gland by submandibular ganglion and its preganglionic fibers. Free the lingual nerve from the gland (Fig. 14.8).

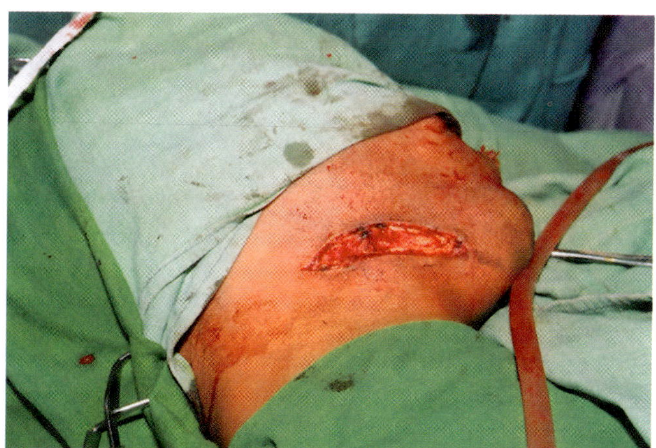

Fig. 14.2 Skin incision

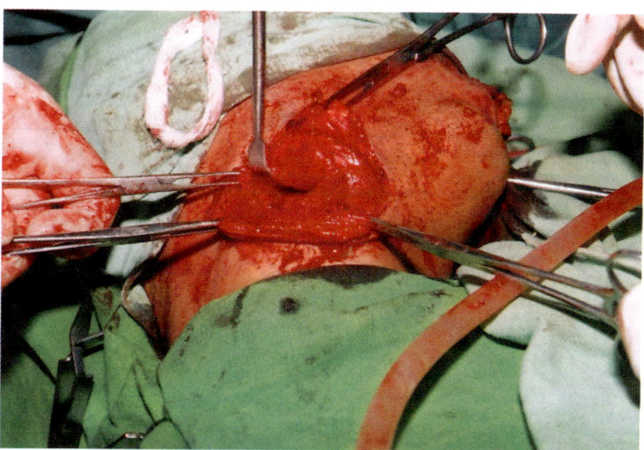

Fig. 14.4 Mobilization of superficial lobe

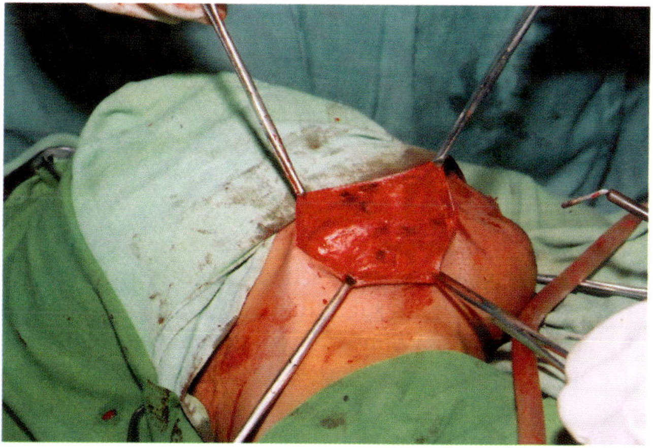

Fig. 14.3 Exposure of superficial lobe

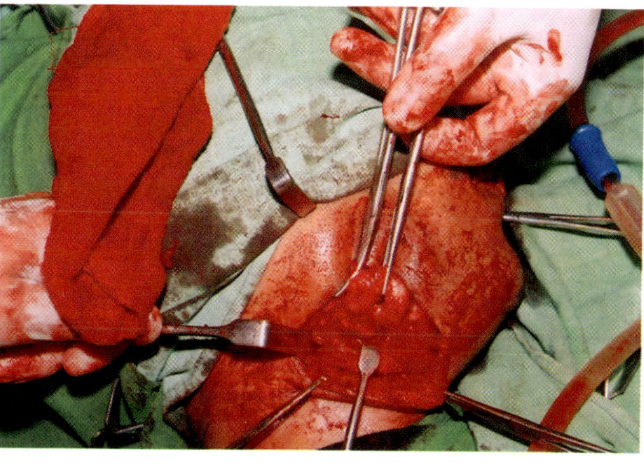

Fig. 14.5 Retraction of tendon of diagastric

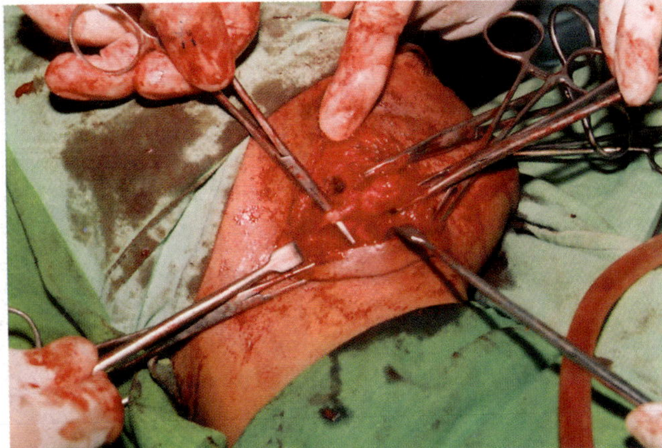

Fig. 14.6 Ligation of facial artery at lower border

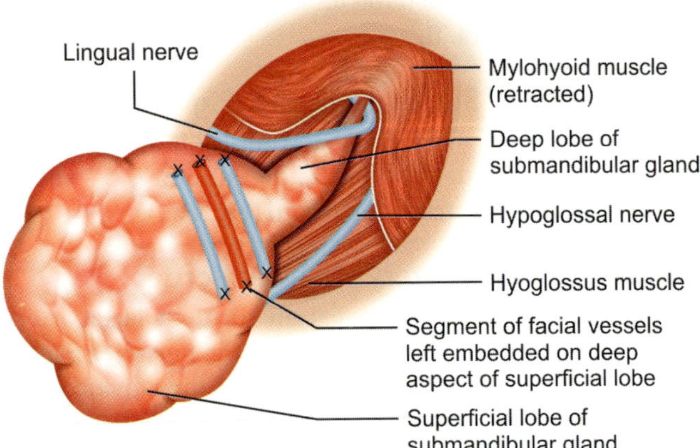

Fig. 14.8 Diagrammatic representation of duct and lingual nerve

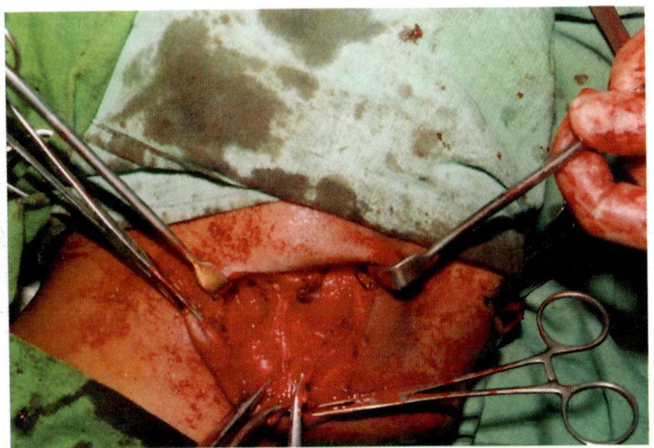

Fig. 14.7A Ligation of facial artery at upper border

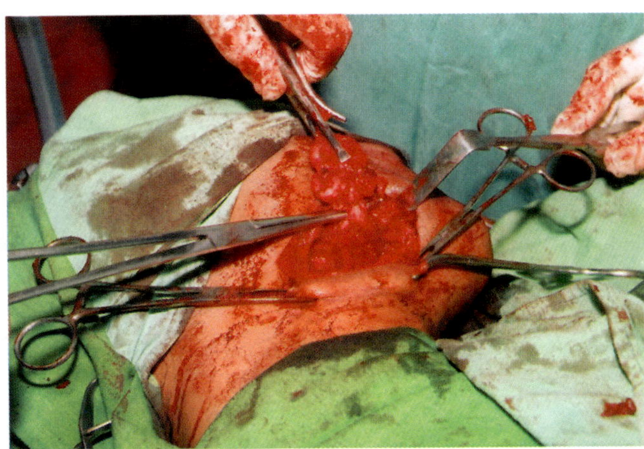

Fig. 14.9 Division of duct

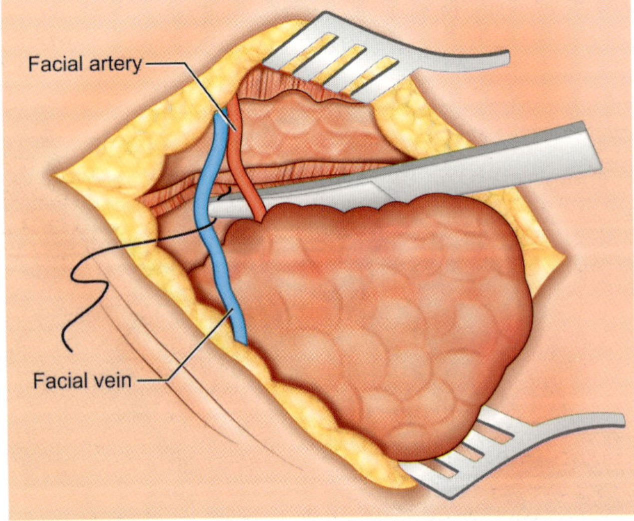

Fig. 14.7B Ligation and division of facial artery at upper border of submandibular gland—Schematic diagram

Division of the Duct (Fig. 14.9)

Blunt dissection will now reveal the duct which runs forward to the papilla in the floor of mouth. Clamp, divide and ligate the duct. Remove the gland and send it for histopathology.

Closure

Hemostasis should be checked carefully. Insert a suction drain and bring it through a separate stab wound. Close the skin with subcuticular suture.

RADICAL EXCISION

Radical submandibular sialoadenectomy with resection of segment of body of mandible and block dissection is popularly known as Commando operation (Chapter 18). In case of neoplastic condition, frozen section histology may be necessary. Full radical resection will often require resection of the hemimandible on the affected side, full clearance of both submandibular triangles and en-block excision of ipsilateral cervical lymph nodes. If involvement of mucosa of the floor of mouth is extensive then repair of the lining may be required.

POSTOPERATIVE CARE

- Continue IV fluid for 24–48 hours
- Maintain oral hygiene
- Systematic antibiotic
- Remove drain after 48–72 hours
- Remove skin stitches after 4 days.

POSTOPERATIVE COMPLICATION

- Injury to mandibular branch of facial nerve
- Hemorrhage reactionary
- Injury to lingual and hypoglossal nerve
- Sepsis.

CHAPTER

15 Operations for Cancer of Face and Lip

Dhiraj Choudhury

BASAL CELL CARCINOMA

Basal cell carcinoma of face (rodent ulcer) can be treated by surgery or radiotherapy.

SURGERY

Indications: Surgery is specially indicated for basal cell carcinoma situated close to eye or over cartilage (nose).

Surgery consists of wide excision (preferably 1 cm wide margin but near eye 0.5 cm) followed by primary closure if possible.

TECHNIQUE: WIDE EXCISION

- *Anesthesia:* General with endotracheal intubation.
- *Skin incision:* An oval-shaped skin incision is marked out.
- *Dissection:* The incision is deepened vertically along the oval line until superficial fat is visible. Deepen the incision at one end and raise the skin with subcutaneous tissue. The plane of cutting should be sufficiently deep to include a wide margin of normal tissue below. The excision is completed by carrying similar dissection at the other end. Secure hemostasis by diathermy.
- *Closure:* If possible primary closure can be carried out. But sometimes skin grafting (full thickness graft) may be necessary. Facial surgeons prefer rotational flaps to cover the defect.

Mohs micrographic surgery is performed by dermatologist under local anesthesia.

CARCINOMA OF LIP

Carcinoma of lip can be treated by surgery or radiotherapy. The decision depends on extent of the lesion, availability of irradiation therapy and experience of the surgeon.

TYPES OF SURGERY

- *Tumor less than 2 cm*: Up to one-third of the lip can be excised by wedge resection of the lesion (Fig. 15.1) with primary closure (Fig. 15.2). The wound is closed in three layers—mucosa, muscle and skin. Correct alignment of vermilion border is top priority.

2. *Large tumors:* If more than one-third of the lip has to be removed it is necessary to utilize local flaps like cross lip flap.
3. *Extensive tumors:* Removal of entire lip requires reconstruction by a forearm flap. Regional lymph node metastasis is treated by a modified radical neck dissection.

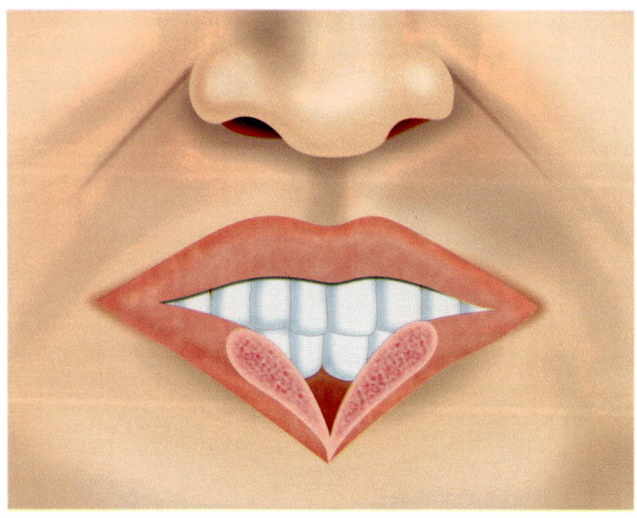

Fig. 15.1 Wedge excision of lip carcinoma

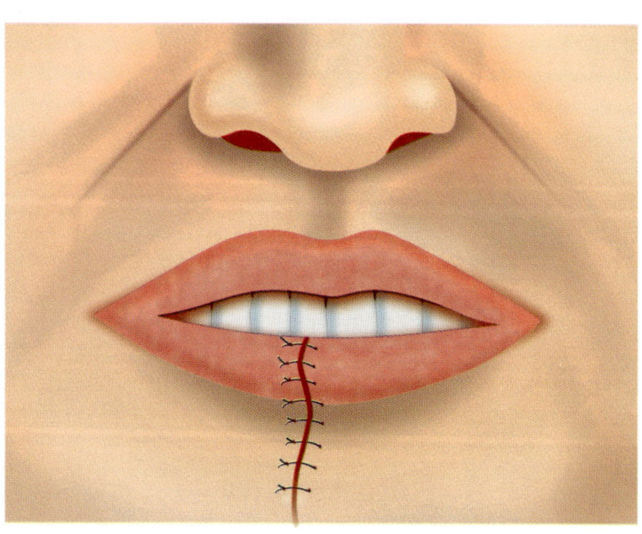

Fig. 15.2 Closure of lip

CHAPTER

16

Operations for Cancer of the Oral Tongue

RS Rao, Satish Rao

INTRODUCTION

Cancer of the tongue is a common malignancy seen in our country. The anterior 2/3rd of the tongue is situated in the oral cavity, while the base of the tongue is in the oropharynx. The clinical course and biological behavior of the two parts are different. Base tongue lesions are usually treated with radiotherapy. Lesions of the oral tongue are treated with surgery, radiotherapy or a combination of surgery and radiotherapy. The choice depends on the stage of the primary lesion. There is a high incidence of lymph node metastases in carcinoma of the oral tongue. Appropriate treatment should be planned for the nodes.

Staging of Carcinoma of the Tongue

The American Joint Committee on Cancer (AJCC)[1] have staged the primary tumors of the tongue as follows.

T1 — Primary tumor less than 2 cm
T2 — Primary tumor between 2–4 cm
T3 — Primary tumor more than 4 cm
T4 — Lesion with ankyloglossia, hypoglossal palsy, invasion of the muscles or bone.

CHOICE OF TREATMENT FOR T1 AND T2 LESIONS

These cases can be treated equally well with either surgery or radiotherapy, depending on the skill and experience of the clinician and the treatment facilities available at the institution. Surgery can be performed either conventionally or with a CO_2 laser. Cancer of the tongue is biologically aggressive. Therefore, the treatment also has to be aggressive, first chance is the best chance. For these reasons, we advocate a hemiglossectomy for T1 and T2 lesions of the oral tongue (Figs 16.1A and B). Some surgeons prefer to do a wide excision of the lesion. In our experience, wide excision is associated with higher rate of local recurrence.[2]

ANESTHESIA AND OTHER PRELIMINARY STEPS

The surgical procedure is done under general anesthesia with nasal endotracheal intubation. In case the patient has trismus or submucous fibrosis, intubation may be achieved under topical anesthesia with the help of a fiberoptic bronchoscope. In advanced cases requiring extensive resection of the tongue, or in cases where a difficult endotracheal intubation is anticipated, it is safer to do a preliminary tracheostomy first, and then induce general anesthesia. A nasogastric tube is passed at this stage. Head end of the table is raised by about ten degrees to reduce venous congestion.

The mouth is opened and a mouth gag is inserted. The jaws of the mouth gag should be placed in the region of the third molar teeth. A mouth gag in the anterior part of the mouth reduces the space for the surgeon to operate. The ideal mouth gag, in our experience, is what the dental surgeons call as dental probe. The pharynx is cleared of secretions by thorough suction. A throat pack is put in the oropharynx to prevent aspiration of blood into the air passages. The surgeon checks with the anesthetist to ensure that the pack is not too tight or too loose.

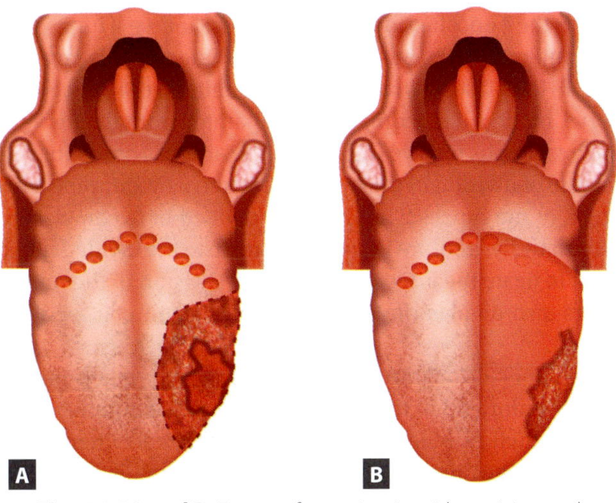

Figs 16.1A and B Extent of resection in wide excision and hemiglossectomy

HEMIGLOSSECTOMY FOR T1 AND T2 LESIONS

Anatomical Basis for the Operation

The oral tongue is like a paired organ. The right and left halves are separated by the median raphe. The midline is an avascular area with scanty vessels and lymphatics. Each half is supplied by the ipsilateral lingual artery and hypoglossal nerve. Lymphatics also drain to the ipsilateral nodes, except in advanced cases. Excision of one-half of the oral tongue surprisingly causes little deformity or dysfunction. The residual tongue undergoes compensatory hypertrophy.

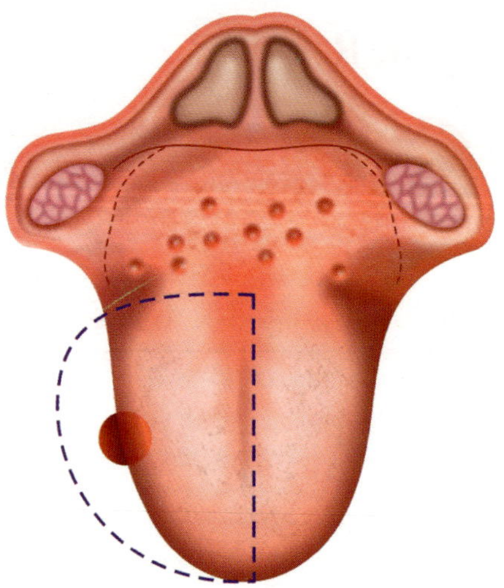

Fig. 16.2 Incision on the dorsum of the tongue

Operative Steps

Incisions

Two stay sutures are taken, one on each half of the tongue, equidistant from the midline. The frenum or under surface of the tongue is incised in midline with number eleven blade. From the tip, the incision is extended backwards with scissors, in midline on the dorsum almost up to the foramen cecum (Fig. 16.2). The incision in the floor mouth extends from midline up to the anterior pillar of tonsil (Fig. 16.3). Care is taken that it is well away from the lateral border of the tumor. At a later stage, a transverse incision is taken posteriorly on the dorsum, joining the anterior pillar to the posterior end of the midline incision.

The two halves of the tongue are separated in midline along the median raphe right up to the posterior end of the mucosal incision. The genioglossus muscle is clearly seen extending from its origin and entering the substance of the tongue. Its lateral border is defined by blunt dissection. The origin of genioglossus is then picked up on a hemostat and divided with cautery (Fig. 16.4).

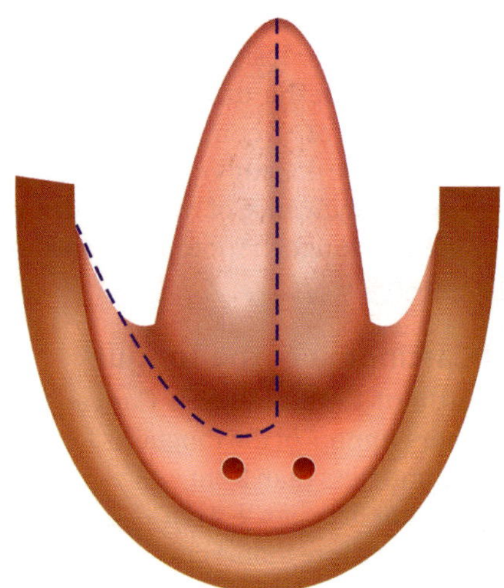

Fig. 16.3 Incision in the ventral surface of the tongue and floor of the mouth

Division of Nerve and Artery

The division of the origin of genioglossus greatly increases the mobility of the tongue. The tongue is pulled upwards and to the opposite side. The hypoglossal nerve with its vena commitants comes in view (Fig. 16.5). The nerve is clamped and divided. The lingual artery runs parallel to the hypoglossal nerve, but in a deeper plane and separated from the nerve by the hyoglossus muscle (Fig. 16.6). The artery is now sought at the site of division of the hypoglossal nerve by snipping a few fibers of the muscle. The artery is divided between clamps. Alternatively, a suture is taken, just deep to the divided nerve, so as to ligate the artery in continuity. Division of the muscle fibers also divides the artery, which is again clamped and ligated.

The posterior transverse incision is now taken joining the posterior end of the dorsal incision to the anterior pillar. The residual muscle fibers connecting the specimen to the base of tongue are divided, taking care to remain in a plane superficial to the divided lingual artery. The specimen is removed and inspected carefully to see whether adequate

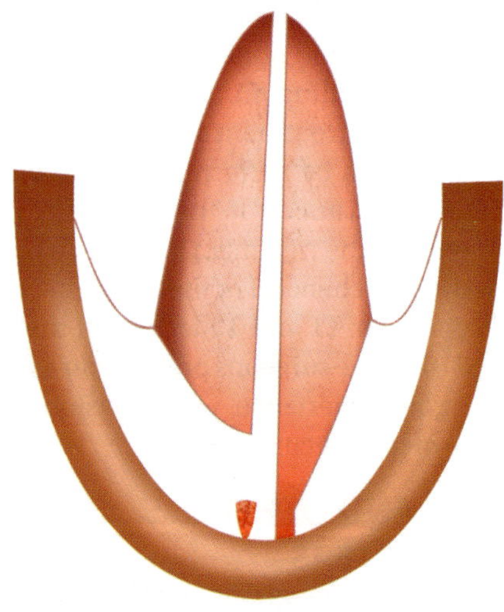

Fig. 16.4 Division of genioglossus muscle

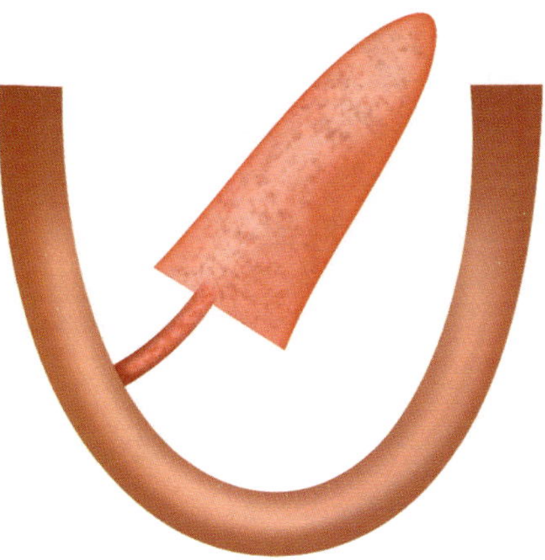

Fig. 16.5 Exposure of hypoglossal nerve

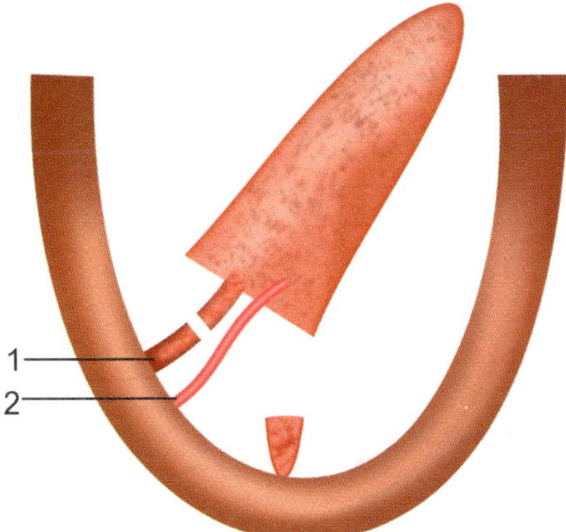

Fig. 16.6 Exposure of lingual artery

margins and depth of excision have been achieved. The residual tongue is inspected and hemostasis achieved (Fig. 16.7). Small bleeding points are cauterized; larger bleeders are underrun with a catgut stitch.

Closure

The medial end of the transverse incision is held in an Allis forceps and pulled forward. This facilitates closure of the wound. Three or four stitches are taken posteriorly, approximating the dorsum to the floor of the mouth. The tip of the tongue is rotated posteriorly by stitching it to the posterior and lateral part of the dorsum. Interrupted sutures are taken to close the gap on the dorsum of the tongue. A few sutures are taken approximating the floor of mouth to the ventral surface of the tongue. Alternately, the tip is not rotated. Some more sutures are taken to approximate the dorsal mucosa to the mucosa on the undersurface of the tongue, right up to the tip. Only absorbable suture material is used in the oral cavity. Rotation of the tip gives a better cosmetic appearance and there is no problem with speech (Fig. 16.8). In the other method, there is a cosmetic defect; but the patient can move the tip to any part of the oral cavity.

Terminal steps: The oral cavity is flushed with saline; all blood clots are removed. The throat pack is taken out. The anesthetist inspects the pharynx with a laryngoscope and sucks out all secretions and blood clots. There should be no blood oozing into the oropharynx from the site of operation.

Postoperative Care

It is our practice to leave the endotracheal tube *in situ* for 24 hours. Therefore the patient is shifted to an intensive care unit. Occasionally, there is reactionary hemorrhage or oozing, requiring intervention. A endotracheal tube greatly facilitates induction of general anesthesia. With bleeding in the mouth, it is dangerous to induce general anesthesia. Attempts to control bleeding under local anesthesia makes

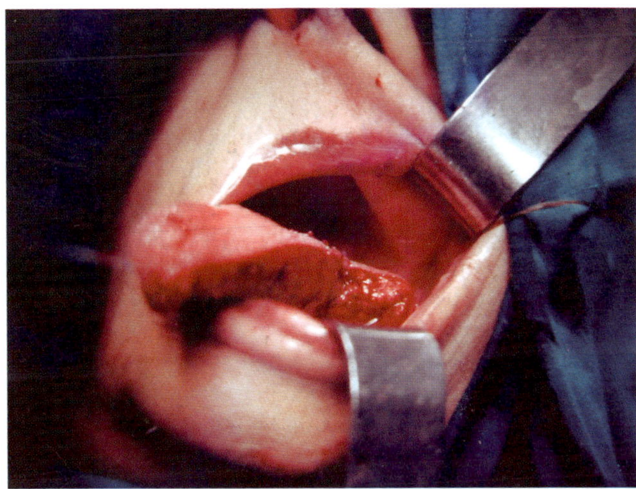

Fig. 16.7 Residual tongue after hemiglossectomy

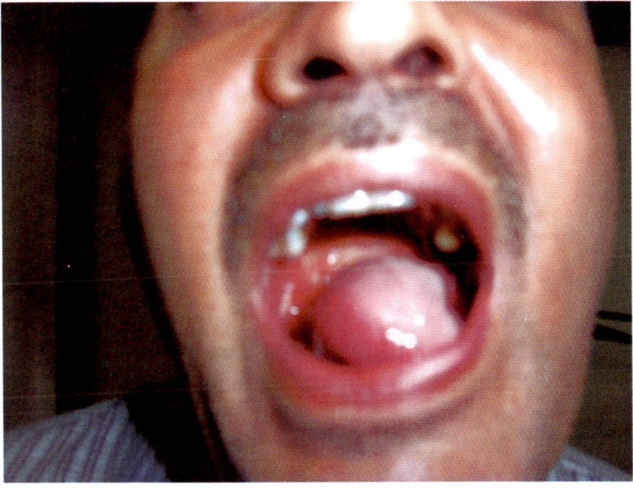

Fig. 16.8 Appearance of the tongue two months after hemiglossectomy

the patient cough and struggle, resulting in more bleeding. Occasionally, there is edema around the glottis resulting in dyspnea. An endotracheal tube can prevent an emergency tracheotomy. The cuff of the tube is, however, kept deflated. The tube is removed next day. Heavy sedation is avoided in these cases. Patients are fed through a Ryle's tube for five days. Oral hygiene is maintained by antiseptic gargles.

Oral feeds are started on the fifth day. By the eighth day, he should be able to take semisolid food. The consistency is gradually increased. The patient should be able to take his normal food by three weeks. After two weeks, patient should be encouraged to speak. At first his speech may be difficult to follow; but in a matter of weeks, it improves rapidly. Patient should be motivated to speak clearly. As a form of speech therapy, he should be asked to read a newspaper loudly for about fifteen minutes. About two months later, the quality of speech is almost normal and acceptable to the patient and his relatives. The residual tongue undergoes compensatory hypertrophy and attains the original volume, giving excellent cosmesis.

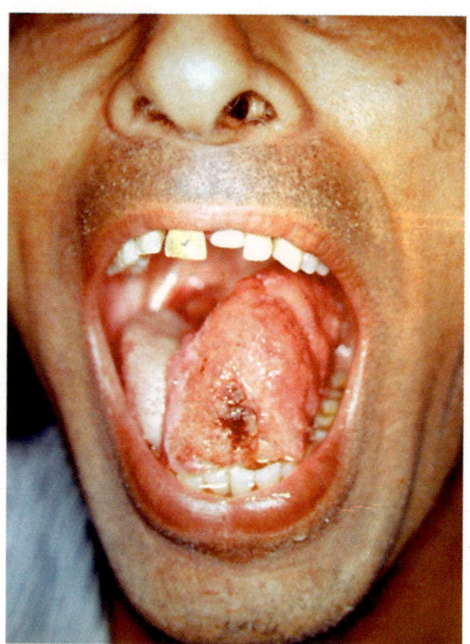

Fig. 16.9 Cancer tongue with extensive involvement of the floor mouth

Complications

- *Intraoperative:* There may be brisk hemorrhage from the lingual artery or its branches. This can be readily controlled.
- *Reactionary hemorrhage:* Under general anesthesia, the bleeding points are caught and securely ligated. In cases of secondary hemorrhage, it is better to ligate the external carotid artery.
- *Hematoma:* There may be a hematoma in the floor of the mouth due to venous bleeding or oozing. One or two stitches in the floor of mouth be removed and the clots evacuated.
- *Dyspnea:* Hematoma or severe edema of tongue can cause respiratory distress. As a preventive measure patient may be put on steroids for 48 hours, to be followed up with oral anti-inflammatory drugs.

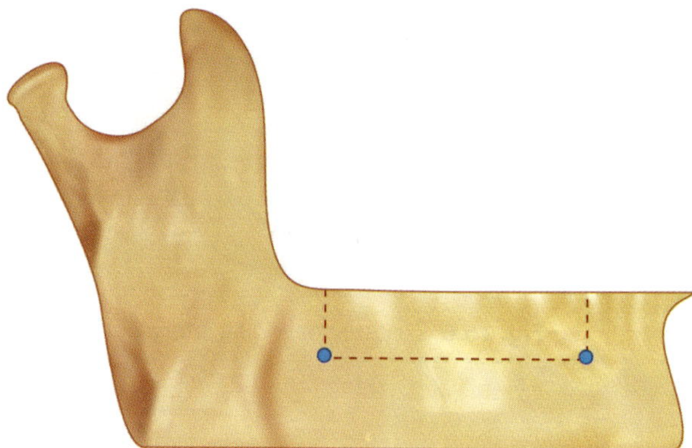

Fig. 16.10 Line of resection in marginal mandibulectomy

SURGERY FOR T3 LESIONS

For T3 lesions, surgery may have to be more extensive than a formal hemiglossectomy. Depending on the spread of the primary, surgery will have to be suitably modified. We may have to cross the midline and remove a longitudinal strip of opposite tongue. Or excision may involve removal of a part of the base tongue. More commonly, the disease extends into the floor mouth, requiring its removal (Fig. 16.9). For these cases, a pure intraoral approach is inadequate.

The incidence of lymph nodes metastases is high in T3 lesions. Hence even in clinical no neck, we advocate a XI nerve sparing neck dissection. After removal of the specimen in the neck, we ligate the lingual artery right at its origin. The hypoglossal nerve is retracted upwards, at the point where it crosses the external carotid artery. The lingual artery arises from the medial wall of external carotid artery, between the origins of superior thyroid and facial arteries. It is identified and ligated in continuity.

GLOSSECTOMY WITH EXCISION OF FLOOR MOUTH

At the conclusion of neck dissection, the upper incision is extended in midline up to the lip; but the lower lip is not divided. The upper neck flap is further raised to expose the lower border of the mandible. An incision is taken in the oral cavity, in the gingiobuccal sulcus from the midline to a point posterior to the 3rd molar tooth. The mucoperiosteum is pushed downwards so that the oral cavity is now in continuity with the neck wound. The proposed line of marginal mandibulectomy is marked out on the bone with cautery (Fig. 16.10). Holes are drilled at the anterior and posterior ends of the incision. The central incisor on the ipsilateral side is

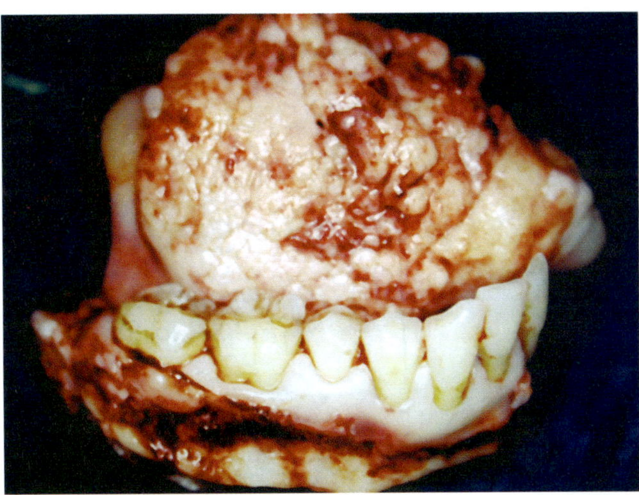

Fig. 16.11 Specimen of the tongue with resected mandible

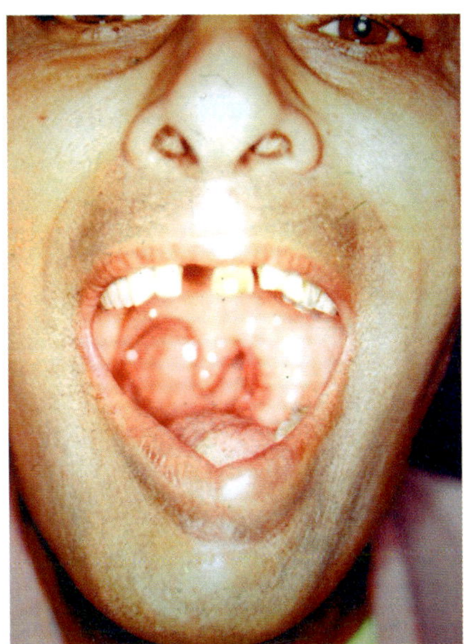

Fig. 16.12 Postoperative appearance of the oral cavity after extension resection

removed. The bone is cut with a dental drill or an AO saw. The vertical cuts are through the socket of incisor teeth and behind the third molar tooth. Care is taken to preserve periosteum of the lower border of the mandible. The genioglossus muscle is detached flush with its bony origin. The mylohyoid muscle is divided. Division of the bone and the muscles greatly increases the mobility of the tongue. The tumor is excised, after obtaining a free margin of 2 cm, particularly along its medial and posterior borders. The specimen consists of the tumor on the tongue, floor mouth with mylohyoid muscle and alveolar part of the mandible in one piece (Fig. 16.11). Adequate hemostasis is achieved. Often, it is possible to get a primary closure (Fig. 16.12). In these cases, the tip of the tongue is not rotated. If the defect is large, then a pectoralis major myocutaneous flap is transposed to close the defect. In cases, where the tongue is removed extensively, a tracheostomy is done to facilitate postoperative respiratory care.

Postoperative care: Patient is started on oral feeds, after about 8–10 days. The tracheostomy tube is removed; when the patient is able to swallow safely without aspiration. Usually, it takes about two weeks to remove the tracheotomy tube.

REFERENCES

1. Staging of oral cancer. AJCC Cancer Staging Manual, sixth edition, Springer-Verlag, Heidelberg, Germany. 2003;23.
2. Parikh HK, Rao RS, Sukhthankar P, Deshmane VH, Parikh DM. Surgery in early cancer of the oral tongue (T1-2). Ind J of Otolaryngol Head and Neck Surg. 1998;50:349-67.

CHAPTER

17

Neck Dissections

RS Rao, Satish Rao

INTRODUCTION

The treatment of metastatic lymph nodes is an important step in the management of carcinomas in the head and neck region. The propensity for lymph node metastases depends on the site of the primary. We have three choices. viz: surgery, radiotherapy, and surgery followed by postoperative radiotherapy. Radiotherapy is the treatment of choice; if the primary is also being treated by radiation, with a curative intent, e.g. in carcinoma of nasopharynx or base of the tongue. Radiotherapy is also given as a palliative measure, when the primary or metastatic node is not resectable. Surgery for radical removal of lymph nodes in the neck is known as radical neck dissection (RND). Postoperative radiation is given as and when indicated. A thorough knowledge of the anatomy of the neck is absolutely necessary for performing this operation.

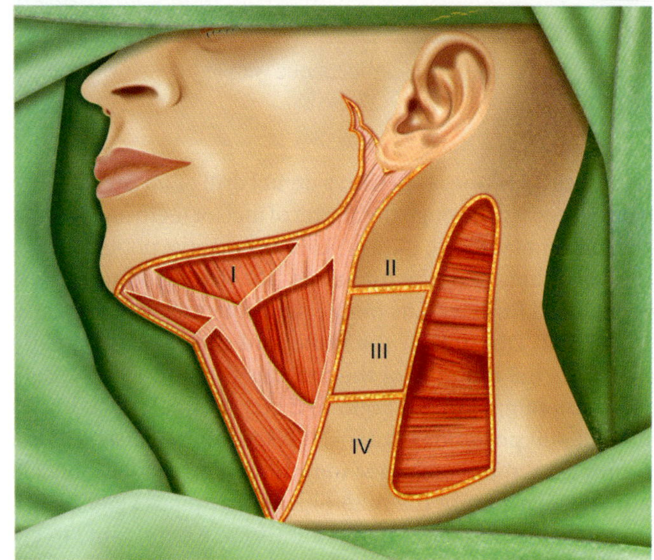

Fig. 17.1 The levels of cervical lymph nodes

INDICATIONS AND CONTRAINDICATIONS

Radical neck dissection is the treatment of choice for the treatment of metastatic nodes provided the following criteria are met.

- The primary is controlled or can be controlled at the time of neck dissection
- There are no distant metastases
- The lymph nodes are clinically mobile. One should not attempt a neck dissection in cases where the nodes are grossly stuck to the sternomastoid muscle, carotid vessels or the skin.

LEVELS OF LYMPH NODES

Surgeons and pathologists have classified the lymph nodes in the neck into well-defined levels (Fig. 17.1).[1]

- *Level I:* The submental and submandibular nodes.
- *Level II:* Vertical chain of upper deep cervical nodes from base skull to the level of the hyoid. These nodes are in intimate relation with the internal jugular vein (IJV). This group is divided by the accessory nerve into two subgroups.
  - 1. II-a, nodes below and medial to the nerve
  - 2. II-b, nodes above and lateral to the XI nerve.
- *Level III:* Nodes along the IJV, from level of hyoid to the lower border of the cricoid.
- *Level IV:* Lower group of nodes up to the clavicle, including the supraclavicular nodes.
- *Level V:* Nodes in the posterior triangle of the neck along the accessory nerve.

VARIANTS OF NECK DISSECTION: DEFINITIONS

Radical Neck Dissection

This is the basic operation. All other operations are modification of this procedure. In radical neck dissection (RND), all the lymph nodes on one side of the neck are removed, from the clavicle to the mastoid process, along with fat, fascia, the submandibular salivary gland, the sternomastoid muscle (SM), the IJV and the accessory nerve (XI nerve). The structures that must be preserved are: the carotid vessels, the vagus, hypoglossal, and phrenic nerves, and the brachial plexus. RND has considerable morbidity; hence the procedure has been modified to reduce the morbidity. In modified neck dissection (MND), the nodes at all the five levels are removed, but with preservation of one or more of the following structures:

- *Accessory nerve:* Division of this nerve causes paralysis of the trapezius muscle, leading to drooping of the shoulder, dragging pain and limitation of shoulder movements.
- *Internal jugular vein:* Its removal causes edema of the ipsilateral face. Bilateral removal of IJV causes severe edema of face and cerebral edema. It can be life-threatening and best avoided. In simultaneous bilateral neck dissection, at least one IJV must be preserved.
- *Sternomastoid muscle:* The morbidity is minimal and only cosmetic.
  - *In MND type 1,* only the XI nerve is preserved.
  - *In MND type 2,* XI nerve and IJV are preserved.
  - *In MND type 3,* all the three structures,viz. XI nerve, IJV and SM are removed. This procedure is also known as functional neck dissection.

Elective or Prophylactic Neck Dissection

When the neck dissection is done in cases where the lymph nodes are clinically not palpable (No neck).

Partial Neck Dissections

In these procedures, only certain group of nodes are removed. They are often performed as a staging procedure and in cases where the nodes are not palpable (No neck).

Supraomohyoid Neck Dissection

In *supraomohyoid neck dissection (SOHD),* lymph nodes at levels I,II and III are removed. In *lateral neck dissection* nodes at levels II, III and IV are removed. In carcinoma of hypopharynx, this procedure may be done bilaterally at the same sitting.

ANESTHESIA AND POSITION OF THE PATIENT

The operation is done under general anesthesia with endotracheal tube *in situ*. The neck is extended by placing a shoulder pad under the upper part of the scapulae. A doughnut ring is placed under the occiput. The neck is turned to the opposite side. The eyes are covered with gauze after putting an eye ointment. The endotracheal tube should be accessible to the anesthetist at all times in any operation in the head and neck region. The head end of the table is tilted upwards by ten degrees to reduce venous congestion.

Operative Steps for MND Type 1 (XI Nerve Sparing Procedure)

Today, this is the most common procedure performed, hence we will describe it, step-by-step.

Choice of Skin Incision

A lot of morbidity in neck dissection is due to wrong choice of incision. As far as possible, the incisions should be transverse, preferably, in one of the neck creases. Vertical incisions should be avoided. They produce contractures, cause limitation in neck movements and are cosmetically unacceptable. If a vertical incision has to be taken, it should be taken in a zig zag fashion, so that it can be closed like a Z plasty. A trifurcate junction of skin flaps, especially over the carotid vessels, should be avoided. Necrosis of skin over the carotid vessels can result in secondary and fatal hemorrhage from the carotid artery. We describe three well-known incisions:

1. *Double trifurcate incision of Hayes Martin:* This was the incision described in the earlier descriptions.
2. *McFee incisions:* Two transverse incisions are taken. Cosmetic results are excellent. The dissection becomes a little tedious as the middle flap has to be retracted repeatedly upwards and downwards.
3. *A transverse incision:* It is taken in the upper part of the neck. A vertical limb is dropped from a convenient point as a lazy S incision.

STEP-BY-STEP OPERATIVE PROCEDURE

1. *McFee incisions (Fig. 17.2):* The upper incision extends from the midline at the chin, downwards up to the hyoid bone; it then extends backwards in one of the skin creases up to the tip of mastoid process. The lower incision starts from the medial end of the clavicle and extends backwards to one cm beyond the anterior border of the trapezius. It should run parallel to the upper incision, and it is placed about 1.5 cm above the clavicle.
2. *The platysma:* It is cut in line with the skin incision. The flaps are raised in the subplatysmal plane. The upper flap is raised up to level of the mandible. The lower flap is raised up to the clavicle. The middle flap is raised up to midline medially and laterally up to the anterior border of trapezius. The two edges of the middle flap are stitched temporarily by a few interrupted stitches to form a tube (Fig. 17.3). This skin tube can be readily retracted during the dissection.
3. *The facial vessels:* These are identified as they hook the lower border of the mandible at the anterior edge of the masseter. The marginal or IV branch of the facial nerve is identified as it crosses the facial vessels (Fig. 17.4). The nerve is carefully identified, retracted upwards and the facial vessels are divided. Usually, a node is seen at this level; it is retracted downwards and included in the main specimen. The external jugular vein is divided at the lower pole of the parotid. The parotid gland is lifted upwards to expose the anterior border of the sternomastoid and the posterior belly of the digastric.

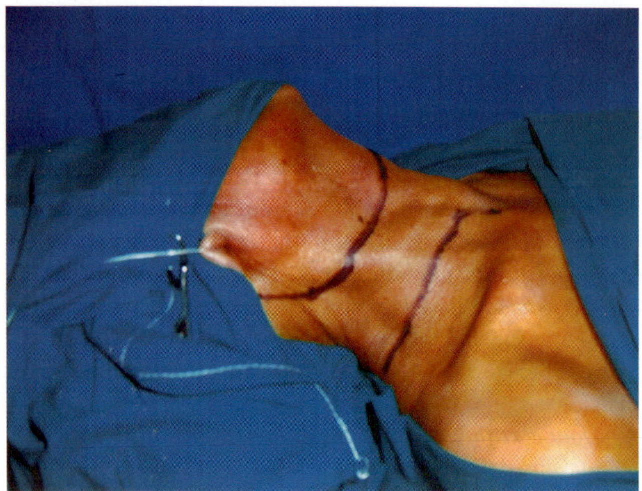

Fig. 17.2 McFee incisions for neck dissection

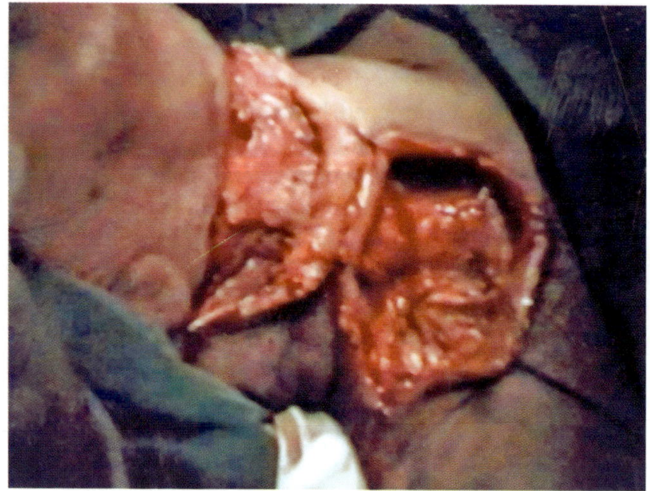

Fig. 17.3 Central bridge of skin has been stitched temporarily to form a tube

4. *Dissection of level I nodes:* The deep fascia is cut along the lower border of the mandible up to the midline. The fascia and adipose tissue with lymph nodes are reflected downwards to expose the anterior belly of digastric and anterior border of the opposite digastric muscle. As the submental and submandibular nodes are reflected down, the mylohyoid muscle is exposed. The posterior border of the mylohyoid is defined and retracted medially. This brings into view, the lingual nerve with the submandibular ganglion, the submandibular duct and deeper part of the submandibular salivary gland. The submandibular duct is divided; the lingual nerve is freed and pushed upwards. The deep part of the salivary gland is delivered from the deep surface of the mylohyoid. The hypoglossal nerve with its venae comitantes now comes into view. The facial artery is identified as we define the upper border of the posterior belly of digastric. The vessel is divided. The dissection of level I nodes is now complete and is attached to the residual specimen by the common facial vein and the investing layer of deep fascia (Fig. 17.5).
5. *Division of sternomastoid muscle*: We now perform our dissection through the lower incision. The deep fascia is incised along the anterior border of the sternomastoid. The sternal origin of sternomastoid is separated from the underlying structures by the index finger and divided by cautery, close to the bone. The clavicular origin is similarly elevated on the finger and divided. The lower end of external jugular vein is divided. The deep fascia is divided along the clavicle and lower part of the anterior border of trapezius. The inferior belly of omohyoid is divided. Its cut medial is held in a hemostat and the fascia along its inferior and medial border is divided right up to its hyoid origin. The muscle is detached from the hyoid bone (Fig. 17.6).

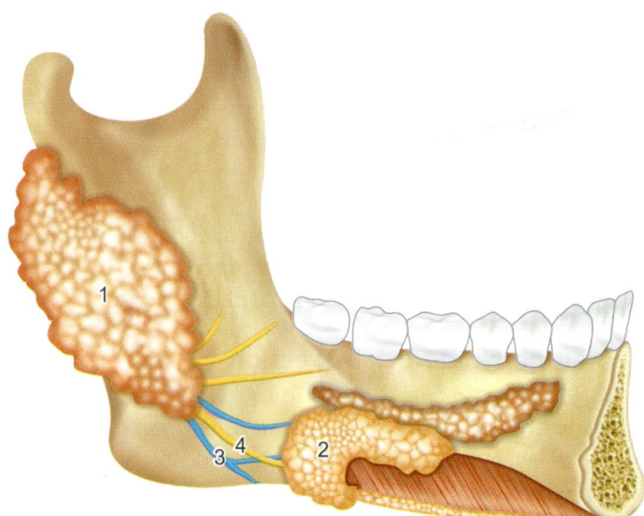

Fig. 17.4 The relation of mandibular branch of facial nerve to facial vessels. (1) Parotid gland; (2) Submandibular salivary gland; (3) Facial vessels; (4) Mandibular branch of facial nerve

6. *Ligation of IJV*: The IJV can now be seen covered by the carotid fascia. The fascia is carefully incised along its medial and lateral border. The anterior surface, medial and lateral borders of the IJV are defined; any tributary seen are divided. The posterior surface is then defined and ligatures passed around the vein. The IJV is retracted laterally; the carotid artery and vagus nerve are identified. Only then is the IJV ligated, transfixed and divided (Fig. 17.7).
7. *Carotid dissection:* The cut upper end of IJV is held in a hemostat. Dissection proceeds upwards between

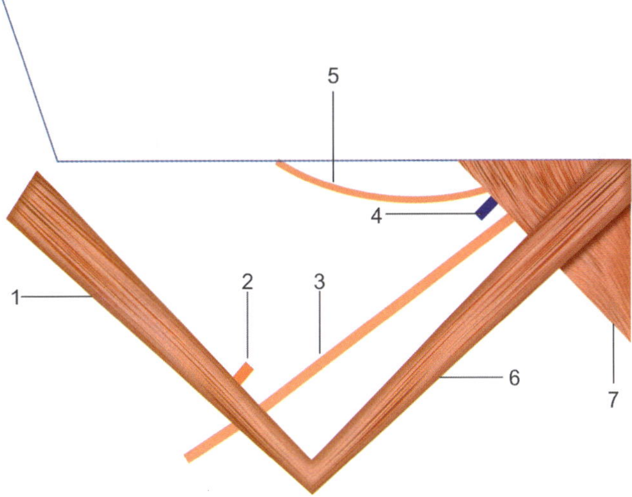

Fig. 17.5 Appearance of upper neck after removal of level I nodes. (1) Posterior belly of digastric; (2) Stump of facial artery; (3) Hypoglossal nerve; (4) Stump of salivary duct; (5) Lingual nerve; (6) Anterior belly of digastric; (7) Mylohyoid

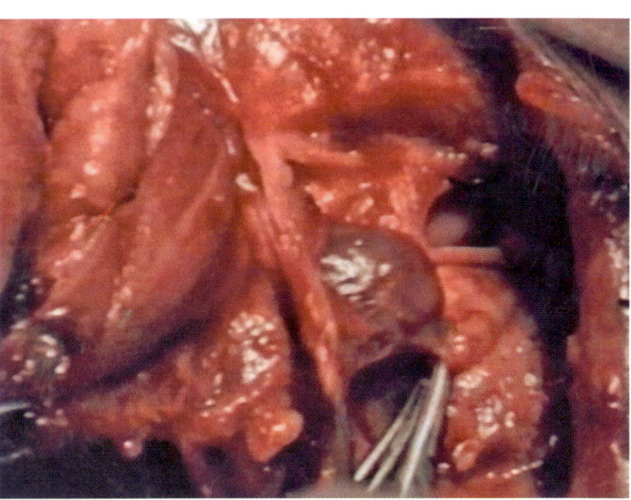

Fig. 17.7 The cut end of IJV held in a hemostat. Vagus is medial and posterior to the vein. A small portion of carotid artery is seen medial to the vagus

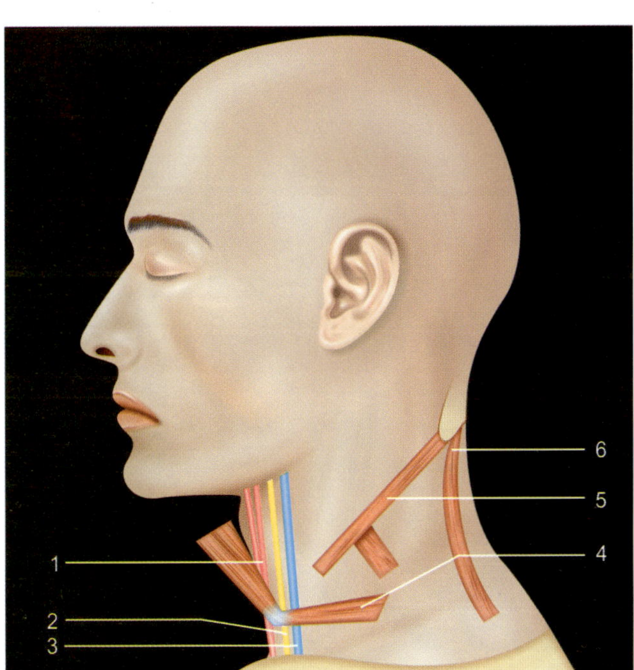

Fig. 17.6 (1) Carotid artery; (2) Vagus nerve; (3) Internal jugular vein; (4) Omohyoid; (5) Sternomastoid with its origin cut; (6) Trapezius

the carotid artery and the IJV, dividing the middle and superior thyroid veins. The IJV is further separated from the carotid vessels by dividing veins entering the IJV along its medial border. An important tributary is the venae comitantes accompanying the hypoglossal nerve. The ansa hypoglossi is also divided at its origin. The IJV can now be separated from the hypoglossal nerve right up to the base skull. Care should be taken not to injure the occipital artery. The IJV is now absolutely free from the carotid vessels. Once the carotid dissection is complete; retraction of the specimen will not cause traction on the carotid bulb. Such traction can cause bradycardia and is best avoided.

8. *Dissection in lower posterior triangle*: We now operate through the lower incision. The fatty tissue posterior to the IJV is divided to expose the scalenus anterior muscle and the phrenic nerve. The fascia covering the muscle and nerve is left intact. At the lower part of this dissection, the areolar tissue behind the carotid artery is divided between hemostats. This is done to take care of any inadvertent injury to the thoracic duct on the left side (Fig. 17.8).
9. *The tissue in the posterior triangle:* It is swept upwards; the brachial plexus is seen emerging between the scalenus anterior and scalenus medius. The fascia covering the plexus must be left intact. The transverse cervical artery and vein is seen in the wound. Some of its branches are divided; the vessels are usually preserved.
10. *The accessory nerve:* It is identified in the inferolateral part of the wound, as it dips into the trapezius. It is isolated and held in tapes. It is traced upwards till it disappears into the sternomastoid muscle. Small veins cross the nerve and are divided. Lymph nodes along the nerve are dissected and removed. The dissected tissue is separated from underlying muscles. The supraclavicular nerves are divided. The specimen is now delivered into the upper

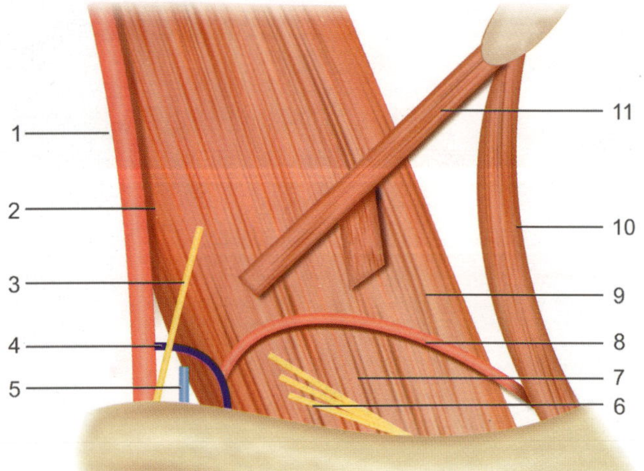

Fig. 17.8 Anatomy of lower neck. (1) Carotid artery; (2) Scalenus anterior muscle; (3) Phrenic nerve; (4) Thoracic duct; (5) Stump of IJV; (6) Brachial plexus; (7) Scalenus medius; (8) Transverse cervical artery; (9) Levator scapulae; (10) Trapezius; (11) Sternomastoid muscle

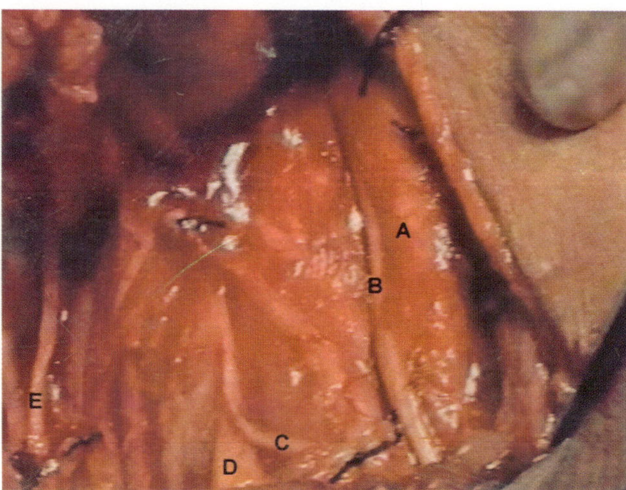

Fig. 17.9 Lower neck after completion of posterior triangle dissection. (A) Carotid artery; (B) Vagus nerve; (C) Transverse cervical artery; (D) Brachial plexus; (E) Accessory nerve

wound. The dissection in the posterior triangle is now complete (Fig. 17.9).

11. *Ligation of IJV at its upper end*: The upper end of sternomastoid is defined and divided. The lateral border of the upper end of IJV is defined. The accessory nerve is identified lateral to the IJV (Fig. 17.10). Lymph nodes above and below the nerve are dissected downwards to expose the underlying muscles. The upper end of IJV is freed all round, ligated, transfixed and divided. Care is taken not to include the X, XI and XII nerves in the ligature. The specimen is lifted from the posterior muscles, viz. levator scapulae and splenius capitis by dividing small vessels and nerve but without disturbing the fascia covering the muscles.
12. *Preservation of the XI nerve:* The specimen hangs around the accessory nerve. The nerve is dissected free from the specimen by dividing its branches to the sternomastoid muscle. The specimen is now removed. Careful hemostasis is achieved.
13. *Inspection of undamaged structure:* The following structures are inspected to make sure that they are not damaged viz. carotid vessels, vagus, accessory, hypoglossal and phrenic nerves, and the brachial plexus (Fig. 17.11). The lower and medial end of the wound is checked to exclude injury to the thoracic duct. The temporary stitches in the middle flap are removed. Suction drains are put in. The wound is closed in two layers, the platysma and then the skin (Fig. 17.12).
14. *Use of healex spray:* It is our practice to leave the sutured wound open and avoid bulky dressings.
15. *Long-term cosmetic result:* Figure 17.13 shows the long-term cosmetic results of neck dissection done through McFee incisions.

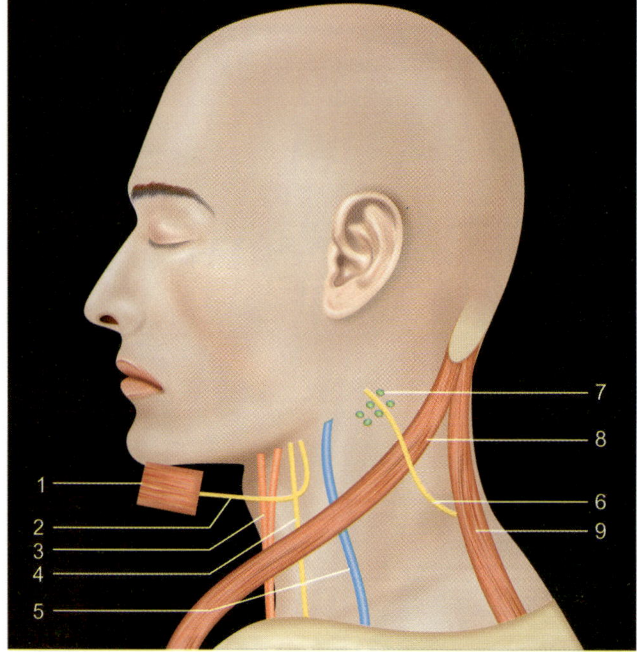

Fig. 17.10 Anatomy of upper neck. (1) Mylohyoid muscle; (2) Hypoglossal nerve; (3) Carotid artery; (4) Vagus nerve; (5) Internal jugular vein; (6) Accessory nerve; (7) Level II nodes; (8) Sternomastoid muscle; (9) Trapezius

RADICAL NECK DISSECTION

In this procedure, all the steps of MND type 1 are repeated, except that the accessory nerve is divided at the skull base, and again, at its junction with the trapezius. RND becomes necessary in cases where there is bulky disease or extranodal spread at level II.

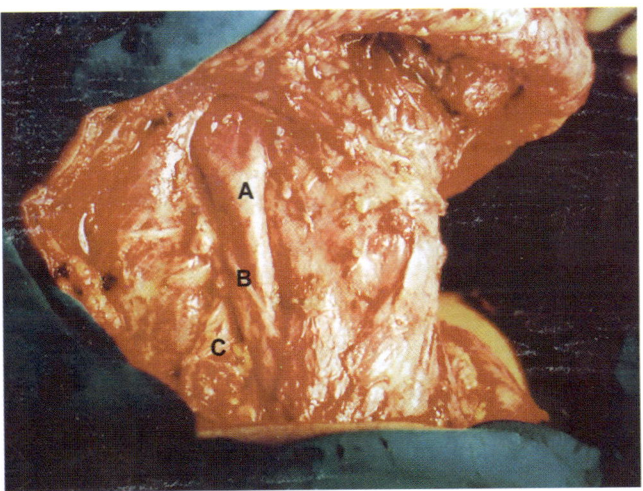

Fig. 17.11 The neck after removal of the specimen. (A) carotid artery; (B) Phrenic nerve; (C) Brachial plexus

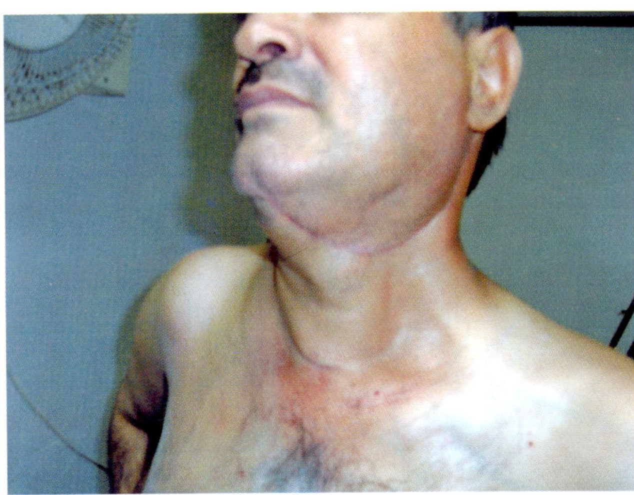

Fig. 17.13 Appearance of neck three months after neck dissection done with McFee incisions

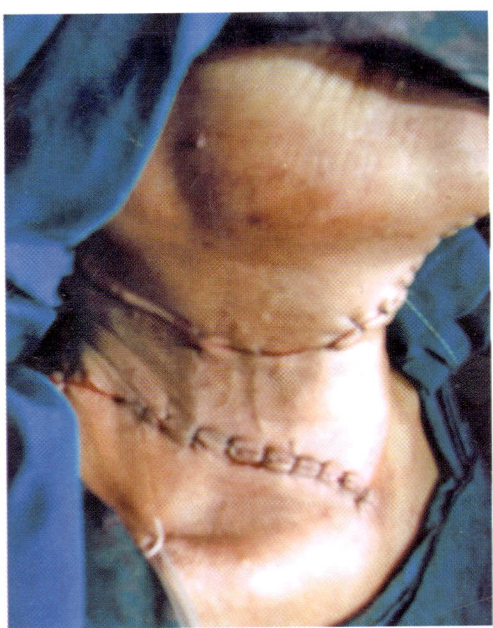

Fig. 17.12 Neck after completion of the operation

POSTOPERATIVE CARE

- Head end of the bed be raised, to reduce venous congestion.
- Oral feeds can be started next day. If neck dissection is combined with excision of the primary, then oral feeds may have to deferred for a few days.

INTRAOPERATIVE PROBLEMS

- *Hemorrhage:* This can be caused by injury to the IJV, carotid artery or its major branches.
- *Injury to the major nerves mentioned above:* If detected, primary suture of the nerves be done.
- *Injury to thoracic duct:* This is detected by collection of chyle in the lower part of the operative field. The site of injury be identified, and the duct sutured or transfixed.

POSTOPERATIVE COMPLICATIONS

- *Hemorrhage:* This can be reactionary from one of the arteries or veins, or due to increased capillary oozing. The cause is identified and appropriate treatment instituted.
- *Respiratory distress:* This could be due to hematoma or collection in the neck. It could be due to edema of larynx or vocal cord palsy due to injury of vagus. Heavy sedation be avoided in cases of neck dissection.
- *Necrosis of skin flaps:* This is usually partial and due to ill-planned skin incision. The incidence is higher in irradiated cases. One of the sequelae of skin necrosis is secondary hemorrhage from the carotid artery. This can prove fatal.

SUPRAOMOHYOID NECK DISSECTION

This is a common procedure done as a staging procedure in cases of oral cancer, hence described below:

1. The operation can be done through a single transverse incision in the upper part of the neck. Flaps are raised in subplatysmal plane.
2. The deep fascia is incised along the anterior border of the sternomastoid. The muscle is retracted laterally. The deep fascia is again incised along the lateral border of the superior belly of omohyoid.
3. The IJV is identified at the lower end of the wound. It is traced upwards right up to the base skull. The lymph nodes and areolar tissue around IJV are stripped upwards. The venous tributaries are divided notably, the common facial vein.
4. Dissection of level I is done as described in the operation of MND.

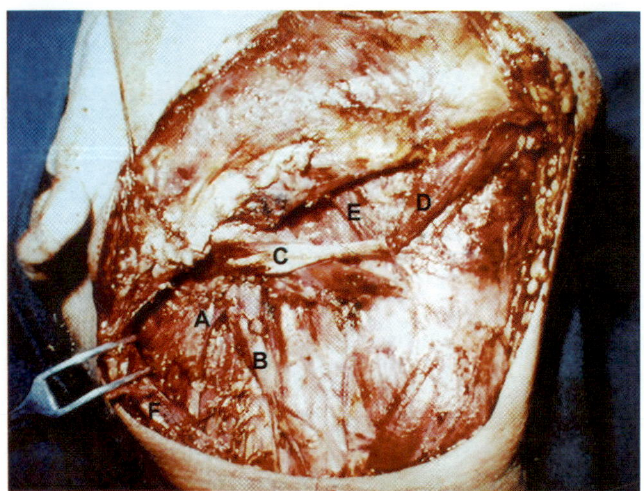

Fig. 17.14 Neck after completion of SOHD. (A) Accessory nerve; (B) IJV; (C) Posterior belly of digastric; (D) Anterior belly of digastric; (E) Mylohyoid

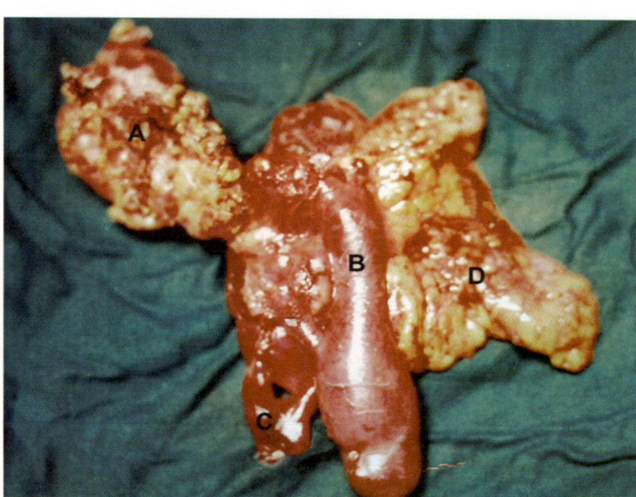

Fig. 17.15 Specimen of neck dissection. (A) Level I nodes; (B) IJV; (C) Sternomastoid muscle; (D) Posterior triangle mass

5. Upper end of the sternomastoid is retracted laterally. The accessory nerve is identified and traced till it disappears into the sternomastoid. All the lymph nodes lateral to the IJV, above and below the XI nerve are dissected and removed (Fig. 17.14).

HISTOPATHOLOGICAL EXAMINATION

The specimen should be properly oriented by the surgeon and the pathologist (Fig. 17.15). The histopathologist should report on the number of nodes examined at each level, the number of histologically positive nodes and evidence of extranodal spread. This information is useful for planning adjuvant treatment.

REFERENCE

1. Levels of cervical lymph nodes AJCC Cancer Staging Manual sixth edition Springer Verlag, Heidelberg, Germany. 2003. pp.18-9.

CHAPTER

18

Commando Operation

RS Rao, Satish Rao

Commando operation denotes excision of tumors of the oral cavity which involve the mandible in continuity with neck dissection.

INDICATION

Locally advanced tumors of oral cavity which involve the mandible and need composite resection of primary, mandible and neck (Fig. 18.1).

PREOPERATIVE PREPARATION

- Anesthetic checkup
- Control of medical problems like diabetes and hypertension
- Special consent regarding extent of excision, reconstruction and tracheostomy if needed
- Shaving of face, neck, anterior chest wall up to nipple and half inch behind ear.

ANESTHESIA

GA, nasal intubation mandatory.

POSITION/DRAPING

After nasal intubation, the neck is extended and turned to the opposite side. As in head and neck surgery draping is done by three towels technique. Skin stitches are given to isolate the sterile area. Sterile cotton plug is put in the ear.

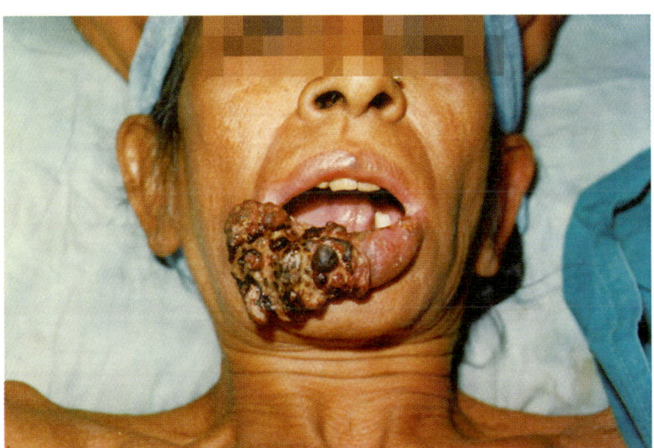

Fig. 18.1 Locally advanced carcinoma lip

INCISION

Marking ink is used to mark the incision. The incision is same as that of neck dissection except that it is to be extended upwards to the midline of the lip or angle of mouth as necessary in the particular case.

PROCEDURE

After completion of neck dissection (refer to Chapter 17 on Neck Dissections) the contents are kept attached to the submandibular gland. The incision is then extended upwards to split the lip either in the midline or angle of mouth as required. A tongue stitch is taken, throat adequately packed and mouth gag placed in position.

- After the lip is split, the upper skin flap is raised beyond the inferior border of mandible carefully preserving the marginal branch of the facial nerve which maintains the function of lower lip and oral competence.
- A mucosal incision is taken in the gingivobuccal sulcus depending on the situation of primary tumor. The upper skin flap of the neck along with the buccal mucosal flap can now be raised along the mandible.
- The masseter muscle can now be detached from the mandible. The coronoid process is now bared after dividing the tendon of temporalis.
- The mandible can now be divided anteriorly and the muscles divided medial to the mandible which include the digastric mylohyoid and pterygoids as necessary in a particular case.
- Adequate mucosal margins are taken while excising the primary tumor. If required frozen section of cut margins are taken.

In case of segment mandibulectomy, the posterior mandibular cut is taken. In case of hemi-mandibulectomy both the medial and lateral pterygoids have to be adequately divided and the mandibular condyle defined and detached from the temporomandibular joint. This allows removal of the specimen (Fig. 18.2). Adequate hemostasis must be achieved

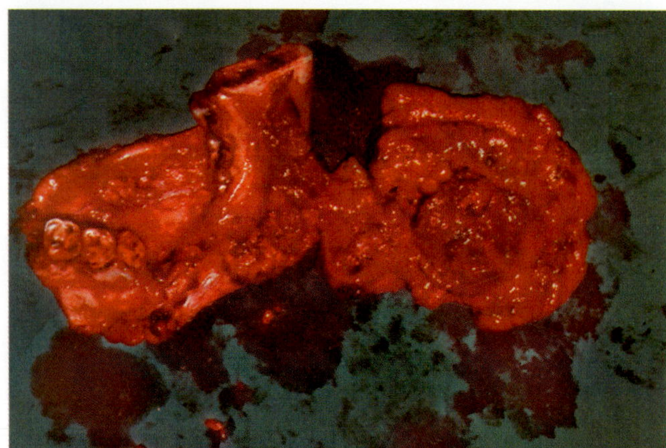

Fig. 18.2 Commando specimen (mandibulectomy neck dissection

both in the neck and oral cavity, especially if the pterygoid venous plexus is opened.

Reconstruction needs to be carried out depending on the extent of excision. It may be in the form of primary closure, tongue flap, pectoralis major myocutaneous flap or microvascular free flap as applicable in a particular case. A nasogastric tube is always inserted prior to reconstruction. If needed a tracheostomy is done. Suction drains are inserted prior to closure.

COMPLICATIONS

- Airway compromise may be a problem and tracheostomy required especially due to postoperative edema in a post-radiated case.
- Bleeding in the immediate postoperative period. If excessive re-exploration is needed.
- Infection is usually unlikely. However, in case of salivary leak from mucosal closure infection may occur. Oral feeding should be discontinued and nasogastric feeding prolonged.

CHAPTER 19

Surgery for Thyroid Cancer

AK D' Cruz

INTRODUCTION

Thyroid cancer is relatively uncommon, accounting for less than 1% of all malignancies. In contrast, nodular thyroid disease is common affecting 4–8% of the population even in developed countries like the USA and UK. A large majority of these present as solitary nodules and a significant proportion will warrant surgery. Therefore, it is not unusual for most surgeons to be often confronted in practice by thyroid patients requiring surgical intervention.

Surgery is the primary treatment modality for thyroid carcinomas. While some of these cancers can be extremely aggressive and lethal, the vast majority are biologically indolent in their course with prolonged survival even with residual or recurrent disease. The morbidity created by a poorly performed thyroid operation can be much worse than that caused by the disease itself even if untreated. Therefore, it is imperative for the surgeon to be aware of the important aspects of the surgical anatomy, pathology and natural history of thyroid disease.

SURGICAL ANATOMY

The thyroid gland is made up of two lateral lobes which extend on either side of the thyroid cartilage to the level of the sixth tracheal ring. These lobes are joined together by the isthmus, which overlies the second to fourth tracheal rings. In addition, there is sometimes a pyramidal lobe which projects up from the isthmus, usually on the left-hand side. The gland is enclosed in pretracheal fascia, covered by strap muscles and overlapped laterally by the sternocleidomastoid muscles. *The relevant anatomical features of surgical importance can be grouped into:*

- The musculofascial coverings
- The vascular supply
- The important close surgical relations of the thyroid gland
- Lymph drainage.

Musculofascial Coverings

Skin lines (of Langer) in the neck seen transversely and are useful in planning the incision. Under the skin is the platysma muscle, which is innervated by cervical branch of facial nerve. The platysma and skin should be mobilized as one layer, exposing the external and anterior jugular veins in the superficial fascia below. The outer layer of deep cervical fascia covers the strap muscles and splits to surround sternomastoid and trapezius muscles. The fascial layer can be incised longitudinally between the strap muscles. The more anterior sternohyoid muscles lie close together, but the midline can be identified between them as a thin line of fat and avascular fascia. As the sternohyoid muscles are elevated, the underlying sternothyroid muscles are exposed.

The sternothyroid muscle is intimately related to the thyroid gland below and care must be taken during dissection to avoid injury to the widely interconnecting venous network in the capsule of the thyroid gland. This is particularly important in a large goiter, where the strap muscles can be splayed out across thyroid lobes, and are deceptively thin. The insertion of sternothyroid muscle into the thyroid cartilage can obscure the superior pole of the thyroid gland and can be partially transected for better exposure. Both the sternohyoid and sternothyroid muscles (as well as omohyoid muscles) are innervated by the ansa cervicalis, derived from the hypoglossal nerve and C1 through C3. The nerve supply enters the strap muscles low down in the neck and when required these should be transected in their upper third to preserve their innervation.

Vascular Anatomy

Each thyroid lobe is supplied by a superior and inferior thyroid artery and drained by three veins.

Superior Vascular Pedicle

The superior vascular pedicle contains the superior thyroid artery, which is the first branch of external carotid, and its accompanying vein, which drains into internal jugular vein. The superior vessels enter the upper pole of the gland at its apex, which branch to the front and back of the gland. The external laryngeal nerve is closely related to this pedicle (discussed below).

Inferior Thyroid Artery

Unlike the superior vascular pedicle, the inferior thyroid artery and vein do not relate to each other at all. The artery arises from the thyrocervical trunk, passes behind the carotid sheath and then runs transversely across the space between the carotid and the thyroid gland to enter deep surface of the gland as several separate branches. These terminal branches are intimately related to the recurrent laryngeal nerve and inferior parathyroid gland.

Inferior Thyroid Veins

The inferior thyroid veins are usually not single, but a plexus which leave the lower border of the gland and pass through the loose fascial space to join the brachiocephalic vein. They are fragile and easily damaged and are best ligated individually.

Middle Thyroid Vein

This vein is usually short stubby and thin-walled leaving the middle of the gland and directly coursing laterally to enter the internal jugular vein.

Thyroidea Ima Artery

The thyroidea ima artery which are direct branches from the aorta are infrequently encountered and are usually only an anatomical curiosity and never of significant surgical relevance.

Important Close Surgical Relations of the Thyroid Gland

These are the recurrent laryngeal nerves, the external laryngeal nerves and the parathyroid glands.

External Laryngeal Nerve

The external branch of superior laryngeal nerve does not usually receive sufficient attention by thyroid surgeons. Injury to this nerve occurs more often than appreciated, resulting in impairment to the quality of voice. The superior laryngeal nerve divides high in the neck into a larger internal branch, which enters larynx through the thyrohyoid membrane to provide sensory innervation to the larynx, and a smaller external laryngeal nerve. The latter descends on the fascia of the inferior pharyngeal constrictor muscle to which it sends a branch, and then passes inferior to the attachment of the sternothyroid muscle to the thyroid cartilage to enter the cricothyroid muscle in the sternothyrolaryngeal (Joll's) triangle (Fig. 19.1).

This is formed laterally by the upper pole of the gland and the vessels, superiorly by the attachment of strap muscles to the thyroid cartilage and medially by the midline (The nerve usually descends medial to the superior thyroid artery). Its floor is cricothyroid muscle.

Several anatomic variations exist that place the external laryngeal nerve at particular risk. These include:

- In 20% of cases, the nerve is located within the inferior pharyngeal constrictor muscle; and therefore may not be visualized.
- In another 20% of cases, the nerve lies lateral to the superior thyroid pedicle.
- In a further 20% of cases the nerve, although medial to the superior thyroid artery, it intertwines between its branches and is therefore difficult to visualize.

There may also be anatomic variations of the external branch of the superior laryngeal nerve on either side. The best way, however, to safeguard it from injury is to stay close to the gland and ligate the branches individually.

Recurrent Laryngeal Nerves

The nerves usually lie in the tracheoesophageal groove and bear a variable relationship to the branches of the inferior thyroid artery before entering the larynx. The nerve can be in front of, pass through or behind the inferior thyroid arteries (Figs 19.2A to C). The right nerve recurs beneath the right subclavian artery while the left recurs beneath the aortic arch, as a result of which the left recurrent laryngeal nerve ascends in a straight longitudinal direction parallel to the border of the trachea in the tracheoesophageal groove while the right nerve follows a shorter course approaching the larynx at a slight angle (Fig. 19.3). The nerve may occasionally divide into 2–3 branches prior to entry into the larynx. The recurrent laryngeal nerve rarely is nonrecurrent, arising in such cases directly from vagus nerve to run in a direct medial course to the inferior lateral aspect of the larynx. This variation usually occurs on the right side.

Parathyroid Glands

The number of parathyroid glands vary from 2 to 6, but, in 80% of cases, there are 4 (2 on each side). The glands are small, the

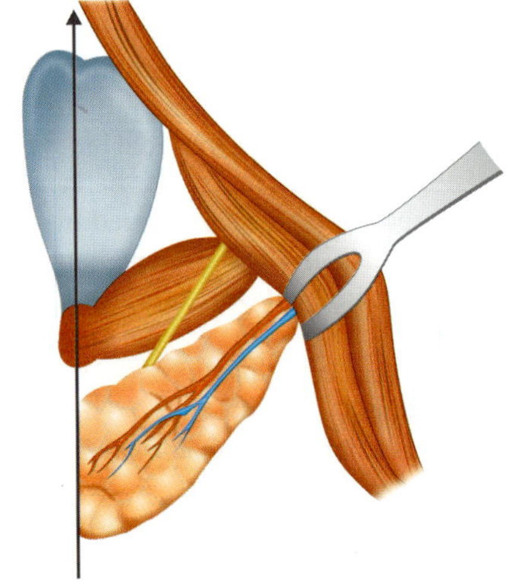

Fig. 19.1 Joll's triangle formed by midline, strap muscles and superior thyroid pedicle. *Note* the external branch of the superior laryngeal nerve in the triangle. The floor is formed by cricothyroid

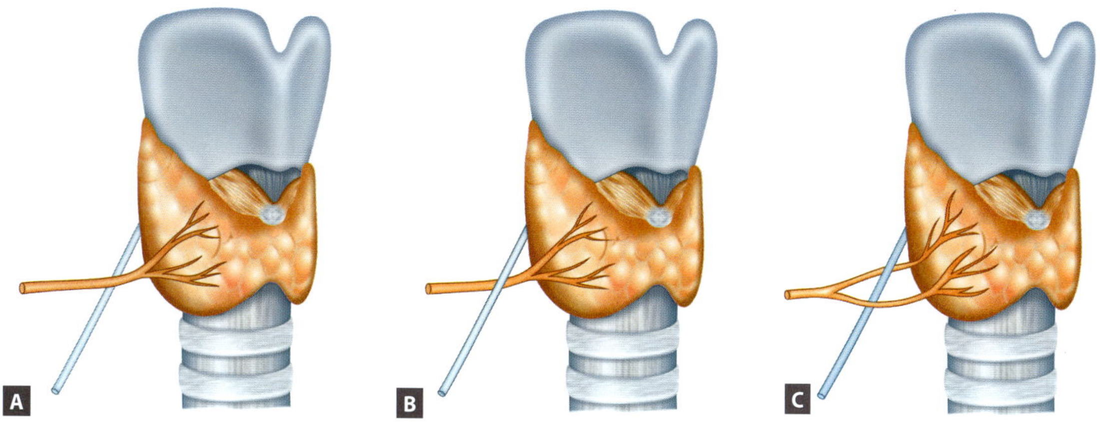

Figs 19.2A to C Relationship of recurrent laryngeal nerve to inferior thyroid artery. (A) Below (most common) the artery; (B) Above the artery; (C) In between the artery

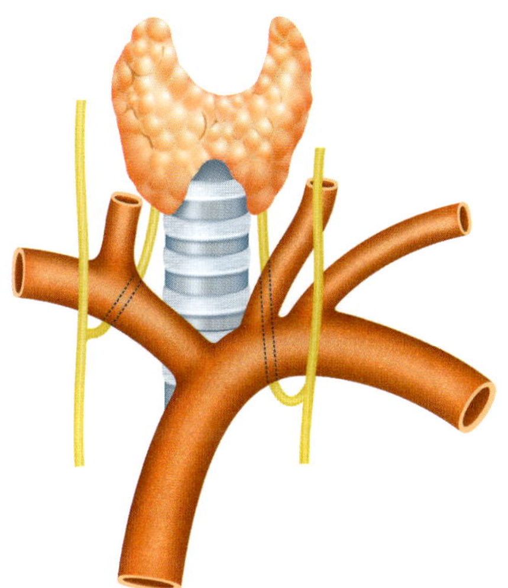

Fig. 19.3 Course of recurrent laryngeal nerve

size of a split pea and are identified by their color, which is darker yellow-brown than fat, as well as by a definite fascial capsule containing minute blood vessels.

The superior glands lie on the posterior surface of the middle third of the thyroid, usually above the inferior thyroid artery. The superior parathyroid glands are most simply found by tracing the course of the recurrent nerve to its penetration of the cricothyroid membrane; it is at this location that they are usually discovered. Because the superior parathyroid glands travel only a minimal distance during embryonic life (derived from fourth pharyngeal pouch), their final location is less varied than that of the inferior glands.

In contrast, the inferior parathyroid glands arise from third pharyngeal pouch with the thymus and travel a longer distance and hence may be more variable in position. They are usually found either on the posterolateral surface of the lower pole of the thyroid gland or at the tip of the cervical thymus or thyrothymic ligament. In fact, this ligament may be helpful as it occasionally points towards the parathyroid gland.

Lymphatics

The thyroid is a gland rich in lymphatics. Numerous lymphatic vessels leave the gland and drain into lymph nodes situated in: The pretracheal, paratracheal and recurrent laryngeal chain (central compartment), the middle jugular chain (level III), lower jugular chain (level IV), posterior triangle nodes (level V) and superior mediastinal nodes (Level VII).

TYPES OF THYROID OPERATIONS

Nodulectomy/lumpectomy (Fig. 19.4A): Removal of nodule with cuff of normal tissue.

Total lobectomy or hemithyroidectomy (Fig. 19.4B): Complete removal of one thyroid lobe and the isthmus.

Isthmusectomy (Fig. 19.4C): Removal of isthmus along with cuff of surrounding normal tissue.

Subtotal thyroidectomy (Fig. 19.4D): Bilateral removal of more than one-half of the thyroid gland on each side plus the isthmus.

Near total thyroidectomy (Fig. 19.4E): Total lobectomy and isthmusectomy with preservation of a small slice of thyroid tissue on the contralateral side to safeguard the recurrent laryngeal nerve or the parathyroids or both.

Total thyroidectomy (Fig. 19.4F): Removal of both lobes of the thyroid as well as the isthmus.

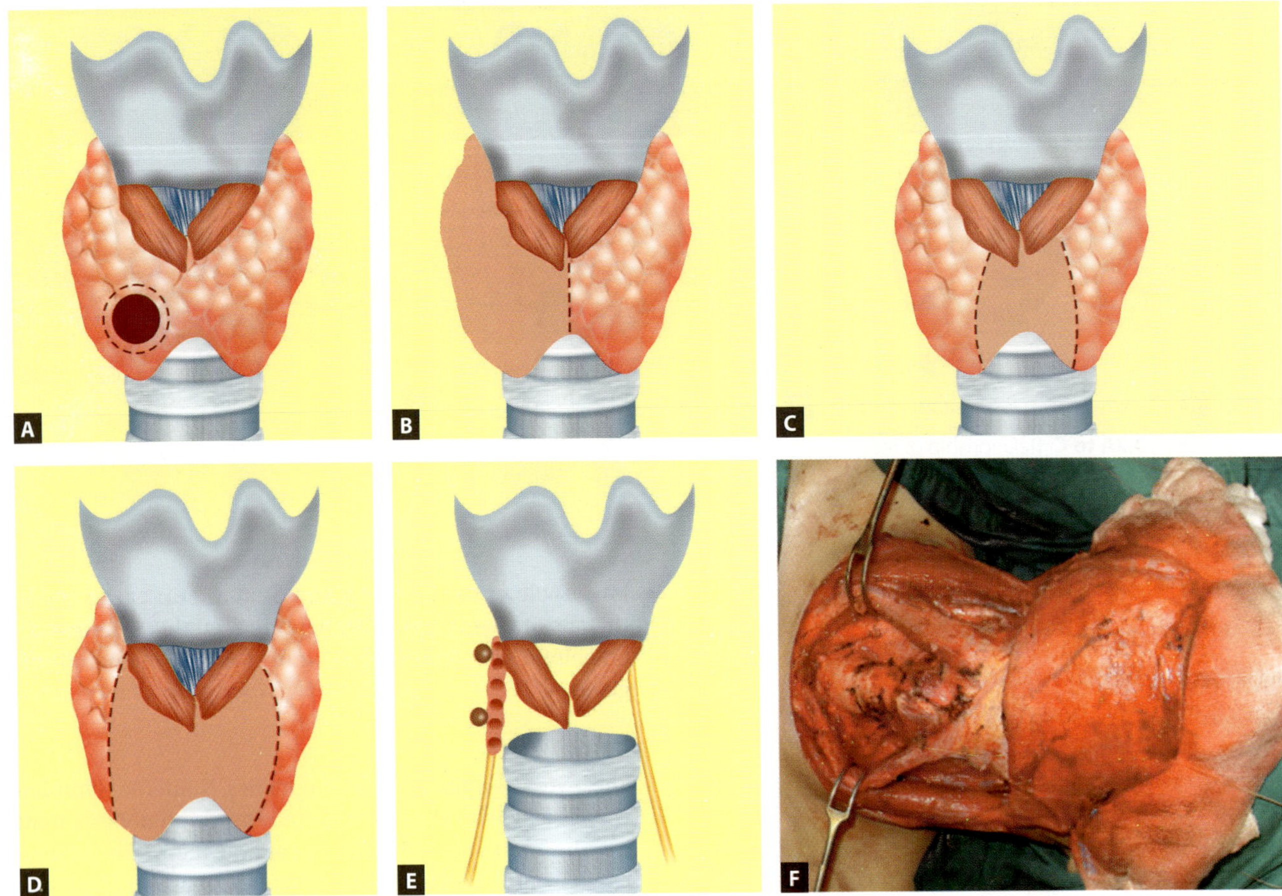

Figs 19.4A to F Types of thyroid surgery: (A) Nodulectomy; (B) Hemithyroidectomy; (C) Isthmusectomy; (D) Subtotal tyhroidectomy; (E) Near total thyroidectomy; (F) Total thyroidectomy

Completion thyroidectomy: A subsequent procedure to convert a lesser operation into a near-total or total thyroidectomy in a case of cancer thyroid.

> The minimum operation which should be done for a suspected or confirmed cancer is a total lobectomy/hemithyroidectomy in low-risk patients and near total or total thyroidectomy in high-risk patients.

PREOPERATIVE PREPARATION

- *Indirect laryngoscopy:* To identify unsuspected recurrent nerve palsy that may be compensated with a near normal voice particularly when longstanding.
- *X-ray neck (AP and lateral):* Particularly if the thyroid swelling is large. This gives an idea of the airway — the lumen and deviation. It may also demonstrate retrosternal extension of the thyroid. In addition, fine stippled calcification (Psammoma bodies) are suggestive of malignancy as opposed to round egg shell calcification which is more commonly observed in benign multinodular goiters.
- *Base line thyroid function tests (T3/T4/TSH):* Most patients with thyroid cancer are normally euthyroid, thyrotoxic patients must be rendered euthyroid prior to surgery.
- *Serum calcium and sonography of the neck:* In patients undergoing completion thyroidectomy, serum calcium levels provide a baseline. Sonography of the neck is also recommended to visualize residual tissue in the thyroid bed. It is not unusual that patients who have supposedly undergone a hemithyroidectomy have significant residual tissue on the operated side.
- *Consent:* Discuss potential complications with the patient specifically mentioning risk to parathyroid glands and recurrent laryngeal nerve.

PREOPERATIVE WORK-UP

- *Fine needle aspiration cytology (FNAC):* Is the investigation of choice for a solitary thyroid nodule. FNAC is safe, cheap and reliable with sensitivity and specificity both approaching 100%. Thyroid conditions that may be diagnosed by FNAC include papillary carcinoma, medullary carcinoma, anaplastic carcinoma, lymphoma, colloid nodules and thyroiditis. However, cytology has its limitations in follicular lesions, as it cannot differentiate follicular adenoma from follicular carcinoma since this distinction is based on the presence of capsular or vascular invasion which are not demonstrated on cytology.

- *Isotope scan:* Popular in past, but largely outdated at present. Its role is limited to a nodule in a patient with clinical signs of toxicity.
- *Tumor markers:*
  - Serum calcitonin—for diagnosis and follow-up in medullary cancer.
  - Serum thyroglobulin—a useful tumor marker for follow-up in differentiated thyroid cancer following total thyroidectomy. It has no role in the preoperative work-up towards establishing a diagnosis of cancer except in a patient with bone metastasis and goiter, when FNAC may be inconclusive. A very high thyroglobulin is indicative of a thyroid cancer.
- *CT scan neck/mediastinum:*
  - In differentiated thyroid cancers—routine imaging is not recommended unless involvement of adjacent structures is suspected.
  - In medullary cancer thyroid, as there is a high propensity for nodal involvement including those in the upper mediastinum.

THYROIDECTOMY TECHNIQUE

Positioning of the Patient

- The patient should be positioned in the supine position with the arms tucked close to the side.
- An inflatable pillow or shoulder roll is placed under the shoulders so that the neck is extended. The head end of the operative table is raised about 15° to reduce venous congestion.

Incision

- The most commonly used incision for thyroid operations is the low "collar" incision (Figs 19.5A and B).
- The incision should be a symmetrical, transverse incision along the skin crease 2 cm above suprasternal notch. Inexperienced surgeons tend to place the thyroidectomy incision too low, particularly in the long-necked patient. In addition to hampering access to the superior poles of the thyroid gland, an incision placed too low tends to fall onto the chest wall when the patient assumes an erect posture and is cosmetically unsatisfactory. This can be avoided if the incision is marked out with the patient sitting prior to induction of anesthesia. This is especially important in women as anatomic orientation changes when the patient is supine with the neck hyperextended.
- The length of the incision depends on the size of the gland. The usual extent of the incision is from the anterior border of one sternocleidomastoid muscle to that of the other. Larger tumors and patients with short thick neck may need larger incisions for better exposure.
- A vertical extension of the incision towards the mastoid may be taken if neck dissection is contemplated and exposure is limited (Fig. 19.5C). A vertical extension of the incision provides optimal exposure for dissection of the upper jugular and posterior triangle nodes particularly when large.

The skin incision is taken and platysma is divided. Skin hooks are applied and the upper and lower flaps are elevated deep to platysma exposing the fascia covering the strap muscles, the external and anterior jugular veins. The flaps are raised up to thyroid notch and the sternal notch. In most patients, the external jugular veins are employed as lateral boundaries for the incision. Flaps are reflected and wound exposed by stay sutures or by Joll's retractor.

Management of Strap Muscles

The thyroid gland is situated deep to the infrahyoid (strap) muscles, which must be retracted or divided in order to expose the gland. The infrahyoid muscles may be managed in a variety of ways depending on the habitus of the patient, the size of the nodule to be removed, and the requirements of resection.

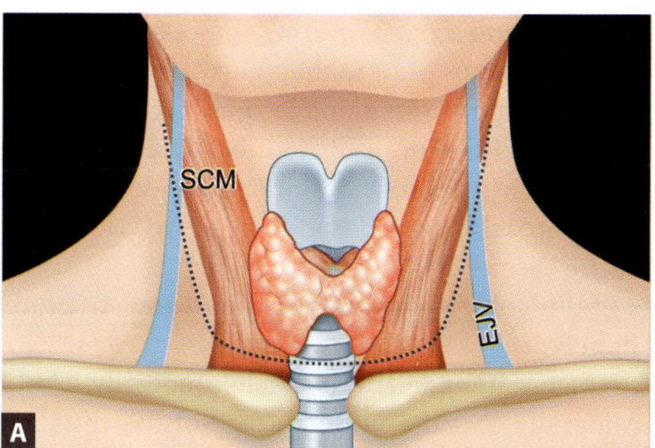

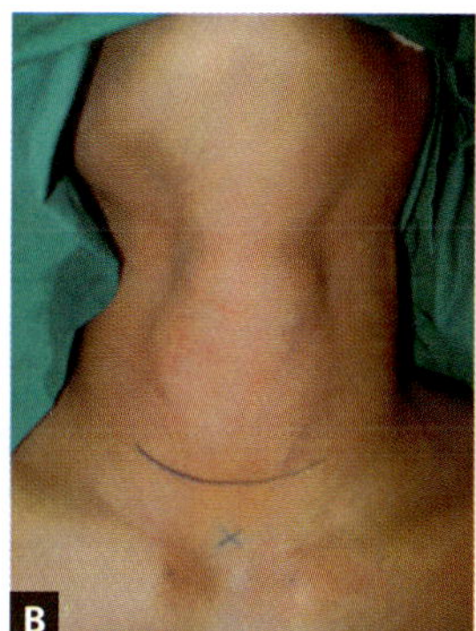

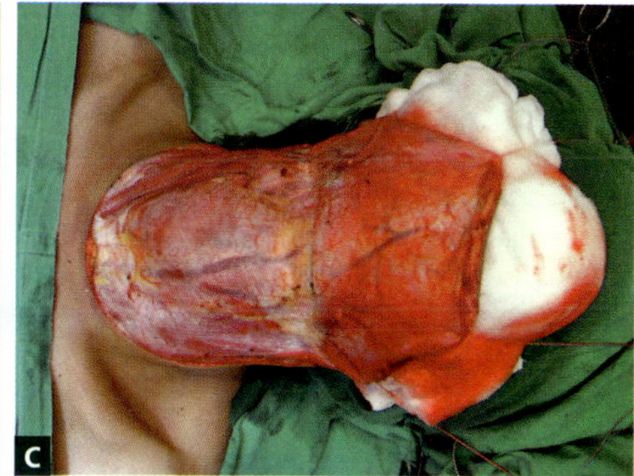

Figs 19.5A to C Incision: (A) Line diagram showing incision for thyroidectomy; (B) Incision for thyroidectomy; (C) Extended incision for thyroidectomy and neck dissection

- The simplest approach to the thyroid gland is by retraction of the sternohyoid and the sternothyroid muscles laterally after separating them vertically in the midline. In order to obtain maximum exposure, the midline should be exposed and the muscles separated throughout their entire length from the hyoid bone to the sternal notch. The deeper sternothyroid is normally slightly adherent to the thyroid capsule, which can be separated by gentle blunt dissection and retracted laterally. If the sternothyroid muscle does not separate easily from the surface of the thyroid nodule, it is left attached to the nodule. Babcock clamps applied to the muscles and elevated superiorly by assistant may help develop plane between gland and undersurface of muscles.
- The sternothyroid muscle inserts on the oblique line of the thyroid cartilage. Because its point of insertion is considerably lower than that of the sternohyoid muscle, the ability to obtain exposure by lateral retraction may be limited, particularly if the lobe or nodule is bulky. Division of a few medial fibers of the sternothyroid muscle helps in better exposure of superior pole.
- In cases of extremely large goiters, both sternohyoid and sternothyroid muscle may be divided. In such cases, it is preferable to commence laterally, separating the sternomastoid muscle from the strap muscles. This permits identification and mobilization of the jugular vein and carotid artery away from a bulky thyroid tumor. The muscles are then transected in a lateral to medial direction to safeguard these structures.
- In cases where malignant invasion of strap muscles is suspected or there is gross extrathyroidal spread of the tumor, the overlying muscle is resected in continuity.
- Having exposed one lobe of the thyroid the same steps are repeated on the opposite side. The opposite thyroid lobe must always be exposed and palpated even if only a hemithyroidectomy is contemplated as malignant thyroid disease is known to be bilateral.

Identify the midline between the straps—it is usually pale white. The anterior jugular veins may also serve as a guide to the midline—the midline is situated between the two veins. The thyroid notch which is a midline structure may also help particularly in large goiters that may cause midline shift. Pick up the fascia on either side of the midline (assistant holds one side) with tooth forceps. Incise the deep cervical fascia longitudinally between the strap muscles superiorly up to hyoid and inferiorly to the sternal notch. Two Babcock forceps are applied to the strap muscles on the side to be retracted and sternohyoid and sternothyroid muscles are lifted off from the thyroid and retracted laterally. When the space is large enough a retractor (Langenbeck) can be used to retract the muscles. Extend the space by blunt dissection either by using the index finger or with the help of a wet cotton pledget around the surface of the lobe.

Initial Mobilization of Gland

The gland is retracted medially by an assistant applying traction using the middle and index fingers. A gauze swab is used to protect the surface of the gland. A Langenbach's retractor retracts the previously dissected strap muscles laterally.

The middle thyroid vein is identified and divided. This is the first structure to be divided in thyroid surgery and ensures adequate mobilization of the gland rendering subsequent dissection easier. The vein is however often short and stubby particularly on the right side and care should be taken to avoid inadvertent damage. It is not constant in position and may occasionally be absent or may consist of two or three small insignificant veins. Loose areolar tissue is dissected up to the posterolateral surface of the gland thus mobilizing the gland further medially.

Identification of the Recurrent Laryngeal Nerve

One of the most crucial steps in thyroid lobectomy is preservation of the recurrent laryngeal nerve—it is first identified and its safety—ensured. The recurrent laryngeal nerve can be inadvertently damaged during division of either the upper or lower poles and must therefore always be identified early in the operation. As mentioned earlier because of differences in their origin the left recurrent laryngeal nerve ascends in a straight longitudinal direction parallel to the border of the trachea in the tracheoesophageal groove while the right nerve follows a shorter course approaching the larynx at a slight angle. The right recurrent laryngeal nerve is therefore more superficial and hence encountered earlier during dissection than the left.

The nerve is best identified first in its infrathyroidal course where it is least prone to injury.

There are various methods to help early identification of the nerve, the most useful of which are:

- *Relationship to inferior thyroid artery:* It is preferable to identify the inferior thyroid artery first which is the only structure to emerge from behind the carotid artery and course horizontally towards the thyroid gland. The nerve usually is below the artery (70%) but may also be above it or within its branches prior to their entry into the thyroid gland; it is used only as a guide to these structures. The artery is never divided prior to identification of the nerve or the parathyroid glands. Once the artery is identified and is traced towards the thyroid gland, the nerve is identified with relative ease.

In case of difficulty identifying the following structures may be of benefit.

- Lore's triangle — bounded by the trachea medially, carotid sheath laterally and the undersurface of the retracted inferior thyroid pole superiorly the apex of the triangle being directed towards the thoracic inlet. The nerve runs in this triangle.

- Beahr's triangle (Fig. 19.6)—bounded by the common carotid artery and the inferior thyroid artery. The recurrent laryngeal nerve forms the third boundary of this triangle.
- If the nerve cannot be identified, it may be nonrecurrent. This occurs in 1-2% of cases, usually on the right side. In this case, the nerve arises in the neck directly from the vagus and is found in the paracarotid tunnel where it runs with the inferior thyroid vessels enroute to the larynx.

Localization and Preservation of the Parathyroid Glands

The parathyroids are not accorded due importance. Their localization and preservation is as important, if not more crucial, as is preservation of the recurrent laryngeal nerve. Failure to safeguard the glands results in severe lifelong morbidity. The location of the glands is discussed in the section on surgical anatomy. The glands are identified by: (1) Their location, (2) the color—darker tan or caramel color compared to surrounding fat, (3) presence of a capsule with a feeding blood vessel. Once identified, it is important to dissect between the parathyroid and the thyroid, the parathyroid being peeled down from the surface of the thyroid. Branches of the inferior thyroid artery are ligated close to capsule of the thyroid preserving the branches to the parathyroid (Capsular ligation—Figure 19.7). The use of bipolar cautery, selectively cauterizing vessels to the thyroid is another option. Use of unipolar cautery is to be avoided.

If the parathyroids have been devascularized or inadvertently removed during surgery they should be auto- transplanted into the sternocleidomastoid muscle or the muscles of the forearm (in medullary cancer associated with the multiple endocrine neoplasia (MEN) syndrome).

The gland is sliced into tiny bits and lodged into a pocket of the muscle.

In case of doubt whether a removed structure is a parathyroid, lymph node or fat—a part of it is sent for frozen section analysis, while the rest is kept in a bowl of sterile isotonic saline. Should frozen section confirm the presence of a parathyroid the preserved portion is transplanted in the manner described.

If frozen section facilities are unavailable, a simple test is to drop the removed structure into a bowl of saline—fat will float while a parathyroid usually sinks.

KEY POINTS

- A careful and meticulous dissection should be done to identify the inferior thyroid artery, the recurrent laryngeal nerve and the parathyroids.
- Do not use unipolar diathermy current close to the nerve and parathyroids. Bipolar diathermy is acceptable or else the bleeding points are carefully ligated.
- Anatomical variations are known, do not divide or remove any structure until the nerve and parathyroids identified.

Mobilization of Superior and Inferior Pole of Thyroid

This part of the procedure requires adequate traction of the strap muscles lateral to and above the upper pole of the thyroid lobe. Great care must be taken not to injure the external branch of superior laryngeal nerve while clamping the superior thyroid vessels.

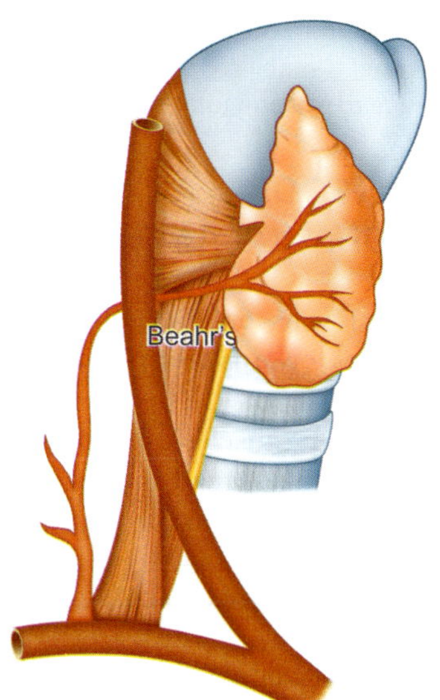

Fig. 19.6 Beahr's triangle. The recurrent laryngeal nerve forms the third side of the triangle. The common carotid artery and inferior thyroid artery form the other two

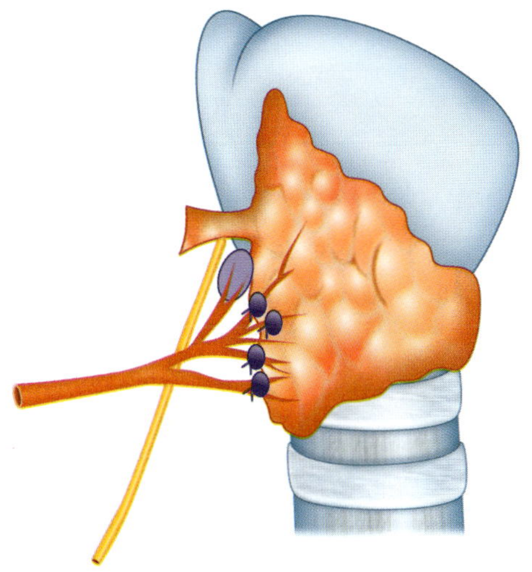

Fig. 19.7 Capsular ligation of inferior thyroid artery. This preserves the blood supply to the parathyroid (parathyroid are shown in brown)

This nerve can be exposed by careful dissection at the upper pole of the thyroid in the Joll's triangle. The nerve descends usually medial to the superior thyroid artery. Often the nerve is not visualized. Injury is best avoided by dissecting the upper pole and thinning the pedicle before transection. The artery clamp is passed from medial to lateral (the nerve is under constant vision) and applied as close to the pole as possible (Figs 19.8 and 19.9). The inferior pole is similarly mobilized after identifying and ligating the inferior thyroid veins. The thyrothymic ligament may need division and this is usually done close to the inferior pole of the gland to avoid damage to the inferior parathyroid which may sometimes be in relation to the upper part of the thymus.

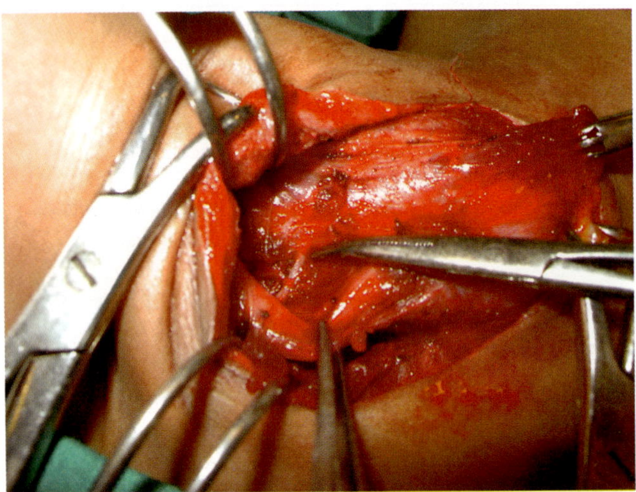

Fig. 19.8 Dissection of upper pole to expose external laryngeal nerve

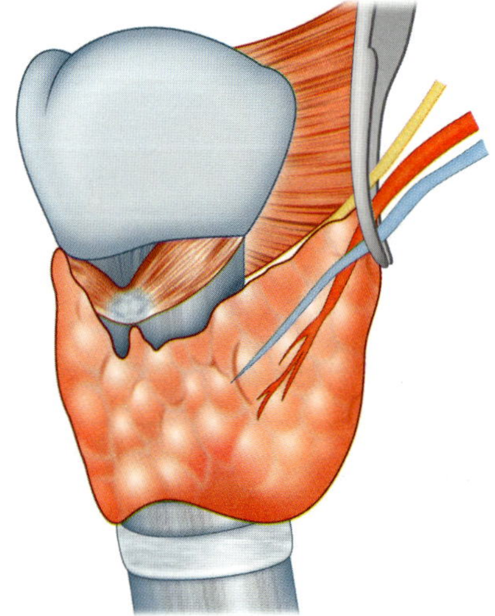

Fig. 19.9 Ligation of superior thyroid pedicle

Final Mobilization of the Gland

The thyroid lobe now remains firmly attached to the trachea by the suspensory (Berry's ligament). The previously identified recurrent laryngeal nerve is followed in its course to its point of entry into the larynx. Branches of the inferior thyroid artery need to be ligated and divided to free the nerve. This is done close to the capsule of the thyroid (Capsular ligation) to safeguard the blood supply to the parathyroids. Truncal ligation of the main inferior thyroid artery away from the gland at its point of emergence below the carotid using non-absorbable suture is a thing of past and not recommended. The most difficult part of the operation is where the nerve is in relation to Berry's ligament and it is here that it is most likely to be damaged. Careful dissection parallel to its course should safely identify and preserve the nerve. Unnecessary traction should be avoided. Should bleeding occur, gentle pressure and use of bipolar cautery is advised. A small portion of the thyroid may be left back to safeguard the nerve if dissection is difficult (near total thyroidectomy). The suspensory ligament may need to be transected after safeguarding the nerve near its point of entry into the larynx. This is usually done using a fine hemostat.

Follow the recurrent laryngeal nerve to its point of entry into larynx. Carefully isolate the inferior thyroid vessels and ligate them close to the capsule of the thyroid preserving vascularity to parathyroids (Capsular ligation—Fig. 19.7).

The thyroid lobe remains firmly attached to the trachea by suspensory (Berry's) ligament. The recurrent laryngeal nerve is particularly vulnerable at this point. One should be very careful in dissecting the thyroid off the ligament. Any bleeding can obscure the nerve and damage can easily occur. Identify the entry of the nerve into the larynx and then the ligament is clamped with a small hemostat and transected.

Once the suspensory ligament has been transected, the thyroid lobe separates easily from the surface of the trachea. Thus the whole lobe of thyroid is mobilized (The same steps are repeated on the opposite side to perform total thyroidectomy).

SPECIAL POINTS FOR THYROIDECTOMY IN CANCER

1. *Incision*: Is the same as for lobectomy but may need to be extended upwards towards the mastoid to facilitate a neck dissection.
2. *Strap muscles*: Strap muscles must be excised if there is doubt of extrathyroidal spread and possible involvement.
3. *Recurrent laryngeal nerves*: Recurrent laryngeal nerve can be sacrificed on one side, if there is a possibility of leaving back gross residual disease in the tracheoesophageal groove.

   However, the nerve should only be sacrificed if its removal will ensure the complete resection R0 (R zero means no malignant tissue left) resection and the other nerve has been saved.

4. *Total versus less than total thyroidectomy*: There is considerable controversy in the literature with regards to the extent of thyroidectomy for a differentiated cancer of the thyroid gland. A detailed discussion for and against a total or less than total thyroidectomy is beyond the scope of this chapter. These cancers are classified into low risk (excellent prognosis) and high-risk groups using various tumor and patient criteria.

   In general, however, all patients with follicular thyroid carcinoma and in those patients with papillary thyroid carcinoma either larger than 1 cm to 1.5 cm or with lymph node metastasis (high-risk group) a total or near total thyroidectomy is the preferred treatment with a decreased likelihood of recurrence and mortality. If the cancer is less than 1 cm to 1.5 cm in a young patient <40 years with no extrathyroidal spread (low-risk group), a hemithyroidectomy is sufficient with a 30 years mortality rate less than 3%.
5. *Dissection*: Non-involved or the less involved side must always be operated first and the recurrent laryngeal nerve and parathyroids saved.
6. *Parathyroids:* An effort to save a minimum of two parathyroids with an intact blood supply must be made. A small slice of thyroid may be left (near total thyroidectomy) to preserve the blood supply to a parathyroid.
7. *Mediastinal split:* A mediastinal split is rarely required. The thyroid usually carries its blood supply from the neck and most retrosternal goiters can be delivered from above. Mediastinal lymph nodes of differentiated thyroid cancer can also usually be removed adequately from the neck. The only real indication for a mediastinal split is to clear mediastinal nodes in medullary thyroid cancer—however, the surgeon must be sure that there is no metastatic spread elsewhere (lung; bone; liver).
8. *Trachea:* Tracheal involvement is not unusual in thyroid cancer. Most often the disease can be shaved off the trachea. However invasive disease particularly if associated with cartilage erosion seen on CT scan requires excision. If localized wedge resection of the trachea is possible, the defect can be closed primarily. If primary closure is not possible then the opening, if anterior, is treated as a tracheostomy and closure is achieved by subsequent decannulation. More extensive resection requires resection and end-to-end anastomosis.
9. *Nodes*: There is no role for prophylactic neck dissection in differentiated thyroid cancer. Typically patients with primary thyroid carcinoma should have an ipsilateral central compartment node clearance (nodes along the recurrent laryngeal nerve). This is because reoperations in this area are more difficult and associated with higher risk of complications. The lateral neck is inspected (jugular nodes) and suspicious nodes sampled and sent for frozen section evaluation. If positive a modified neck dissection preserving the internal jugular vein, sternocleidomastoid muscle and the spinal accessory nerve is performed. There is no role for "Berry picking", i.e. removal of only grossly positive nodes. This is because inadequately treated neck metastasis increases the risk for subsequent nodal recurrences, necessitating surgery and thereby contributing to increased morbidity
10. *Medullary cancer*: Given the higher frequency of microscopic tumor spread in medullary carcinomas (50%) and the inability of these tumors to take up iodine, elective central compartment lymph node dissection is performed. Central compartment clearance in this case differs from that for differentiated thyroid cancers with fibrofatty and lymphatic tissues being cleared from the hyoid to the innominate artery below and laterally from one carotid artery to the other. Ipsilateral modified neck dissection/radical neck dissection is performed for lateral cervical adenopathy depending on the size of the nodes and involvement of surrounding structures.

POSTOPERATIVE COMPLICATIONS

- *Hemorrhage:* Bleeding is a serious complication following thyroidectomy. Significant hemorrhage usually occurs due to the slipping of a ligature. With the advent of suction drainage, a hematoma causing pressure on the trachea with respiratory obstruction is rarely seen. Nevertheless it should be treated as an emergency and the patient returned to the operating rooms for evacuation of the hematoma and control of the bleeding.
- *Vocal cord palsy:* Unilateral iatrogenic cord palsy usually requires no active intervention manifesting as a hoarse or breathy voice. The opposite cord compensates with time and voice usually returns to normal in a couple of months. Occasionally, a medialization procedure may be required in cases where opposite cord compensation is inadequate. Bilateral cord palsy is rarely seen but must be kept in mind in infiltrative thyroid cancers involving both tracheoesophageal grooves. This manifests as respiratory stridor and may necessitate an emergency tracheostomy.
- *Respiratory obstruction:* Is a rare complication these days and is usually seen in patients who have significant tracheal compression prior to surgery. The denuded trachea may collapse or kink following surgery. If this complication is anticipated, the patient is left intubated following surgery. An attempt at extubation is made 48–72 hours later taking all precautions and keeping the tracheostomy as standby.
- *Hypocalcemia:* This is the most morbid of all complication following thyroid surgery with an incidence of 0 to 25% depending on the expertise of the operating surgeon. It is largely preventable with meticulous dissection during surgery. It is usually transient due to vascular insufficiency

to the parathyroid glands. This commonly occurs 24 to 48 hours following total thyroidectomy and infrequently requires treatment. Symptomatic patients should be treated with intravenous calcium initially which can be gradually tapered off. Permanent hypoparathyroidism would require calcium supplementation along with vitamin D over longer periods of time. Hypocalcemia beyond 6 months is likely to be permanent. Patients with refractory hypocalcemia may require magnesium supplementation as well.

- *Hypocalcemic tetany:* Is a medical emergency that is treated with slow intravenous administration of 10 mL of 10% calcium gluconate over 10 minutes. Subsequently a continuous infusion of calcium gluconate at the rate of 1 mL/kg is started to maintain the serum calcium level at 8–9 mg/dL.

CHAPTER

20

Subtotal Thyroidectomy

Dhiraj Choudhury

INDICATIONS

- Thyrotoxicosis
- Multinodular goiter
- Hashimoto's disease.

PREOPERATIVE PREPARATIONS

- Patients who are euthyroid requires routine preparations
- Patients who are thyrotoxic should be rendered euthyroid with carbimazole
- Indirect laryngoscopy is done to evaluate the mobility of the vocal cord.

OPERATIVE PROCEDURE

1. *Anesthesia:* General with endotracheal intubation.
2. *Position:* Supine with sandbag behind shoulders, neck extended and head supported on ring. The Surgeon usually stands on the right side of the patient.
3. *Draping:* Usual three towels method.
4. *Incision:* Mark a collar incision 1" or two fingers above the suprasternal notch extending from posterior border of one sternomastoid to posterior border of other sternomastoid (Fig. 20.1).
5. *Exposure:* The incision is deepened through skin, subcutaneous tissue and platysma.

   The upper skin flap is raised by working horizontally with knife blade, superficial to anterior jugular vein, picking up small vessels with hemostat and coagulating them. The dissection is completed bluntly with finger and gauze, reaching up to the thyroid prominence.

   The lower flap is raised down to suprasternal notch.

   The skin flaps subplatysma are held retracted with Jolls' self-retaining thyroid retractor.

   The anterior jugular veins are divided between ligatures.

   The investing layer of the deep cervical fascia is incised vertically in the midline and the interval between the infrahyoid (Strap) muscles is opened up to expose the sheath of the pretracheal fascia covering lobe of thyroid.
6. *Dealing with one lobe (Fig. 20.2)*
   a. Retraction of infrahyoid muscles will expose the anterolateral surface of the lobe. Improved access can be obtained by division of the infrahyoid muscles, sternohyoid and sternothyroid (high up to avoid damage to their nerve supply).
   b. At this point, loose facia over the thyroid gland is picked up with forceps and incised with scalpel to

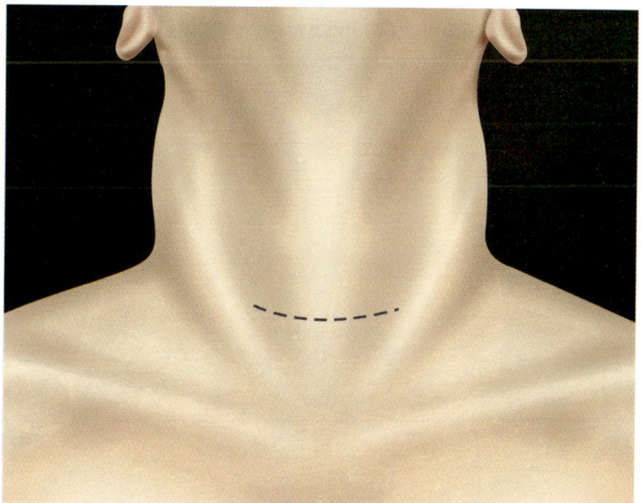

Fig. 20.1 Skin incision

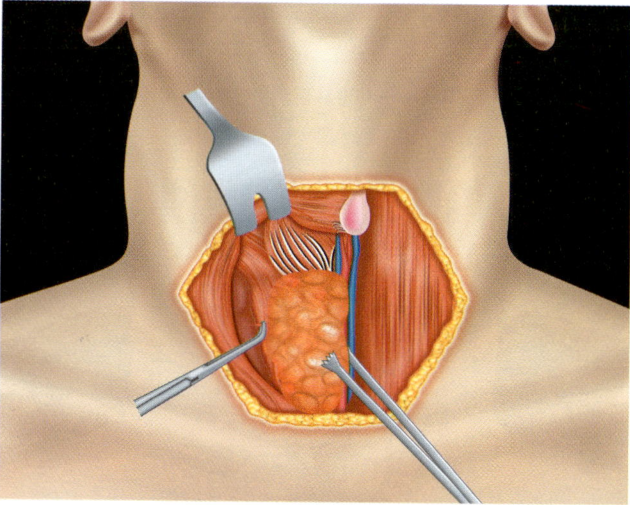

Fig. 20.2 Dealing with middle thyroid vein

develop a cleavage plane between thyroid lobe and sternothyroid muscle. This is an important step to make the operation bloodless. Now the blood vessels in capsule of the thyroid gland becomes visible. The strap muscles can be pulled away from the gland with retractor for better visualization.

c. The middle thyroid vein is divided between ligatures at this stage with great care, to improve mobility and exposure of upper pole vessels.
d. The superior pole is mobilized and delivered at the wound. The superior vascular pedicle consisting of superior thyroid vessels are dissected and clamped carefully to avoid injury to external laryngeal nerve. The second clamp is applied in substance of the gland (about 1 cm below upper pole) if thyroid tissue can be left in upper pole, or upper limit of the gland (Fig. 20.3).

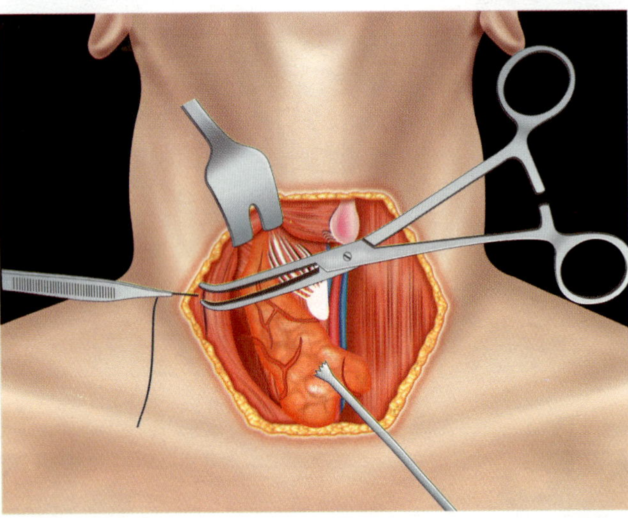

Fig. 20.3 Ligating superior thyroid vessles

e. Mobilization of the upper pole, downwards and forward will bring the inferior thyroid artery in view. Traction is maintained medially to expose inferior thyroid artery on the lateral inferior surface of the gland. The inferior thyroid artery is visualized clearly by gauze dissection on the lateral surface of the gland. Ligate the inferior thyroid artery in continuity at the level of cricoid cartilage where it emerges from behind the carotid sheath. The recurrent laryngeal nerve runs in the tracheoesophageal groove and should be carefully identified and preserved (Fig. 20.4).
f. A finger is then swept around the lower pole of the lobe which is delivered forwards and inferior thyroid veins are ligated and divided.
g. Now, select the line of section of the lobe and apply several pairs of Kocher's hemostatic forceps. The lobe is then sectioned using scalpel from lateral to medial side in a plane towards front of the trachea. Clamp any bleeding vessels encountered and do suture ligation (Fig. 20.5).

7. *Dealing with isthmus:*
   - Separate the isthmus from the trachea and divide it between forceps applied at its junction with the opposite lobe. The isthmus is then ligated. In freeing isthmus, care should be taken to avoid injury to thin tracheal fascia.
8. *Dealing with opposite lobe:*
   - The opposite lobe of the gland is then dealt in a similar manner, and an equal amount of gland being left behind.
9. *Closure:*
   - Check hemostasis and put a suction drain
   - Anesthetist checks vocal cords
   - Close the wound with interrupted ethilon sutures or Michel's clips.

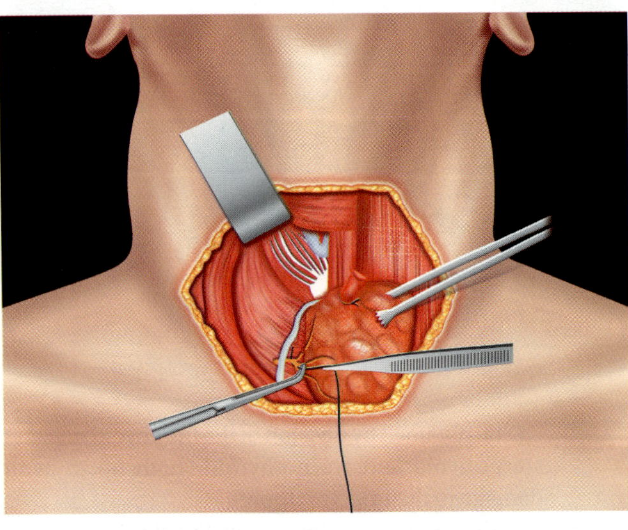

Fig. 20.4 Dealing with inferior thyroid artery

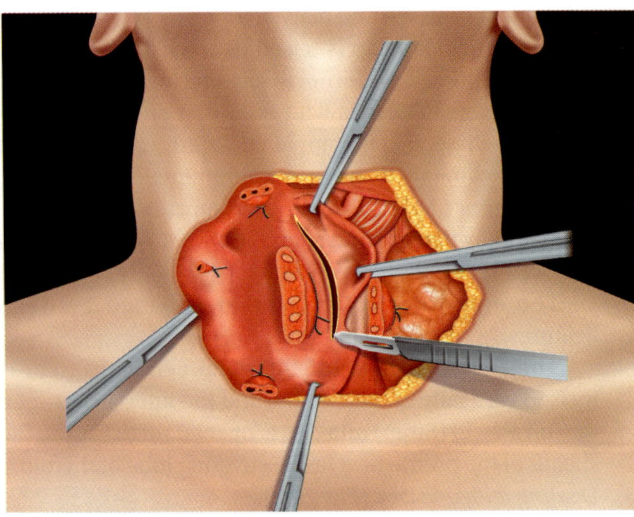

Fig. 20.5 Division of the gland

CHAPTER

21 Excision of Thyroglossal Cyst and Fistula

Dhiraj Choudhury

Thyroglossal cysts are congenital tubuloepidermoid cysts resulting from persistent remnant of the thyroglossal duct. They are commonly (75%) found at the lower border of the hyoid bone (subhyoid). The other less common sites being at the level of the thyroid or cricoid cartilage, suprahyoid, in the floor of the mouth or foramen cecum of the tongue.

EXCISION OF THYROGLOSSAL CYST

Indications

- Cosmetic
- Complications
  - Particularly infection
  - Rarely thyroglossal duct carcinoma.

Operative Procedure

1. *Position of patients:* The patient is placed on supine position with neck extended by sandbag under shoulder.
2. *Anesthesia:* General anesthesia with endotracheal intubation is used.
3. *Incision:* A transverse incision is made over the cyst. In case of fistula, an elliptical incision is made (Fig. 21.1).
4. *Exploration:* The incision is deepened through subcutaneous tissues, platysma and deep cervical fascia. Raise the skin and platysma flaps upwards at least half way between hyoid bone and symphysis menti and downwards for 2 to 3 cm. Divide and ligate the anterior jugular veins as they pass over midine. Identify the cyst and dissect it from surrounding tissues (Fig. 21.2).
5. *Technique:* Apply self-retaining retractor. Now hold the cyst with tissue forceps and apply traction to define the track (Fig. 21.3).

   Dissect the track up to hyoid bone and free muscular attachment and thyrohyoid membrane. Excise the central part of the body of hyoid bone in continuity with the track (Sistrunk's operation), 5 cm on either side of the midline. The hyoid bone may be steadied with Kocher's artery forceps to facilitate division with strong Mayo's scissors or bone cutting forceps: Figure 21.4 shows schematic diagram of division of central part of body of hyoid bone.

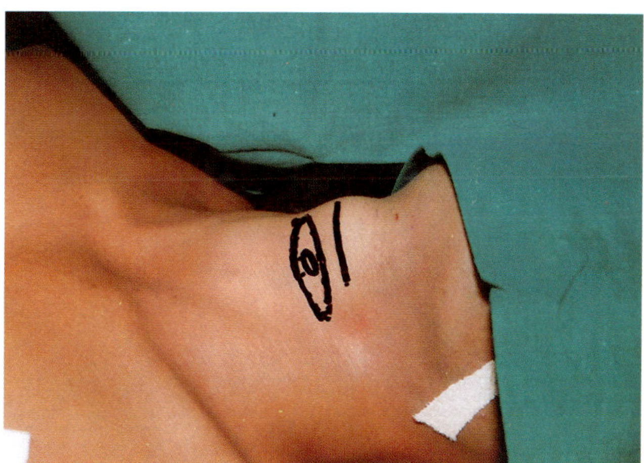

Fig. 21.1 Skin incisions

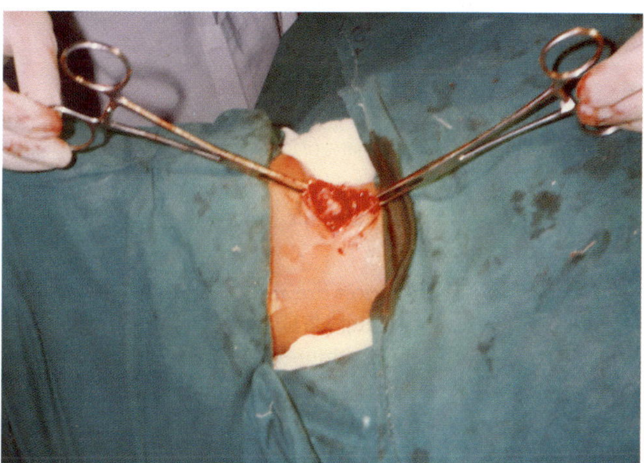

Fig. 21.2 Exploration

Above the hyoid bone excise a core of myelohyoid muscle with diathermy extending for 2 cm deep to the muscle. This part of dissection may be facilitated by introduction of a finger of the assistant into mouth to push posterior part of tongue downwards and forwards. Hemostasis should be perfect. Cyst excised (Fig. 21.5) is sent for histopathology.

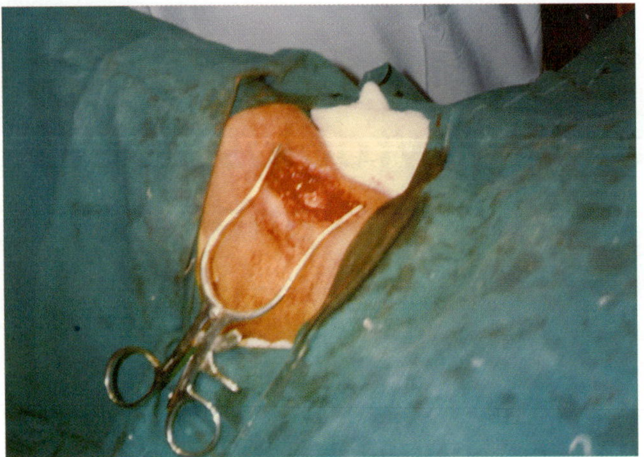

Fig. 21.3 Application of self-retaining retraction

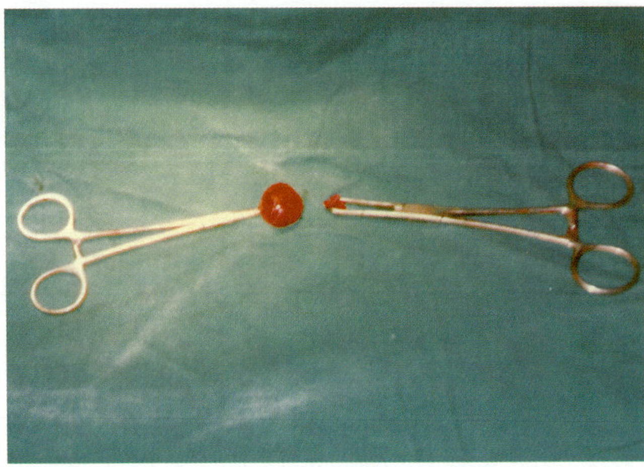

Fig. 21.5 Cyst and excised central part of body of hyoid bone

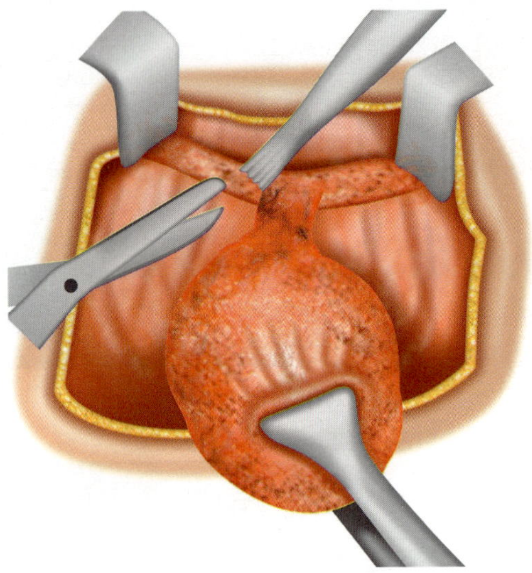

Fig. 21.4 Schematic diagram of division of central part of hyoid bone

Fig. 21.6 Excision of core of genial muscles along with fistula tract and part of hyoid bone—schematic diagram

6. *Closure:* Insert a suction drain. Muscles are closed with interrupted sutures using 3/0 chromic catgut. The platysma is approximated by continuous suture with 3/0 chromic catgut. The skin is closed with subcuticular stitches.

EXCISION OF THYROGLOSSAL FISTULA

Thyroglossal fistula is always an aquired fistula (better called median cervical sinus) which develops from an infected thyroglossal cyst discharging spontaneously or being incised.

1. *Incision:* An elliptical incision is made around the orifice of fistula (sinus).
2. *Exposure:* The ellipse of the skin is dissected through the subcutaneous tissues towards the hyoid bone.
3. *Excision:* The central part of body of hyoid bone is excised with fistulous tract.

   A core of geniohyoid and genioglossus muscles, including fistulous tract is excised up to the level of foraman cecum of tongue (Fig. 21.6).
4. *Closure:* The wound is closed in layers.

POSTOPERATIVE CARE

- Take care of airway
- Administer systemic antibiotic.

POSTOPERATIVE COMPLICATION

- Hemorrhage
- Airways obstruction
- Sepsis.

CHAPTER 22

Parathyroidectomy

Dhiraj Choudhury

The parathyroid glands lie behind the lateral lobes of the thyroid gland. They are four in numbers—superior glands two in number are constant in position, the inferior glands two in number are variable in position.

INDICATIONS

Primary hyperparathyroidism caused by an adenoma (85%). Parathyroidectomy is the gold standard in the treatment of symptomatic parathyroid adenoma.

- Primary hyperparathyroidism due to hyperplasia (15%). Excision of three glands and one-half of the fourth gland, leaving half carefully marked or autotransplanted is the common surgical treatment for hyperplasia.
- The indications for parathyroidectomy in symptomless hyperparathyroidism include high calcium levels, high urinary calcium (excretion of >10 mol/day), reduced creatinine clearance, significant osteoporosis, deteriorating renal function.
- Tertiary hyperparathyroidism may occasionally require surgery. Full exploration of the neck with either subtotal excision of parathyroids or total parathyroidectomy is carried out.

PREOPERATIVE PREPARATIONS

Attempts to localize the glands are justified. Procedures used to localize adenoma include—ultrasound and radionuclide imaging. Ultrasound is noninvasive and should identify 75% of adenoma. Computerized tomography (SPECT) can give three dimensional image which is helpful during operation. Cross-sectional MRI may be helpful in evaluation of retrosternal and mediastinal location.

TECHNIQUE

1. *Anesthesia:* General with endotracheal intubation.
2. *Position:* The patient is placed in supine position with head resting on a head ring 30 degree.
3. *Incision:* A collar incision is made 1 cm above sternal notch.
4. *Exposure:* It is similar to that in subtotal thyroidectomy (Chapter 20).

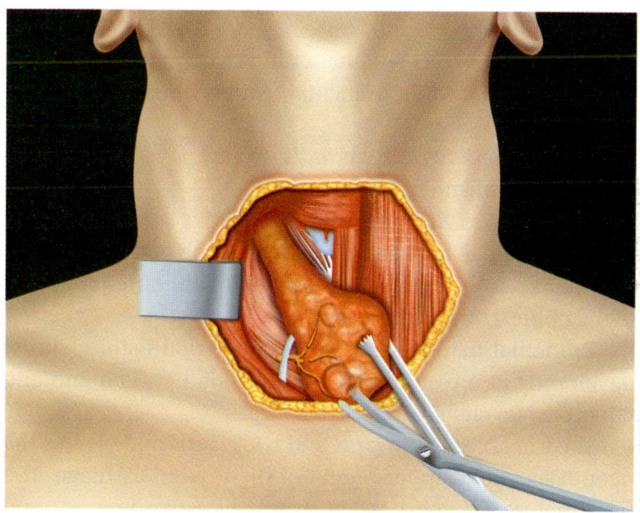

Fig. 22.1 Localization of parathyroid

5. *Mobilization of muscles:* The sternomastoid and strap muscles are retraced to expose the lobe of the thyroid gland.
6. *Localization of parathyroids (Fig. 22.1):* The thyroid lobe is lifted medially and anteriorly. The middle thyroid vein is divided and ligated. Lift the lobe of the thyroid to opposite side to identify inferior thyroid artery and recurrent laryngeal nerve. Dissect a thin fascia covering the thyroid and parathyroid. The parathyroids are identified by their color (brown), shape and soft texture. The inferior glands are most likely to be found in cervical tongue of the isthmus while superior glands along pharynx.
7. *Excision;* Ideally all four glands are identified and subjected to frozen section. The adenoma is removed. Three adenomas can be safely removed. In four glands hyperplasia three and a half glands can be removed. If a tumor is adherent to muscle, en-block excision of the muscle can be done.
8. *Closure:* The wound is closed in layers with a suction drain.

CHAPTER

23

Excision of Branchial Cyst and Fistula

Dhiraj Choudhury

ANATOMY

Branchial cyst is a congenital cystic swelling on the lateral side of the neck while branchial fistula is better termed as lateral cervical sinus.

Developmentally, a branchial cyst may be:

- Remnant of 2nd pharyngeal pouch
- Persistent cervical sinus of His
- An epithelial inclusion in cervical lymph node.

Anatomically, the cyst appears behind the anterior border of the upper 1/3rd of the sternomastoid muscle.

Branchial fistula is usually a congenital fistula (sinus) developing as a result of failure of fusion between 2nd and 6th branchial clefts.

The tract passes upwards and backwards and pierces the deep fascia near upper border of the thyroid cartilage. The proximal part when present passes between internal and external carotid artery to open into supratonsillar fossa of Rosenmüller.

A branchial cyst probably develops from persistent cervical sinus. The commonest site supper 1/3rd of sternomastoid muscle along its anterior border.

INDICATIONS

- Cosmetic
- *Complications:*
  - It is prone to infection and may give rise to fistula
  - Rarely bronchogenic carcinoma may develop.

PREOPERATIVE STEP

A sonogram may be helpful in case of a cyst and lipoidol or hypaque sonogram in case of fistula.

OPERATIVE PROCEDURE

1. *Position of patient:* The patient is placed in supine position with head tilted to opposite side and a sandbag beneath the shoulders.
2. *Anesthesia:* General anesthesia with endotracheal intubation.
3. *Incision:* A horizontal crease incision is made at the level of the cyst at the junction of upper and middle 1/3rd of sternomastoid (Fig. 23.1).
4. *Exposure:* Deepen the incision through subcutaneous tissue and platysma and raise the skin flaps.

   Display the wall of the cyst by blunt dissection after retracting the flaps.

   The deep cervical fascia is divided next to anterior border of sternomastoid muscle.

   Retract the muscle to display the cyst anteriorly and medially.

   Expose the cyst wall by careful blunt dissection avoiding rupture of the cyst. Particular care should be taken during deep dissection because jugular vein and carotid arteries are intimately related (Fig. 23.2).
5. *Excision:* The pedicle of the cyst passes between external and internal carotid arteries.

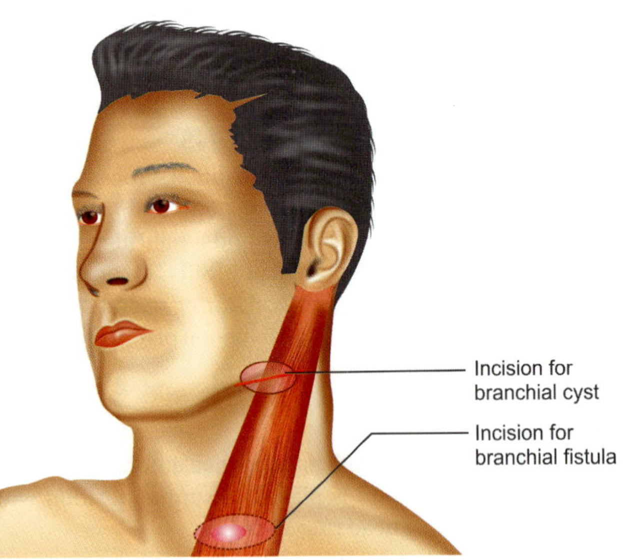

Fig. 23.1 Incision for branchial cyst and fistula

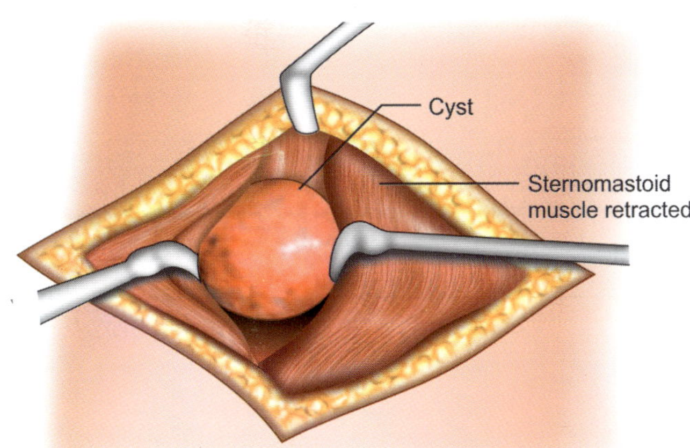

Fig. 23.2 Dissection of cyst

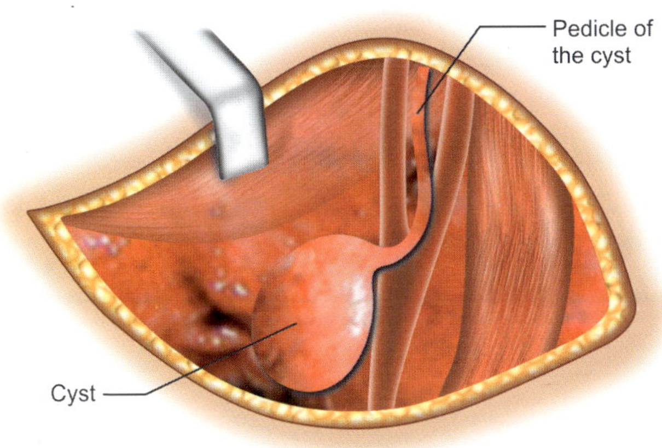

Fig. 23.3 Dissection of pedicle of the cyst

It is dissected towards tonsillar pillar, clamped, divided and ligated with nonabsorbable suture. Secure the hemostasis (Fig. 23.3).

6. *Closure:* The platysma is closed with interrupted catgut sutures. The skin is apposed with subcuticular stitches.

EXCISION OF BRANCHIAL FISTULA

A branchial fistula is usually a congenital fistula (lateral cervical sinus) developing as a result of failure of fusion between second and sixth branchial cleft. But, it can be acquired also. The external opening of the congenital fistula is situated in the lower third of the neck along the anterior border of the sternomastoid.

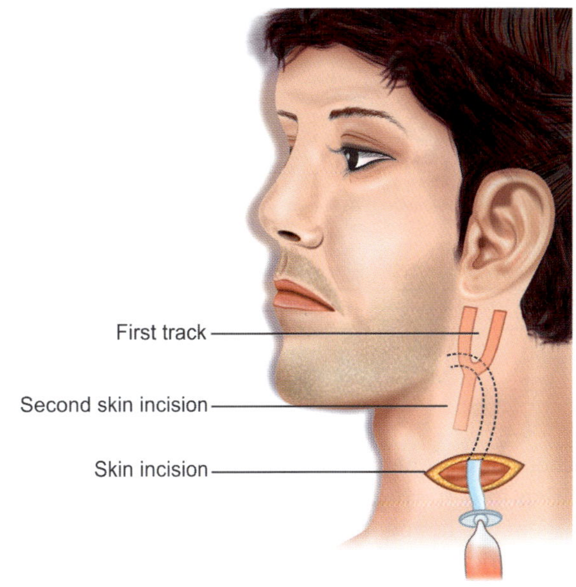

Fig. 23.4 Fistulectomy

1. *Incision:* Apply an elliptical incision around the fistula opening. A second incision is better made at a higher level to avoid unsightly scar (Fig. 23.4).
2. *Exposure:* Hold the skin ellipse containing fistulous opening with tissue forceps to apply traction and dissect it from below upwards as far as possible. A second skin crease incision (staircase) is made at the junction of middle and upper third of sternomastoid muscle. The track is followed carefully as it passes between external carotid and internal carotid artery above. Follow the track upwards as it merges with the fascia covering the middle constrictor muscle.

   The glossopharyngeal and hypoglossal nerves run between the tract and middle constrictor muscle.

   Apply two pairs of artery forceps to the track where it blends with middle constrictor muscle and cut in between. Tie the pharyngeal end.
3. *Closure:* Put a suction drain and close the wound in layers.

Postoperative Care

- Systemic antibiotic
- Analgesic.

Postoperative Complications

- Hemorrhage
- Sepsis.

CHAPTER

24

Tracheostomy

Dhiraj Choudhury

Tracheostomy is the procedure of constructing an artificial opening into trachea through the neck. During serious emergency a laryngotomy by a horizontal stab incision between cricoid and thyroid cartilage is preferred, as the quickest method.

INDICATIONS

Upper Airway Obstruction

- Foreign bodies
- Faciomaxillary trauma
- Tumors of head and neck
- Ludwig's angina
- Major reconstructive facial surgery.

Prolonged Ventilatory Support

- Flail chest
- Acute respiratory distress syndrome
- Guillain-Barré syndrome, tracheobronchial toilet.

Neurological Impairment

Coma, stroke, motor neuron disease.

Preoperative Steps

Keep suction apparatus and tracheostomy tube ready.

PREOPERATIVE PROCEDURE

Position

The patient is placed in supine position with extension of neck by placing a sandbag behind the shoulders (Fig. 24.1).

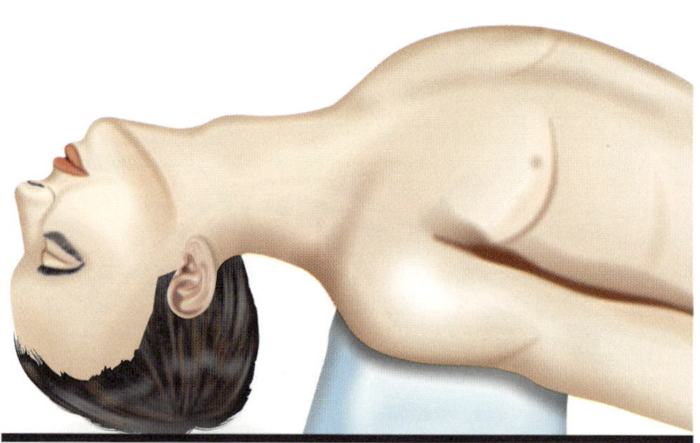

Fig. 24.1 Position of patient

Emergency Procedure

Anesthesia: Local infiltration with 1% lignocaine with 1:300,000 adrenaline may be sufficient or general anesthesia may be given if time is permitted.

1. *Incision:* A vertical incision is made in the midline from the lower border of the thyroid cartilage to suprasternal notch (Fig. 24.2).

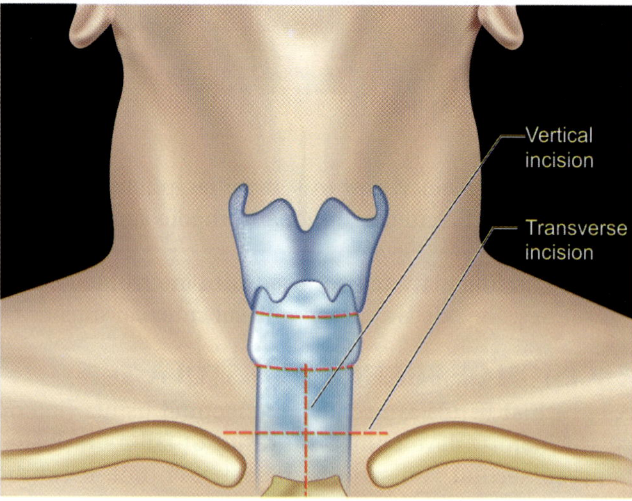

Fig. 24.2 Skin incision

2. *Exposure:* The incision is carried through platysma and deep fascia. The anterior jugular veins are either avoided or divided and ligated.

   The strap muscles are retracted laterally to expose the rings of the trachea. Divide the thyroid isthmus between

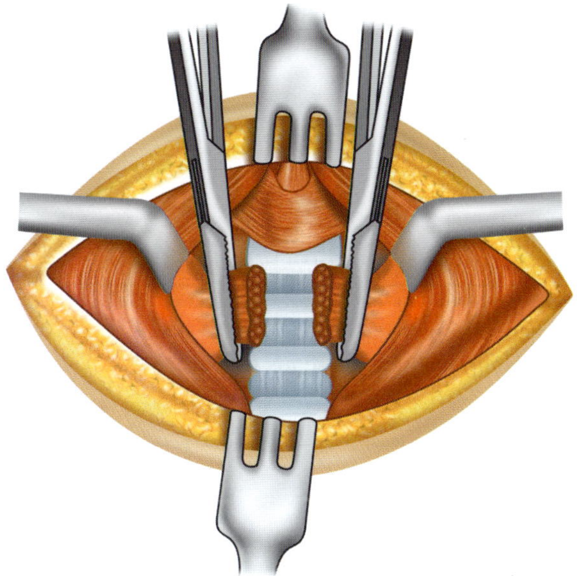

Fig. 24.3 Exposure of trachea

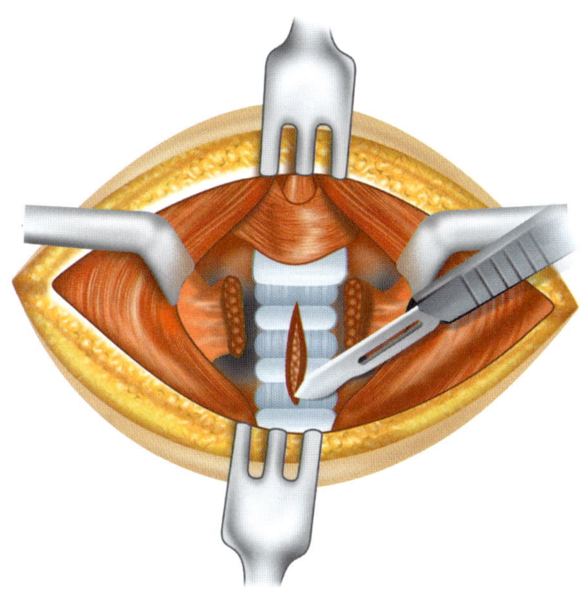

Fig. 24.4 Incision of trachea

hemostats to expose the anterior wall of the trachea. If time is permitted ligate the bleeding point (Fig. 24.3).

3. *Tracheal entry:* Incise the trachea vertically through 2nd and 3rd rings. Insert a tracheal dilator to secure an airway (Fig. 24.4).
4. *Inserting the tracheostomy tube:* A cuffed plastic tracheostomy tube is inserted which allows complete control of the airway and prevention of aspiration. The time between incising trachea and inserting tracheostomy tube should be as minimal as possible (Fig. 24.5).

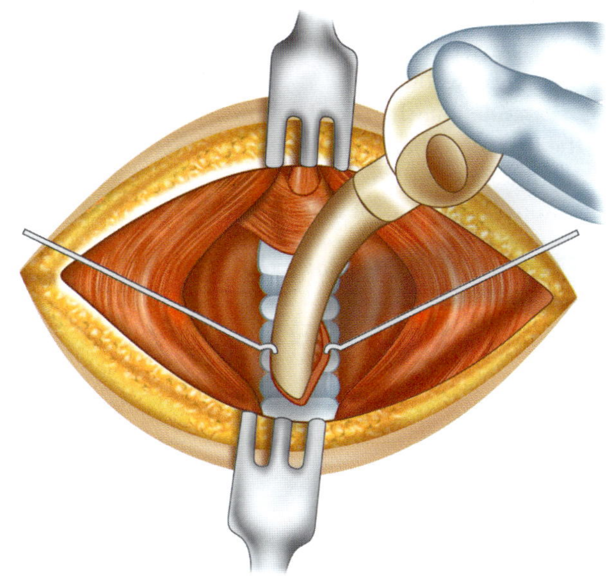

Fig. 24.5 Insertion of tracheostomy tube

5. *Tracheal toilet:* Tracheal suction must be immediately started.
6. *Closure:* The skin incision is closed loosely around the tube. A gauze dressing is placed at the side of tracheostomy tube.

Elective Procedure

Elective Procedure is easier to perform as the patient is adequately prepared and anesthetized.

1. *Anesthesia:* General endotracheal anesthesia may be used.
2. *Incision:* A transverse crease incision is made half way between cricoid cartilage and suprasternal notch.
3. *Exposure:* The incision is deepened through subcutaneous tissue and deep cervical fascia. Strap muscles are retracted laterally to expose rings of the trachea. The thyroid isthmus is divided and ligated to expose anterior wall of the trachea.
4. *Tracheal entry:* A vertical or U-shaped incision is made on the 2nd and 3rd rings of trachea. The margins are retracted with dilator.
5. *Inserting tracheostomy tube:* A cuffed plastic tracheostomy tube is inserted.
6. *Tracheal toilet:* Tracheal suction must be started immediately.
7. *Closure:* The skin incision is closed loosely around the tube. A gauze dressing is placed at the site of tracheostomy tube.

POSTOPERATIVE CARE

- Humidification of the inhaled air is required for proper ciliary function and can be carried out by humidifier

- Aseptic suction of tracheostomy tube (tracheobronchial toilet) must be carried out with a septic precaution
- Dressing of wound
- Decannulation when need for tracheostomy is over
- The first tube change can take place after 3–4 days when the track has sterilized
- A proper nourishment is necessary.

POSTOPERATIVE COMPLICATIONS

Short-term

- Hemorrhage from cut end of the thyroid isthmus
- Sepsis
- Subcutaneous emphysema
- Injury to adjacent structures
- Tube displacement
- Tracheal ulceration
- Mucus plugging
- Aspiration.

Long-term

- Tracheal stenosis
- Tracheomalacia
- Tracheoesophageal fistula (1%)
- Persistent tracheocutaneous fistula.

SECTION

3

Breast

CHAPTER

25

Operation for Benign Breast Lesions

Dhiraj Choudhury

INCISION AND DRAINAGE OF BREAST ABSCESS

Acute breast abscess occurs most commonly during lactation and pregnancy resulting from bacterial invasion through cracked nipple (puerperal). May be nonpuerperal.

Indication

Incision and drainage is reserved for larger abscess (75 cm).

Preoperative Preparation

Systemic antibiotic should be started.

Operative Procedure

- *Position:* The patient is placed in supine position.
- *Anesthesia:* General anesthesia is preferred.
- *Incision*: The incision should allow full drainage and be cosmetically acceptable. A curve transverse incision is made over the most fluctuant part of the abscess, after antiseptic dressing and draping.
- *Procedure.* Deepen the incision into the abscess cavity. Obtain pus for culture and sensitivity test. Explore the abscess cavity with fingers and break the loculi, to from a single cavity (Fig. 25.1).
- *Counterincision:* If the abscess cavity is large or if the incision is not in the dependent part, a counterincision in the dependent part is advisable after introduction of a hemostat (Fig. 25.2). The abscess cavity may be filled with roller gauze (particularly when bleeding is considerable) or drained by corrugated rubber drain (Fig. 25.3).
- *Closure:* If the margin are healthy, few interrupted skin stitches may be applied. The wound may be packed lightly and left open.

Postoperative

Breastfeeding should continue from nonaffected breast. Affected breast is emptied either manually or with a breast pump.

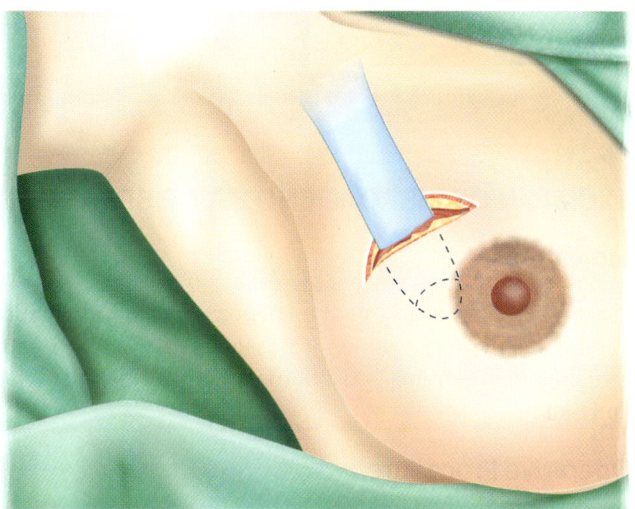

Fig. 25.1 Skin incision and exploration of abscess

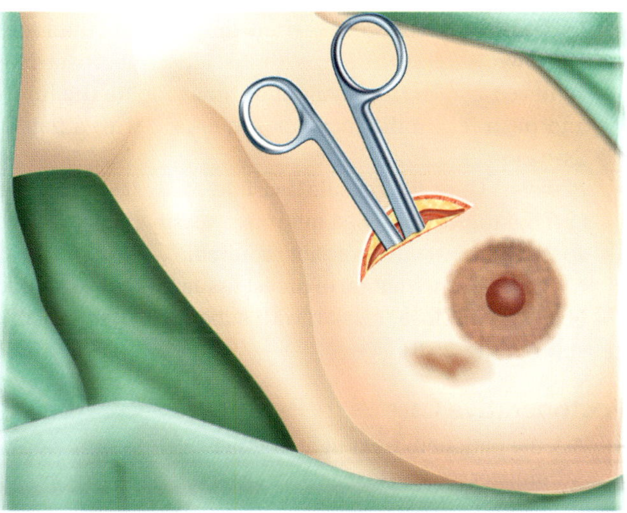

Fig. 25.2 Counterincision

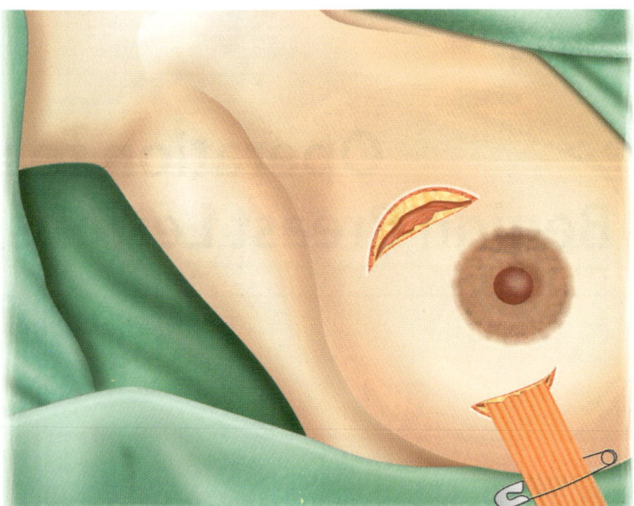

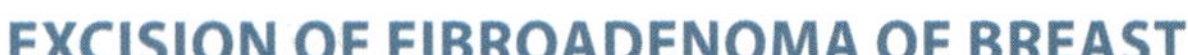

Fig. 25.3 Corrugated rubber drain

EXCISION OF FIBROADENOMA OF BREAST

Indications

Surgery is indicated for large fibroadenomas or fibroadenomas having suspicious, cytology or associated with patient's anxiety and symptoms. Most fibroadenomas are superficial and mobile.

Operative Procedure

- *Position:* The patient is placed in supine position.
- *Anesthesia:* General anesthesia is preferred.
- For lesion near the nipple a periareolar incision (Fig. 25.4) gives excellent cosmetic results. For others, a transverse curved incision over the lump is satisfactory (Fig. 25.5).
- *Exposure:* Dissection is carried through subcutaneous fat down to breast tissue with a scalpel. Hemostasis is achieved by electrocoagulation. Now palpate the lump, and push it into the incision and hold it with a pair of tissue forceps.
- *Removal:* Once the capsule is visible, incise it with scalpel and the tumor is shelled out mostly easily (Figs 25.6 and 25.7). Drainage is usually not required.
- *Closure:* Reconstruction of breast tissue by sutures should be avoided. Close the skin with subcuticular absorbable sutures (Fig. 25.8).

Postoperative Care

- Ask the patient to wear tight brassier
- Administer analgesic.

Postoperative Complication

- Hematoma
- Infection.

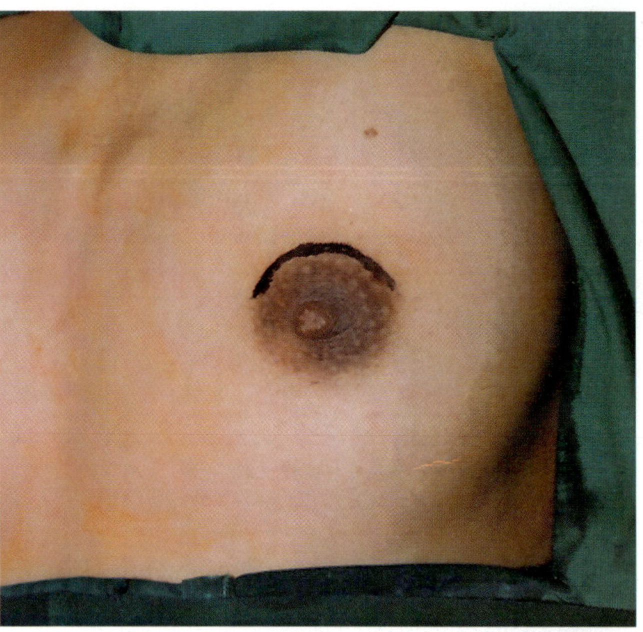

Fig. 25.4 Circumareolar or periareolar incision

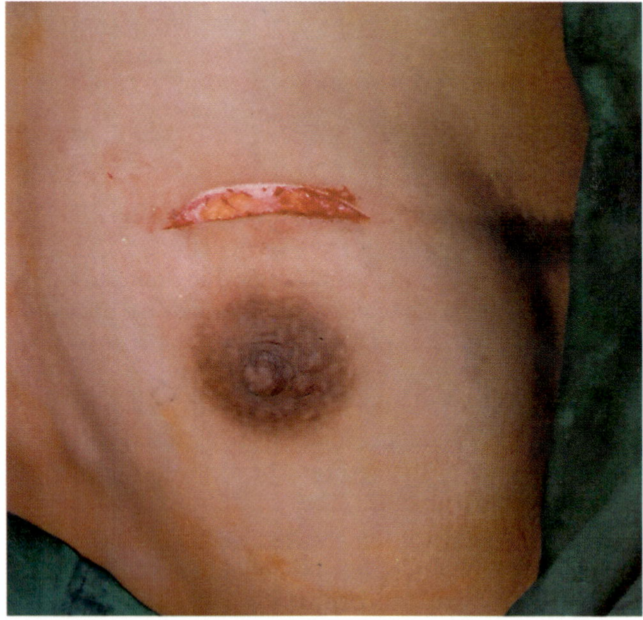

Fig. 25.5 Transverse curved incision directly over the lump

EXCISION OF GIANT FIBROADENOMA

A giant fibroadenoma (more than 5 cm in diameter and usually in deeper plane) in young patients can be removed by a Galliard Thomas incision (Fig. 25.9). When a giant fibroadenoma occupies the greater part of breast, simple mastectomy may be required.

Operative Procedure

- *Position:* The patient is placed in supine position.
- *Anesthesia:* General anesthesia is preferred.

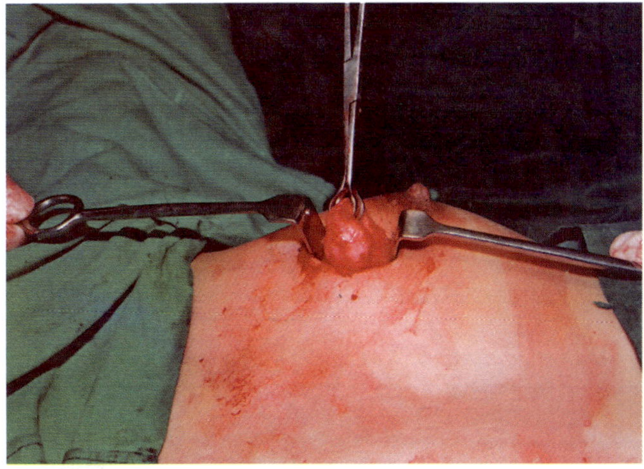

Fig. 25.6 Lump

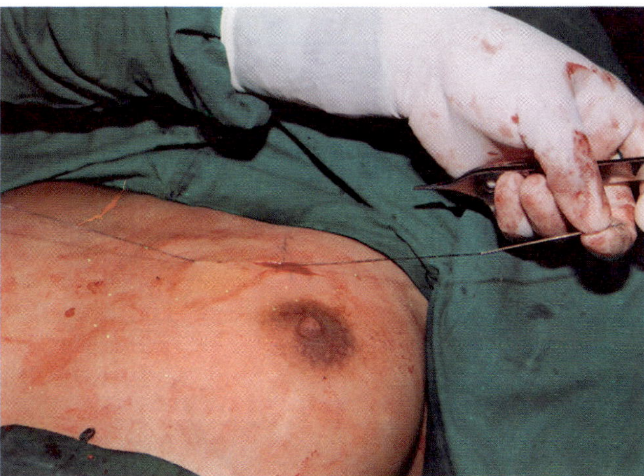

Fig. 25.8 Subcuticular suture

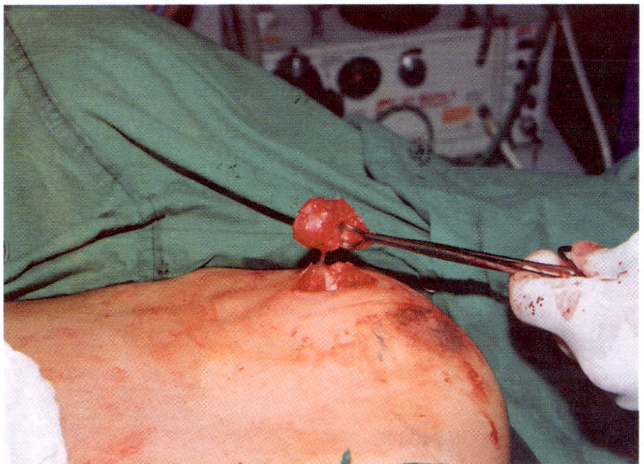

Fig. 25.7 Removed lump

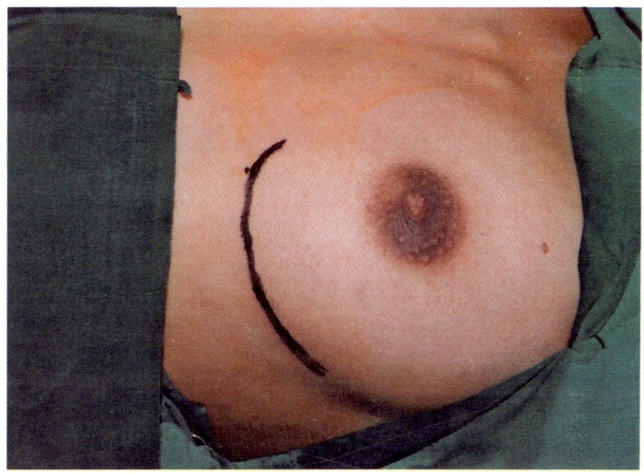

Fig. 25.9 Galliard Thomas incision

- *Incision:* An incision is made in the submammary crease (Galliard Thomas incision) (Fig. 25.9).
- *Exposure:* A blunt dissection, almost bloodless is carried between breast tissue and fascia.
- *Removal of the mass:* The fibroadenoma is pushed into the wound and removed. Hemostasis should be meticulous.
- *Closure:* Put suction drain. The subcutaneous tissue is closed with interrupted 3/0 catgut sutures. The skin is closed with interrupted 3/0 ethilon sutures.

EXCISION OF DUCTS

Excision of Single Duct Microdochectomy

Microdochectomy is both diagnostic and therapeutic procedure. The patient is advised not to express the discharge for at least a week prior to surgery.

Indication

Blood-stained discharge from a single duct:

The discharge is usually caused by duct ectasia, intraduct papilloma.

- *Position:* The patient is placed in supine position, with both arms at the side.
- *Anesthesia:* General anesthesia is used.
- *Procedure:* Localize the affected duct opening by observing discharge of blood while squeezing the breast and nipple by gentle digital pressure. Cannulate the duct opening using a lacrimal probe. Make a radial incision into the skin of the nipple along the line of probe, encircling the duct orifice.

  Dissect the skin of the areolar area from the underlying breast tissue for approximately 1 cm on each side of the probe (Fig. 25.10).

  Excise the breast segment containing the probe with scissors behind the duct orifice.
- *Closure:* Secure hemostasis. Close the breast tissue starting behind the duct orifice. Skin is closed with subcuticular absorbable sutures.

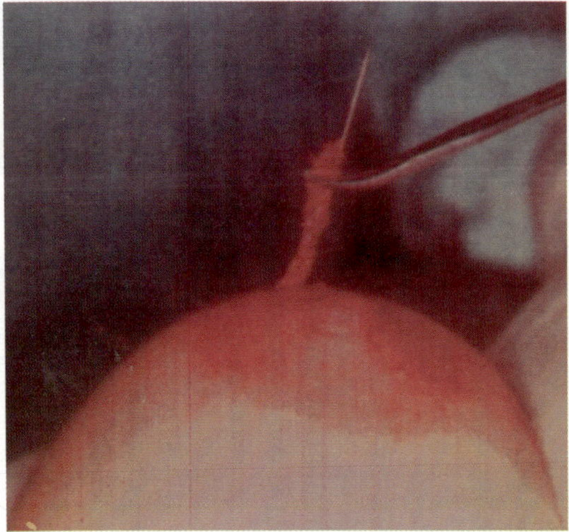

Fig. 25.10 Microdochectomy

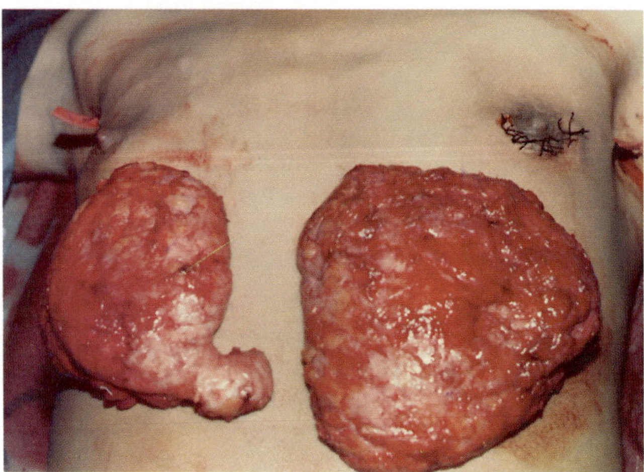

Fig. 25.12 Excised breast tissue

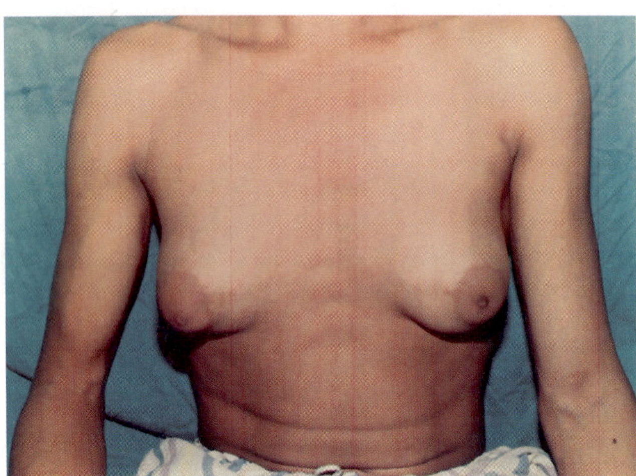

Fig. 25.11 Gynecomastia

Excision of Major Duct System: Hadfield's Operation

Indications

- Blood-stained discharge from two or more ducts in women above 40 years
- Duct ectasia with discharge causing discomfort
- Major duct excision is the procedure of choice for recurrent periductal mastitis and its complication like mamillary fistula.

Operative Procedure

- *Position:* The patient is placed in supine position.
- *Anesthesia:* General anesthesia.
- *Incision:* A periareolar (circumareolar) incision is made.
- *Exposure:* Deepen the incision through subcutaneous tissue and ligate all vessels with 3/0 chromic catgut.
  The plane of dissection should lie between fat lobules of breast and areola. Lift the areola to expose the main ductal system and create a tunnel by passing curve artery forceps behind the nipple.
- *Excision of duct tissue :* Hold the ductal tissue which looks like a conical mass with artery and cut it close to vessels before they retract. Check hemostasis.
- *Closure:* A suction drain may be inserted. Close the skin with interrupted 3/0 absorbable sutures (Subcuticular).

OPERATION FOR GYNECOMASTIA

Indications

Cosmetics (Fig. 25.11).

Operative Procedure

- *Position:* The patient is place in supine position.
- *Anesthesia:* General anesthesia is used.
- *Incision:* A curved incision in submammary area or a periareolar incision may be made.
- *Exposure:* Raise an upper flap by dissecting between skin and the breast tissue. It is better to leave a little duct tissue beneath the nipple. Proceed with the dissection in the subcutaneous plane above the nipple.
- *Procedure:* Excise the breast tissue until the deep fascia overlying pectoralis muscle is encountered and removed it. Secure hemostasis by controlling bleeding with diathermy (Fig. 25.12).
- *Closure:* Leave a suction drain. Close the skin with interrupted 3/0 ethilon sutures.

Postoperative Care

- Patient can be discharged
- Remove drain when it stops draining
- Analgesic.

Postoperative Complications

- Hematoma
- Sepsis

CHAPTER

26

Surgery for Breast Cancer

RA Badwe, Vani Parmar

INTRODUCTION

Anatomy of the Normal Breast

The breast is a modified apocrine gland in origin and lies in the superficial fascia of the chest wall, extending vertically between the 2nd and 6th ribs and horizontally from the sternal edge to the midaxillary line. The axillary tail of Spence extends upwards and laterally into the axilla and is the only part of the breast entering the deep fascia. The functional unit of the breast is the terminal ductal lobular unit (TDLU). These aggregate into lobules drained by ducts, which converge and open at the nipple. Fibrous tissue bands extend from the deep fascia across the stroma to the skin (ligaments of Cooper) with accompanying lymphatics implicated in the spread of cancer.

The main blood supply of the breast is from the lateral thoracic artery, perforator branches from the internal mammary and the intercostal (2nd to 4th) arteries. The glandular lymphatics drain into the subareolar plexus and into the plexus under the deep fascia underlying the breast. From here the lymph drains into the regional lymph nodes in the axilla and into nodes along the internal mammary lymph vessels. The efferent lymphatics from the regional lymph nodes are received into the supraclavicular nodes.

Surgery in Breast Cancer

The role of surgery in breast cancer varies on one end from the diagnostic incision biopsy or excision biopsy to the therapeutic radical mastectomy at the other end of the spectrum. Women with operable breast cancer are offered surgery first (either breast conservation or modified radical mastectomy) followed by adjuvant therapy (chemotherapy, radiation therapy and hormonal therapy based on the histopathological and receptor status). In the adjuvant settings, bilateral oophorectomy can be performed in premenopausal women (above 40 years age) with hormone-responsive tumors.

Women with large operable tumors and locally advanced breast cancer receive neoadjuvant chemotherapy followed by surgery after downsizing of tumor. In metastatic breast cancer, local surgery is mainly palliative in presence of a fungating tumor or bleeding ulcer. In estrogen receptor positive tumors, oophorectomy can be offered to premenopausal women with metastatic breast cancer as a hormonal manipulation.

Surgery in bone metastasis encompasses spinal decompressive surgery and long bone fixation (in fractures). Solitary bone, visceral (lung, liver, brain) metastasis has also been considered for excision followed by radiation therapy (in brain/bone metastasis) or chemotherapy (lung/liver metastasis). There is, however, not much of long-term evidence so far regarding the benefits of such an intervention, though an overall better prognosis in presence of solitary distant metastasis is the basis for offering radical treatment in these cases.

Introduction

For several decades, there has been a steady rise in the incidence of invasive breast cancer, which has become one of the leading causes of cancer mortality in women between 40 to 45 years of age. Surgery for breast cancer has evolved over a period of time from the radical mastectomy of the Halstedian era to the current era of conservatism. Breast conservation surgery followed by radiotherapy has now become the standard of care in early breast cancer and is also feasible in select cases of locally advanced breast cancer after downsizing with neoadjuvant chemotherapy.

Between 1970 to 1980, six prospective randomized trials were carried out comparing mastectomy with conservative surgery and radiation[1] for stage I and stage II breast cancer. In all these trials, adjuvant systemic chemotherapy was used in node positive patients. Whole breast irradiation was administered with a boost to the primary tumor site in all except the NSABP B-06 trial.[2] The results of these trials showed that radical mastectomy and breast conservation surgery (with radiotherapy) have equivalent therapeutic benefits in terms of overall survival. The incidence of ipsilateral breast tumor recurrence (IBTR) after conservation and irradiation was 3–19%, as compared to 4 to 14% incidence of chest wall recurrence after mastectomy (p = NS). All the trials had a pre-requisite of clear resection margins excepting the National Cancer Institute trial[3] in which only a tumorectomy was practiced and which reported the highest local recurrence rate of 19% in the conservation group.

A more recent meta-analysis of nine prospective randomized trials[4] comparing mastectomy with conservative surgery and radiation published in 1995, again showed no difference in overall survival at 10 years in seven of these trials. There was a 6.2% local recurrence rate in mastectomy patients and 5.9% in breast conservation. Morris et al. have published a meta-analysis of 10 years survival following BCT as compared to modified radical mastectomy[5] in which the pooled odds ratio was 0.91. When more than 50% of node-positive patients received adjuvant RT in both mastectomy and BCT arms, both arms had similar survival rates. When less than 50% of node-positive patients in both arms received adjuvant nodal irradiation, the odds ratio was 0.69, and patients receiving BCT had a survival advantage. In particular, mastectomy without adjuvant RT appears to be inferior to BCT for node-positive patients.

There have been six randomized trials in the past comparing radiation vs no radiation in breast conservation.[1] A clear benefit from radiation therapy was noted with an average reduction in rate of local recurrence by 84% (range 73–97%). The NSABP B-06 trial (total mastectomy vs. lumpectomy vs. lumpectomy with radiation) showed that the cumulative incidence of recurrence of tumor in the ipsilateral breast was 35% in the group treated with lumpectomy alone as compared to 10% in the group treated with lumpectomy and breast irradiation ($p < 0.001$) at 12 years of follow-up.[6] These studies clearly showed that BCT was an appropriate treatment for early breast cancer and that radiation therapy was an integral part of this treatment.

The current standard of care for extent of surgery of axillary nodes in invasive breast cancer is a complete clearance of level I to III nodes. Leaving behind positive nodes in the axilla results in a 5% detriment in survival.[7] Sentinel node biopsy in clinically node negative breast cancer is still under study and awaits the results of larger randomized trials (NSABP B32 and American College of Surgeons Oncology Group Z0010/Z0011) comparing SNB with standard axillary clearance to show that leaving behind disease in the axilla as a result of a false negative sentinel node is not detrimental to disease-free or overall survival before being adopted as the standard of care.

The advent of mammography has resulted in detection of higher number of cases of *in situ* cancers (Ductal carcinoma *in situ* or DCIS) with its associated controversies in extent of surgery necessary and nature of adjuvant therapy required after adequate local surgical excision in these cases. The incidence of axillary node metastases in pure DCIS is 0–1%, but in situation of associated palpable mass with high suspicion of microscopic invasion level I clearance should be performed. DCIS is detected mammographically due to presence of microcalcification though 10% of DCIS may not be associated with calcification. The significance of such localized screen-detected *in situ* carcinoma is a matter of debate.

Before the widespread use of mammography, DCIS was an infrequently encountered entity that was routinely managed by mastectomy. Duct carcinoma *in situ* (DCIS) treated by mastectomy alone carries a small risk (0–2%) of relapse. With its evident success in invasive breast carcinoma, breast conservation surgery is also being considered for management of localized *in situ* carcinoma of breast. Palpable DCIS is managed on lines of invasive carcinoma. Impalpable DCIS presenting only as focal microcalcification on mammogram has to be localized by image-directed biopsy and confirmed pathologically to rule out the presence of invasive cancer.

The NSABP protocol B-17 trial[8] was a prospective randomized trial evaluating the role of radiotherapy after lumpectomy for patients with DCIS and clearly confirmed a reduction in ipsilateral breast tumor recurrence of both invasive and noninvasive cancer by radiotherapy. The trial showed a 26.8% incidence of recurrence in DCIS treated by excision alone with 50% of these recurrences being of invasive nature. With reduced from 13.4 to 8.2% ($p = 0.007$) and invasive IBTR reduced from 13.4 to 3.9% ($p < 0.0001$). Other randomized trials have also confirmed benefit of RT in DCIS treated by conservative surgery.[9] The role of tamoxifen in DCIS is still under study. The NSABP B-24, which randomly assigned patients undergoing excision of DCIS and irradiation to either placebo or tamoxifen, has shown that tamoxifen further reduces recurrence of DCIS.[10]

Contraindications to Breast Conservation Surgery

The decision to perform a breast conservation therapy in any patient has to be individualized based on various factors including compliance to RT, feasibility to obtain a satisfactory cosmesis, and patients' motivation.

Absolute contraindications: Pregnancy (first and second trimester), multicentric tumors, and presence of extensive microcalcification on mammogram (indicating presence of DCIS) are absolute contraindications for breast conservation surgery. Conservation can be offered in small tumors in third trimester of pregnancy with radiation therapy starting after the delivery. Multifocal tumors may be treated conservatively if limited to a single quadrant.

Relative contraindications: Collagen vascular disorders, ataxia telangiectasia, postburn scarring and previously irradiated skin tolerate radiation poorly and are relative contraindications for radiation treatment and are not suitable for breast conservation treatment. Relatively large tumors compared to breast size in early breast cancer can be widely excised and breast reconstructed with autologous myocutaneous pedicled flaps like the latissimus dorsi myocutaneous flap.

SURGERY IN BREAST CANCER

The common surgical interventions in breast cancer are as follows:

Excision Biopsy

In a suspicious lesion with inconclusive fine needle aspiration cytology, an excision biopsy with 1.0–1.5 cm rim of grossly normal breast tissue is performed to confirm the histological diagnosis.

The placement of incision (Fig. 26.1) should be directly over the palpable lump with no elevation of flaps or tunneling. In the upper half of the breast, incisions are placed circumferentially while lower half incisions give cosmetically better results if placed radially, especially so if they also require excision of skin.

Breast tissue is not reapproximated after the excision. Meticulous hemostasis is a must and no drains are kept at the lumpectomy site.

The lumpectomy specimen should always be oriented with sutures (standard labeling technique being short superior suture, long lateral suture and black silk for anterior surface) to enable pathologists to clearly indicate status of margin (Fig. 26.2).

Routine frozen section reporting is not advised for assessment of margin. The histological diagnosis may be established by frozen section examination and the specimen is then sent for histopathological reporting after paraffin section.

Needle Localization Biopsy

Needle localization biopsy is performed for mammographically detected suspicious nonpalpable lesions. Presurgical mammography in craniocaudal and mediolateral views should be performed with localization of the suspicious lesion or microcalcification using a hook wire (Figs 26.3 and 26.4). The patient is shifted to the operation theater with the wire in place.

The exact location of the lesion should be assessed by triangulation based on the position, angle of wire and depth of penetration of wire as estimated by the labeled mammography films.

The incision for biopsy of the lesion is placed closest to the tip of the wire avoiding any tunneling or undermining of skin. The specimen should be labeled as for invasive cancers. The entire specimen should also be radiographed (Figs 26.5A and B) to confirm complete removal of the suspicious lesion. Radio-aided grossed specimen is bread-loafed (Figs 26.5A and B) to exactly localize and section areas with microcalcification.

Frozen section reporting of the needle-localized calcification is not advisable as it is difficult to distinguish between atypical ductal hyperplasia and DCIS on frozen section preparations and areas of microinvasion may be completely missed. Margin assessment of needle-localization specimens is also necessary to ensure complete excision of lesion.

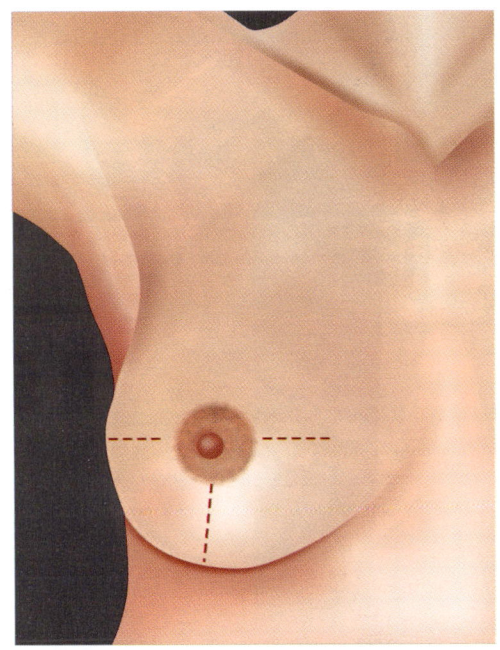

Fig. 26.1 Site of incisions of lumpectomy

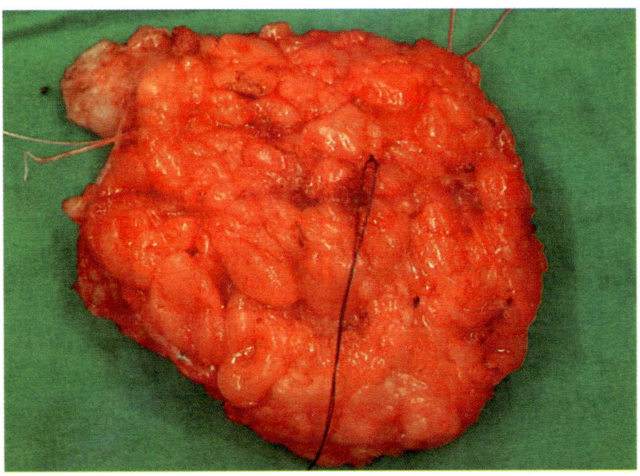

Fig. 26.2 Lumpectomy specimen is oriented with sutures—long lateral and short superior. Anterior surface is identified by skin ellipse or by a black silk suture

Breast Conservation Surgery

It includes wide excision of primary tumor (or the lumpectomy scar, if prior excision biopsy done) plus a complete axillary clearance.

Under aseptic precautions, with patient in supine position and ipsilateral arm abducted at 90° position the operating surgeon stands on the same side.

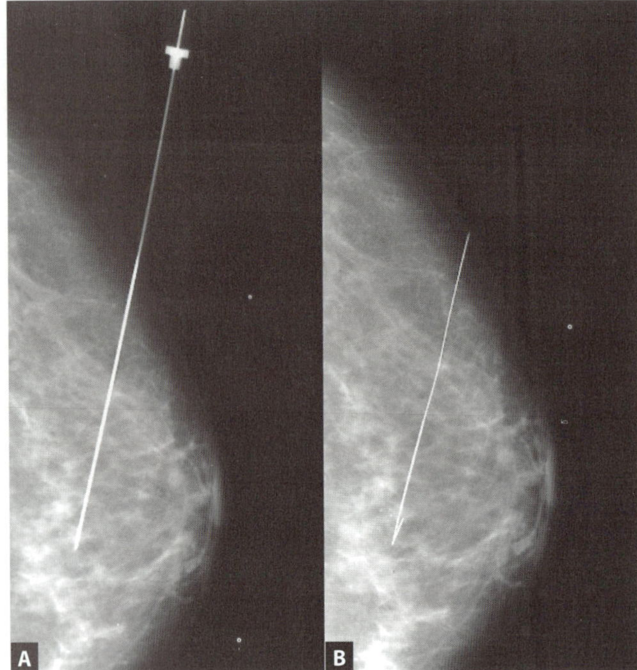

Figs 26.3A and B Mammogram showing suspicious microcalcification in a clinically normal breast with wire-localization of the microcalcification under mammography guidance

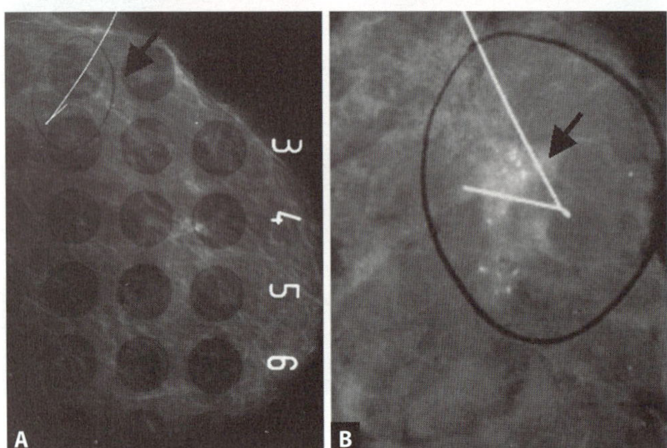

Figs 26.4A and B Wire-localization of the microcalcification under mammography guidance

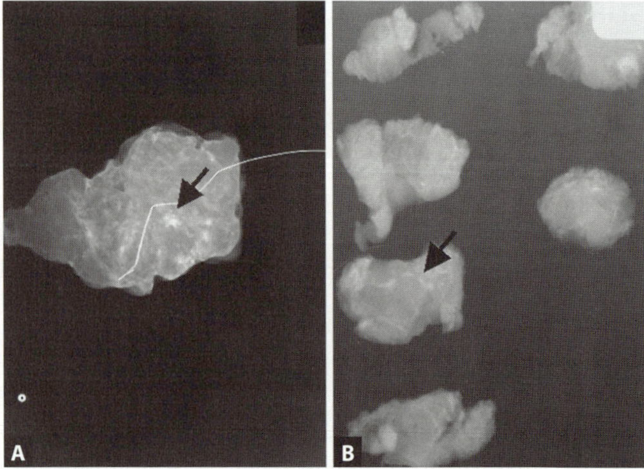

Figs 26.5A and B Radio-aided localization of area with microcalcification

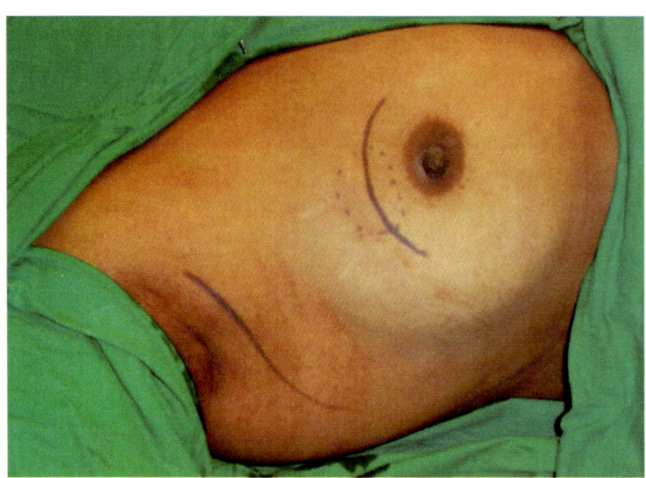

Fig. 26.6 Incision for lumpectomy and axillary clearance

The goal of conservative surgical treatment in breast cancer is complete removal of all suspicious or known malignant tissue with a gross clear margin by excising a 1.0–1.5 cm rim of grossly normal breast tissue with a minimal resultant cosmetic deformity. Where a previously biopsied site with unknown margin status is re-excised, a 1.0–1.5 cm rim of breast tissue is removed around the previous biopsy site incorporating the previous biopsy scar.

The placement of incision should be directly over the palpable lump (Fig. 26.6) with no elevation of flaps or tunneling (Figs 26.7 to 26.9). In the upper half of the breast, incisions are placed circumferentially while lower half incisions give cosmetically better results if placed radially, especially so if they also require excision of skin. The dissection is completed down to the pectoralis major muscle with excision of the fascia (Figs 26.10 and 26.11).

Breast tissue is not reapproximated after the excision. Meticulous hemostasis is a must and no drains are kept at the lumpectomy site. Wound is closed in a single layer.

The lumpectomy specimen should always be oriented with sutures (standard labeling technique being short superior suture, long lateral suture and black silk for anterior surface) to enable pathologists to clearly indicate status of margin (Fig. 26.12). Routine frozen section reporting is not advised for assessment of margins. Entire specimen is sent for histopathological examination.

Fig. 26.7 Wide excision of primary tumor by a circumferential incision

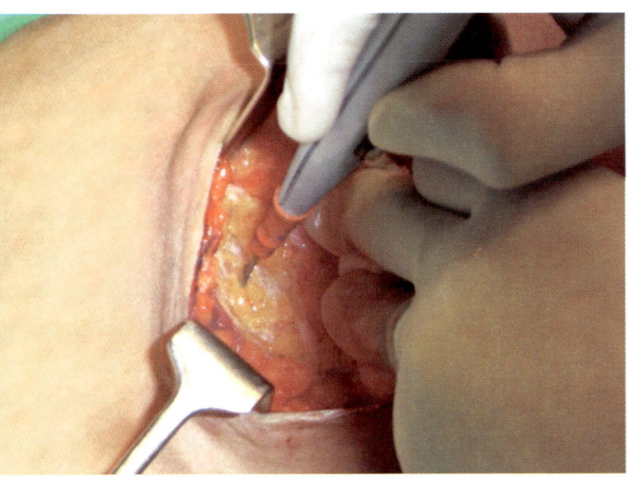

Fig. 26.8 Depth of excision reaching pectoralis major muscle including fascia

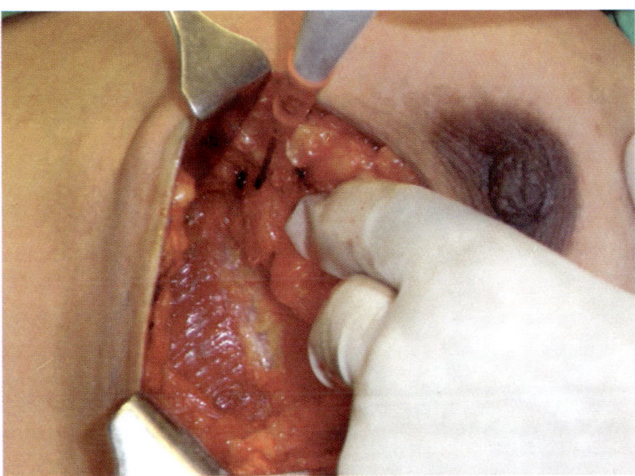

Fig. 26.9 Excision depth is muscle deep

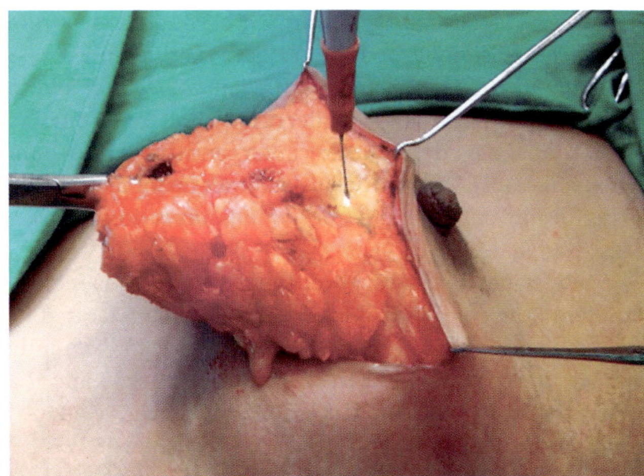

Fig. 26.10 Lower skin incision deepened till muscle. Margin of excision is grossly 1.0–1.5 cm

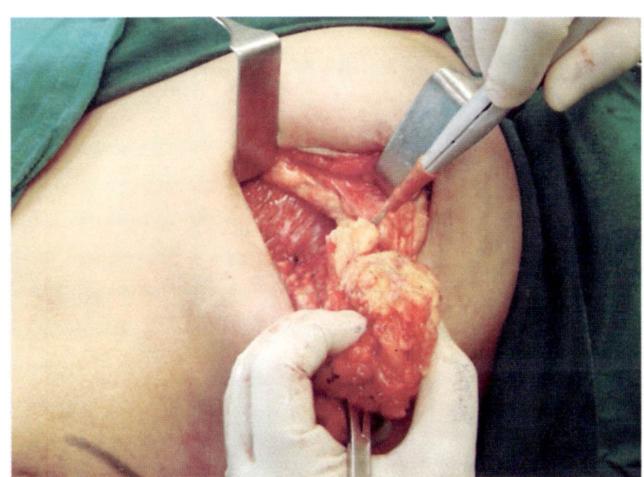

Fig. 26.11 The pectoralis fascia is excised together with the lump and forms the base of excision

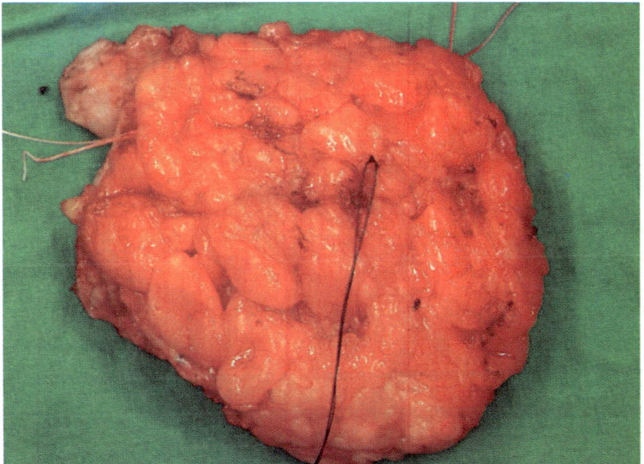

Fig. 26.12 Lumpectomy specimen is oriented with sutures—long lateral and short superior. Anterior surface is identified by skin ellipse or by a black silk suture

Axillary clearance is performed through a separate transverse incision at the lower axillary hairline in a *lazy-S* fashion (Fig. 26.13) starting from the lateral pectoral fold to the fold raised by the lateral border of latissimus dorsi muscle. Incision is deepened with electrocautery and the anterior limit of dissection till lateral border of pectoralis major muscle and posterior limit till lateral border of latissimus dorsi muscle (Figs 26.14 and 26.15).

The clavipectoral fascia over the axillary vein is incised parallel to the vein and all level I and II axillary fat and its contents are dissected downwards off the vein. The long thoracic nerve of Bell to serratus anterior muscle and the latissimus dorsi pedicle and its accompanying thoracodorsal nerve are identified and preserved (Figs 26.16 and 26.17).

Axilla is completely cleared with removal of level III nodes with laying bare of the axillary vein (but not stripping the whole vein to minimize postoperative arm edema). The medial pectoral nerve should also be preserved and, if feasible, the intercostobrachial nerve may also be preserved.

The apical nodes are addressed separately through the interpectoral plane, at the same time excising any interpectoral fat tissue with any node present in the same. The medial extent of excision (apex of axilla) is the costoclavicular ligament of Halsted.

Hemostasis should be ensured. A thorough wound lavage is then performed. The cavity of the axillary dissection is isolated from that of the primary tumor cavity if the latter is in the upper outer quadrant for a subsequent better cosmesis. Axillary wound is closed in a single layer after placing a 14-G closed suction drain brought out near the inferior end of axillary incision (Fig. 26.18). A closed suction drainage of the axilla is always recommended. Early postoperative mobilization should be encouraged to minimize a frozen shoulder.

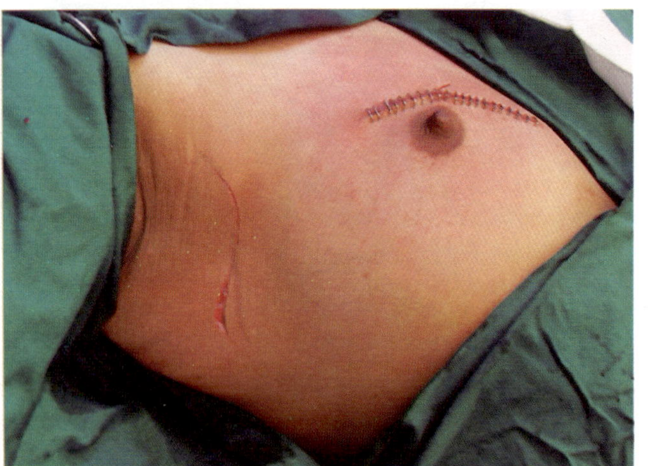

Fig. 26.13 Axillary clearance incision site

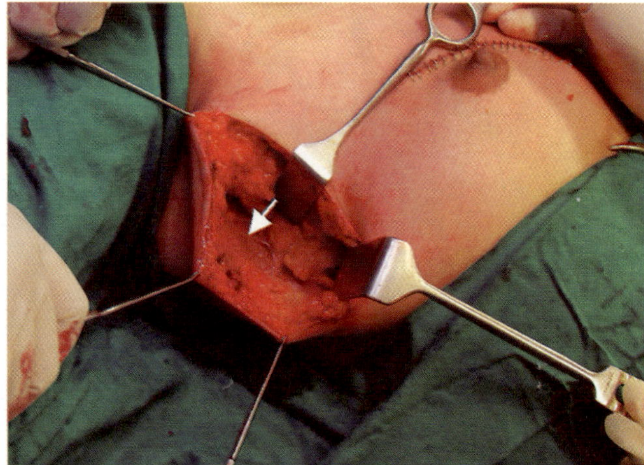

Fig. 26.15 Axillary clearance: Posterior dissection till the lateral border of latissimus dorsi muscle

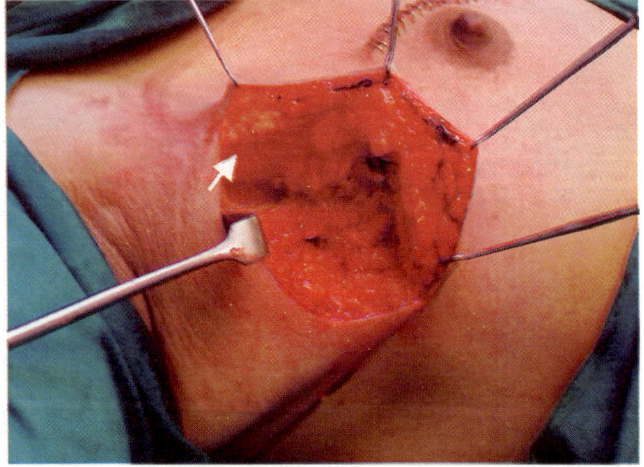

Fig. 26.14 Axillary clearance: Anterior dissection till the lateral border of pectoralis major muscle

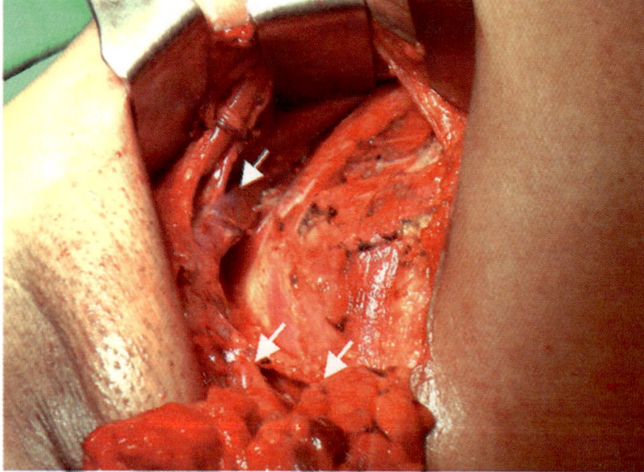

Fig. 26.16 Axillary clearance: Axillar vein exposed along its entire length with complete apical clearance

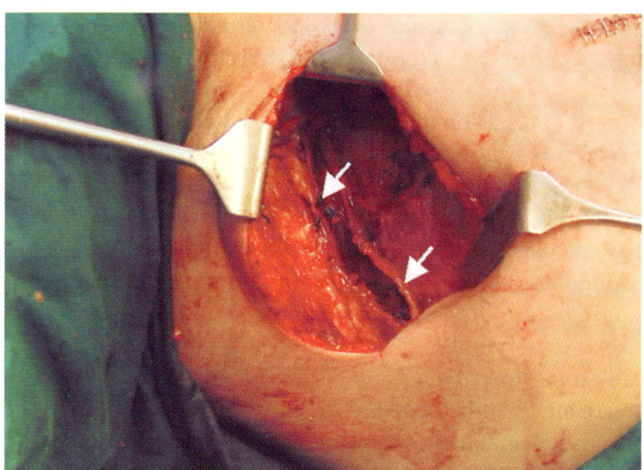

Fig. 26.17 Axillary clearance: Thoracodorsal nerve, LD pedicle preserved and long thoracic nerve to serratus anterior muscle preserved

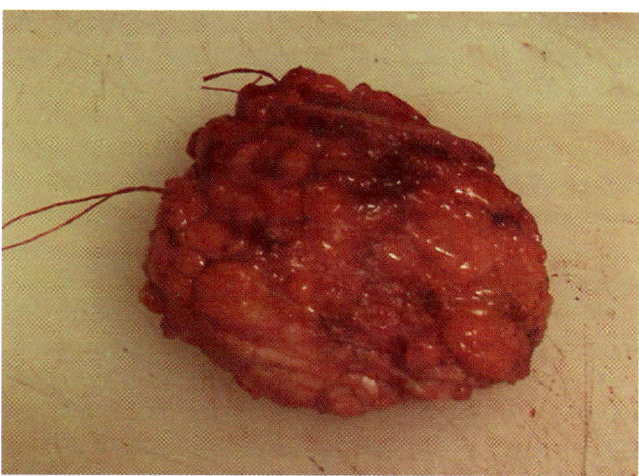

Fig. 26.19 Lumpectomy specimen is oriented with sutures—long lateral and short superior. Anterior surface is identified by skin ellipse or by a black silk suture

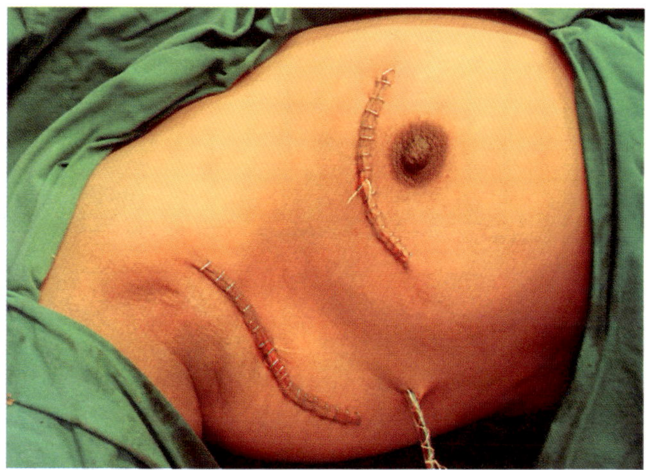

Fig. 26.18 Breast conservation surgery: Incision closed in single layer with placement of single suction drain in the axilla

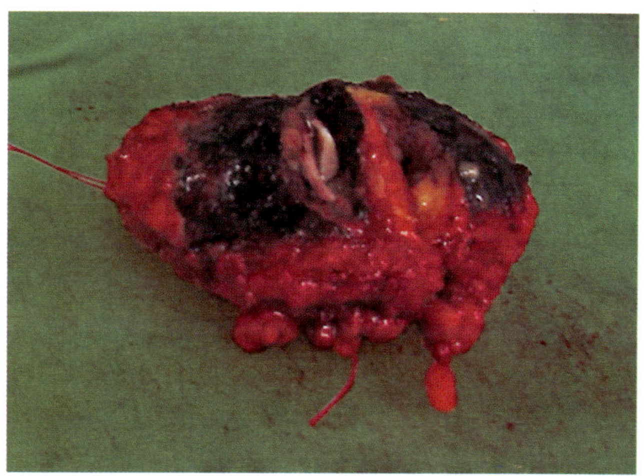

Fig. 26.20 Surface is inked at grossing and processed for evaluation of margin status

Histopathological Evaluation

The lumpectomy specimen should be oriented by sutures to identify corresponding margins after excision and inked on the outer surface before processing (Figs 26.19 and 26.20). Gross examination should document size of specimen, size of tumor in three-dimensions, distance of all margins from tumor. Microscopic evaluation should report the histologic type and grade of tumor, presence and extent of DCIS and presence of extensive intraductal carcinoma (EIC), the microscopic presence or absence of tumor at the margins (shave cut margins or radial cut margins to be specified), presence or absence of lymphovascular invasion, perineural and perinodal invasion, lymph node status (total dissected and positive nodes). Immunohistochemistry with reporting of estrogen receptor and progesterone receptor status is also necessary to decide adjuvant systemic therapy.

The term *extensive intraductal component* (EIC) was coined by Schnitt et al[11] for moderate or marked intraductal cancer in the primary tumor and intraductal cancer involving grossly normal surrounding breast tissue. Lindley et al[12] studied histological features in locoregional relapses in 293 patients with BCT and reported that when intraductal carcinoma comprised 25% or more of the tumor, there was an increased risk of LR failure (p = 0.003). Holland et al.[13] concluded that higher rates of recurrences occurred in patients with breast conservation with EIC positive tumors due to a larger subclinical tumor burden in the remainder of the breast as compared to tumors that do not contain EIC. The residual tumor was predominantly DCIS.

At the annual meeting of the American Society for Therapeutic Radiology and Oncology at Florida in October 1995, a consensus was arrived at defining a *'positive margin'*. Any amount of tumor at the margins in a low-power field was considered positive. Positive margins were further classified as *focally positive* (if invasive or *in situ* ductal carcinoma was present at the margin in ≤3 low-power fields) or *more than focally positive* (if invasive or *in situ* ductal carcinoma was present at the margins in > 3 low-power fields).

The 5 years IBTR for patients with focally positive margins was 9% (9% for EIC-negative and 7% for EIC-positive patients) and for patients with greater than focally positive margins was 28% (19% for EIC-negative and 42% for EIC-positive patients). A re-excision of close, indeterminate, or positive margins with final attainment of negative margins resulted in a significant improvement in local control.[14,15] By univariate and multivariate analysis, margin status was found to be a significant predictor (P = 0.009) for local recurrence while EIC was not significant (P = 0.20) in presence of clear surgical margins.

Modified Radical Mastectomy

Under aseptic precautions, with patient in supine position and ipsilateral arm abducted at 90° position, a transverse elliptical incision (Stewart's) including the nipple and skin over the tumor is taken. The lateral limit of incision should stop at the anterior axillary line and the anterior limit is the midline (Fig. 26.21).

Upper flap is raised in the subcutaneous plane between the superficial fascia of the breast and the subdermal fat using electrocautery, superiorly up to the clavicle, medially up to the sternum, laterally up to the lateral border of latissimus dorsi muscle.

Breast tissue including the pectoralis fascia is raised off the pectoralis muscle completely (Fig. 26.22) taking care to ligate or cauterize the perforators from internal mammary vessels. Pectoralis major muscle is retracted to visualize the lateral border of pectoralis minor muscle. The deeper aspect of breast is dissected off the fascia covering the serratus anterior muscle on the lateral chest wall preserving the nerve to serratus anterior and the chest wall perforator vessels from the latissimus dorsi pedicle. The axillary tail is maintained in continuity with the axillary fat.

The clavipectoral fascia over the axillary vein is incised parallel to the vein and all level I and II axillary fat and its contents are dissected downwards off the vein. The long thoracic nerve of Bell to serratus anterior muscle and the latissimus dorsi pedicle and its accompanying thoracodorsal nerve are identified and preserved.

The lower flap is now raised similarly in the subcutaneous plane till the rectus sheath is reached inferiorly. The entire breast, along with level I and II axillary nodes (and fat), is thus excised (Figs 26.23 and 26.24).

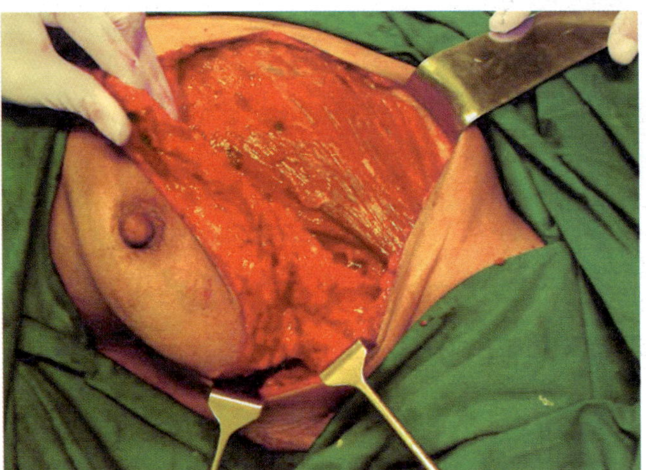

Fig. 26.22 Breast tissue with the pectoralis fascia dissected off the pectoralis muscle

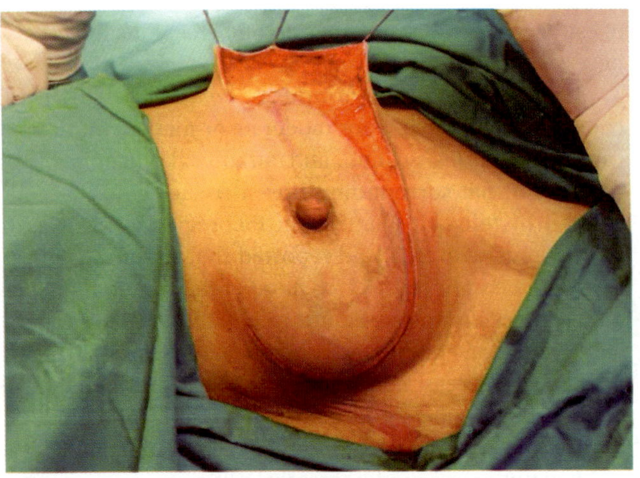

Fig. 26.21 Upper flap being raised beginning at the medial end of incision

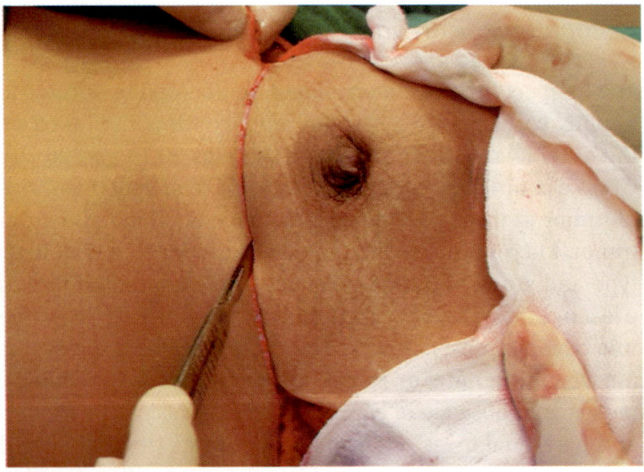

Fig. 26.23 Lower flap incision being taken

The apical nodes are addressed separately through the interpectoral plane, at the same time excising any interpectoral fat tissue with any node present in the same. The medial extent of excision is till the costoclavicular ligament of Halsted (Fig. 26.24).

Hemostasis ensured. A thorough wound lavage is then performed. Wound is then closed in a single layer after placing 14-G suction drains under the mastectomy flaps and in the axilla. The drains are brought out laterally at the mid-axillary line (Figs 26.25 to 26.27).

Entire specimen is sent for histopathological examination.

Radical Mastectomy

Under aseptic precautions, with patient in supine position and ipsilateral arm abducted at 90° position, a transverse elliptical incision (Stewart's) or classical Halsted incision including the nipple and skin over the tumor is taken.

Upper flap is raised in the subcutaneous plane using the electrocautery, superiorly up to the clavicle, medially up to the sternum, laterally up to the lateral border of latissimus dorsi muscle.

Pectoralis major muscle is divided at its insertion along with detachment of the pectoralis minor muscle from the coracoid process of clavicle. The acromiothoracic vessels that pierce the costocoracoid membrane are secured as they enter the posterior surface of the pectoralis major muscle. The medial and lateral pectoral nerves along with lateral thoracic artery and vein are also secured and divided.

Breast tissue with the underlying pectoralis muscles is then dissected off the chest wall attachment completely till rectus sheath inferiorly.

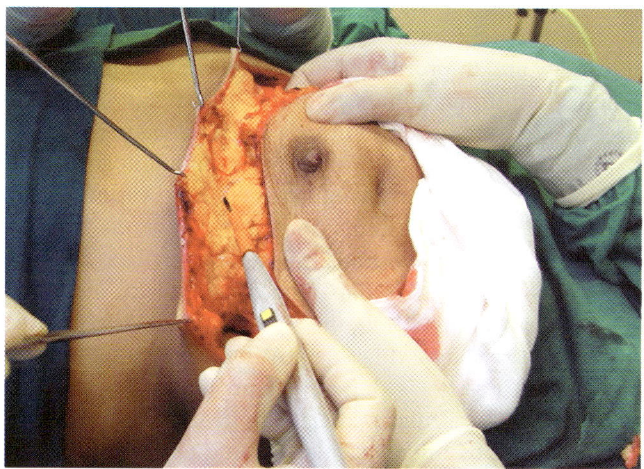

Fig. 26.24 Lower flap raised using electrocautery

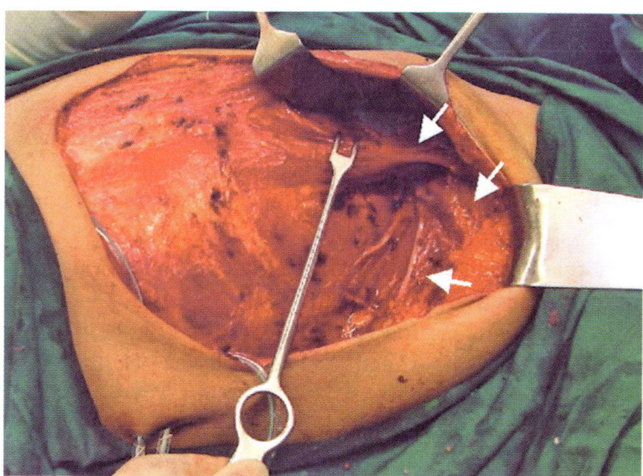

Fig. 26.26 Completed mastectomy with preserved pectoralis minor muscle, axillary vein, nerve to serratus anterior and thoracodorsal nerve along with the LD pedicle

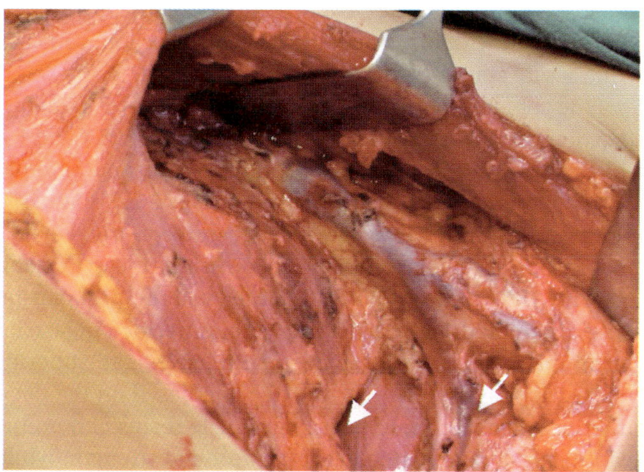

Fig. 26.25 Thoracodorsal nerve, latissimus dorsi pedicle and nerve to serratus anterior preserved

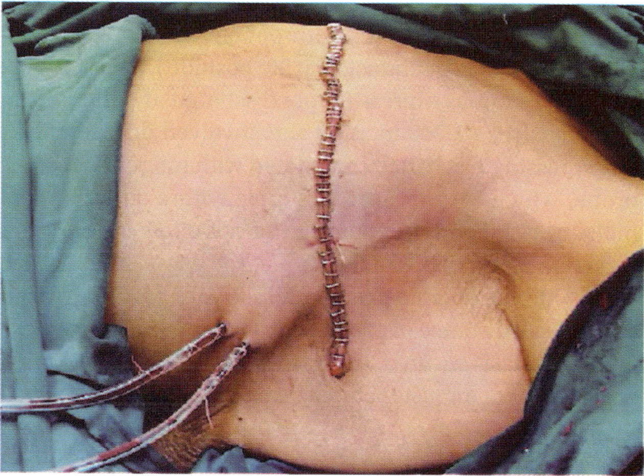

Fig. 26.27 Primarily closed mastectomy wound after excision of primary and complete axillary clearance

The clavipectoral fascia over the axillary vein is incised parallel to the vein and all level I to level III axillary fat and its contents are dissected downwards off the vein. The medial extent of excision is the costoclavicular ligament of Halsted. The long thoracic nerve of Bell to serratus anterior muscle and the lattissimus dorsi pedicle and its accompanying thoracodorsal nerve are identified and preserved.

The lower flap is now raised similarly in the subcutaneous plane till the rectus sheath is reached inferiorly. The entire breast with attached pectoralis muscles and axillary lymph nodes are removed in continuity.

Hemostasis ensured—A thorough wound lavage is then performed. Wound is then closed in a single layer after placing a 14-G suction drain under the mastectomy flaps and in the axilla. The drains are brought out laterally at the mid-axillary line.

Entire specimen is sent for histopathological examination.

Simple Mastectomy

Under aseptic precautions, with patient in supine position and ipsilateral arm abducted at 90° position, a transverse elliptical incision (Stewart's) including the nipple and skin over the tumor is taken. Upper flap is raised in the subcutaneous plane using the electrocautery, superiorly up to the clavicle, medially up to the sternum, laterally up to the lateral border of latissimus dorsi muscle.

Breast tissue including the pectoralis fascia is raised off the pectoralis muscle completely.

The lower flap is now raised similarly in the subcutaneous plane till the rectus sheath is reached inferiorly. The entire breast is thus excised.

Hemostasis ensured. A thorough wound lavage is then performed. Wound is then closed in a single layer after placing two 14-G suction drains under the mastectomy flaps. The drains are brought out laterally at the mid-axillary line.

Entire specimen is sent for histopathological examination.

Microdochectomy

Under general anesthesia, with patient in supine position (with arm by side or abducted at 90° position), area scrubbed taking care not to express nipple discharge. If patient is not hypertensive, a 1:200 incision site. Involved duct identified by expressing discharge, cannulated with microdochectomy probe, which is then fixed to nipple with a suture. Radial incision is taken by including the pathological duct in a racket-shaped incision at the nipple. The entire ductal system along with the ductuloglandular tissue with probe in place is excised to a distance of about 2 cm.

Hemostasis ensured. Incision closed in single layer. Entire specimen sent for histopathological examination.

POSTOPERATIVE CARE

In the immediate postoperative period, antiemetics and analgesics are necessary. Arm exercises are taught and should be followed diligently to prevent pain and stiffness in the ipsilateral shoulder joint. Seroma formation is common sequelae to raising of flaps and should be managed by repeated aspirations after removal of suction drain on the 11th to 14th day. The patient has to be counseled for proper exercises and postoperative sequelae in the form of pain, paresthesia and numbness or even hyperesthesia on the medial aspect of upper arm and axilla. Mild lymphedema occurs in nearly 70–80% of patients in the upper arm but significant lymphedema is seen in only 5–7% cases. The importance of care of the arm on the operated side should also be stressed to avoid late sequelae of arm edema.

BREAST RECONSTRUCTION

Breast reconstruction can be performed following a partial mastectomy or after a modified radical mastectomy. Based on timing, immediate or late reconstruction may be contemplated. There is an increasing trend towards an immediate reconstruction in select patients, offering an advantage of improved esthesis, decreased cost, less morbidity and improved quality of life. For an optimal end-result, the inframammary fold and breast skin should be preserved without compromising surgical clearance.

Reconstruction may be performed using autologous tissue (skin, subcutaneous tissue and muscle) from various donor sites such as the latissimus dorsi myocutaneous flap (LD flap), transversus abdominis myocutaneous flap (pedicled or free vascular TRAM flap), the deep inferior epigastric perforator free flap (DIEP), the superior gluteal flap (SGAP), and the anterolateral thigh flap (ALT). Reconstruction from the distant tissues is dependent on harvesting the flap with its intact vascular pedicle. The free vascular flaps are anastomosed by microvascular technique to the recipient vessels at the mastectomy site (to the thoracodorsal or internal mammary vessels). Breast reconstruction using saline-filled or silicone implants can be placed in a subpectoral pocket. The advantage of using internal implants is its simplicity, reliability and avoidance of donor site morbidity. However, it is associated with increased incidence of infection, capsular contracture and occasional rejection of implant.

The commonest flap is the latissimus dorsi myocutaneous flap along with an overlying skin island (Figs 26.28A and B). It has the advantage of simplicity in harvesting and minimal donor site morbidity or disfigurement (Figs 26.29 to 26.34). However, it is insufficient for a total breast reconstruction and may require an additional augmentation using a breast implant.

The TRAM flap provides a larger volume and can be single pedicled (based on opposite superior epigastric) or double pedicled (with both recti muscles and superior epigastric vessels), or used as a free flap based on the deep inferior epigastric vessels. Use of a single rectus abdominis can result in nearly 10% loss of abdominal strength, while using both recti can result in as much as 40% loss of abdominal wall strength and require repair using a mesh. The

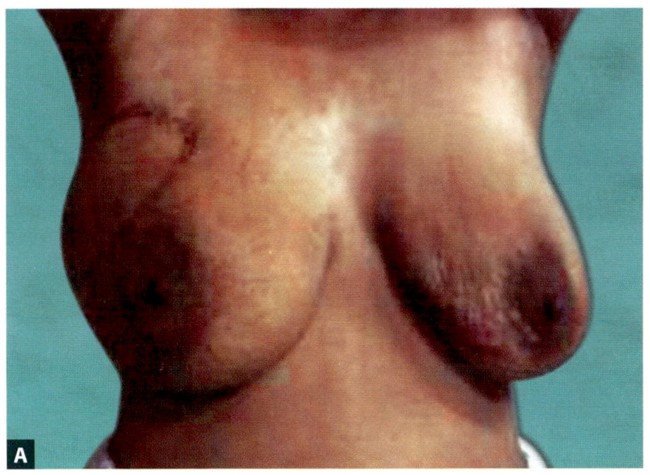

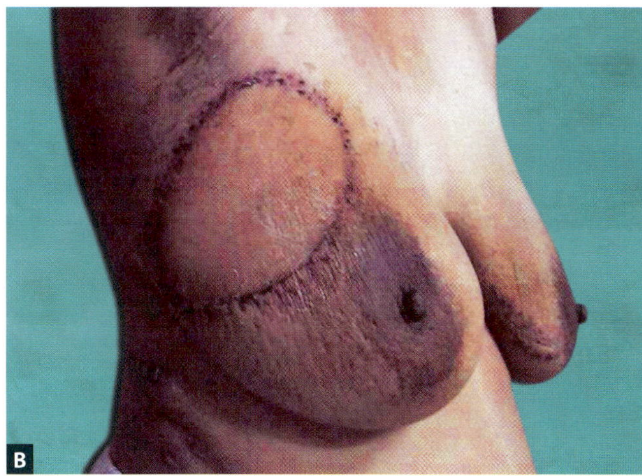

Figs 26.28A and B Breast reconstruction using an autologous latissimus dorsi myocutaneous flap

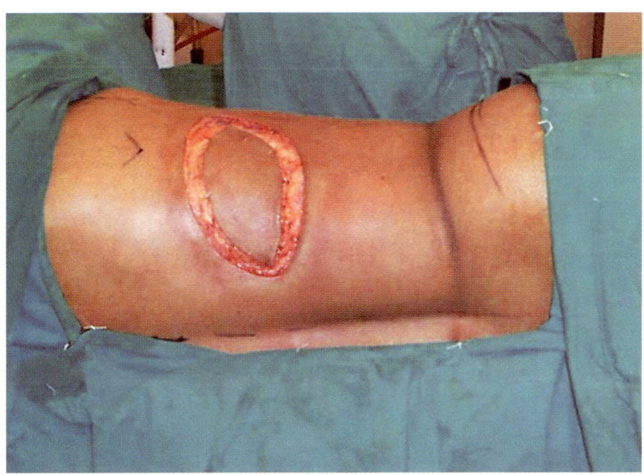

Fig. 26.29 Marking of skin island on posterior chest wall for LD reconstruction

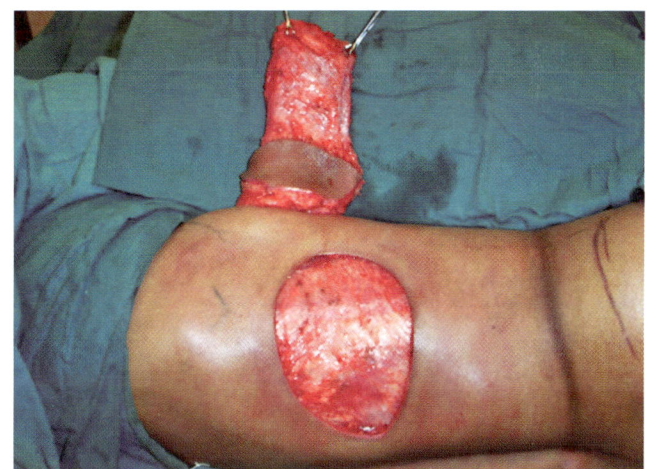

Fig. 26.31 LD flap raised completely and transposed anteriorly to fill the defect in breast

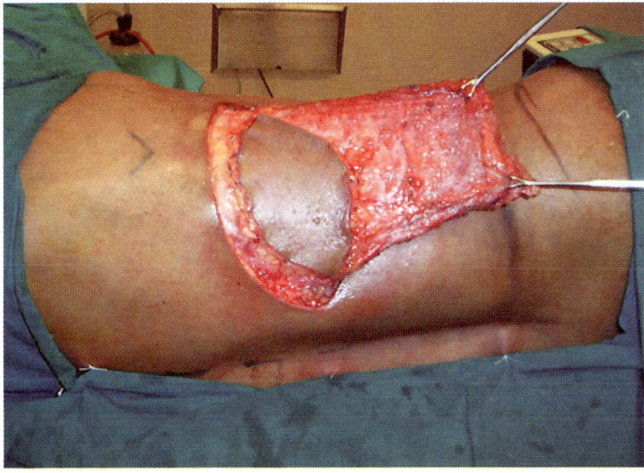

Fig. 26.30 Skin island with LD muscle being raised

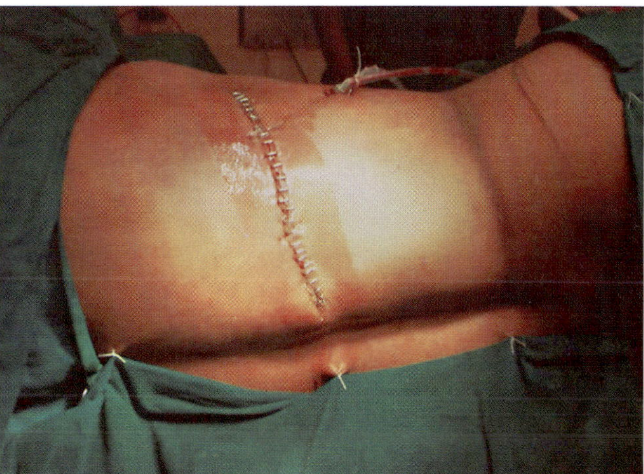

Fig. 26.32 Donor site closed in single layer with suctions

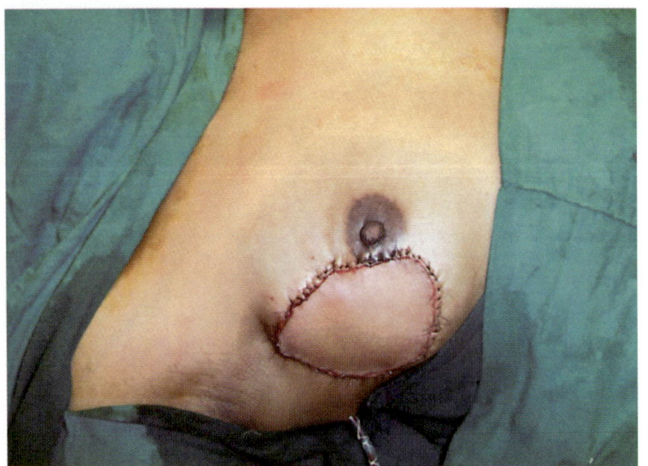

Fig. 26.33 Flap inset into the defect in the breast created after wide excision of primary

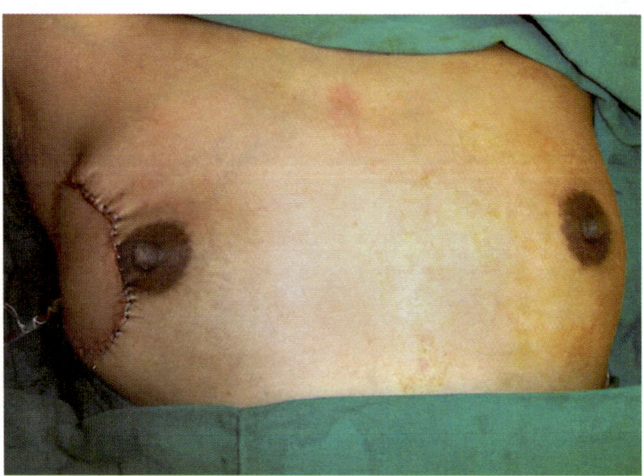

Fig. 26.34 Final cosmetic result after inset of LD flap

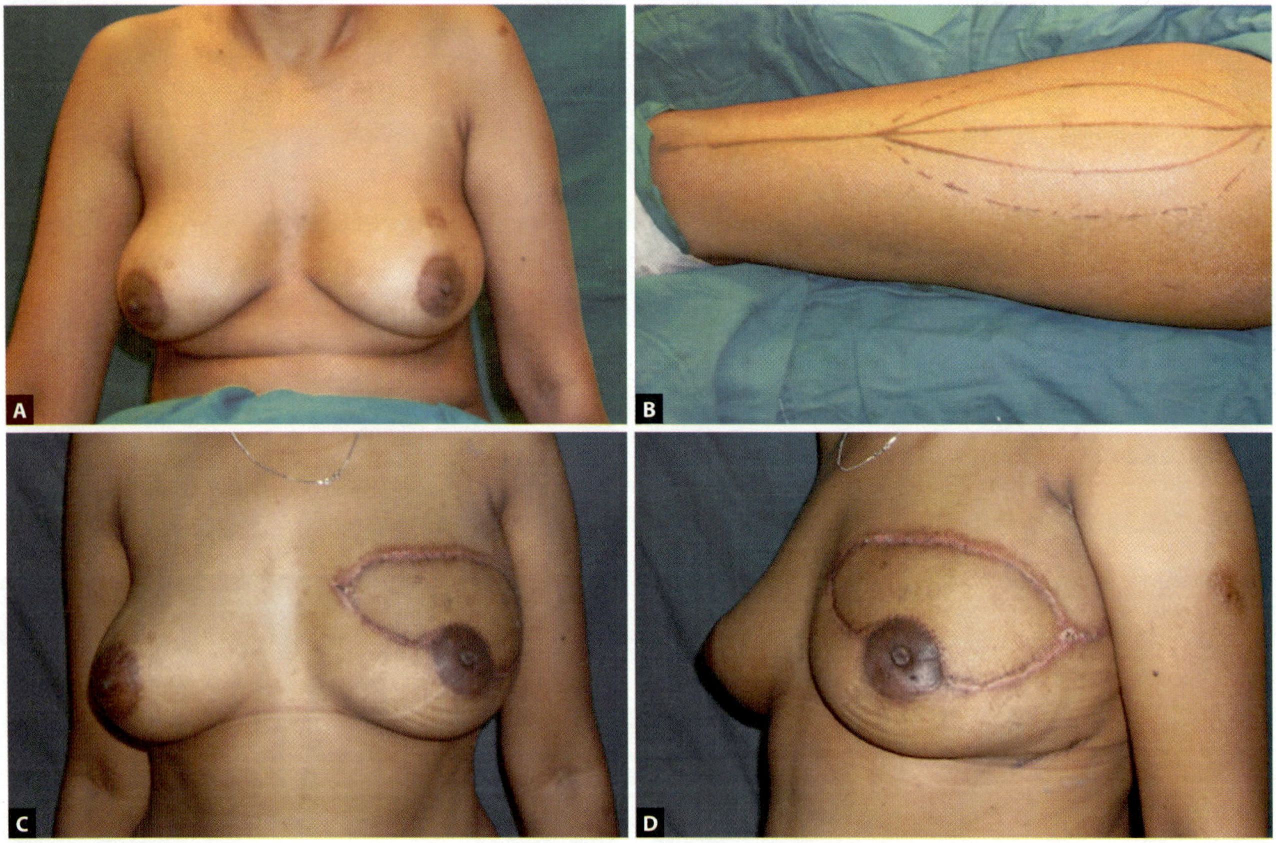

Figs 26.35A to D Immediate breast reconstruction using autologous free anterolateral thigh flap

anterolateral thigh flap (ALT) is a suitable flap for larger breast defect reconstruction or total reconstruction of breast (Figs 26.35A to D).

Breast reconstruction performed after completion of adjuvant therapy, especially postirradiation is better using autologous tissue as the skin characteristically loses its elasticity, undergoes fibrosis and is relatively less vascularized after radiation. Ski-sparing mastectomy is an option to be considered in early multicentric breast cancer (with or without nipple sparing) with no reporting of increased local failure rates. Late nipple-areola reconstruction can be performed in those where the nipple has been sacrificed.

REFERENCES

1. Winchester DP, Cox JD. Standards for diagnosis and management of invasive breast carcinoma. CA Cancer J Clin. 1998;48:83-107.
2. Fisher B, Redmond C, Poisson R, et al. Eight-year results of a randomized clinical trial comparing total mastectomy and lumpectomy with or without irradiation in the treatment of breast cancer. N Eng J Med. 1989;320:822-8.
3. Jacobson JA, Danforth DN, Cowan KH, et al. Ten-year results of a comparison of conservation with mastectomy in the treatment of stage I and stage II breast cancer. N Eng J Med. 1995;332:907-11.
4. EBCTCG—Effects of radiotherapy and surgery in early breast cancer: An overview of randomized trials. N Eng J Med. 1995;333(22):1444-55.
5. Morris AD, Morris RD, Wilson JF, White J, Steinberg S, Occunief P, et al. Breast conserving therapy versus mastectomy in early stage breast cancer: A meta-analysis of 10 years survival. Cancer J Sci Am. 1997;3(1):2-3.
6. Fisher B, Anderson S, Carol K, et al. Reanalysis and results after 12 years of follow-up in a randomized clinical trial comparing total mastectomy with lumpectomy with or without irradiation in treatment of breast cancer. N Eng J Med. 1995;333(22):1456-61.
7. Orr RK. The impact of prophylactic axillary node dissection on breast cancer survival—A Bayesian meta-analysis. Annals of Surg Oncol. 1999;6(1):109-16.
8. Schnitt SJ, Harris JR, Smith BL. Developing a prognostic index for ductal carcinoma *in situ* of the breast. Are we there yet? Cancer. 1996;77:2189-92.Editorial.
9. Julien JP, Bijker N, Fentiman IS, et al. Radiotherapy in breast conserving treatment for ductal carcinoma *in situ*: First results of the EORTC randomised phase III trial 10853. The Lancet. 2000;3555:528-33.
10. Wolmark N, Dignan J, Fisher B. The addition of tamoxifen to lumpectomy and radiotherapy in the treatment of ductal carcinoma *in situ* (DCIS): Preliminary results of NSABP protocol B-24. Breast Cancer Res Treat. 1998;50:227.
11. Schnitt SJ, Connolly JL, Harris JR, et al. Pathologic predictors of early local recurrence in stage I and II breast cancer treated by primary radiation therapy. Cancer. 1984;53:1049-57.
12. Lindley R, Bulman A, Parsons P, et al. Histologic features predictive of an increased risk of early local recurrence after treatment of breast cancer by local tumor excision and radical radiotherapy. Surgery. 1989;105:13-20.
13. Holland R, Connolly JL, Gelman R, et al. The presence of an extensive intraductal component following a limited excision correlates with prominent residual disease in the remainder of the breast. J Clin Oncol. 1990;8(1):113-8.
14. Gage I, Schnitt SJ, Nixon AJ, et al. Pathologic margin involvement and the risk of recurrence in patients treated with breast conservation therapy. Cancer 1996;78(9):1921-8.
15. Smitt MC, Nowels KW, Zdeblick MJ, et al. The importance of the lumpectomy surgical margin status in long-term results of breast conservation. Cancer. 1995;76(2):259-67.

SECTION

4

Thorax

CHAPTER

27

Basic Surgical Procedures

Dhiraj Choudhury

CHEST DRAINS

Indications

- Pneumothorax due to chest trauma
- Hemothorax due to chest trauma
- Pneumothorax in ventilated patient
- Bilateral pneumothorax
- Pleural effusion malignant or infective
- Postoperative thoracotomy for surgery of esophagus, lungs.

Technique

As an emergency, a *wide bore needle* is introduced into pleural cavity through second intercostal space 4 cm from sternum.

Intercostal Tube Drain (Closed Drainage)

An intercostal tube connected to underwater seal is central to management of pneumothorax, hemothorax and pleural effusion.

- *Technique:* The safest site for insertion of a tube drain into chest is in the triangle of safety. It lies:
  - Anterior to midaxillary line
  - Above the level of nipple
  - Below and lateral to pectoralis major muscle, it indicates the fifth intercostal space
- *Position*: The patient lies on the back with arms abducted
- *Anesthesia*: Local infiltration with 1% xylocaine
- An incision 1 cm in length is made in the overlying skin. The trocar and cannula are introduced by steady thrusting movement accompanied by rotation. The instrument is kept as close as possible to rib below. The trocar is withdrawn and stretched catheter is introduced. The cannula is now removed.
- *Underwater seal*: Connect the outer end of the drainage tube to a long tube passing well below the level of a measured amount of water in the bottle so that the water acts as seal preventing entry of air into the chest (Fig. 27.1). After completion, check the position of drain by taking chest X-ray.

DRAINAGE BY RIB RESECTION

This is indicated when pus is thick or when there is organized fibrin. It is preferably carried out under general anesthesia.

THORACOTOMY

Thoracotomy may be done as an emergency or elective procedure.

Emergency thoracotomy: This is indicated in case of chest injury for the following situations:

- Persistent shock
- Hemothorax with massive or persistent bleeding
- Cardiovascular injuries
- Thoracoabdominal injuries.

Elective thoracotomy is indicated for lesions of lung, heart, esophagus and blood vessels.

According to route of approach thoracotomy may be:

- Posterolateral thoracotomy
- Anterolateral thoracotomy
- Median sternotomy.

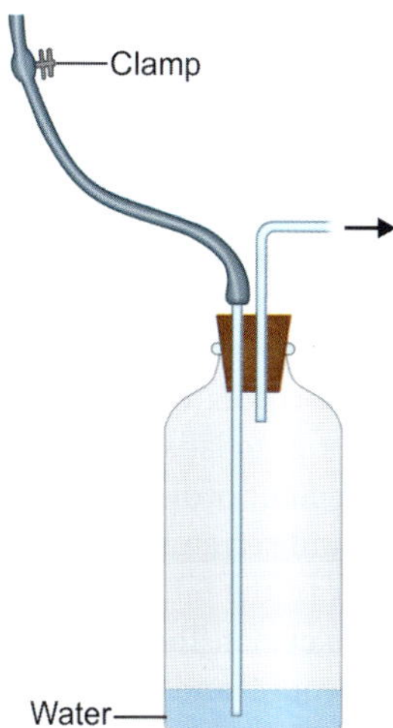

Fig. 27.1 Underwater seal drainage

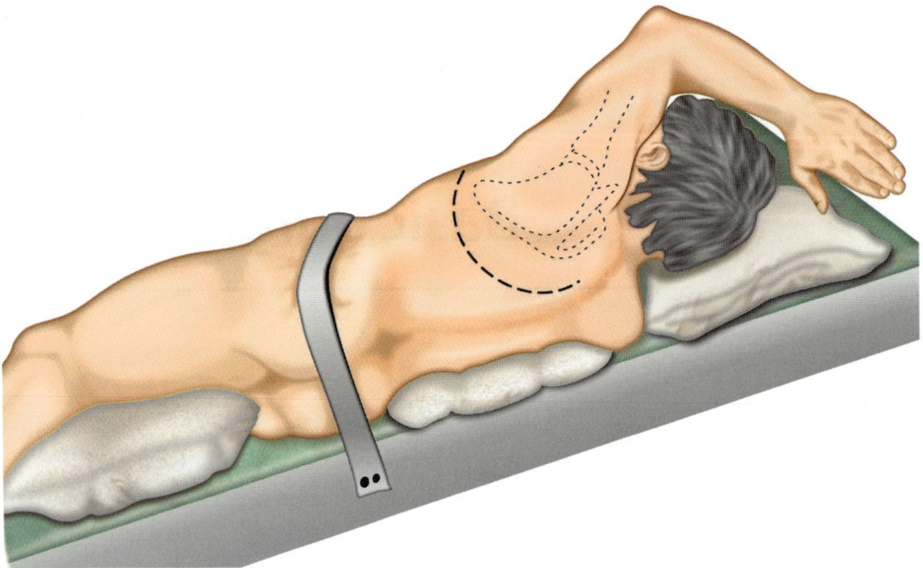

Fig. 27.2 Position and incision for posterolateral thoracotomy

POSTEROLATERAL THORACOTOMY

The standard route into thoracic cavity is through posterolateral thoracotomy.

Indications

- Lung operation
- Esophageal operation
- Operation for posterior and middle mediastinum
- Repair of coarctation of aorta, division of patent ductus arteriosus and thoracic aneurysm.

Steps

1. *Position* of the patient lies in the lateral position with affected side up. The lower leg is flexed at hip and knee with a pillow between legs.
2. *Anesthesia:* General anesthesia with endotracheal intubation.
3. *Incision:* The standard incision is through 5th interspace running from midway between the midline and medial border of scapula posteriorly and passing forward to anterior axillary line (Fig. 27.2).
4. *Dissection:* The incision is deepened thorugh subcutaneous tissues to latissimus dorsi which is divided with diathermy. A plane of dissection is developed by hand deep to scapula and serratus anterior. The periosteum of the upper border of the 6th rib is divided and stripped with periosteum elevator. The pleura is now opened along the length of the wound and a rib spreader is inserted and opened gently. Divide any adhesions and proceed with the procedure.

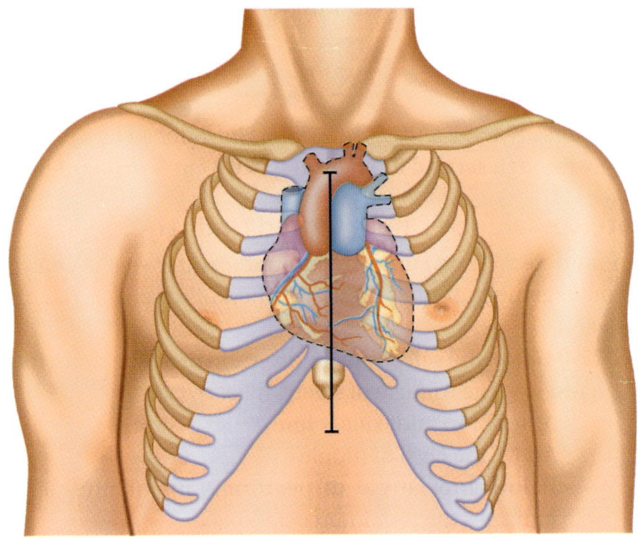

Fig. 27.3 Median sternotomy

5. *Insertion of drain:* Large caliber (24–28F) intercostal drain is inserted at the end of procedure and brought out through seventh or eighth intercostal space anterior to midaxillary line.
6. *Closure:* Close the intercoastal layer with continuous suture using vicryl.

ANTEROLATERAL THORACOTOMY

Indications

- Operations on heart, pericardium and lungs
- Rarely used for closed mitral vavotomy

- May be used for open cardiac massage
- May be used for open pericardial drainage.

Steps

1. *Position:* Patient lies obliquely rotated with ipsilateral hip and shoulder supported on pillows.
2. *Anesthesia:* General anesthesia endotracheal intubation.
3. *Incision:* An incision is made following the line of fifth rib starting close to midline and extending to axilla.
4. *Dissection:* The pectoralis major muscle is divided in the line of incision while the serratus anterior muscle is split along the line of rib. The periosteum is stripped from the upper border of the rib posteromedially.
5. *Procedure:* It depends on the indication.

Closure: Insert a drainage tube through a separate incision laterally below the main wound. The intercostals layer is sutured with vicryl. Skin is closed with ethilon.

MEDIAN STERNOTOMY

This is the best thoracotomy approach for cardiac operations using cardiopulmonary bypass. The sternum is split in midline (Fig. 27.3).

SECTION

5

Esophagus

CHAPTER

28

Open Esophagocardiomyotomy: Heller's Operation for Esophageal Achalasia

Dhiraj Choudhury

Esophageal achalasia is a primary motility disorder of unknown etiology characterized by absence of esophageal peristalsis and increased resting pressure of the lower esophageal sphincter, which fails to relax completely in response to swallowing.

The treatment is elimination of outflow resistance at the level of gastroesophageal junction caused by the abnormal lower esophageal sphincter (LES) function.

There are several therapeutic options once achalasia is definitely diagnosed.

PNEUMATIC DILATATION

Pneumatic dilatation has been for many years the first line of treatment for esophageal achalasia. Pneumatic dilatation is not as effective as surgery in relieving symptoms. The success rate is between 70% and 85%. Abnormal gastroesophageal reflux following dilatation is as high as 23–35%. About 5% of patients suffer perforation at the time of dilatation.

INTRASPHINCTERIC INJECTION OF BOTULINUM TOXIN

In achalasia, there is loss of inhibitory nerve impulse resulting into hypertensive and nonrelaxing LES. Intrasphincteric injection of botulinum toxin results in blocking the acetylcholine release and tries to restore the balance.

In this process, the symptomatic relief is achieved in only 60% of patients after 6 months, and only 30% are still symptom-free after one year. This injection causes inflammation and fibrosis in the muscle planes, making future laparoscopic myotomy more difficult. So this procedure is reserved for elderly and high-risk patients who are poor candidates for surgery or dilatation.

Both pneumatic dilatation and intrasphincteric injection of botulinum toxin are nonsurgical therapeutic options.

SURGICAL METHODS

The aim of cardiomyotomy is to weaken the lower esophageal sphincter enough to allow food to pass without allowing gastroesophageal reflux.

Open Surgery

The principle of Heller's myotomy involves the longitudinal division of the musculature of the distal 6 cm of the esophagus, extending onto the gastric wall for 0.5–2 cm. The procedure is performed through the left chest wall or the abdomen alone on a thoracoabdominal approach. Around 90–94% of patients gets good results. But there is postoperative pain of long incision and a long hospital stay is required.

But today open-surgery has been almost completely replaced by minimally invasive surgery.

INDICATIONS

This operation is indicated for cardiospasm, when:

- Conservative treatment fails to relieve dysphagia
- Secondary or organic changes (ulceration) occur in esophagus
- There is worsening of achalasia
- Young patients—patients under age of 40 do not respond well to pneumatic dilatation.

Preoperative Preparations

- Nasogastric tube
- Prophylactic antibiotic
- Deep vein thrombasis (DVT) prophylaxis
- Correction of nutritional status
- Chest physiotherapy.

Operative Procedure: Transabdominal

- *Position:* The patient is placed on supine position.
- *Anesthesia:* General anesthesia with endotracheal intubation is used.
- *Incision:* An upper midline incision is made to open abdomen.
- *Exposure:* The left lobe of the liver is mobilized and retracted by division of left triangular ligament.

  A transverse incision is made over the peritoneum covering the esophageal hiatus and the esophagus is

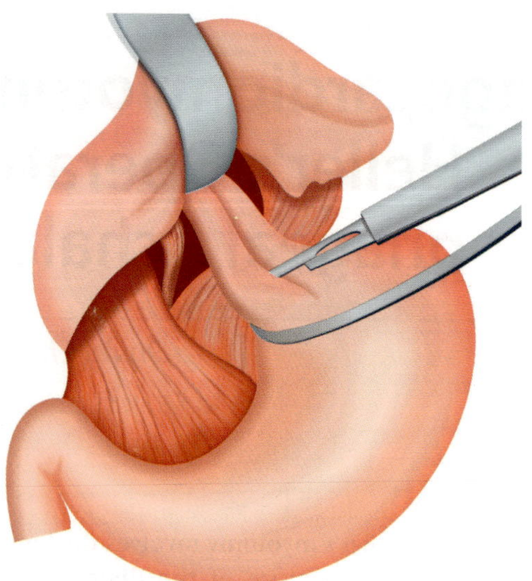

Fig. 28.1 Seromyotomy being done

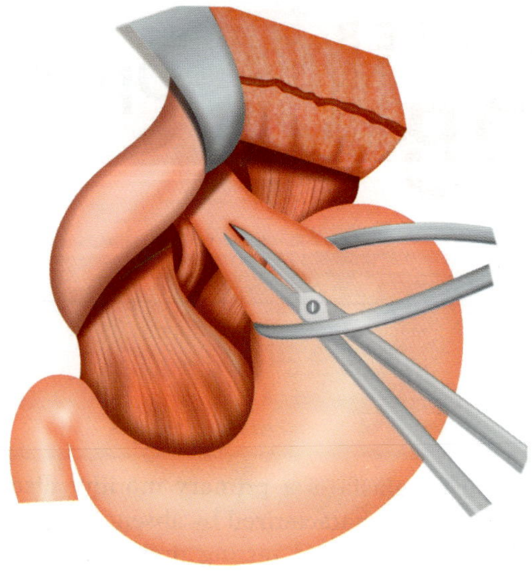

Fig. 28.2 Seromyotomy: Further dissection of muscles

mobilized by finger dissection. The mobilized esophagus is pulled gently by a tape passed around it.

- *Procedure:* A longitudinal incision is made on the constricted part of the esophagus extending at least 5 cm proximally and 2 cm distally on to stomach (Fig. 28.1).

  The incision is deepended through muscle coat (seromyotomy) until submucosa is reached (Fig. 28.2). The muscle fibers are carefully dissected apart with artery forceps, so that intact mucosa bulges out. Hemostasis is achieved. Repair of associated hiatus hernia is recommended. Stomach is gently compressed to push up air and demonstrate any air leak due to perforation.
- *Closure:* Abdomen is closed enmass.

Postoperative Care

- Oral fluid can be started after 48 hours provided there is no pain on swallowing.
- Systemic antibiotic for five days.
- Normal diet can be started by 5–7 days.

COMPLICATIONS

Intraoperative

Mucosal tear: If it is detected during the procedure, it should be repaired immediately with fine vicryl sutures.

Postoperative

- Peritonitis
- Chest complications
- Persistent dysphagia.

CHAPTER

29

Laparoscopic Cardiomyotomy

Kalyan Kar

Minimally Invasive Surgery (Laparoscopic Heller's Myotomy)

Laparoscopic Heller's myotomy involves shorter hospital stay, minimal postoperative discomfort and faster return to work. The result is as good as the open technique. So today, the laparoscopic surgery is preferred as the primary treatment modality.

Indications: Same as described under open method.

PREOPERATIVE PREPARATION

- Preoperative fasting of 8 hours is recommended because esophagus retains food and secretions.
- Some surgeons evacuate the esophagus with esophagoscope.
- Oral antifugal therapy given preoperatively decreases *Candida albicans* colonizing in the lower end of esophagus.

OPERATIVE PROCEDURE

Anesthesia

General anesthesia (GA) with endotracheal intubation.

Patient Positioning and Room Setup

- Patient lies supine with legs spread apart on the operation table. Patient is placed in a step reversed Trendelenburg's position.
- An orogastric tube is passed to decompress the stomach.
- The surgeon stands between the patient's legs facing the monitors. The camera operator stands on the patient's right side. The first assistant and scrub nurse stand on the patient's left.

Trocar Position

- The supraumbilical trocar (10 mm) is placed 15 cm from the xiphoid in the midline. This is used for the laparoscope which is preferably 30° one.
- Right subcostal trocar (5 mm) is placed 15 cm from the xiphoid in the right midclavicular line and is used for liver retraction.
- A 5 mm epigastric port and a 10 mm left subcostal port are the working trocars of the surgeon.
- A 5 mm trocar in left midclavicular line is used to retract the stomach.

The Hiatal Dissection

- With scissors or hook diathermy, the avascular area of the gastrohepatic omentum above the hepatic branch of the vagus is incised. This exposes the caudate lobe of the liver and the right crus. Preserve the hepatic branch of the vagus nerve and accessory hepatic artery if present.
- Right crus is dissected from the esophagus with blunt dissection.
- Peritoneum overlying the esophagus at the hiatus, i.e. the phrenoesophageal ligament and the epiphrenic fat pad are dissected with electrocautery or ultrasonic shear.
- Left crus of the diaphragm is feed from the esophagus by blunt dissection.
- Anterior vagus nerve is properly identified and preserved.

The Myotomy

- The myotomy can be performed at 11 o'clock position (i.e. right of the anterior vagus) or at the 2 o'clock position (i.e. the left of the anterior vagus), on the anterior surface of the esophagus.
- Myotomy is started just proximal to the gastroesophageal junction and extends proximally for about 5 cm and distally 2 cm into the stomach wall.
- Myotomy is done with dissecting scissors, carefully separating the outer longitudinal fibers. A hook may be employed for myotomy after creating a small groove in seromuscular layer of the esophagus to allow its introduction.
- With the help of the blunt dissection, inner circular fibers are separated from the mucosa. Ultrasonic shear (Harmonic scalpel) helps in achieving hemostasis as well as in the dissection. Once the concerned plane is reached, the mucosa can be seen bulging (Figs 29.1 and 29.2).

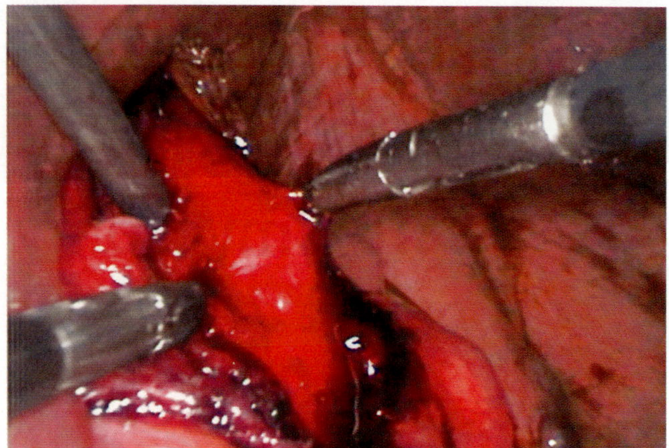

Fig. 29.1 Blunt dissection separating circular muscle fibers from mucosa

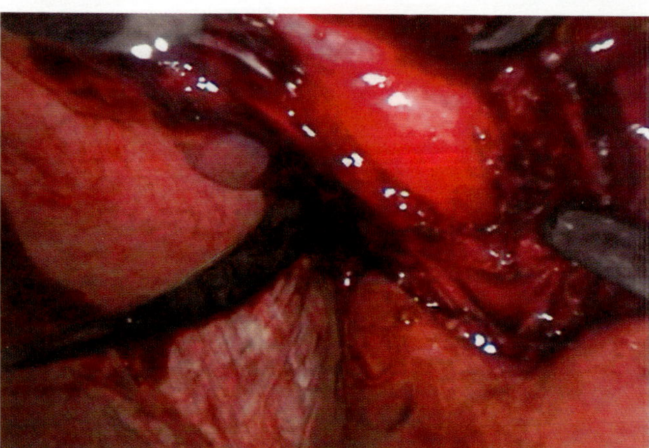

Fig. 29.2 Mucosal bulging

- The muscle fibers are to be separated from the underlying mucosa for approximately 40% of the circumference of the esophagus.
- Adequacy of the myotomy can be checked by passing a upper GI endoscope.

Antireflux Procedure

Dorprocedure (Anterior Fundoplication)

The redundant fundus is rolled over the exposed mucosa. Two or three interrupted sutures are placed between the left margin of the myotomy and the fundus. The second row of sutures are placed between the fundus and the anterior crural arch.

Postoperative Care

These are identical to those described in Chapter 28.

Complications

- *Mucosal perforation:* This is the most common complication and easily recognized during installation of methylene blue inside the esophagus. They are repaired with interrupted stitches.
- Pneumothorax
- Dysphagia.

CHAPTER

30

Nissen Fundoplications for Gastroesophageal Reflux Disease: Open Method

Dhiraj Choudhury

Majority of patients with gastroesophageal reflux disease (GERD) can be treated successfully by conservative methods. About 10–15% patients will require antireflux surgery.

INDICATIONS

- Failure of medical treatment to control symptoms
- Development of complications like peptic ulcer, peptic stricture, hemorrhage, aspiration
- High grade esophagitis from the beginning
- Atypical symptoms like respiratory, pharyngeal.

PREOPERATIVE PREPARATIONS

- Apart from routine preoperative preparation, reduction of bodyweight should be given priority in obese patient.
- A nasogastric tube is introduced.

OPERATIVE PROCEDURE

- *Position:* The patient is placed in supine position.
- *Anesthesia:* General anesthesia with endotracheal intubation.
- *Incision:* An upper middle incision is made.
- *Exposure:* After opening abdomen full laparotomy is done. Now retract the left lobe of the liver after dividing the left triangular ligament.
- *Dissection of the crura:* The stomach is pulled downward and to the left. This reduces the hernia and create an intra-abdominal segment of the esophagus. The peritoneum overlying the esophagus is incised and the incision is carried on to the crus of the diaphragm. The operator's finger is inserted in the groove between exposed esophagus and crus of the diaphragm. By blunt dissection, the right and the left crus of the diaphragm are exposed. The esophagus can be retracted by a sling around it.
- *Crural closure:* The crura are approximated by 2–3 interrupted sutures using 1-0 silk (Fig. 30.1).
- *Mobilization of fundus and fundoplication:* The reflection of peritoneum from gastroesophageal junction over the spleen is incised and 2 or 3 short gastric vessels may be ligated. This will provide mobility of the fundus. It is easier to perform Nissen fundoplication if the fundus of the stomach is mobilized first. The mobilized fundus is passed behind the esophagus and grasped with tissue forceps. A portion of the anterior fundus is rotated over the anterior aspect of the esophagus. The fundoplication sutures are inserted from the anterior fundus through the muscles of the esophagus and through the posterior fundus. About 3–4 sutures are placed until a 3–4 cm length of intra-abdominal esophagus is completely wrapped by gastric fundus. The vagus nerves remain within the wrap. The operator's finger is passed through the tunnel to be sure that it is loose (Figs 30.2 and 30.3).

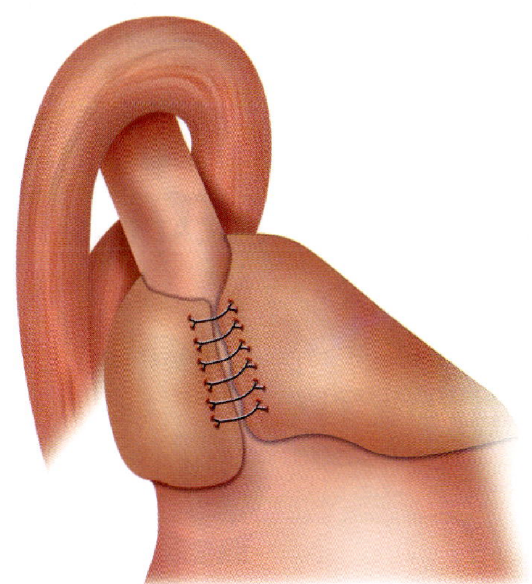

Fig. 30.1 Crural closure

- *Closure:* Check hemostasis and close the abdomen en masse.

POSTOPERATIVE CARE

- Remove nasogastric tube after 24 hours
- Start oral fluid after 24 hours
- Administer systemic antibiotic
- Chest physiotherapy.

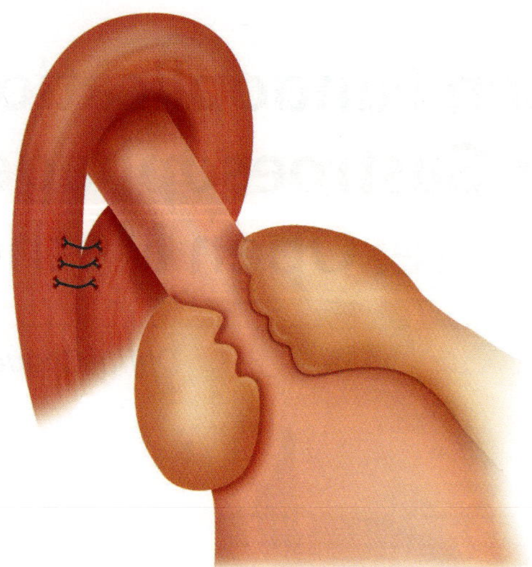

Fig. 30.2 Creation of fundal wrap

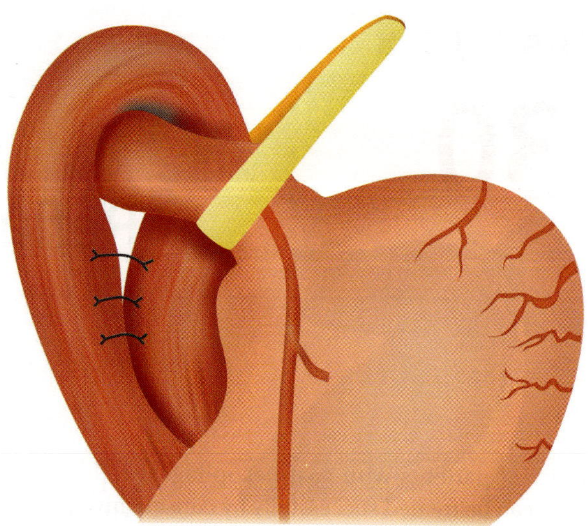

Fig. 30.3 Completion of fundoplication

POSTOPERATIVE COMPLICATIONS

Early

- Pneumothorax and surgical emphysema
- Reactionary hemorrhage.
- Acute gastric dilatation
- Transient dysphagia.

Late

Recurrent gastroesophageal reflux.

CHAPTER

31

Laparoscopic Repair of Gastroesophageal Reflux and Hiatus Hernia

Kalyan Kar, Dhiraj Choudhury

INDICATIONS

Indications are identical to those described under conventional method in Chapter 30, page 120. Operation is indicated for symptomatic GERD (refractory to medical treatment), complications of GERD (ulcer, stricture, aspiration) and Barrett's esophagitis.

AIMS OF OPERATION

- Reduction of a hiatal hernia and resection of a sac if present
- Fixation of the lower esophageal sphincter in the abdomen
- Closure of the crura behind the esophagus
- Ensuring an adequate length of the intra-abdominal sphincter.

PREOPERATIVE PREPARATION

Routine preparation is required.

OPERATIVE PROCEDURE

Anesthesia

GA with endotracheal intubation.

Patient Position

The patient is placed in a supine position. Patient is to be apart in a modified lithotomy position with the knees slightly flexed.

Surgeon to stand between two legs so that he is able to work with both hands.

A 30–45° reverse Trendelenburg's position to displace the small intestine and transverse colon inferiorly is also required.

Trocar Position (Fig. 31.1)

Five 10 mm ports are utilized.

- Camera port is placed above the umbilicus, one-third of the distance to xiphoid process
- Two lateral retracting ports in the right and left anterior axillary lines, respectively

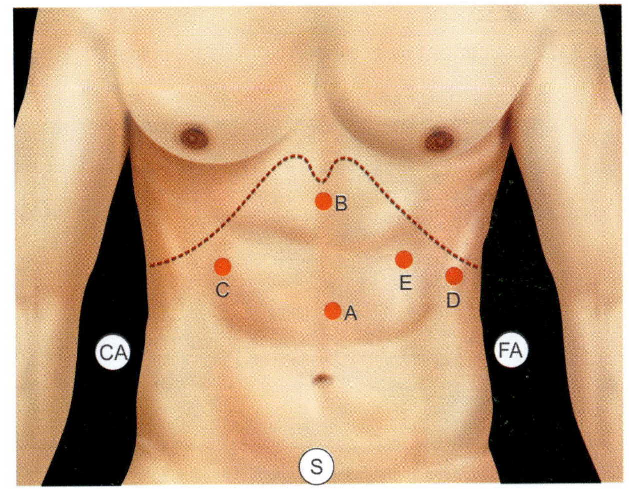

Fig. 31.1 Port positions for Nissen fundoplication (Schematic diagram)
A = Supraumbilical video laparoscope
B = Xiphoid trocar for liver retraction
C = Grasper in surgeon's left hand (right axillary port)
D = Grasper for first assistant (left axillary port)
E = Operating port
S = Surgeon
FA = First assistant
CA = Camera assistant

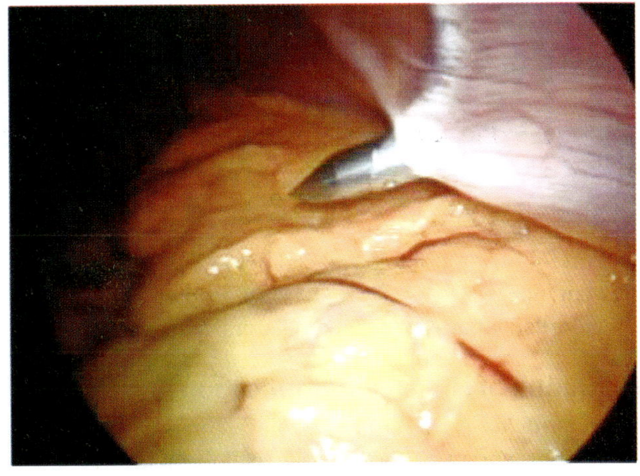

Fig. 31.2 Introduction of xiphoid trocar

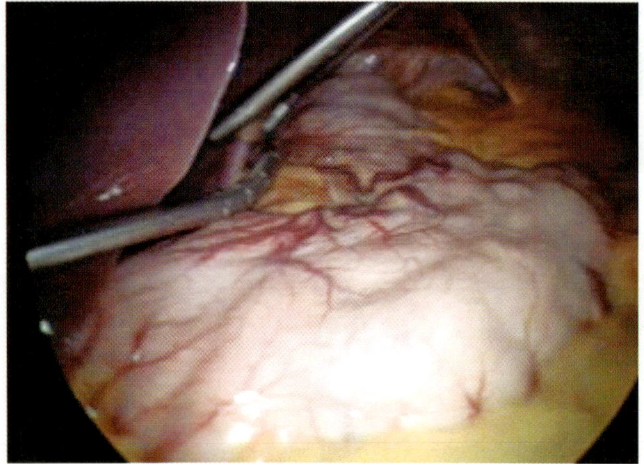

Fig. 31.3 Liver retraction of exposed esophagus (initial retraction)

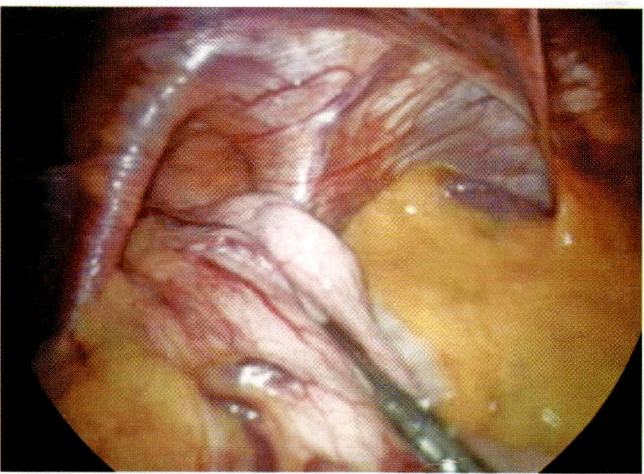

Fig. 31.4 Downward traction of stomach

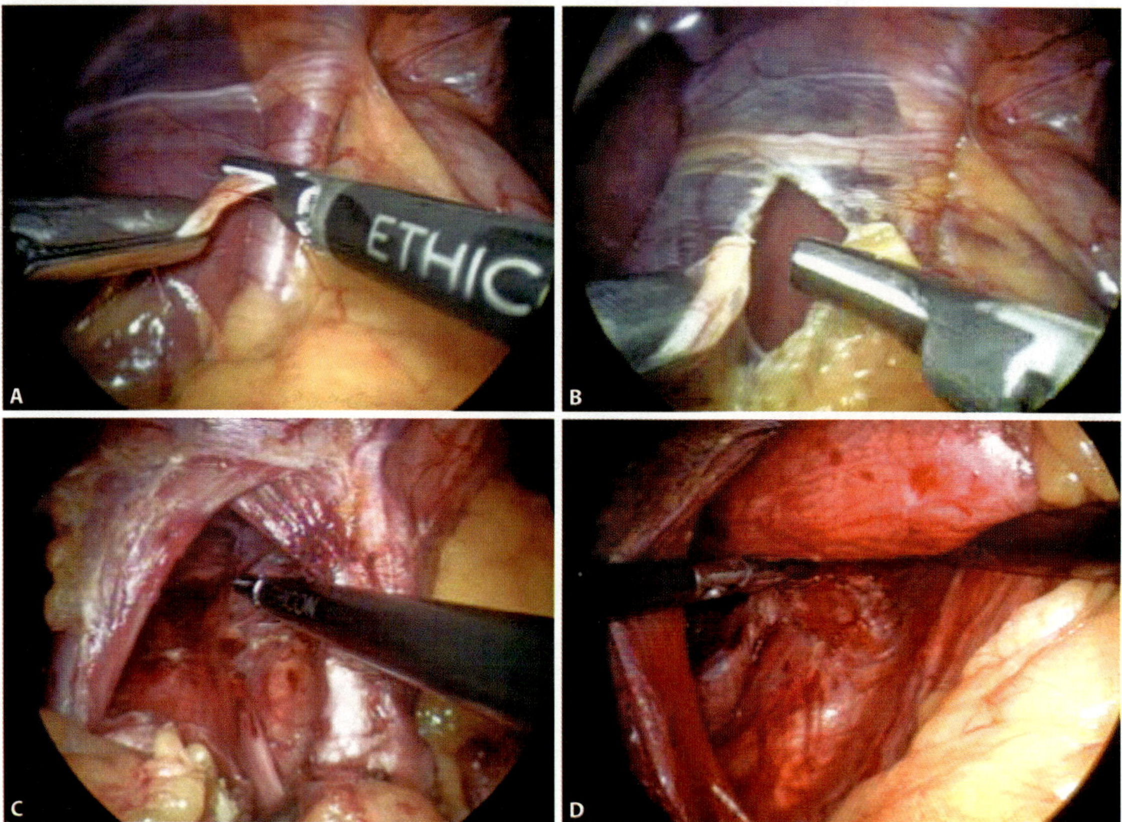

Figs 31.5A to D Crural dissection (dissection of crura)

- Port for liver retractor is placed below xiphoid process
- Main operating port (Fig. 31.1) is placed midway between the video laparoscope and left lateral trocar.

Technique of Nissen Fundoplication

Initial retractor: A fan retractor is placed on the right anterior axillary port and used to retract the left lobe of the liver gently (Figs 31.2 and 31.3).

A Babcock forceps is passed through the left anterior axillary port which helps in pulling the stomach towards the patient's feet. This exposes the esophageal hiatus (Fig. 31.4).

Dissection of the Crura (Figs 31.5A to D)

- The portion of the gastrohepatic omentum overlying the caudate lobe of the liver is incised, and this exposes the anterior aspects of the right crus.

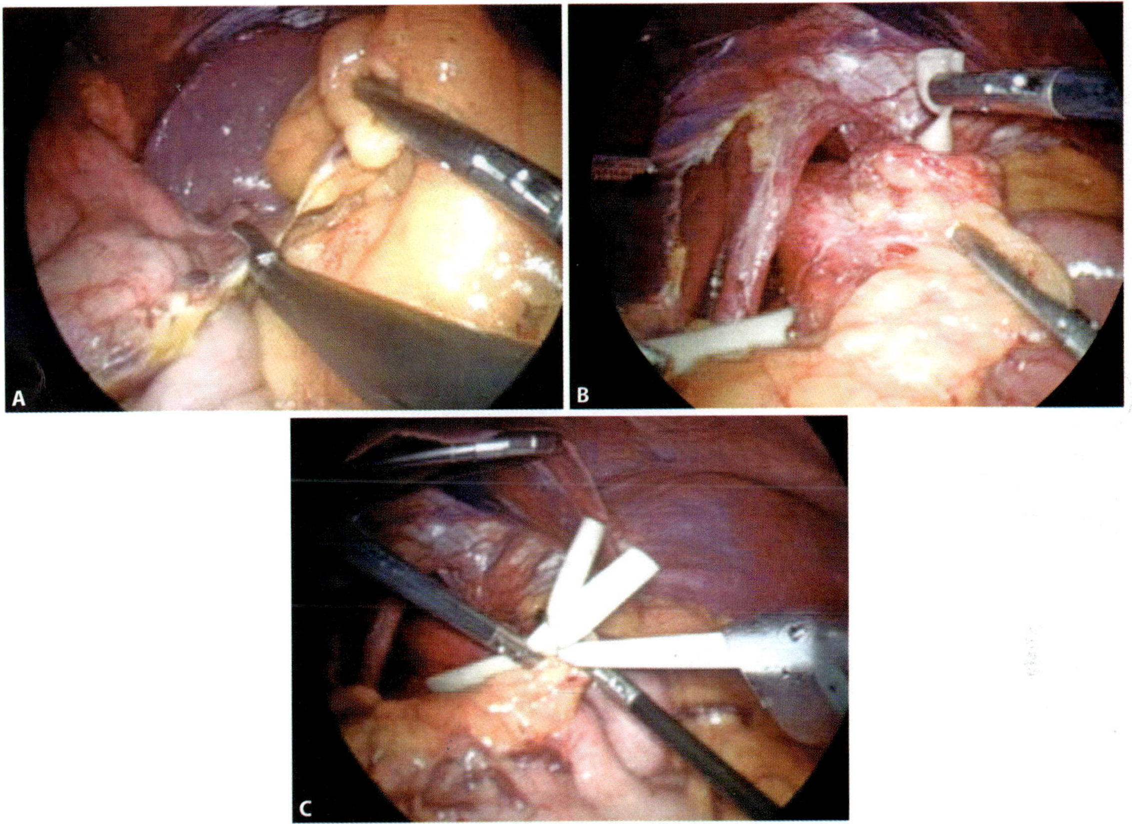

Figs 31.6A to C Fundic mobilization

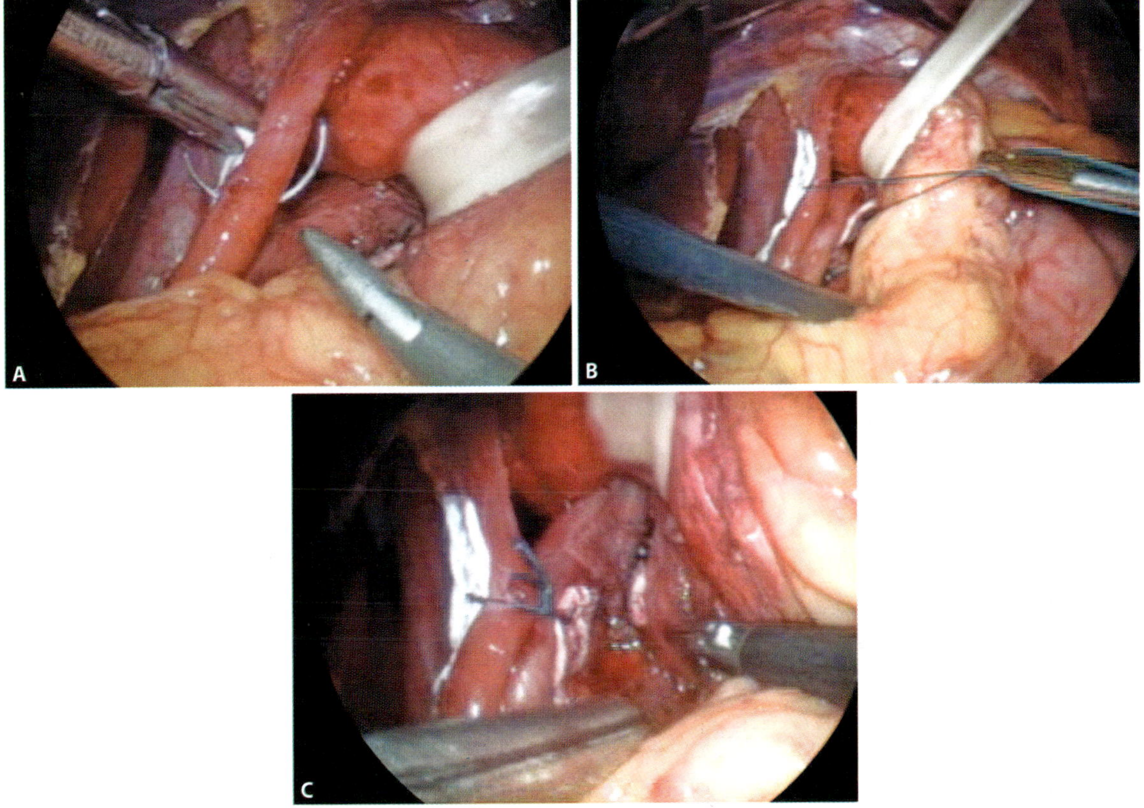

Figs 31.7A to C Closure of crura

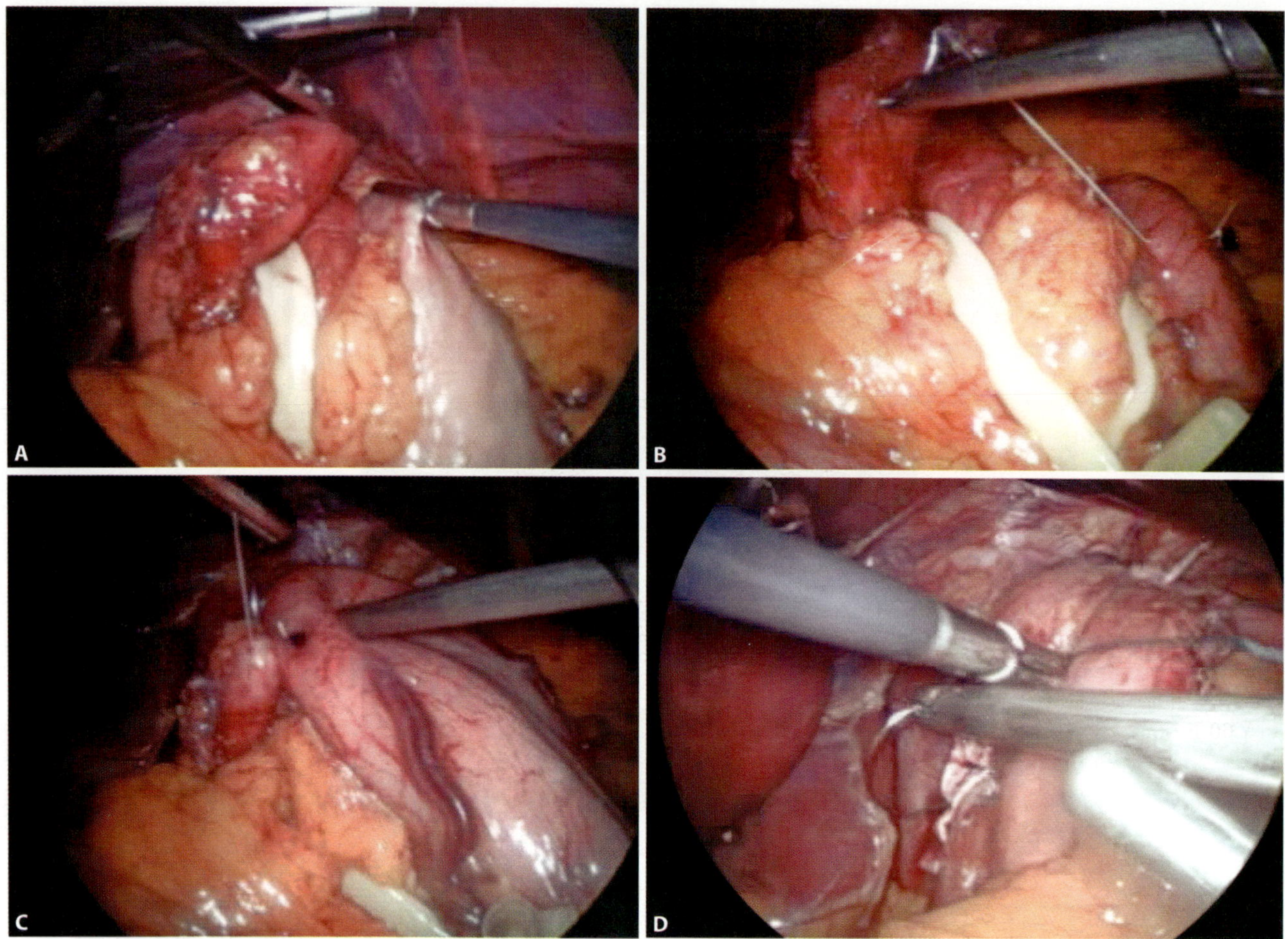

Figs 31.8A to D Fundoplication

- The peritoneum covering the right crus is incised and the right crus is dissected from anterior to posterior as far as possible.
- Right crus is retracted laterally and modest dissection of tissues posterior to the esophagus is performed.
- With the help of the left hand grasper, the tissues anterior to the esophagus is dissected downward and separated from the left crus.
- Anterior crural tissues are divided and left crus is identified.
- Left crus is dissected as completely as possible including taking down the angle of His and attachment of fundus to the left diaphragm.

After completing the posterior dissection, a grasper is passed behind the esophagus and over the left crus. A penrose drain is passed around the esophagus and used as esophageal retractor (Fig. 31.6B).

Fundic Mobilization (Figs 31.6 A to C)

Complete fundic mobilization allows construction of a tension-free fundoplication.

A second Babcock is passed through the right anterior axillary port to facilitate retraction during division of the short gastric vessels.

Short gastric vessels are sequentially dissected and divided with the help of ultrasonic shears. This starts at one-third the distance down the greater curvature of the stomach. The dissection includes the pancreaticogastric branches posterior to the upper stomach. Mobilization is complete when right crus and caudate lobe can be seen from the left side.

Crural Closure

The esophagus is retracted to the left. The crura are approximated from below upwards with 1-0 interrupted silk sutures 4–6 are required (Figs 31.7A to C).

Fundoplication (Figs 31.8A to D)

After complete mobilization, posterior fundus is grasped and passed to the left behind the esophagus.

Anterior wall of the fundus is brought anterior to the esophagus.

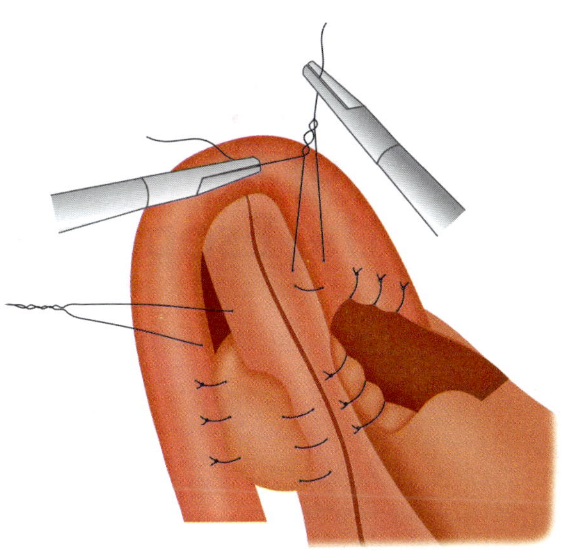

Fig. 31.9 Toupet posterior partial fundoplication (schematic)

Both anterior and posterior fundic lips are manipulated, so that they completely envelope the lower end of the esophagus without any twisting.

A 60 F bougie is passed through the esophagus before suturing the two fundic lips. This ensures that the envelope does not become too tight.

Fundoplication is completed by suturing the two lips with nonabsorbale suture material (2-0 prolene) (Fig. 31.9).

The suture line of fundoplication should be facing in the right anterior direction.

Laparoscopic Partial Fundoplication

(Modified Toupet procedure—a 270° posterior fundoplication).

In this procedure, initial dissection is same as that of Nissen's fundoplication. Here the right limb of the fundoplication is sutured to the esophagus at 11 o'clock and the left at 1 o'clock, thus leaving the anterior portion of the esophagus uncovered.

POSTOPERATIVE CARE

- Patient is kept nil orally for 24 hours
- After 24 hours liquid diet is started and if the patient tolerates then soft diet is given
- Systemic antibiotics are given for first 24 hours only
- Patient is mobilized out of bed after 24 hours and discharged after 72 hours.

COMPLICATIONS

- *Perforation of the esophagus or stomach*: This occurs during hiatal dissection. Intraoperative recognition and repair has to be done
- Splenic injury rarely occurring during the dissection of the short gastric vessels. If the bleeding does not stop on pressure or diathermy then splenectomy is required
- Pneumothorax and surgical emphysema occurs in 1-2% of the patients
- Dysphagia in the postoperative period following tight or twisted fundic wrap.

CHAPTER

32

Surgery for Carcinoma of the Esophagus

Rajesh Mistry, CS Pramesh

Carcinoma of the esophagus is one of the common sites of malignancy in the gastrointestinal tract. Worldover, the incidence of esophageal cancer, particularly adenocarcinoma, is on the rise. In the US, the incidence has increased five-fold. Unlike in the west, in India, the majority of esophageal cancers are squamous carcinoma. The standard treatment of operable cancer of the esophagus in the absence of medical contraindications is surgery. Radiation, chemoradiation and combination of radiation and chemotherapy with surgery are other treatment options. However, the overall five years survival remains far from satisfactory, ranging from 5 to 30%.

The first step in planning the treatment for a patient with esophageal carcinoma is accurate staging of the disease. It determines whether the intent of treatment will be curative or palliative. It is based on clinical examination and information obtained by imaging: CT scan and/or EUS. The TNM staging is one of the most important and reliable prognostic variables.

TNM STAGING

T-stage (primary tumor):

- TX: Primary tumor cannot be assessed
- T0: No evidence of primary tumor
- Tis: Carcinoma *in situ*
- T1: Tumor invades lamina propria or submucosa
- T2: Tumor invades muscularis propria
- T3: Tumor invades adventitia
- T4: Tumor invades adjacent structures.

N-stage (regional lymph nodes):

- NX: Regional lymph nodes cannot be assessed
- N0: No regional lymph node metastasis
- N1: Regional lymph node metastasis.

M-stage (distant metastases):

- MX: Distant metastasis cannot be assessed
- M0: No distant metastasis
- M1: Distant metastasis.

Tumors of the lower thoracic esophagus:

- M1a: Metastasis in celiac lymph nodes
- M1b: Other distant metastasis.

Tumors of the midthoracic esophagus:

- M1a: Not applicable
- M1b: Nonregional lymph nodes and/or other distant metastasis.

Tumors of the upper thoracic esophagus:

- M1a: Metastasis in cervical nodes
- M1b: Other distant metastasis.

For tumors of midthoracic esophagus use only M1b.

Stage Grouping

Stage 0: Tis, N0, M0
Stage I: T1, N0, M0
Stage IIA: T2, N0, M0/T3, N0, M0
Stage IIB: T1, N1, M0/T2, N1, M0
Stage III: T3, N1, M0/T4, any N, M0
Stage IV : Any T, any N, M1
Stage IVA: Any T, any N, M1a
Stage IVB : Any T, any N, M1b

The current staging system for esophageal cancer is most applicable to patients with squamous cell carcinomas of the upper- and middle-thirds of the esophagus, as opposed to distal esophageal and gastroesophageal junction adenocarcinomas. The present system of classifying celiac lymph node metastases as M1 seems to be unreasonable. The prognosis of patients with positive abdominal lymph nodes is considerably better than those with metastases to distant organs. Patients with regional and/or celiac axis lymphadenopathy should not necessarily be considered to have unresectable disease and treated with palliative intent. Complete resection of the primary tumor and appropriate lymphadenectomy should be attempted when possible. The Japanese system of lymph nodal staging which takes into consideration location of the primary tumor in relation to the involved lymph nodes appears more reasonable.

INVESTIGATIONS

Diagnostic Investigations

- *Barium swallow:* This continues to be the first investigation in patients presenting with dysphagia. It gives information regarding the:

  - Site
  - Length of lesion
  - Morphology (proliferative/stricturous/ulcerative or combination)
  - Extraesophageal spread (axis deviation, sinuses and fistulation)
- *Esophagoscopy:* Fiberoptic esophagoscopy is essential for exact localization and biopsy/cytology.

Staging Investigations

- *CT scan:* Chest and upper abdomen
- Endoscopic ultrasonography (EUS)
- *Fiberoptic bronchoscopy:* For tumors located at and above the level of carina.

CT scan and EUS are complimentary for assessing the lateral extension of disease and lymph node status. EUS scores over CT scan in assessment of the depth of tumor invasion, particularly in early cancer, and status of regional lymph node. However in stricturous lesions EUS may not always be possible. CT scan is equally accurate in assessment of T3/T4 lesions; abdominal CT scan in addition scans liver and celiac lymph nodes. Bronchoscopy is an essential investigation for assessing the tracheobronchial tree for early or frank invasion. It is recommended prior to surgery or radiation for carcinoma of the upper and mid-esophagus and in patients with recent onset change in voice.

PET scan, thoracoscopy and laparoscopy are investigational modalities for staging the disease and not done as a routine.

Routine investigations for assessing fitness for treatment include:

- Hemogram
- Liver function test/renal function test
- Chest X-ray
- Pulmonary function test
- ECG.

TREATMENT OPTIONS

Two Factors Determine the Treatment

- General condition or performance status is an important factor in determining the treatment of a patient with esophageal cancer. Dysphagia, particularly if long standing and complete, leads to chronic dehydration and malnutrition. Such patients do not tolerate surgery, radiation or chemotherapy. Supportive care to optimize the general condition should be the priority. Subsequently, if the performance status improves, definitive treatment can be contemplated depending on the stage of the disease.
- *Stage:* If the disease appears operable based on imaging and other investigations discussed earlier, surgery should be the treatment of choice provided there are no medical contraindications. Presence of abdominal or celiac lymph nodes is conventionally classified as M1 disease along with patients with disseminated disease. However, the prognosis of patients with abdominal or celiac lymph node metastasis is not the same as that with systemic distant metastasis. Hence, the authors consider fit patients with operable disease for surgery with radical lymphadenectomy.

Surgical Approaches

- Transthoracic total esophagectomy with cervical anastomosis
- Transthoracic esophagectomy with intrathoracic anastomosis (Ivor-Lewis procedure)
- Transhiatal esophagectomy with cervical anastomosis.
- Esophagogastrectomy through left thoracoabdominal approach.

Transthoracic Esophagectomy with Cervical Anastomosis

This procedure is suitable for carcinoma of the thoracic esophagus. The advantages of this approach are:

- The entire esophagus is dissected and mobilized under direct vision, improving circumferential clearance
- The esophagus is divided in the neck and hence adequate proximal tumor free margin is available even for carcinoma of the mid and upper thoracic esophagus
- The anastomosis is in the neck and hence consequences of a small leak are not very grave
- Radical lymph node dissection in the upper mediastinum (and lower neck) which is often the site of metastases in carcinoma of the thoracic esophagus is feasible.

Radical lymph node dissection can lead to significant fluid shift in the postoperative period and is generally associated with higher pulmonary morbidity. Hence patients should be selected carefully. Patients should have normal pulmonary and cardiac functions. Age above 70 years is only a relative contraindication for this procedure.

Anesthesia

The surgery is routinely performed under general anesthesia. The insertion of an epidural catheter for postoperative analgesia is invaluable in alleviating postoperative pain and facilitating aggressive physiotherapy. A central venous catheter is not routinely necessary, but if required, should be introduced through the right subclavian or internal jugular veins. In patients where a three-field lymphadenectomy is planned, the catheter should be passed through the right subclavian vein as the right neck will be explored for infraomohyoid lymph node dissection. An arterial line is optional for intraoperative blood pressure monitoring. A nasogastric tube is also passed to decompress the stomach and to facilitate esophageal dissection.

The procedure is performed through three incisions:

1. Thoracotomy for mobilization of the esophagus and mediastinal lymph node dissection.
2. Laparotomy for gastric mobilization and abdominal lymph node dissection.
3. Neck exploration for bilateral infraomohyoid lymph node dissection and anastomosis of cervical esophagus to the gastric tube.

Thoracotomy

The patient is given a left lateral decubitus position with the right thorax up. Posterolateral thoracotomy is performed. The skin incision starts an inch behind the scapula, skirts around its angle and is extended anteriorly up to the midclavicular line along the curvature of the rib. The incision is deepened, preferably with diathermy, and the latissimus dorsi muscle divided. The posterior edge of the serratus anterior muscle is defined and the auscultation triangle identified. The scapula is retracted up and the operator's hand introduced from the auscultation triangle up along the chest wall. The topmost rib to be felt by the palpating fingers is the second rib. The fifth rib is identified. The serratus anterior muscle is divided along the fifth rib. Alternatively it can be mobilized and retracted anteriorly (muscle sparing thoracotomy). The thorax is opened by stripping off the intercostal muscles from the upper border of the fifth rib. The wounds are isolated and a self retaining thoracic retractor applied for adequate exposure. Gradual opening of the self-retaining chest wall retractor gives adequate exposure without fracturing the rib(s).

Esophageal Mobilization

The lung is retracted towards the heart with a lung retractor and the esophagus identified in the posterior mediastinum. The diseased segment is identified and operability assessed by examining its mobility. The parietal pleura on either side of the esophagus is incised longitudinally starting from the apex of the thorax down to the phrenoesophageal reflection. The azygous vein is identified, dissected and divided between the ligatures. Alternatively a segment of the azygous arch overlying the esophagus may be transected. The right bronchial artery is usually located below and behind the azygous vein. Preservation of the artery is reported to reduce the postoperative pulmonary complications. However, if the disease is in close proximity of the artery, it should be resected. The esophagus is mobilized above and below the diseased segment and looped with a tape. Applying upward traction on both the tapes, the diseased segment of the esophagus is dissected from the posterior mediastinum. While dissecting the esophagus from the posterior mediastinum, one should identify direct branches from the descending aorta (usually two to four) and divide them between ligatures or clips. In the upper mediastinum, esophageal branches of the vagus nerve are divided few centimeters below the level of the carina after it has given off the pulmonary branches.

Caudally at the level of the inferior pulmonary vein, an avascular plane between the esophagus and pericardium is developed. The dissection is continued upwards in this plane and lymph nodes in the subcarinal region are dissected. The dissection in this region should be meticulous proceeding from the right pulmonary hilum to right main bronchus, carina and finally, the left main bronchus. This will avoid troublesome bleeding from the carina. The authors do not routinely resect the thoracic duct which is found between the aorta and vertebral column. However, if it is involved or close to the disease or inadvertently injured during the esophageal mobilization, it should be resected and the cut ends secured carefully.

Lymph Node Dissection

The mediastinal lymph node dissection has been classified in Table 32.1.

The paraesophageal lymph nodes along the entire length of the esophagus are dissected with the specimen. This will include the mid and lower paraesophageal lymph nodes, and nodes around the hiatus. The subcarinal and bronchial lymph nodes are dissected as described. In the upper mediastinum the upper paraesophageal, right and left recurrent lymph nodes are dissected. The right recurrent nerve can be identified by following the vagus nerve up to the subclavian artery. The recurrent nerve will be seen curving around the artery; nodes around the nerve are dissected. The left recurrent nerve loops around the arch aorta and ascends in the mediastinum along the left paratracheal border. The left recurrent nerve is identified and nodes along its length dissected carefully. Nodes in the left tracheobronchial angle and the aortopulmonary window are dissected by retracting the left main bronchus anteriorly.

Table 32.1 Types of lymphadenectomy

Types of lymphadenectomy	*Extent of lymphadenectomy*	*Lymph nodes resected*
Standard	Infracarinal	Subcarinal, left and right main bronchial, middle and lower paraesophageal, posterior mediastinal and supradiaphragmatic
Extended	Standard + right upper mediastinal	Standard + upper paraesophageal, right recurrent ± pretracheal
Total	Extended + left upper mediastinal	Extended + left recurrent, left tracheobronchial, aortopulmonary window
Three-field	Total + bilateral infraomohyoid	Total + bilateral medial and lateral supraclavicular

The thorax is closed after confirming hemostasis. The ribs are approximated with three pericostal sutures and the chest closed in layers with an intercostal drain in place.

Abdomen

The abdomen is opened by a midline vertical supraumbilical incision. The incision should extend superiorly at least up-to the xiphoid which may be resected for better exposure. A self-retaining Balfour retractor is then positioned to retract the abdominal wall. A thorough abdominal examination is done to rule out metastases in the liver, pelvis, peritoneum, omentum, retroperitoneum and para-aortic regions. Any suspicious area should be biopsied and sent for frozen section examination. The abdominal part of the surgery consists of gastric mobilization and lymph node dissection.

Gastric Mobilization

The first phase of the surgery is gastric mobilization. The gastric substitute is based on the right gastroepiploic artery (the arcade along the greater curvature of the stomach). The right gastric artery is preserved wherever possible but is not mandatory. The stomach is held up gently and the gastroepiploic arch along the greater curvature of the stomach identified in the gastrocolic ligament of the greater omentum. Keeping a safe distance of atleast an inch from the gastroepiploic arch, a small opening is made in an avascular portion of the gastrocolic ligament at a point midway along the greater curvature. This opens the omental bursa. The greater curvature of the stomach is mobilized on either side of the initial opening from the pylorus to the gastrosplenic ligament. The vessels in the ligament are divided between ligatures. While ligating the vessels towards the stomach side care should be taken to stay away from the vascular arch. The vascular arcade is interrupted precisely at the junction where it meets the left gastroepiploic artery. The short gastric vessels are then divided between ligatures, staying close to the stomach. After mobilizing the entire greater curvature right up to the gastroesophageal junction on the left side (Fig. 32.1), mobilization of the lesser curvature is begun. The lesser omentum is largely avascular. The stomach is retracted inferiorly and lesser omentum divided close to the inferior surface of the liver by an incision which is extended onto the anterior surface of the abdominal esophagus. The phrenoesophageal ligament is divided and the esophagus mobilized all around. The right and the left vagus nerves can be identified as cord-like structures on the esophagus. These should be divided between ligatures or with diathermy. The mobilized stomach is gently lifted up to expose the posterior aspect. This will make the left gastric pedicle prominent. The fibrofatty tissues along with lymphatics and nodes are dissected from the root of the left gastric pedicle towards the lesser curvature. The artery and the vein are then divided separately between ligatures at its origin. It is advisable to double ligate or transfix the proximal segment of the artery.

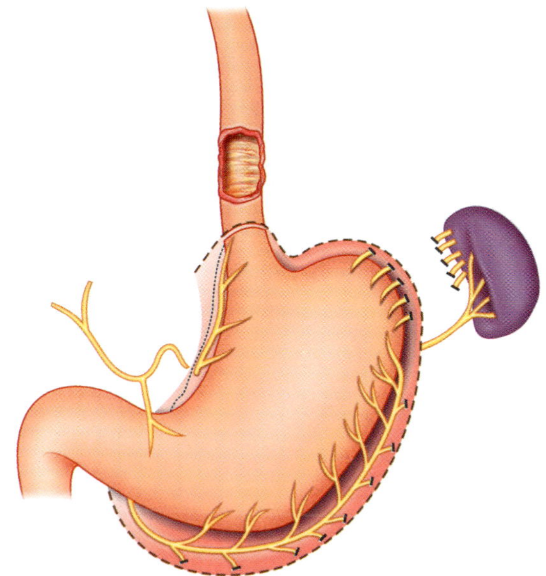

Fig. 32.1 Gastric mobilization

A Kocher maneuver is not always necessary for adequate gastric mobilization but may be done if there is concern about the length of the stomach tube. The need for a pyloric drainage procedure is also controversial with some authors advocating no drainage. Some surgeons recommend some form of pyloric drainage ranging from a finger fracture to a myotomy to a formal pyloroplasty.

The abdominal part is concluded by mobilizing the cardioesophageal junction all around and dilating the hiatus, if necessary by dividing one of the diaphragmatic crus with diathermy.

Lymph Node Dissection

The lymph nodes along the celiac trunk and its branches (common hepatic, left gastric and splenic arteries) are dissected to complete D2 lymphadenectomy. The limits of retroperitoneal lymph node dissection are the diaphragm above, splenic hilum laterally, common hepatic and splenic arteries inferiorly. The lesser curvature of the stomach has lymph nodes around the branches of the left gastric artery. Adequate clearance of this is achieved by clearing the upper half of the lesser curvature. This will ensure that the right gastric artery and its branches along the lesser curvature are preserved.

Gastric Tube

The esophagus (after division in the neck) is retrieved in the abdomen. The mobilized stomach along with the esophagus is brought out of the abdominal wound. The highest point on the fundus of the stomach is grasped with an atraumatic Babcock forceps. An adequately broad gastric tube is fashioned out of the stomach using 75 mm linear staples (Figs 32.2A and B).

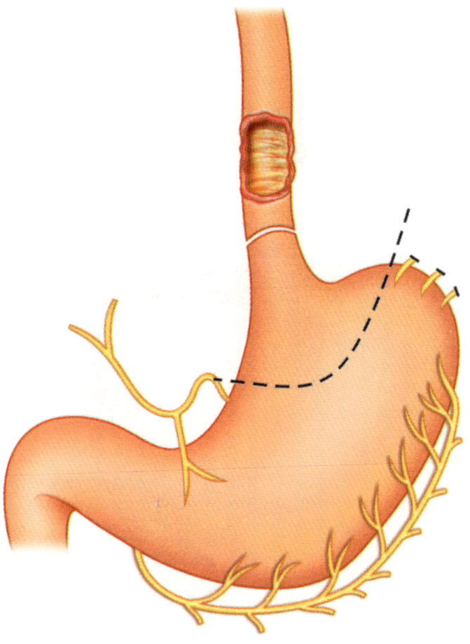

Fig. 32.2A Fashioning of gastric tube

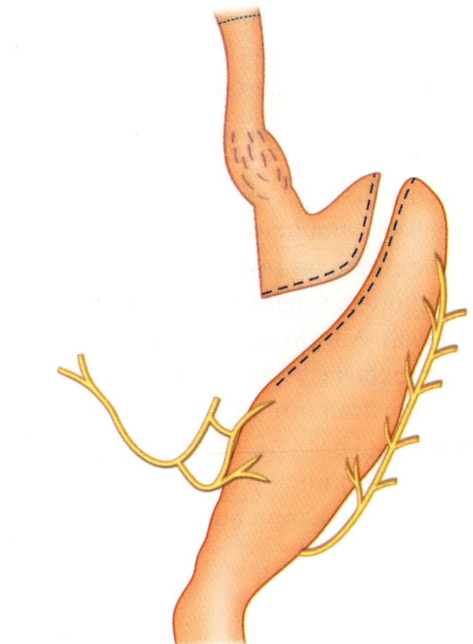

Fig. 32.2B Formation of gastric tube using linear stapler

The stapled line is reinforced with 3-0 silk suture. The surgical specimen should include the esophagus, cardia and proximal half of the lesser curvature. This will ensure removal of all the lymph nodes along the lesser curvature that are at highest risk of metastases.

Conduit Route

The posterior mediastinum is the shortest route for the gastric tube. However, it may advisable to use the retrosternal route if the bronchial artery alone is preserved. The retrosternal route is also preferred when the circumferential resection margins are not satisfactory or where there is residual disease in the esophageal bed (posterior mediastinum).

Neck

Conventionally the cervical esophagus is approached through the left neck. A transverse incision is made in the left lower neck (Fig. 32.3). The sternal head of the sternomastoid muscle may be divided. The internal jugular vein and common carotid are identified and retracted laterally. The trachea is retracted medially taking care of the left recurrent laryngeal nerve. The esophagus is identified and dissected all around beginning in the prevertebral space. The esophagus is taped and brought out in the neck wound. It should be transected at a level such that the esophageal end can be brought out of the neck wound for tension-free anastomosis with the gastric tube. Two stay sutures are placed proximal to the proposed line of transection. The muscle is transected all around up to the mucosal tube. The mucosal tube is transected a centimeter below the muscular tube. The stomach tube is brought in the neck using the railroad technique and an end to end, single-layer interrupted anastomosis with 4-0 vicryl is performed (Figs 32.4A and B). Alternatively a double layered

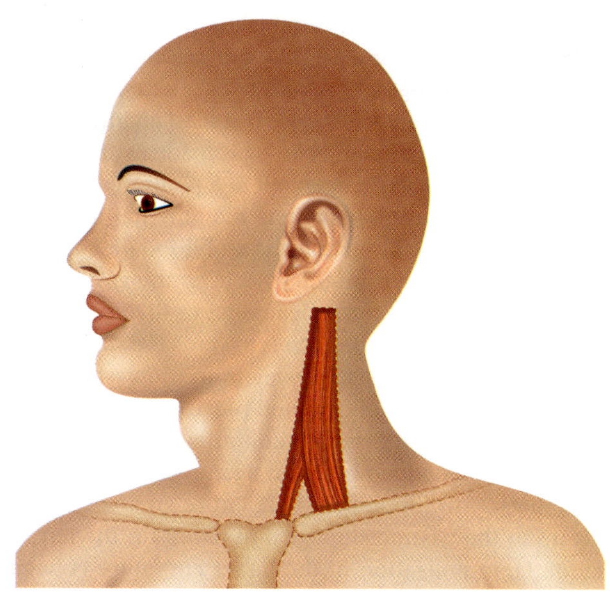

Fig. 32.3 Approach to cervical esophagus through left neck

anastomosis can be performed. The neck is closed in layers with a suction drain in place.

Infraomohyoid Neck Dissection

The lower neck is opened by bilateral collar incisions. The skin flaps are raised along with the platysma. The posterior belly of the omohyoid muscle is identified. The lymph nodes lateral to the internal jugular vein along with the fibro-fatty tissue below the level of the omohyoid muscle are dissected. The recurrent nerve is identified in the tracheoesophageal groove and lymph nodes along the nerve dissected. This along with dissection done in the thorax clears all the lymph nodes along the entire length of the nerve.

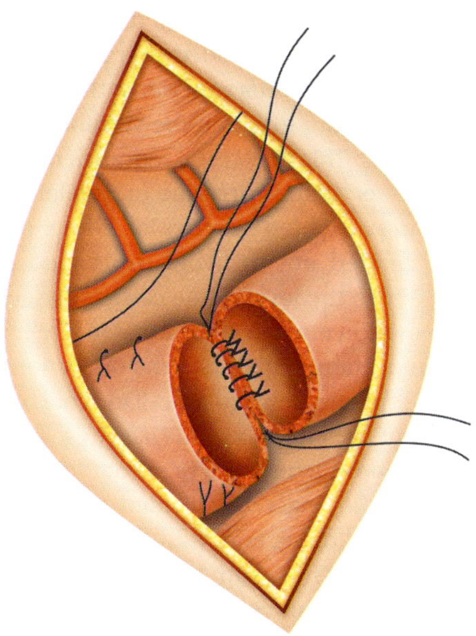

Fig. 32.4A Anastomosis of esophagus with gastic tube

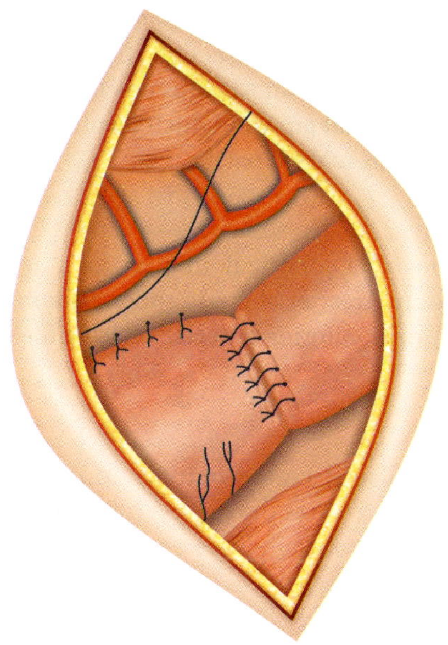

Fig. 32.4B Esophagogastric anastomosis completed

Ivor–Lewis Procedure

The procedure is suitable for disease of the lower and mid-esophagus. It is not suitable for carcinoma of the upper (thoracic) esophagus as it may not be possible to get an adequate tumor-free proximal surgical margin.

Operative Steps

The procedure is carried out under general anesthesia through two incisions: Laparotomy followed by thoracotomy.

Abdomen

This is the first step in the Ivor-Lewis procedure. The abdominal part of the surgery which consists of gastric mobilization and lymph node dissection is identical to that described in the transthoracic procedure.

Thorax

The thoracic part of the surgery which consists of esophageal mobilization and lymph node dissection is similar to the transthoracic procedure described above with few differences. The esophageal mobilization and lymph node dissection is limited to a level just above the arch of the azygous vein. The aim is to achieve adequate tumor-free proximal margin of the esophagus.

After having dissected the esophagus two stay sutures are taken one centimeter above the proposed level of transection. The nasogastric tube is withdrawn and esophagus divided with scissors keeping the mucosal tube 5 mm longer than the outer muscular layer. The mobilized stomach is then pulled into the chest. The upper half of the lesser curvature along with the cardioesophageal junction and a portion of the fundus is divided using a linear stapler. The staple line of the gastric tube is oversewn with continuous seromuscular suture. The distal most end of the gastric tube is transected transversely to match the lumen of the proximal end of the esophagus.

Anastomosis

An end-to-end interrupted single layer anastomosis with 4-0 vicryl is performed. Alternatively a two layered anastomosis may be performed. A mechanical stapled anastomosis may also be performed using an end-to-end anastomosis (EEA) circular stapler. The important thing is to have an anastomosis between well vascularized tubes which is 'tension-free'. The nasogastric tube is advanced beyond the anastomosis into the gastric tube. The stomach tube is positioned in the posterior mediastinum. The chest is closed in layers after approximating the ribs with pericostal sutures and an intercostal tube in placed.

Transhiatal Esophagectomy

Indications and Patient Selection

Transhiatal esophagectomy may be done for benign and malignant conditions of the esophagus. This approach is safe and well tolerated in properly selected patients. This approach would be ideal for patients with lower third esophageal and cardioesophageal junction growths who are borderline candidates for thoracotomy. An important requisite for this surgery is that the part of the esophagus which is mobilized blindly (at the level of the carina) should either be normal or have no extraesophageal disease. Patients who have bulky disease at this level are at risk for intraoperative injury to adjacent vital structures. Another prerequisite is that there should be adequate length of the esophageal substitute, i.e. the residual stomach after resection should be sufficient to reach the neck for anastomosis. This precludes the use of this surgery for junctional growths which involve a considerable portion of the proximal stomach.

Anesthesia

The anesthesia is identical to that in a transthoracic esophagectomy. An arterial line is optional for intraoperative blood pressure monitoring especially during the mediastinal dissection.

Procedure

The patient is placed supine with the arms by the side and the head is tilted towards the right. A roll placed transversely behind the shoulders extends the neck and improves cervical exposure.

Gastric Mobilization

The gastric mobilization and abdominal lymphadenectomy is identical to the transthoracic procedure. The actual transhiatal dissection time should be kept to a minimum and hence is done after mobilization of the stomach in the abdomen and the cervical esophagus in the neck.

Cervical Dissection

A modified left collar incision is taken either as a transverse incision parallel to the medial one-third of the clavicle or as a hockeystick-shaped incision along the anterior border of the sternomastoid. The sternomastoid muscle is retracted laterally and the thyroid retracted medially. The avascular plane between the carotid sheath and the thyroid is entered and dissected posteriorly to reach the prevertebral fascia. The same avascular plane is developed posteriorly by blunt digital dissection to separate the esophagus from the prevertebral fascia. The anterior dissection to create the plane between the trachea and esophagus is done with sharp dissection. A retractor is used medially to improve exposure taking care not to injure the recurrent laryngeal nerve in the tracheoesophageal groove. The distal cervical esophagus is dissected and looped. Once the esophagus is looped in the neck, transhiatal dissection may then be commenced.

Transhiatal Esophageal Dissection

The major part of the esophageal dissection is performed from below, i.e. through the esophageal hiatus. The hiatus is enlarged by a vertical incision on the diaphragm (Pinotti maneuver) and if necessary transverse incisions on the diaphragmatic crurae. A malleable retractor or a Deaver retractor is used to retract the pericardium and heart anteriorly and the lower half of the periesophageal dissection is done under direct vision. Posteriorly, a plane is developed between the esophagus and the aorta and anteriorly between the esophagus and the pericardium. The lateral periesophageal attachments are now separated under vision by a combination of blunt and sharp dissection. Any blood vessels encountered may be divided after applying clips.

As the dissection proceeds superiorly, the surgeon's hand enters the mediastinum between the vertebral column and the heart (Fig. 32.5). This may result in transient hypotension and arrhythmias as there is pressure on the left atrium and consequently impaired left ventricular filling. Intermittent dissection is carried out to avoid prolonged periods of hypotension. Above the level of the carina, dissection is not possible under vision and has to be done in a relatively blind manner. It is important to maintain the dissection in a plane strictly on the esophageal muscular wall to avoid bleeding and injury to adjacent structures, viz. the azygous vein, recurrent laryngeal nerve and trachea. The vagus nerves on either side are hooked on to the finger and divided as high as possible. Simultaneous digital dissection through the hiatus inferiorly and the cervical incision superiorly facilitates complete dissection of the intrathoracic esophagus.

Stay sutures are taken on the cervical esophagus and the esophagus divided in the neck between clamps. The esophagus is delivered in the abdomen through the hiatus. An area is selected in the lesser curve and cleared of omentum. The authors prefer to select this point at the juncture between the left and right gastric arterial territories. If the growth involves the lesser curvature of the stomach, the right gastric artery may also have to be ligated to get an adequate margin. The specimen is separated and the stomach tube formed by multiple (three or four) firings of a linear stapler. The staple line is then oversewn with a continuous suture to prevent the staples from eroding into the tracheobronchial tree. Radical lymphadenectomy (D2 type) is done in the abdomen, specifically removing the lesser curve, greater curve, splenic,

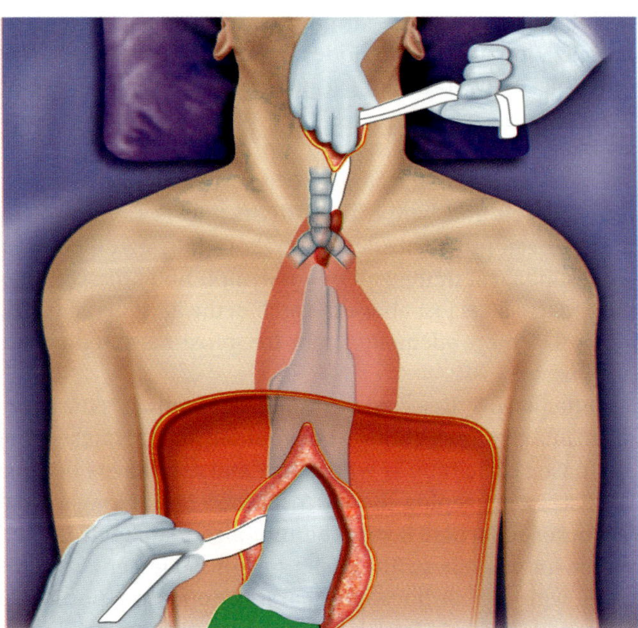

Fig. 32.5 Manual mobilization of esophagus in mediastinum

hepatic, left gastric and celiac groups of nodes. The stomach tube is then taken along the posterior mediastinal or retrosternal routes to the neck for anastomosis to the cervical esophagus. It is important to manually guide the stomach tube in the mediastinum to prevent twisting of the tube and the gastroepiploic pedicle.

Anastomosis

The esophagogastric anastomosis is as described in the transthoracic esophagectomy and is done using a single layer of interrupted Vicryl or PDS sutures. A nasogastric tube is placed under direct vision across the anastomosis in the stomach tube for decompression.

Esophagogastrectomy Through Left Thoracoabdominal (Garlock) Approach

Indications and Patient Selection

A left thoracoabdominal (Garlock) approach may be used for selected patients with cardioesophageal junction tumors. The authors use this approach only for the pure cardioesophageal junction (Siewert type II) and Siewert type III cancers. The type I tumors are better treated using a transthoracic or transhiatal approach as the proximal margin would be compromised through a left thoracoabdominal approach.

Anesthesia

The anesthesia is similar to that for a transthoracic or transhiatal approach.

Procedure

The patient is positioned in a semilateral (using a sandbag to lift the left side) and supported on the operating table using straps (Figs 32.6A and B). The incision is taken obliquely starting from the midline at a point midway between the xiphisternum and the umbilicus and curving to the left along the seventh or sixth intercostal space. Initially, the incision is limited to the abdominal part; the thoracic part of the incision is taken only after ruling out liver metastases, peritoneal dissemination and confirming local operability.

The abdominal part of the incision is deepened and the peritoneum opened. The liver is palpated and metastases ruled out. The peritoneum is thoroughly inspected and palpated (including the pelvis) to rule out peritoneal and omental disease. Infracolic para-aortic lymph nodes are palpated and suspicious nodes biopsied and sent for frozen section. The lesser sac is entered by opening the gastrocolic omentum to assess local operability. Adherence to the body of the pancreas and encasement of the celiac axis are obvious signs of inoperability. Once metastases are ruled out and local operability is confirmed, the incision is extended to the thoracic part.

A sixth or seventh intercostal space thoracotomy is done in continuity with the abdominal incision. The diaphragm is divided radially using the shortest route from the thoracotomy incision to the esophageal hiatus. Some diaphragmatic vessels may need to be underrun and ligated while incising the diaphragm. Self-retaining chest and abdominal retractors are now placed to optimize exposure. The gastric mobilization is similar to that of a transthoracic or transhiatal esophagectomy. The lower esophagus is dissected off the aorta, ligating or clipping the direct branches from the aorta to the esophagus. Stay sutures are taken on the esophagus proximal to the proposed level of esophageal transection, which is decided depending on the site of disease and ensuring an oncologically safe margin. The esophagus is then transected and the specimen is removed using multiple firings of a linear stapler (which also forms the remnant stomach substitute). D2 lymphadenectomy is done and a pyloric drainage procedure (pyloroplasty, myotomy or fracture) is carried out.

The authors prefer a stapled anastomosis though a handsewn technique may also be done. In the stapled technique, an end-to-end anastomosis stapler is used to create the esophagogastric anastomosis. A purse string is placed on the esophageal stump taking care that the suture does not get interlocked inadvertently. The anvil of the EEA stapler (with a long artery forceps holding the tip to prevent proximal migration into the esophagus) is introduced into the esophagus and the purse string tightened and tied around it. An anterior gastrotomy is done to introduce the stapler and brought out through a puncture along the posterior wall of the remnant stomach a little away from the tip. The stapler ends are then engaged and the stomach approximated to the esophagus, taking care that there is no extraneous tissue in between. The stapler is then fired and the anastomosis created. The authors prefer to test the anastomotic integrity on table by clamping the stomach distal to the anastomosis and introducing saline through the nasogastric tube. Any defect in the anastomosis will be recognized immediately as saline will be seen trickling out through the anastomosis.

A 'hypnotic' stitch is taken through the diaphragm, the anterior wall of the stomach to prevent bowel herniation into the thorax. The diaphragm is closed using No 1 Vicryl and a feeding jejunostomy performed. The thorax is closed with an intercostal drain and the abdomen closed.

POSTOPERATIVE CARE AND COMPLICATIONS

Postoperatively, patients may need to be electively ventilated overnight, especially if the surgery is prolonged or in patients with borderline fitness. Fit patients with no comorbidities with an uneventful intraoperative course may be extubated on table. The authors follow a protocol of jejunostomy test feeds (Ringer's lactate at 20 mL per hour) on the first postoperative day, half jejunostomy feeds on the second postoperative day and full jejunostomy feeds by the third postoperative day. Routine antithrombosis prophylaxis is carried out with low molecular weight heparin. Prophylactic antibiotics

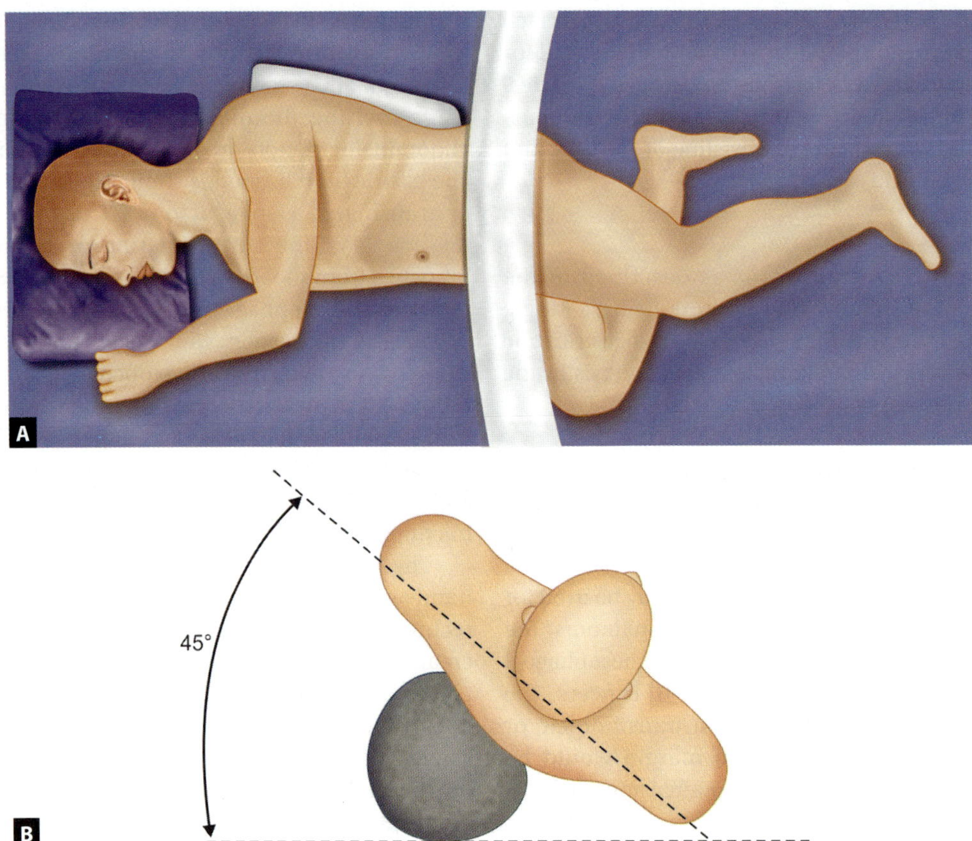

Figs 32.6 A and B Position of the patient

are given as per the unit protocol (the authors administer antibiotics for five days, unless there is overt evidence of sepsis, in which case, antibiotics are changed as dictated by culture and sensitivity reports and clinical response). Aggressive chest physiotherapy is important to reduce the incidence of chest complications and should be started soon after extubation. Deep breathing exercises, active and passive chest physiotherapy, incentive spirometry should be performed every hour to prevent postoperative atelectasis and bronchopneumonia. Active mobilization should also be started, preferably from the first postoperative day.

Early recognition of complications and their management is important to improve postoperative outcome after surgery. Judicious use of bronchoscopy for tracheobronchial toilet with resort to tracheostomy in case of persistent pulmonary secretions is advocated. Any unexplained tachycardia, cardiac arrhythmias, bronchospasm, fever, acidosis, etc. should raise the suspicion of an anastomotic leak and should be further investigated with upper gastrointestinal endoscopy, neck exploration or CT scan. In the authors' experience, a contrast swallow examination is of limited value and a normal report cannot rule out a leak. The authors start patients on oral feeds around the sixth to eighth postoperative day. Patients should be instructed to take small, frequent meals and avoid lying down soon after a meal. The follow-up protocol in the authors' institute is four monthly for the first two years, six monthly for the next three years and annually after five years.

PALLIATIVE PROCEDURE FOR CARCINOMA OF THE ESOPHAGUS

1. Palliative resection of the esophagus by combined transhiatal abdominal and cervical approaches is not suitable when expected survival of the patient is short.
2. Surgical bypass with stomach, jejunum or colon is also a major procedure, and not ideal for patients with limited expectancy of life.
3. Stenting: Intubation with Soutter tube, Celestin tube is an alternative to bypass surgery. Celestin tube is safer to insert and offers better quality of swallowing. The technology of intubation has advanced with invention of various types of expanding metal stents. These can be inserted under radiography or endoscopic control.
4. Endoscopic laser may be used to core a channel through tumor for feeding.
5. Brachytherapy is a method of delivering intraluminal radiation with short penetration distance.
6. Palliation can be attempted with bipolar diathermy bipolar circumactive probe (BICAP), argon-beam plasma coagulator or alcohol injection.

SECTION

6

Abdomen: General

CHAPTER

33

Abdominal Incisions and Closure

Dhiraj Choudhury

VERTICAL INCISIONS

Midline Incisions

A midline incision provides:

- Speed of access
- Ease of closure
- Unrestricted access
- Less blood loss.

Upper Midline Incision (Fig. 33.1)

This extends from xiphisternum to umbilicus and is suitable for exposure of esophagus, stomach, duodenum, gallbladder, left lobe of liver.

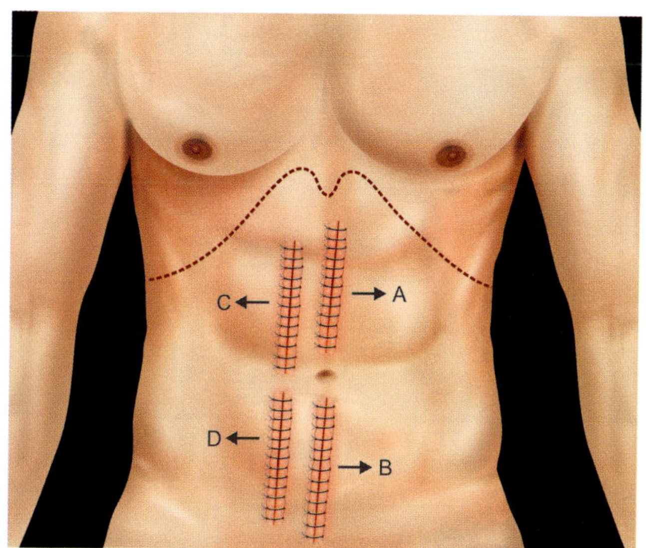

Fig. 33.1 *Vertical incisions*: (A) Upper midline incision; (B) Lower midline incision; (C) Upper right paramedian incision; and (D) Lower right paramedian incision

Steps

- A vertical incision is made from xiphisternum to umbilicus, but can be extended downwards skirting umbilicus. The incision is deepened through subcutaneous tissue to line a alba which is also incised in the line of incision.
- The peritoneum is picked up with two artery forceps away from abdominal contents and incised with scalpel. Introduce two fingers upwards and downwards while dividing peritoneum.

Lower Midline Incision (Fig. 33.2)

This is suitable for exposure of pelvic organs. The incision extends from umbilicus to symphysis pubis. Put a self-retaining catheter to empty the bladder before making incision.

A long midline incision-skirting umbilicus may be required for laparotomy and aortic surgery.

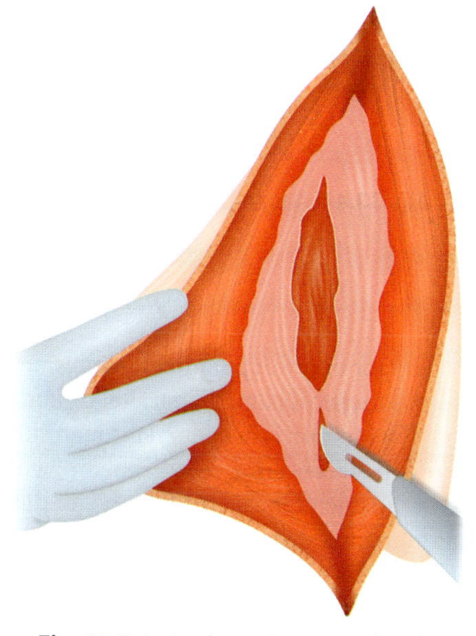

Fig. 33.2 Incised anterior rectus sheath

Paramedian Incision (Figs 33.3 and 33.4)

This is a time honored incision through anterior rectus sheath which is less used nowadays. It permits access to organs located in different quadrants of abdomen according to its position.

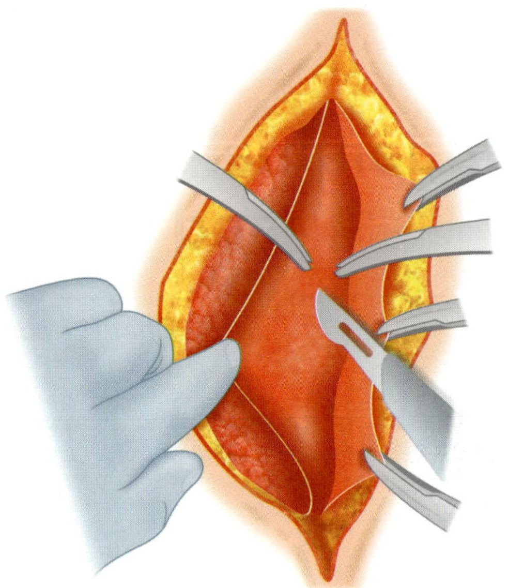

Fig. 33.3 Opening posterior sheath and peritoneum

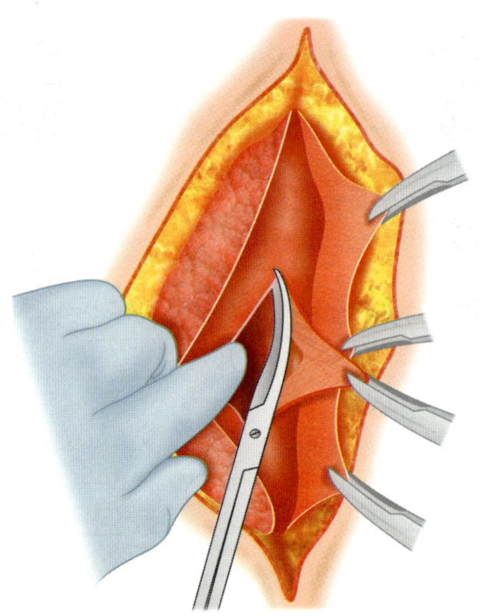

Fig. 33.4 Enlarging peritoneal incision

Steps

- It may be upper or lower paramedian incision on right or left side. An incision is made parallel to and 2 cm from mid-line. The incision is deepened through subcutaneous tissue to expose anterior rectus sheath which is also divided in the line of incision. Hold the medial margin of the anterior rectus sheath with artery forceps.
- The rectus muscle is freed from the sheath by dissecting with scalpel and securing hemostasis with diathermy. Retract the rectus muscle laterally to expose posterior sheath and peritoneum (Figs 33.2 to 33.4) and open it as in case of mid-line incision.

Rectus Splitting

Sometimes the rectus muscle is split to gain access to posterior rectus sheath which is relatively quicker. Theoretically, the medial part of the muscle is denervated and may be atrophied, but in practice the wound heals strongly.

OBLIQUE INCISIONS

Kocher's Subcostal Incision (Fig. 33.5A)

On the right side, it provides good access to gallbladder, bile duct and liver.

On the left side, it is indicated for splenectomy.

Steps

- An oblique incision is made 2 cm below and parallel to costal margin extending from midline to lateral margin of the rectus muscle. Medially the incision is deepened to divide the anterior rectus sheath and muscle. Laterally, the flat muscles are divided in the line of incision. It is safer to introduce a long straight artery forceps under the muscles to emerge at mid-line and divide the muscle with diathermy over the forceps.
- Bleeding point should be caught and coagulated or ligated. Pick-up peritoneum with hemostats and incise it.

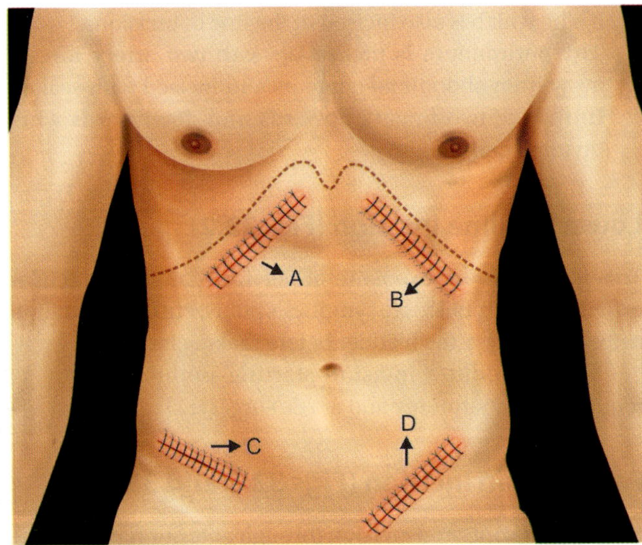

Fig. 33.5 *Oblique incisions*: (A) Kocher's right subcostal incision; (B) Left subcostal incision, A+B roof-top incision; (C) McBurney Gridron's incision; and (D) Rutherford Morrison left oblique incision

Roof-Top (Bilateral Subcostal) Incisions (Figs 33.5A and B)

This provides better exposure of pancreas, liver and adrenals.

Steps

A curved skin incision is given below and parallel to both costal margins. The incision is deepened through recti and part of oblique muscle of the anterior abdominal wall.

McBurny's Gridiron Incision (Fig. 33.5C)

This is oblique muscle-splitting incision. This is indicated for appendicectomy.

Steps

- An oblique incision is made at right angle to spinoumbilical line passing through McBurny's point (junction of medial 2/3rd and lateral 1/3rd of spinoumbilical line), joining anterior superior iliac spine and umbilicus.
- The incision is deepened through subcutaneous fat and fascia. The external oblique is divided in the line of incision. The internal oblique and transversus abdominis are split in the line of fiber to expose the peritoneum.
- The space created by retraction of internal oblique and transversus abdominis by Langenbach's retractor, resembles Gridiron.
- The peritoneum is picked up with hemostats and incised. In case of difficulty in exposure of appendix, this incision can be extended laterally and upwards by muscle cutting.

Rutherford-Morrison Incision (Fig. 33.5D)

This is indicated for exposure for lower ureter, colon and iliac arteries. The approach can be extraperitoneal or intraperitoneal.

Steps

- An oblique skin incision is made from above the anterior superior iliac spine to a point 1 inch above the pubic tubercle medially.
- The subcutaneous tissues and muscles of the anterior abdominal wall are divided in the same line. The peritoneum is then pushed anteriorly to approach ureter.

TRANSVERSE INCISIONS

Upper Transverse incision (Fig. 33.6A)

This can be used for pyloromyotomy in infants, for exposure of biliary tree and adrenals.

Steps

The transverse incision divides skin and subcutaneous tissues, anterior rectus sheath, rectus muscles and posterior rectus sheath and peritoneum.

Lanz Transverse Incision (Fig. 33.6B)

This offers the best cosmetic result following appendicectomy.

Steps

A transverse skin incision is made centered over McBurny's point. The rest of the steps are similar to Gridiron incision.

Pfannenstiel Incision (Fig. 33.6C)

This incision is extensively used for operations on female pelvic organs and for operations on bladder and prostate in males.

Steps

A transverse crease incision is made above the pubis.

The incision is deepened through subcutaneous tissue to anterior rectus sheath. The sheath is divided in the line of incision and reflected upwards and downwards.

Hemostasis is achieved with diathermy. The recti are separated in the midline and retracted laterally. The peritoneum is picked up, incised and opened.

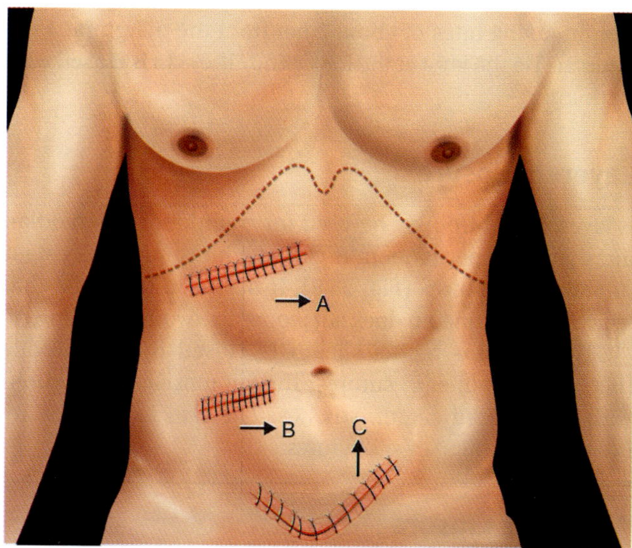

Fig. 33.6 *Transverse incisions*: (A) Upper transverse incision; (B) Lanz transverse incision; and (C) Pfannenstiel incision

Thoracoabdominal Incision

This joins the pleural cavity with the peritoneal cavity.

Indications

Right side, for exposure of liver and portal vein. Left side, for exposure of esophagus, stomach and spleen.

Steps

Position: The patient lies on lateral position.

Incision: An incision is made in the line of 8th or 9th rib from lower border of the scapula.

The thoracic incision is given on the 8th interspace which is continued across the costal margin as oblique upper abdominal incision. Alternatively, abdominal incision may be midline or left upper paramedian.

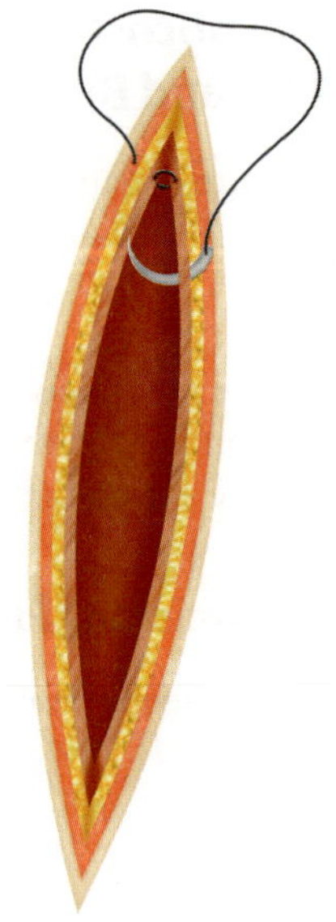

Fig. 33.7 Mass closure–I

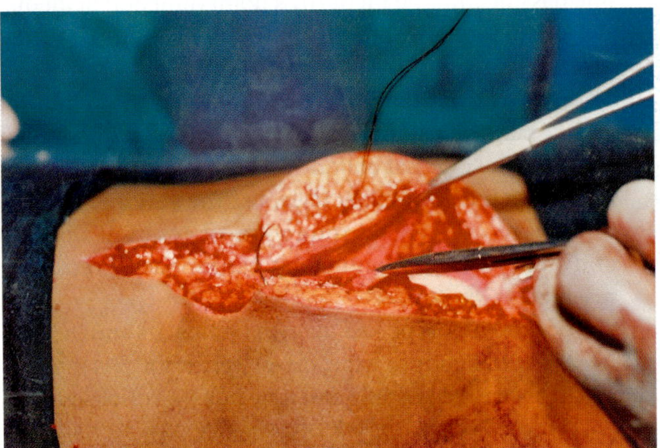

Fig. 33.8 Mass closure–II

CLOSURE OF ABDOMINAL WOUNDS

Mass Closure

This is a continuous full thickness closure (except skin) of abdominal wounds using nonabsorbable sutures like 1 proline or loop ethilon (Figs 33.7 and 33.8). This is ideal for closure of midline incisions. Starting at the upper end of the incision, take a comfortable 1 cm bite through all layers, (except skin) with large a needle. The needle is passed from within out and outside in and the knot is tied on the inside. Now bring the needle out through left side of the wound and pull the thread through and ask the assistant to hold it. Now, apply continuous suture along the full-length of the wound taking bites of about 1 cm from the margin at 1 cm interval. Tie the knot at the lower end. The skin is closed with 0 ethilon.

Layered Closure

A layered closure may be used for traditional paramedian incisions. The peritoneum is closed with continuous catgut (0 chromic) sutures (Fig. 33.9). It has been observed that tearing of peritoneum does not jeopardize wound healing.

The anterior rectus sheath is closed by continuous (Fig 33.10) proline (0) sutures. The cut muscles are sutured with interrupted catgut, stitches. The skin is apposed by interrupted ethilon or silk sutures.

All Layers Closure

Sometimes mass closure incorporating skin, anterior rectus sheath (linea alba) and peritoneum is done, if there is genuine need for quicker closure. Usually interrupted stitches with 1 proline or silk are applied.

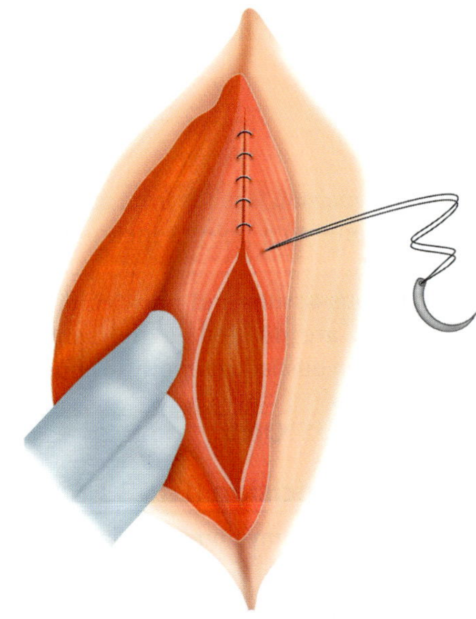

Fig. 33.9 Closure of anterior rectus sheath

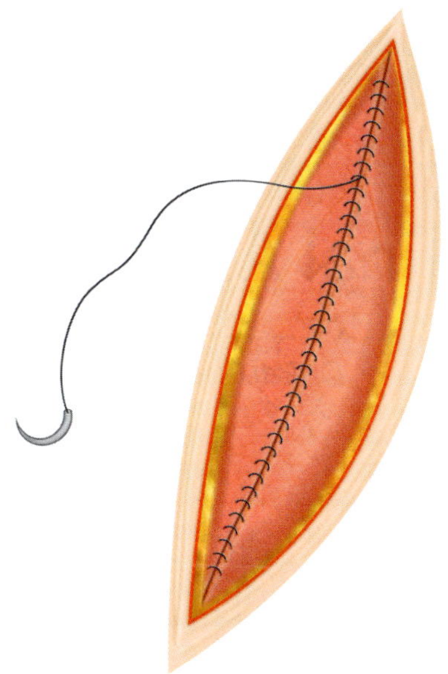

Fig. 33.10 Closure of posterior sheath and peritoneum

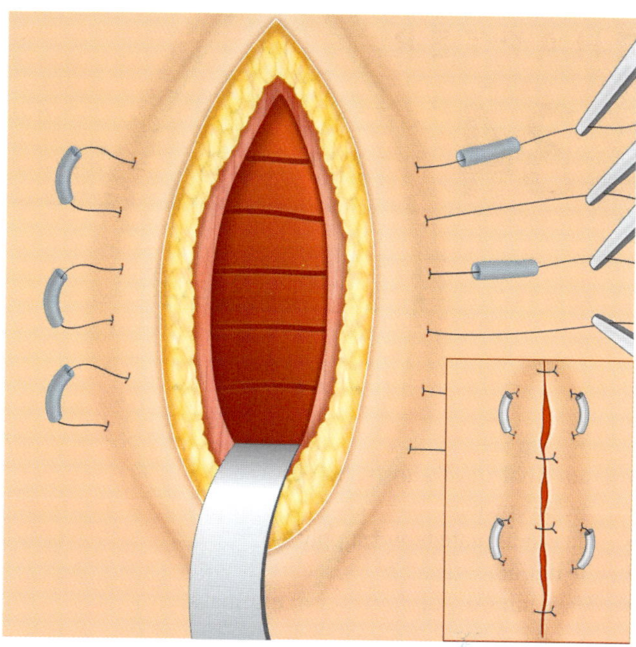

Fig. 33.11 Method repairing a disrupted abdominal wound by means of through-and-through mattress stitches of strong silk, stainless steel wire or nylon. The stitches are made to pass through all layers of the abdominal wall about 2.5 cm from the wound edge, and are passed through pieces of rubber tubing to prevent them from cutting into the skin. A few additional sutures are inserted to coapt aponeurosis and skin

Method of Closure of Burst Abdomen (Fig. 33.11)

The protruding abdominal contents are wrapped in fresh packs soaked in saline. Repair of the wound is carried out by use of through-and-through stitches of thick silk. Traversing all layers of abdominal wall about 2–3 cm from the wound margin. Mattress sutures are used and may be tied over small swabs or rubber tubing. Additional sutures apposing skin and aponeurosis may be applied.

CHAPTER

34

Intestinal Anastomosis

Dhiraj Choudhury, Abir Banerjee

An intestinal anastomosis should:

- Be leak proof
- Have adequate blood supply
- Be under no tension
- Have minimal discrepancy in luminal size.

METHODS: SEW OR STAPLE

Intestinal anastomosis may be hand sewn or stapled, the choice lies with the surgeon. Stapled anastomosis has the advantage of speed but has the disadvantage of being expensive.

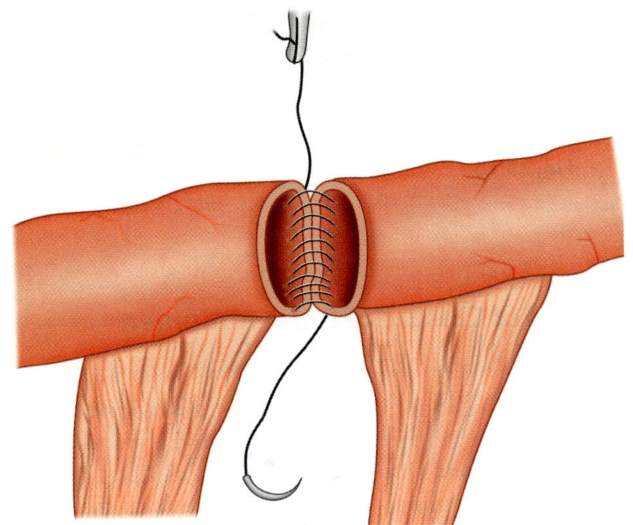

Fig. 34.1A Application of continuous full-thickness sutures posteriorly

HAND-SEWN METHODS

End-to-end Anastomosis: Between Two Mobile Segments

For example, Small bowel anastomosis
Ileocolic anastomosis
Colocolic anastomosis.

Technique: Traditionally, anastomoses were hand sewn.

Two-layered anastomosis: The two cut ends of the bowel is united first by a continuous through-and-through suture with 2/0 chromic catgut or vicryl. Starting from the antimesenteric border, the suture is applied first posteriorly and then continued anteriorly until the starting point is reached where it is tied to the short end (Figs 34.1A and B).

In case of the double-ended suture, the anastomosis is started mid-posteriorly and ended mid-anteriorly (Fig. 34.1C).

Now apply few interrupted seromuscular stitches with 2/0 silk (Fig. 34.1D).

Continuous single layer extramucosal anastomosis: Presently, this technique of anastomosis is favored because it is associated with less chance of anastomotic leakage. This is particularly useful in upper gastrointestinal tract, and is quicker than interrupted single layer technique.

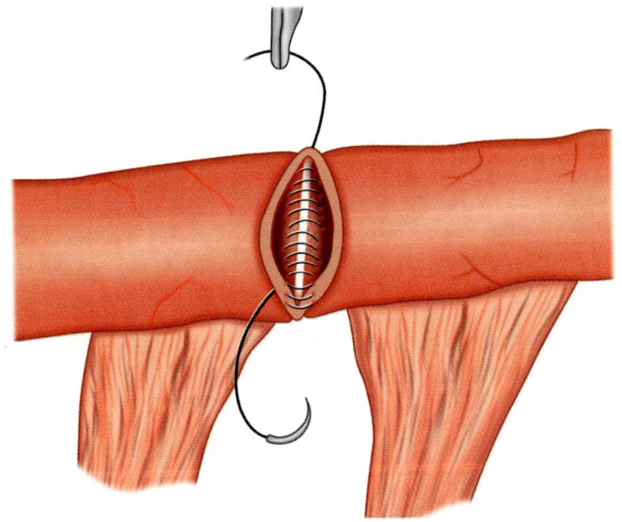

Fig. 34.1B Application of continuous full-thickness sutures anteriorly

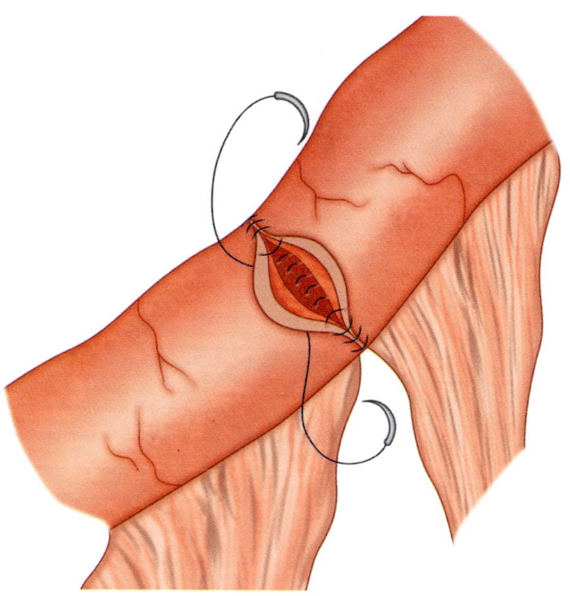

Fig. 34.1C Application of continuous full-thickness sutures with double-ended suture

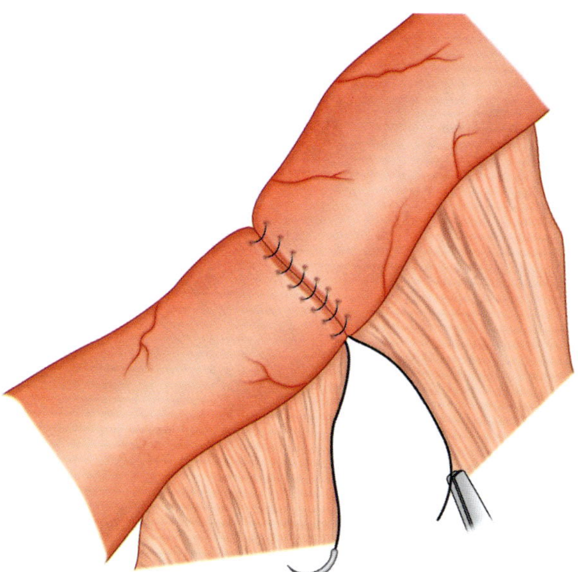

Fig. 34.1D Seromuscular sutures

Technique: Apply two stay sutures on the mesenteric and antimesentric aspect of the gut. A continuous suture technique is used taking serosa, muscle fibers and submucosa, but omitting mucosa (Fig. 34.2).

Apply the sutures first posteriorly starting from the antimesenteric border and continue anteriorly till starting point is reached when it is tied to short end.

Interrupted single layer extramucosal anastomosis: A series of interrupted sutures are applied between bowel ends taking submucosa, muscle coat and serosa but omitting

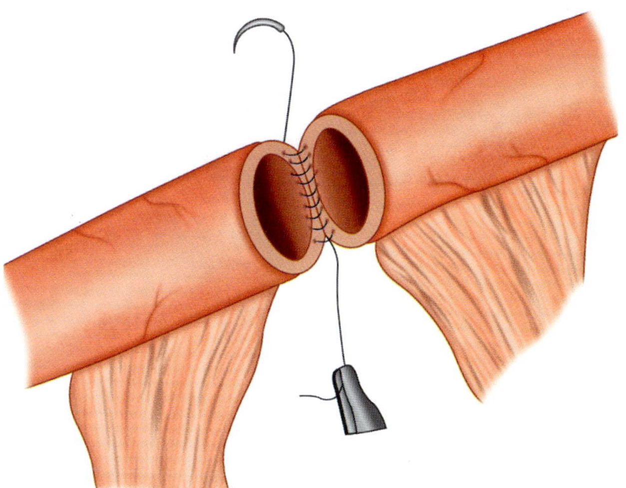

Fig. 34.2 Continous extramucosal sutures posteriorly

mucous membrane. This is considered to be the 'gold-standard' for intestinal anastomoses and is the preferred hand-sewn technique. Interrupted serosubmucosal sutures allow accurate tissue apposition, incorporate the strongest layer of the gut (submucosa), cause minimal damage to the submucosal vascular plexus and minimize the risk of malignant implantation.

Discrepancy in luminal size can be overcome by creating a Cheatle luminal diameter by making a longitudinal incision along antimesenteric border of narrower segment (Fig. 34.3).

End-to-end Anastomosis (Between Mobile and Fixed Segments)

For example, Ileorectal anastomosis
Colorectal anastomosis

Techniques

Interrupted, single layer, full thickness anastomosis: A single layer anastomosis is simpler and satisfactory method for ilo-rectal or colorectal anastomosis. The author prefers 2/0 silk suture material but 2/0 PDS is also being used.

Apply first a series of through-and-through sutures incorporating full thickness of bowel posteriorly (Fig. 34.4).

A full thickness bite of the proximal bowel is taken from within and full thickness bite of rectum from outside so that at completion of anastomosis, the knots lie on mucosa (Fig. 34.5).

The sutures are held by series of hemostats and tied when the layer is complete. Now, the full thickness interrupted suture are applied anteriorly in similar manner (Fig. 34.6).

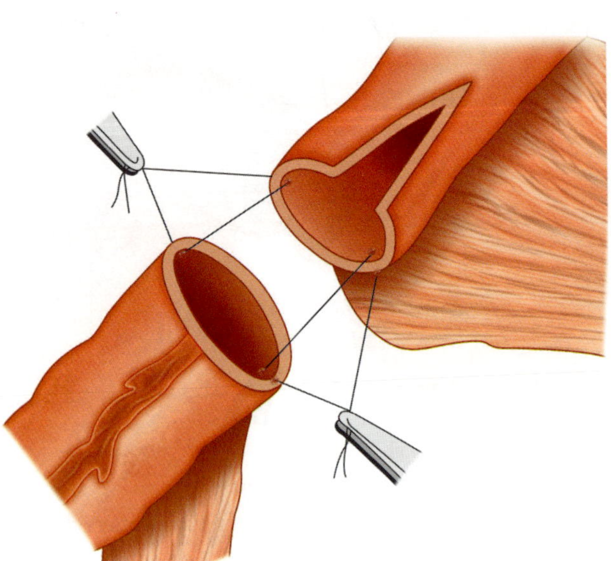

Fig. 34.3 Creation of chelate slide

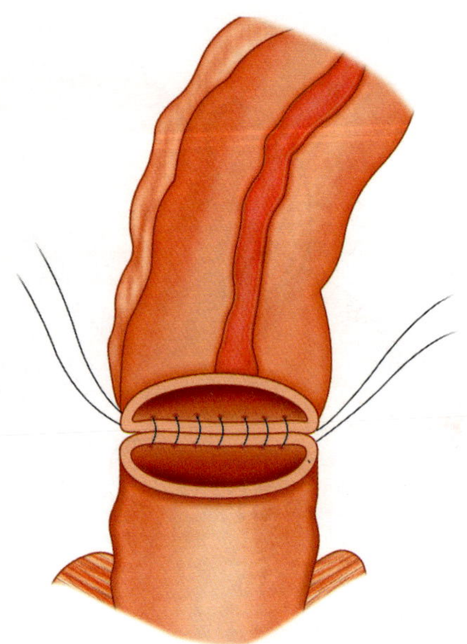

Fig. 34.5 Completion of knots

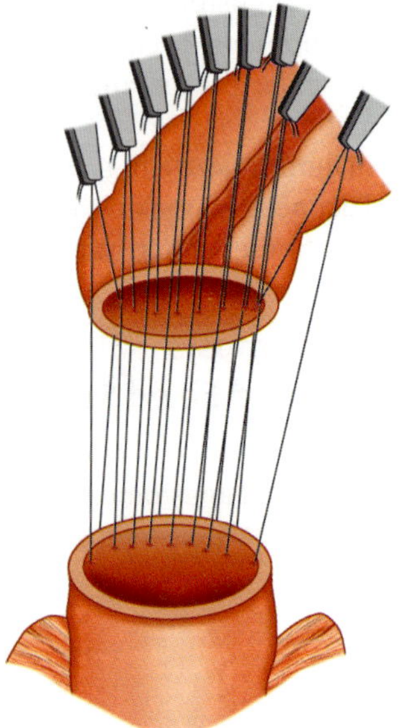

Fig. 34.4 Application of posterior full thickness sutures

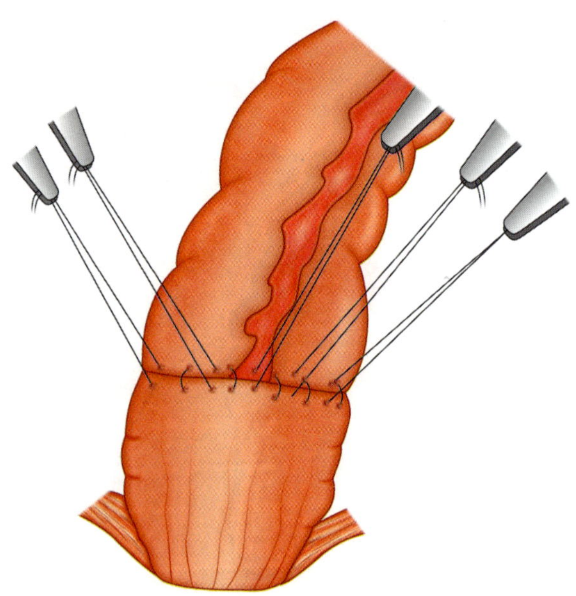

Fig. 34.6 Application of anterior full thickness interrupted suture

Continuous single layer extramucosal anastomosis: This technique is possible if the site of anastomosis is at the level of pelvic brim and if there is no gross disparity between luminal diameters of bowels.

End-to-side Anastomosis

This is preferred if there is discrepancy in the luminal diameter of the bowel ends, e.g. ileocolic anastomosis. The end of the narrow-diameter bowel is closed with sutures of staples.

An antimesenteric enterotomy is made in the that loop. Now an end-to-side anastomosis is constructed using two layer suture technique (Fig. 34.7).

Side-to-side Anastomosis

If both bowel lumina are narrow, it is desirable to construct side-to-side anastomosis. The bowel ends are closed either with staples or sutures.

Enterotomy is made on the antimesenteric side of both bowels. A side-to-side anastomosis is created using either two

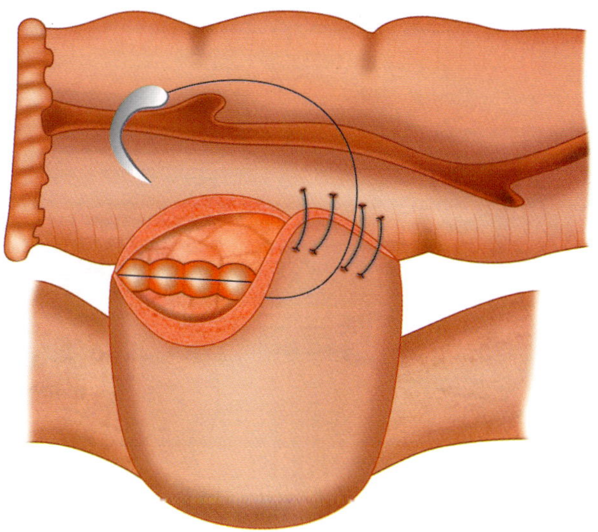

Fig. 34.7 End-to-side anastomosis

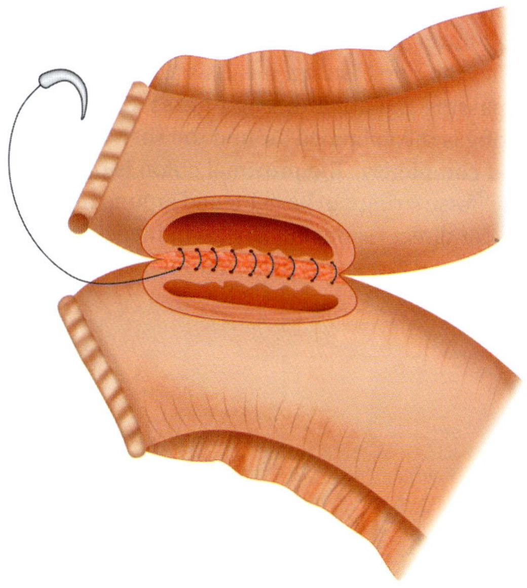

Fig. 34.8 Technique of side-to-side anastomosis

layer anastomosis or extramucosal continuous single layer anastomosis (Fig. 34.8).

STAPLED ANASTOMOSIS

The development of surgical tools, essential for modern surgery resulted in standardization of the surgical technique, the shortening of operative times and an important support to the new mini-invasive approach digestive surgery.

The first surgical stapler was invented in 1908 and the two people who were responsible for this invention were Victor

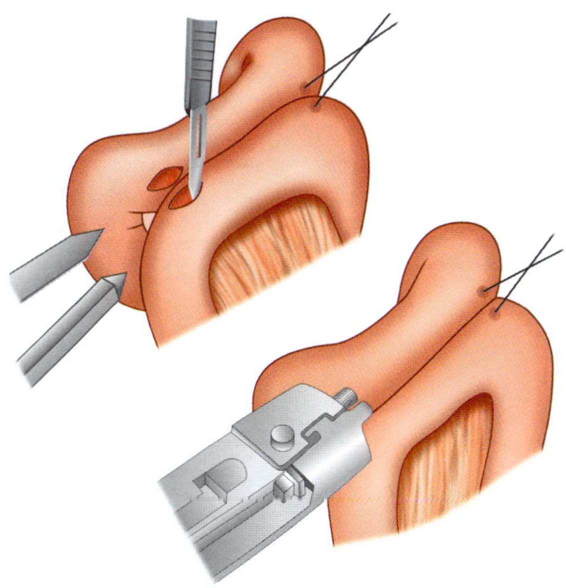

Fig. 34.9 Linear cutting staplers being used for side-to-side small bowel anastomosis

Fisher and Hummer Hultl, although it is the latter who is popularly known as the "*Father of Surgical Staplers*".

Staplers of various types are now used increasingly in various surgical procedures and have become quite well established in gastrointestinal surgery. The chief advantage of these devices is that they can cut down by up to 80% the time taken for bowel anastomosis. This can be very important in a moribund patient where anesthetic/operative time can be cut down substantially. They are also useful for anastomosis in inconvenient/awkward regions, for instance ultralow anterior resection of rectum.

On the other hand, these devices are fairly expensive and in a developing country, this factor has been responsible for the relatively infrequent use. However, it must be noted that most of these devices now available are of "presterilized, single use and discard" types and more widespread use will probably bring down their cost.

The anatomy of the stapled intestinal anastomosis resembles that of the traditional two-layer hand-sewn anastomosis. The bowel ends are inverted and serosal surfaces are held in apposition by staples while healing occurs.

Anastomosis can be made with linear or circular stapling devices used alone or in combination. Linear stapling devices are used for side-to-side and functional end-to-end anastomosis. Circular stapling devices are required for end-to-end anastomosis.

Stapled side-to-side anastomosis: The antimesenteric borders of the bowel to be anastomosed are approximated with traction sutures (Fig. 34.9). Small (1 cm) enterotomies are

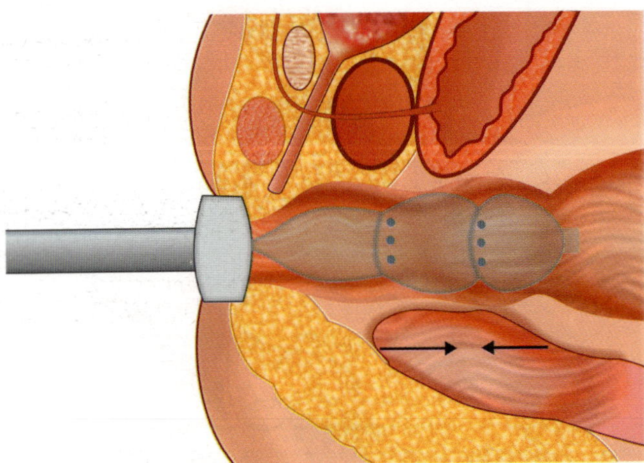

Fig. 34.10A Application of circular stapler

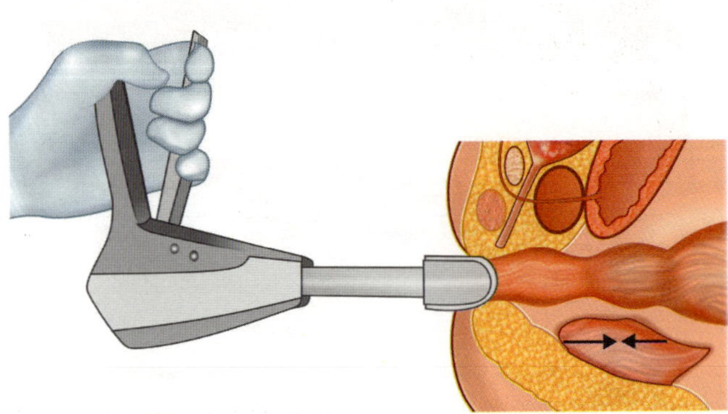

Fig. 34.10B Circular stapler being used for colorectal anastomosis during anterior rectal resection

made with a blade or cutting diathermy. One limb of the linear stapler is inserted into each lumen and the tissue is aligned evenly on each side so that the full length of the stapler is used. The instrument is closed and the staples are fired. The residual enterotomy is closed using staples or sutures.

Stapled colorectal anastomosis (Figs 34.10A and B): End-to-end anastomosis: The end-to-end anastomosis is most commonly created with circular stapler. Such anastomosis is created in pelvis to restore continuity between sigmoid colon and rectum. A noncrushing bowel clamp is applied across to distal bowel which is transected. A purse-string suture is placed around the open rectum. Proximally, the colon is transacted and a purse-string suture applied. Now, the circular stapler is inserted through anus and advanced through rectum. As it approaches the purse-string, the assistant opens the stapling device, passing the anvil through purse string suture. The purse string is the tightened around the shaft and instrument is opened completely. The proximal colon is placed over the anvil. The purse string can be tightened around the shaft of the anvil. Under direct vision, the anvil is tightened and stapler is fired. The stapler is then withdrawn from the anus.

CHAPTER

35

Intestinal Stomas

Dhiraj Choudhury

Intestinal stomas are surgically made openings that connect parts of gastrointestinal tract to the anterior abdominal wall. Functionally they may be:

- Input stomas—feeding gastrostomy or jejunostomy.
- Temporary stomas to allow diversion of fecal matter.
- Permanent stomas when large gut has been resected.
- May be end or loop stomas.

GASTROSTOMY

Indication

A gastrostomy can be used for:

- Gastric decompression without nasogastric intubation
- Feeding patients who are unable to swallow because of esophageal obstruction
- Treating duodenal fistula.

Percutaneous Endoscopic Gastrostomy

The percutaneous endoscopic gastrostomy (PEG) is the method of choice. It can be used for feeding, gastric decompression in patients with carcinomatosis and for the recycling of bile. This is safe and convenient.

Steps

A topical anesthesia is needed for oropharynx to introduce endoscope. Pass the gastroscope and transilluminate anterior abdominal wall. Determine the optimum place of insertion. Under local anesthesia, pass a needle or canula through a small skin incision into lumen of stomach. A wire is passed through needle and grabbed by a snare passed through endoscope. The endoscope is withdrawn until wire comes out of the mouth. The wire is then fixed to gastrostomy tube and pulled down esophagus into stomach and out of abdominal wall where it is secured.

Stamm Gastrostomy

This is the most commonly performed temporary gastrostomy.

Steps

- *Position*: The patient is placed in supine position.
- *Anesthesia* : General or local.
- *Incision*: An upper mid-line incision is made.
- *Procedure*: Two concentric purse string sutures are placed 2.5 cm apart in anterior wall of body of stomach after abdomen has been opened.

A gastrotomy opening is made and a Malecot catheter is inserted into stomach.

A stab wound is made in the upper left quadrant through which catheter is brought out. The anterior wall of stomach is fixed to abdominal wall with four sutures.

ENTEROSTOMY

Feeding Jejunostomy

Enterostomy in high jejunum may be utilized for feeding either before or after major surgery.

Indications

- Following major esophageal surgery for cancer
- Trauma
- Corrosive injury
- Gastroparesis
- Duodenal atresia
- Pre- and postoperative nutritional support.

Methods

Stamm Enterostomy

Select a point in a loop of upper jejunum, a few centimeters distal to duodenojejunal flexure and apply a purse string catgut suture. Introduce a tube or a Foley's catheter through a tiny enterotomy in the center of the purse string suture. Now apply knot snugly around the catheter. The tube or the catheter is brought outside the abdomen through a separate stab wound. Nowadays needle catheter jejunostomy tube is also available (Fig. 35.1).

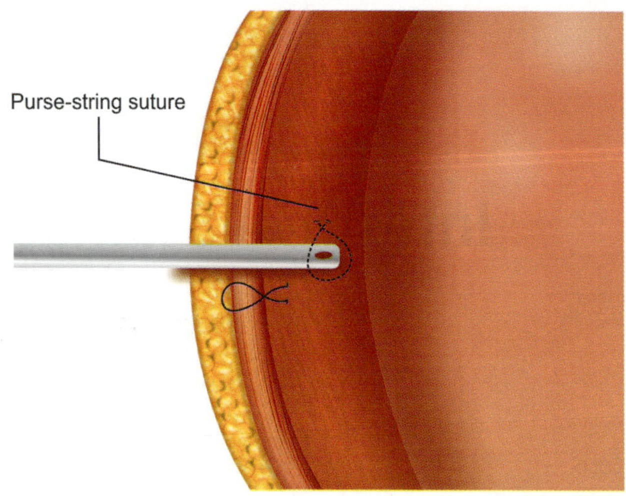

Fig. 35.1 Feeding (catheter) jejunostomy

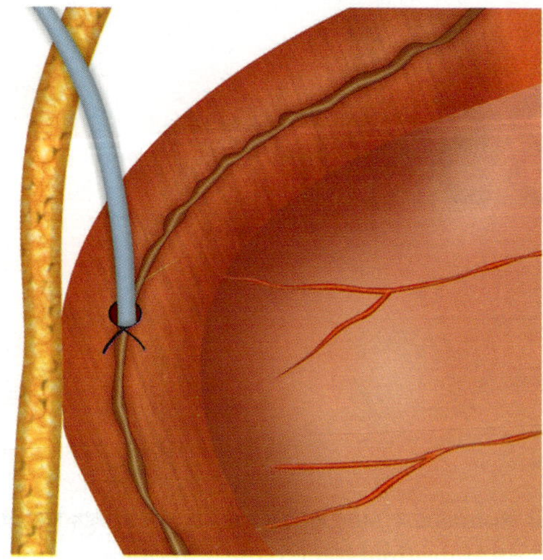

Fig. 35.2A Witzel method: catheter introduction

Witzel Method

Witzel enterostomy provides a valve like protection to opening into jejunum. It is preferred when long-term enterostomy is needed.

- Select a loop of jejunum 30 cm distal to ligament of Treitz.
- A noncrushing clamp may be applied.
- Make a enterotomy through which catheter or jejunostomy tube to be introduced, and fastened at the point of entry (Fig. 35.2A).
- The catheter in then tunneled in a seromuscular groove.
- The tunnel is then closed by seromuscular suture (Fig. 35.2B). The catheter is brought through anterior abdominal wall.
- The jejunostomy is sutured to the anterior abdominal wall.
- Apply a purse-string suture opposite to the mesenteric border at the planned site of entrance.

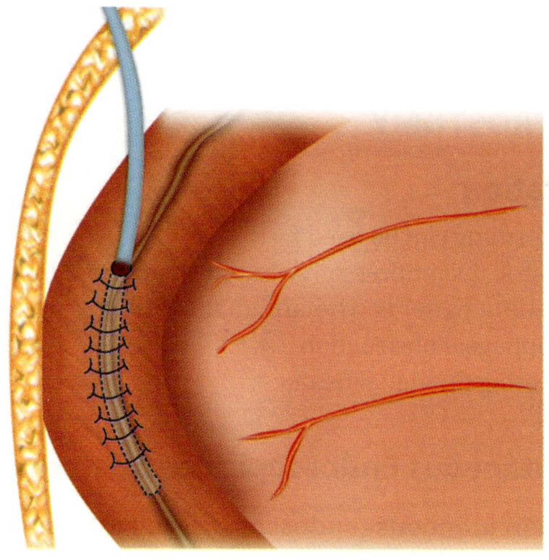

Fig. 35.2B Witzel method: seromuscular sutures

Recent Methods

Following methods of feeding jejunostomy are also available now:

- Laparoscopic-assisted jejunostomy
- Endoscopic percutaneous jejunostomy
- Fluoroscopic-assisted jejunostomy.

LOOP ILEOSTOMY

A distal loop ileostomy is indicated for temporary diversion of gastrointestinal contents to protect a colonic anastomosis. It has replaced conventional transverse colostomy in many occasions as it is easier to construct and close.

Operative Procedure

- *Position*: The patient is placed in supine position.
- *Anesthesia*: General anesthesia with endotracheal intubation.
- *Incision and exposure*: Initial steps consist of laparotomy and resectional surgery for the primary condition. Once decision to defunction distal colorectal anastomosis is taken, proceed to form loop ileostomy.

Formation of Loop Ileostomy

- Incise a 2 cm circle of skin over predetermined site, usually the right quadrant (rectus muscle) (Fig. 35.3)
- Continue the dissection down to the rectus sheath
- Make a cruciate incision in the sheath (Fig. 35.4) and split the muscle fibers down to peritoneum and open it (Fig. 35.5)

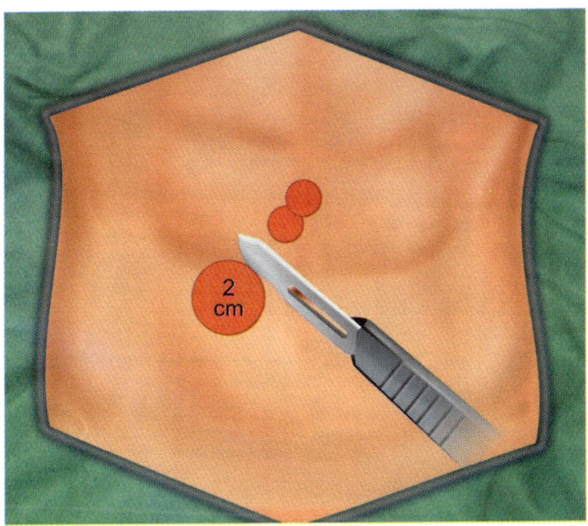

Fig. 35.3 Skin incision for ileostomy

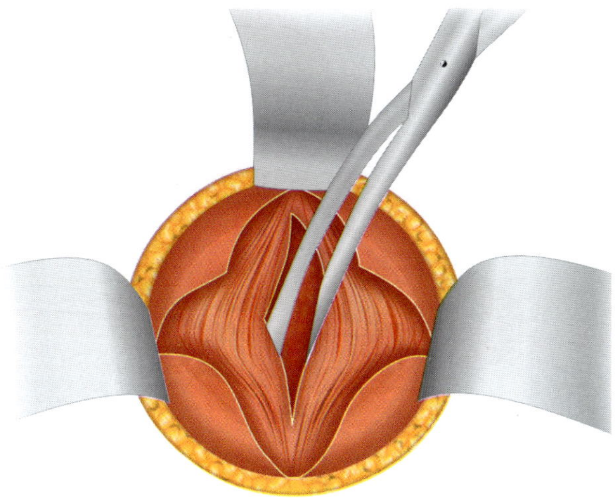

Fig. 35.5 Splitting of muscle fibers

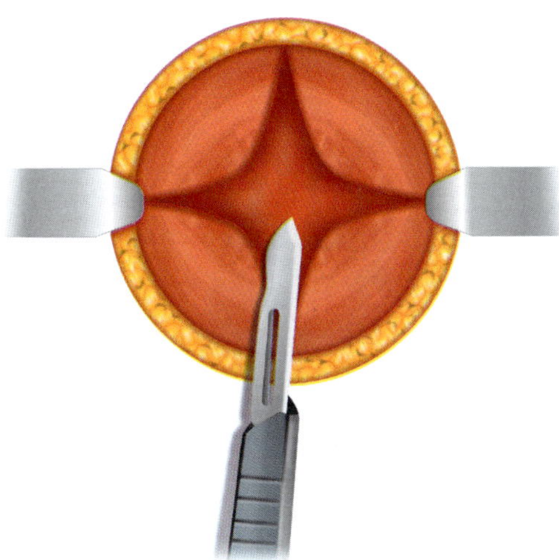

Fig. 35.4 A cruciate incision over (rectus) sheath

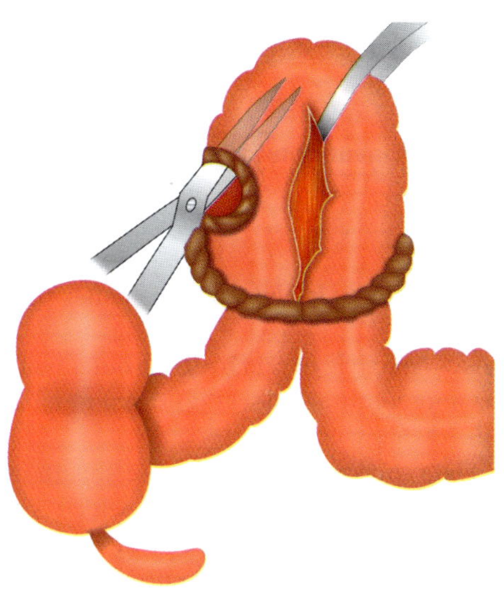

Fig. 35.6 Enterotomy in distal limb

- Select a loop of ileum that will form the stoma without tension, and open a window in its mesentery to pass a rubber tubing through it
- Hold the loop of ileum with a tissue forceps introduced through the opening and gently manipulate the loop through abdominal wall. The rubber tube can be replaced by ileostomy rod
- Open the ileum by incising the bowel for half its circumference at a point 2 cm from the level of skin in distal limb (Fig. 35.6)
- A spout can be formed from the longer proximal loop by everting it following insertion of a pair of tissue forceps into its lumen gently.

  Insert three or four interrupted absorbable sutures to secure the defunctioned side, and six to eight on functioning side (Fig. 35.7)
- Apply ileostomy bag.

Closure of Loop Ileostomy

- *Anesthesia*: General anesthesia is used.
- *Incision*: Incise around the stoma about 0.5 cm from mucocutaneous margin.
- *Exploration*
  - Deepen the incision to free the two limbs of terminal ileum with their mucocutaneous junction.
  - Continuity can be established by end-to-end anastomosis between two ends by stapling technique or hand sewn methods.
  - A linear stapler is used to produce a side-to-side anastomosis.
- *Closure*: Close the abdominal wall with a nonabsorbable sutures and skin with interrupted nonabsorbable sutures.

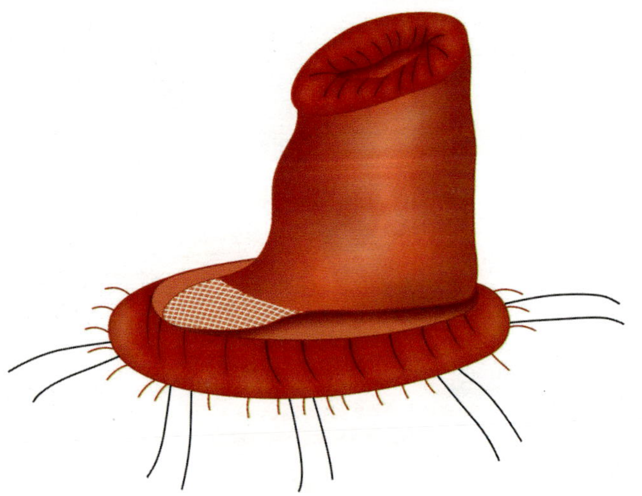

Fig. 35.7 Mucocutaneous sutures

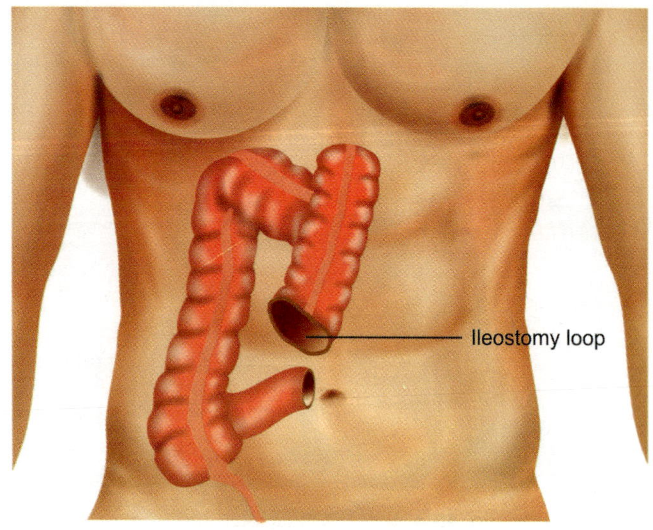

Fig. 35.8 Terminal loop of ileum

END ILEOSTOMY (BROOKE)

Indication

To create a permanent stoma after total colectomy.

Procedure

1. An end ileostomy is always formed after pancolectomy (Fig. 35.8)
2. Incise a 2 cm circle of skin over, the outer half of the right rectus and continue dissection down to anterior rectus sheath.
3. A cruciate incision is made in the sheath and muscle fibers are split down to peritoneum, which is opened.
4. Introduce a tissue forceps through the peritoneal opening to grasp the ileum, and bring it outside (Fig. 35.9).
5. At least 6–8 cm of ileum should protrude beyond skin surface to create a spout-ideal length of which is should be 2–3 cm (Fig. 35.10). The use of spout was originally advocated by Bryan Brooke.
6. Suture the ileal serosa and mesentery to anterior abdominal wall to close mesenteric defect.
7. Insert 6–8 anchoring sutures between the ileum and external oblique aponeurosis to prevent stomal prolapse.
8. Apply mucocutaneous interrupted stitches with absorbable sutures (Fig. 35.11).

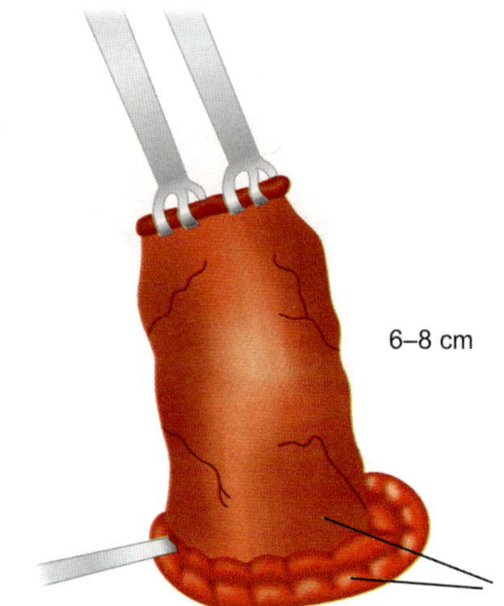

Fig. 35.9 Delivery of ileum

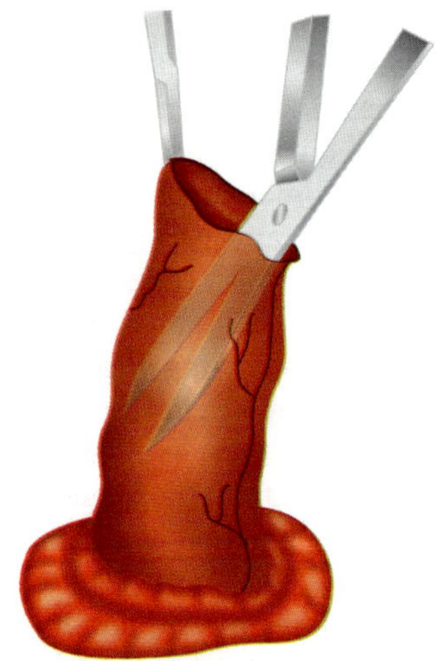

Fig. 35.10 Creation of spout

Complications of Ileostomy

- Prolapse
- Retraction
- Stenosis
- Bleeding
- Fistula
- Paraileostomy hernia.

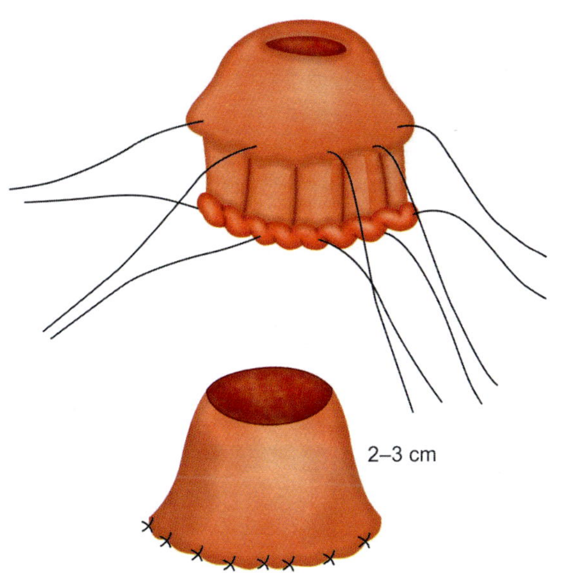

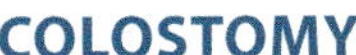

Fig. 35.11 Mucocutaneous sutures

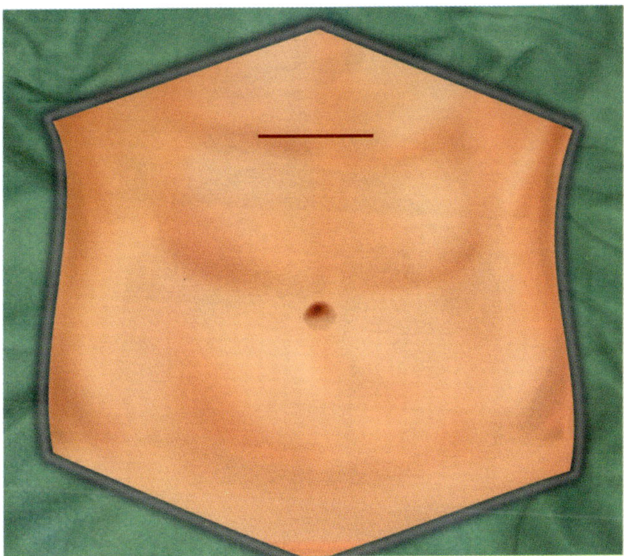

Fig. 35.12 Skin incision for transverse colostomy

COLOSTOMY

Colostomy is operative drainage of colon.

Indications

- *Congenital:* High anorectal anomalies
- *Acquired:*
- *Traumatic:* Colorectal injuries
- *Inflammatory:* Diverticulitis
- *Neoplastic:* Colorectal malignancies
- *Miscellaneous:*
  - Colonic obstruction
  - Rectovesical/Rectovaginal fistula
  - Intractable fistula in ano.

Types

- Temporary or permanent.
- According to technique:
  - *Loop colostomy*: This is the most common type of temporary colostomy.
  - *Double barreled colostomy*: A spur is constructed between the two limbs of the colostomy which can subsequently be necrosed by application of crushing enterotome. This is the type of colostomy used in the Paul-Mikulicz operation.
  - *Devine divided colostomy*: The colostomy is made with a of bridge of skin between the two stomas (defunctioning colostomy).
  - *End or terminal colostomy*: This is part of abdomino-perineal excision of rectum or Hartmann's procedure. Type b, c and d are defunctioning colostomy
- According to anatomical site:
  - Transverse colostomy
  - Pelvic colostomy.

Loop Colostomy

This is the most usually formed temporary colostomy. It may be either in transverse colon or sigmoid colon, depending on indication. Most loop colostomies are performed during emergency laparotomy.

Transverse Colostomy (Loop)

In the past, transverse loop colostomy was frequently used to defunction an anastomosis done on left colon. But nowadays it is less advocated as it offers unpleasant stoma.

Indications:
- Malignant obstruction of distal colon or rectum as emergency procedure
- Volvulus sigmoid colon
- Perforated diverticulitis
- Rectal injury.

Procedure:
- *Position:* The patient is lies in supine position.
- *Anesthesia:* General with endotracheal intubation is used.
- *Incision:* A transverse incision is made midway between umbilicus and costal margin placed over the rectus abdominis muscle (Fig. 35.12) or right upper quadrant.
- *Division of rectus abdominis muscle:* The incision is deepened dividing the rectus abdominis muscle.

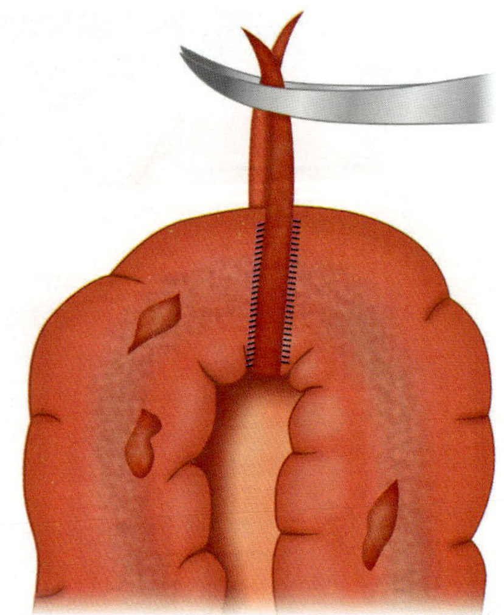

Fig. 35.13 Delivery of loop of transverse colon

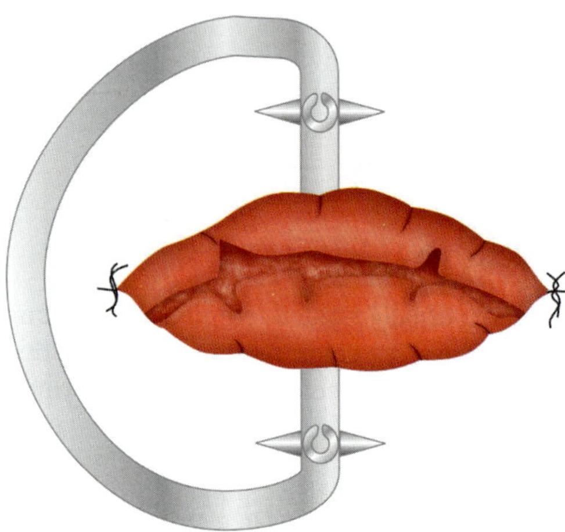

Fig. 35.14 Securing the loop

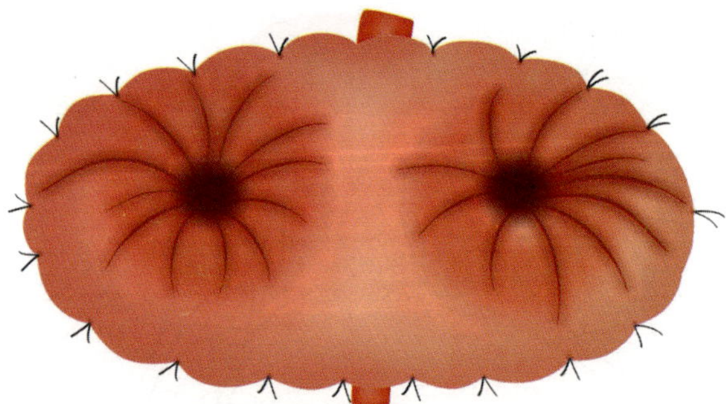

Fig. 35.15 Mucocutaneous sutures

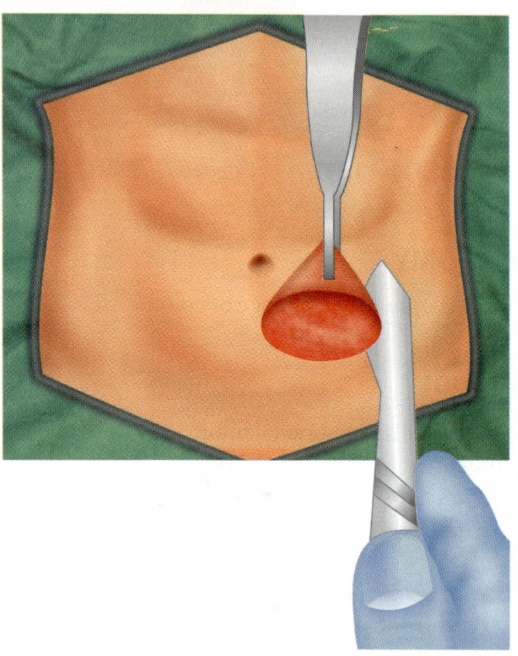

Fig. 35.16 Skin incision for pelvic colostomy (circular disc of skin)

- *Preparation of the colon:* The transverse colon is prepared by incising the greater omentum. A small hole is made in transverse mesocolon, by the edge of the bowel wall and a rubber tube is passed through it to facilitate delivery of the colon (Fig. 35.13).
- *Securing the colostomy:* Once the loop of transverse colon has been delivered through the wound, it is held on the surface either with the help of rubber tubing and glass rod (Fig. 35.14).
- *Opening colostomy:* In case of acute of obstruction, the colon is immediately opened along a taenia (Stronger part) and mucocutaneous sutures are applied with catgut or vicryl (Fig. 35.15).

In nonemergency cases, colon is opened 2–3 days after operation to allow adhesion between bowel and wound margins.

Pelvic (Loop) Colostomy

Operative Procedure

- *Incision:* Left grid-iron muscle splitting incision is made.
- *Procedure: Identification:* Pelvic colon (Mobile) is identified and withdrawn.
- *Selection of loop:* The site of stoma should be in proximal part of the mobile loop of pelvic colon in order to prevent prolapse.
  The loop is brought out and retained by glass rod.
- *Opening colostomy:* See transverse colostomy.

End/Terminal Colostomy

- *Incision*
- *Removal of skin disk:* Remove a circular disk of skin (1″ diameter) from the left iliac fossa just above the

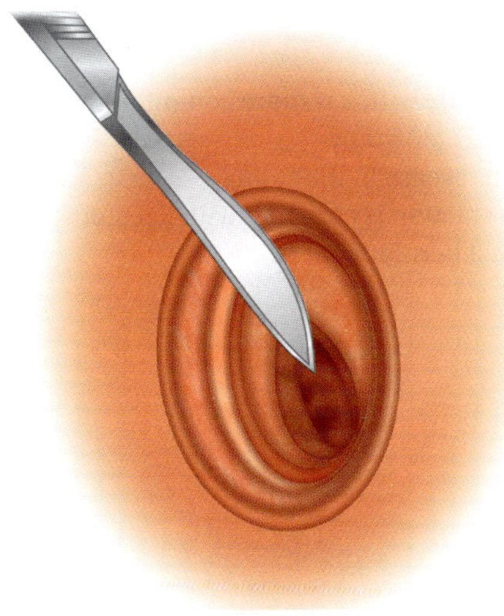

Fig. 35.17 Division of muscle layer

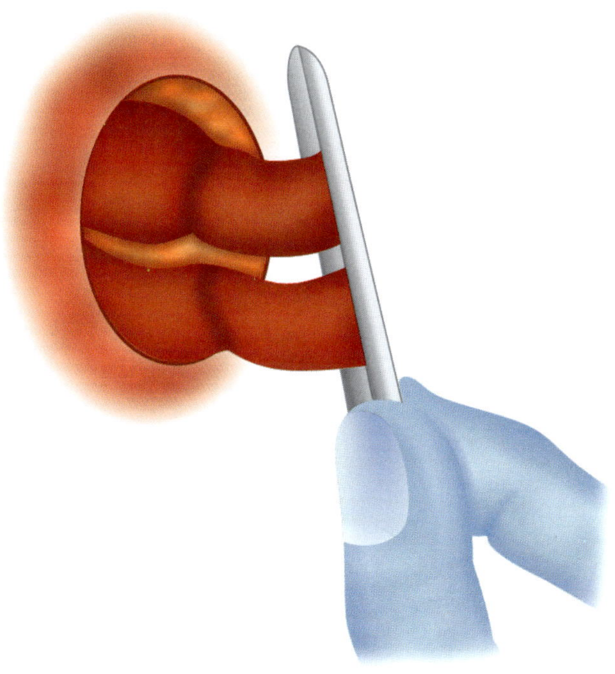

Fig. 35.18 Delivery of colon

mid-point between umbilicus and anterior superior iliac supine (Fig. 35.16).

- *Division of muscle layers:* Incise the external oblique aponeurosis in a crucial manner and the underlying muscle is split (Fig. 35.17).
- *Division of peritoneum:* The peritoneum is incised and the loop of colon is brought out. Obliterate the space lateral to colostomy to prevent herniation by giving interrupted stitches with 2/0 chromic catgut (Fig. 35.18).
- *Mucocutaneous sutures:* Apply mucocutaneous sutures with 3/0 chromic catgut or vicryl (Fig. 35.19) to fashion the stoma.

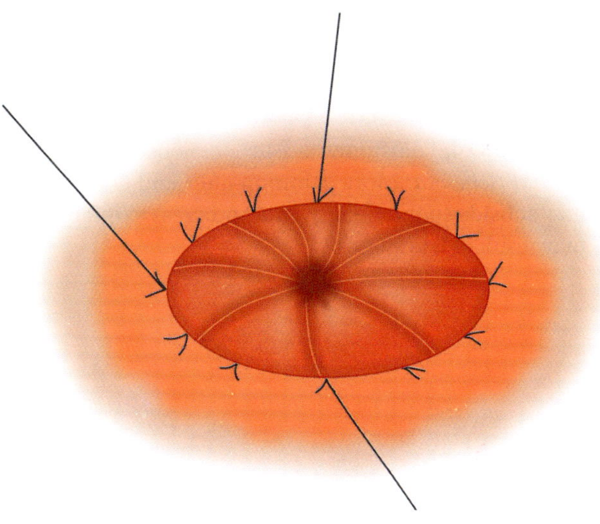

Fig. 35.19 Fashioning end colostomy

OTHER STOMAS

Cecostomy

A cecostomy decompresses the bowel rather than defunctions it. The only indication of cecostomy may be pseudo-obstruction not responding to medical treatment.

Paul-Mikulicz Type

In this procedure, parts of bowel are brought outside. It is indicated in case of ischemic bowel.

Closure of Colostomy

Preoperative

Assess the integrity of distal colon by barium enema.

Methods

Intraperitoneal closure:

- A circumstomal incision is made to mobilize the loop of colon from the skin, subcutaneous tissue and muscle.
- It is essential to free the colon from the muscle on all sides and to enter the peritoneal cavity before attempting closure.
- *Closure:* This can be achieved by single layer full thickness interrupted sutures or by continuous full thickness closure reinforced by seromuscular sutures or by stapling.

Extraperitoneal closure: The colostomy is closed in subcutaneous plane after defining the margins.

COMPLICATIONS OF STOMA

- About 20% for colostomy and 40% for ileostomy
- *Stomal ischemia:* More common after end colostomy. It may subside spontaneously, may progress to infarction or may result in late stenosis
- Peristomal abscess
- Stomal stenosis
- *Stomal prolapse:* This is more common in loop colostomy than in end colostomy
- Recurrent disease in the stoma
- Stomal retraction is common with ileostomy
- Parastomal herniation.

CHAPTER

36

Laparotomy for Abdominal Trauma

Dhiraj Choudhury

Exploratory laparotomy is required for 'acute abdomen' which includes abdominal trauma, intestinal obstruction and peritonitis. About 15% of all trauma patients have abdominal injuries of which over 25% require laparotomy.

Immediate management of abdominal trauma should be based on attention to:

- Airway
- Breathing
- Circulation

Correction of circulatory failure should get top priority in these cases before definitive (laparotomy) treatment is planned.

INDICATIONS OF LAPAROTOMY

- *Blunt trauma abdomen:* Laparotomy is indicated for the following situations:
  - When patient is hemodynamically unstable despite resuscitation
  - When there is unequivocal clinical evidence of peritonitis
  - When there is evidence of air under the diaphragm
  - When there is positive diagnostic peritoneal lavage (DPL)
  - When CT scan reveals rupture of solid viscera.

DIAGNOSTIC PERITONEAL LAVAGE

The diagnostic peritoneal lavage (DPL) is 98% sensitive for intraperitoneal bleeding.

Contraindications of DPL

- Absolute contraindication: When there is an indication for laparotomy.
- Relative contraindications include previous abdominal operation, morbid obesity, advanced pregnancy, advanced cirrhosis and pre-existing coagulopathy.

Technique (Open Method)

Decompress urinary bladder and stomach. After skin preparation, inject 1% lignocaine with adrenaline in midline for one-third distance from umbilicus to symphysis pubis. Now incise skin and subcutaneous tissue till fascia is exposed. Lift the fascial edge and incise peritoneum. Insert dialysis catheter into peritoneal cavity and advance the catheter into pelvis.

Results

- Positive peritoneal lavage:
  - Aspiration of frank blood
  - Aspiration of frank bowel contents
  - Aspirate red cell count > 100,000/mm^3
  - Aspirate white cell count > 500/mm^3
  - Aspirate amylase > 175 units/mL
  - Detection of bile, bacteria or fecal matter
- Penetrating injuries of the abdomen require urgent laparotomy.

PREOPERATIVE PREPARATIONS

- *Fluid resuscitation*: Intravenous administration of normal saline, Ringer's lactate, plasma volume expander and whole blood should be done urgently
- Nasogastric suction
- *Prophylactic antibiotic:* Metronidazole plus third generation cephalosporin like ceftroxime
- Indwelling catheterization.

OPERATIVE PROCEDURE: LAPAROTOMY

- *Position:* The patient lies in supine position.
- *Anesthesia:* General anesthesia with endotracheal intubation is used.
- *Skin preparation and drapping:* This should extend from chin to knees.
- *Incision:* A generous midline incision is made from xiphisternum to symphysis pubis
- *Exploration:* On opening, the abdomen blood and clots are thoroughly evacuted. Bleeding is controlled by packing four quadrants and removing pack in a fashion that the most likely area of hemorrhage is exposed last. Control of bleeding is top priority. Life-threatening bleeding

(ruptured aortic aneurysm) may require opening chest and cross-clamping aorta. The contents of the peritoneal cavity are systematically explored and injuries noted. The lesser sac is explored through the greater omentum to expose pancreas and posterior wall of the stomach. The under surface of the diaphragm is examined along with liver and spleen. The retroperitoneal structures can be inspected by reflection of the left colon, medially.

This allows good exposure of left kidney, aorta and inferior vena cava. On the right side reflection of cecum, ascending colon and duodenum allows examination of right kidney and vena cava.

MANAGEMENT OF SPECIFIC INJURIES

Diaphragm

Diaphragmatic injury following blunt trauma is frequently missed. When identified, small injuries can be repaired with interrupted, nonabsorbable sutures, while larger injuries may require a prosthetic mesh to cover defect.

Liver

Liver injuries occur in 30–40% of patients with blunt trauma abdomen. There is wide spectrum of injury, ranging from simple tear-to-tear of retrohepatic vena cava associated with bilobar parenchymal disruption.

Nonoperative management of blunt liver trauma has been shown to be safe in selected patients. Hemodynamic stability has become the decisive factor in favor of undertaking non-operative management.

Operative management: A significant number of patients will require urgent surgical intervention.

Simple tear can be treated by application of surgicel, fibrin glue or suture hepatorrhaphy. Bleeding wounds of such nature should be managed by suturing. Classically, horizontal mattress sutures with 0 chromic catgut is used.

Expanding subcapsular hematoma should be evacuated.

Major Liver Injuries: Gross Lacerations, Vena Caval Injuries

Immediate steps: Hemostasis/control of bleeding.

Pringle maneuver: Digital compression of the portal triad in hepatoduodenal ligament (free border of the lesser omentum) can be used and compression maintained with atraumatic vascular clamp for 10–15 minutes.

Hemostasis can be also achieved by packing the wound particularly if the bleeding is from hepatic veins.

Atrial caval shunting: A shunt placed between infrahepatic inferior vena cava and right atrium allows for exclusion, visualization and subsequent repair of major hepatic vein injuries.

Definitive procedures: Primary procedures for major liver injuries includes: Resectional debridement with selective vascular ligation (tracheotomy), hepatotomy and vessel ligation, segmentectomy, lobectomy, selective hepatic artery ligation, perihepatic packing, omental pack and deep liver sutures. Mortality from liver injuries is about 10 percent. The most common cause of death is shock and transfusion coagulopathy.

Complications of Liver Injuries

- Rebleeding
- Biloma
- Hepatic duct injury
- Coagulopathy
- Hepatic sepsis
- Hemobilia.

Gallbladder and Extrahepatic Biliary Track

Injury of these organs are relatively rare. Perforation of gallbladder is best treated by cholecystectomy. Duct injury should be repaired with vicryl suture with or without T-tube drainage.

Spleen

In blunt abdominal trauma, spleen is the solid organ most commonly injured (about 40 to 50% cases). In view of its important immunological and reticuloendothelial functions, attempts should be made to salvage and preserve spleen, particularly in children and young adults.

Conservative Treatment

The increase use of CT scan in blunt abdominal trauma has made nonoperative treatment of splenic injury more and more possible, particularly in hemodynamically stable patients.

Operative: Splenectomy

Indications:

- Splenic injury with hypotension inspite of resuscitation
- Shattered or avulsed spleen
- Associated with multiple intra-abdominal injuries
- Failure of splenorrhaphy

The details of splenectomy has been described in See Chapter 57 for details.

Splenorrhaphy (Splenic Salvage)

Indications:
- Splenic injury in stable patients (Grade I to Grade III injuries).

Contraindications: Pathological spleen.

Stomach

Rupture of stomach secondary to blunt trauma is uncommon. Gastric injuries can be safely sutured with absorbable materials in two layers. More severe injuries may require resection and anastomosis. It is important to look for posterior wall injuries by opening the lesser sac through gastrocolic omentum.

Duodenum

About 75 percent of duodenal injuries result from penetrating trauma and 25 percent from blunt trauma. The duodenum should be examined carefully by Kocher's maneuver for identification of duodenal injuries. In presence of retroperitoneal hematoma or biliary discoloration, duodenum should be explored.

Classification

Duodenal injuries have been classified into:

Mild: Injury to less than 75 percent of circumference of duodenum.
- Third and fourth part injuries
- Upto 24 hours delay to repair
- No injury to CBD or pancreas.

Severe
- Injury to 75 percent or more of the circumference of the duodenum
- First and second part injuries
- More than 24 hours delay to repair.

Options for Treatment of Duodenal Rupture or Perforation

Closure

- *Simple closure:* Simple closure is performed in two layers with full thickness continuous inner sutures with 2/0 vicryl and an interrupted seromuscular sutures with 2/0 silk sutures
- *End-to-end anastomosis:* End-to-end anastomosis is recommended for total circumferential separation, if ampulla is not involved
- *Serosal patch:* A loop of jejunum can be used to act as a patch over a large defect in duodenum (Figs 36.1A to C).
- Roux-en-Y duodenojejunostomy.

Diversion

- Duodenal diverticulization
- Pyloric exclusion with gastrojejunostomy
- Tripple tube.

Indications

- Duodenal perforations diagnosed late
- Large duodenal perforation
- Devascularizing injury to duodenal wall
- Combined pancreatoduodenal injuries.

Duodenal diverticulization: This technique is described for combined pancreaticoduodenal injuries and includes repair of injury, oversewing of duodenal stump with insertion of a tube duodenostomy, a gastrojejunostomy, T-tube drainage of CBD and external drainage.

Pyloric Exclusion with Gastrojejunostomy

The first step is closure of pyloric muscular ring with polypropylene suture through a dependent gastrotomy. The second step consists of creation of an antecolic gastrojejunostomy at the site of gastrotomy.

Tripple tube: This is a useful adjunct in patient with severe duodenal injury. It involves primary repair of duodenal injury, insertion of gastrostomy tube, insertion of a retrograde jejunostomy tube and an antegrade jejunostomy tube for entered feeding.

Resection: The most common complications are duodenal fistula, dehiscence of repair and sepsis.

Pancreas: Though pancreatic injuries are uncommon, they have high morbidity. In case of pancreatic injury, it is important to assess the integrity of pancreatic duct by on-table pancreaticography. Complications of pancreatic injury are—fistula formation, acute pancreatitis, pseudocyst, intra-abdominal abscess.

Options for treatment of pancreatic injury:
No ductal transection: This can be treated by drainage or pancreaticorrhaphy or omental plug.

Ductal transection in head: This can be treated by Roux-en-Y pancreatic jejunostomy, anterior Roux-en-Y

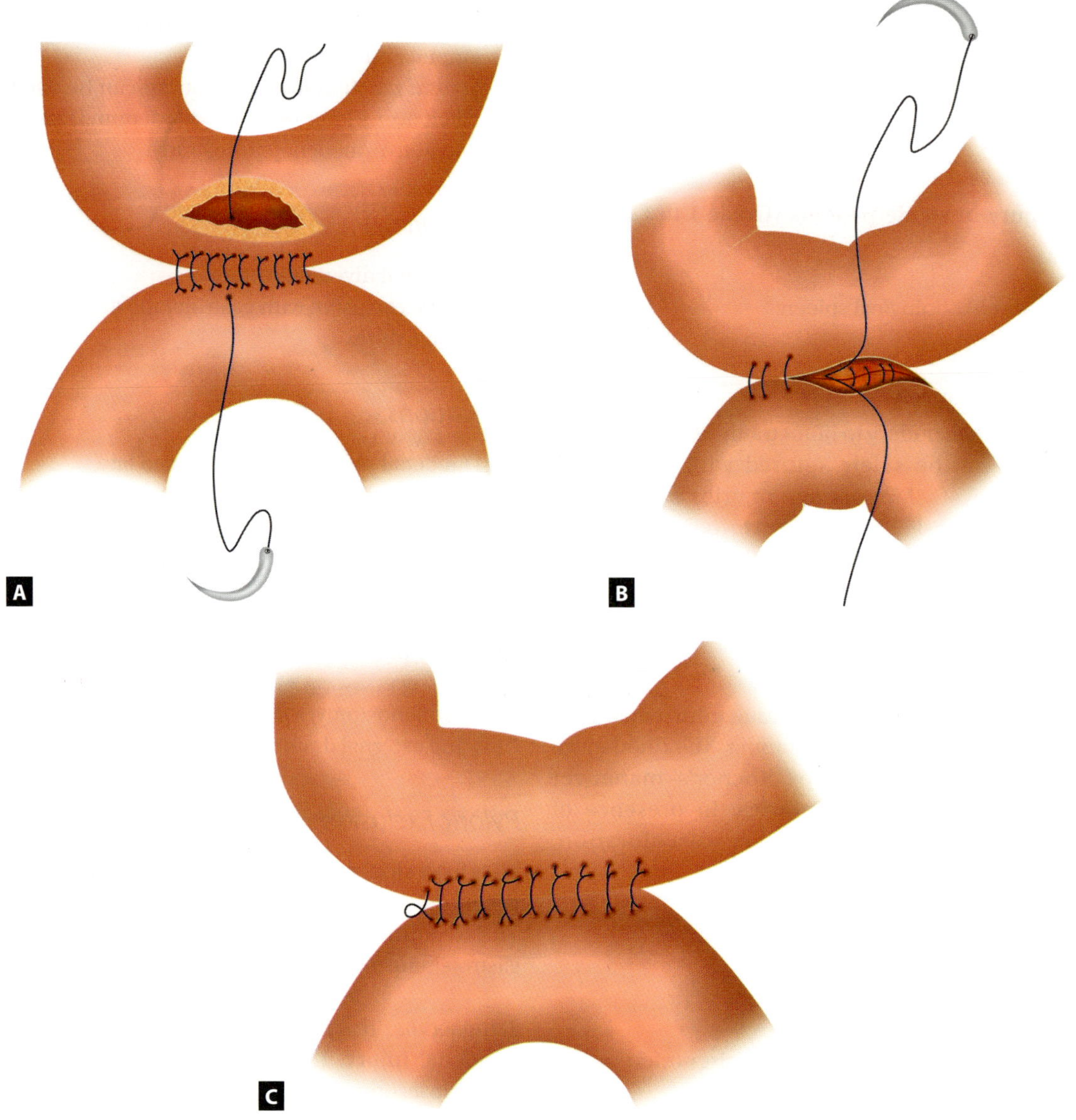

Figs 36.1A to C Serosal patch

pancreaticojejunostomy or pancreaticoduodenal resection. Pancreaticoduodenal resection in indicated for:

- Proximal pancreatic duct injury.
- Injury to head of the pancreas involving the ampulla or the distal bile duct that precludes reconstruction.
- Combined devascularizing injury to pancreas and duodenum.

Small bowel: Simple injuries are repaired in two layers while multiple perforation and laceration to bowel and mesentery are best treated by resection and primary anastomosis. Nonviable gut must be excised.

Mesenteric tear: A clean tear in the area of the vessels can be treated by ligation of bleeding point and closure of the rent. A laceration along the axis of the bowel measuring more than 5 cm requires intestinal resection and anastomosis (Fig. 36.2).

Colon: Treatment of colorectal injuries should depend on nature of injury, degree of contamination, severity and number of associated injuries, stability of the patient and interval between injury and operation. Injury to right colon can be treated by resection and anastomosis (Right hemicolectomy) in stable patient. Left-sided colonic injuries were previously treated by exteriorization. Nowadays primary

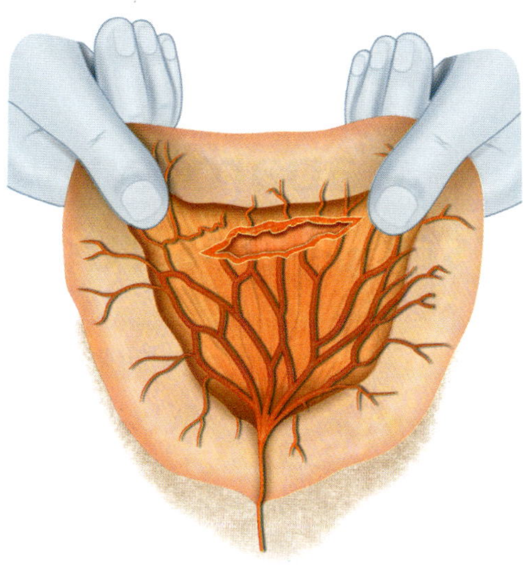

Fig. 36.2 A tear of the mesentery

repair is advocated for wounds that have no risk factor. If injury is considered to be high-risk, mucus fistula or Hartmann's procedure should be preferred.

Rectum: All injuries of the rectum should be treated with:

- Defunctioning colostomy
- Repair of injury
- Drainage of presacral space
- Irrigation of distal segment of bowel

Genitourinary: Hematuria should be investigated by IVU. At laparotomy, kidneys can be approached by reflecting right or left colon. Nephrectomy is indicated for gross renal injuries. Ureteric injury can be corrected by single layer suture and double 'J' stent.

Vascular injuries: These should be treated with the help of vascular surgeon when available.

Retroperitoneal hematoma: Retroperitoneal hematomas in the pelvis and lower abdominal region are best not explored unless they are actively expanding or an arterial source has been identified. Many of these are associated with pelvic fractures and are not controllable by surgical means. However, retroperitoneal hematomas in the upper abdomen, particularly those in proximity to duodenum, pancreas and renal pedicles should be explored.

Pelvic fracture: These may require internal fixation by orthopedic surgeon.

Closure: Abdomen is closed en-masse after putting one or more drains.

CHAPTER

37

Laparotomy for Intestinal Obstruction

Dhiraj Choudhury

INDICATIONS

- Immediately in case of strangulation
- After failure of conservative treatment for 72 hours in case of simple obstruction.

PREOPERATIVE PREPARATIONS

- Nasogastric suction
- Intravenous fluid and electrolytes
- Systemic antibiotic
- Blood grouping and cross-matching.

OPERATIVE PROCEDURE

- *Position*: The patient is placed in supine position.
- *Anesthesia*: General anesthesia with endotracheal intubation is used.
- *Incision*: A liberal midline incision (skirting umbilicus) is preferred.
- *Exploration*: On opening peritoneum exploration of whole of abdomen should be carried out systematically, starting from ileocecal region.
  - If cecum is collapsed, it is small bowel obstruction
  - If cecum is distended, it is large bowel obstruction.

  Trace the site and cause of obstruction.

Decompression of Bowel

In presence of distended loops of bowel (small or large) following steps can be undertaken to decompress the bowel.

- Bowel small or large distended with gas can be deflated with an aspirating needle attached to a mechanical suction apparatus. The needle (0.7 to 0.9 mm) is inserted obliquely through the bowel wall when dealing with small intestine, but in case of colon, the needle is introduced through a *Taenia coli.*
- Decompression of small bowel can be done through a distal enterotomy which was once a popular method but it has the risk of contamination.
- *Retrograde stripping*: Intestinal contents can be emptied back into stomach to be removed through nasogastric or wide bore tube. Alternately the tube can be manipulated into second or third part of duodenum for aspiration. The bowel is held lightly in fingers of the left hand and index and middle finger of the right hand are applied across it to act as an occlusion clamp. The pressure applied is sufficient to prevent escape of intestinal contents. The bowel is decompressed by progressive stripping through finger of the right hand.

Irrigation of Bowel

- On-table irrigation or bowel wash: A Foley's catheter can be introduced through the appendicular stump or terminal ileum and bowel wash can be given through the catheter with Hartmann's solution.

MANAGEMENT OF SPECIFIC CAUSES

Bands

Congenital or acquired bands should be divided and tied.

Adhesiolysis

Should be done gently, and all adhesions should be divided.

Noble's Plication

In case of extensive adhesions short-circuiting of small bowel by multiple side-to-side anastomosis is a better procedure than attempting to free adhesions (Fig. 37.1).

Stricture

The surgical management of small bowel strictures is governed by the underlying pathology.

- Short fibrous strictures and short stricture secondary to Crohn's disease should be treated by stricturoplasty.
- Long (75 cm) or multiple Crohn's strictures require resection and anastomosis.
- Malignant strictures should be widely excised.

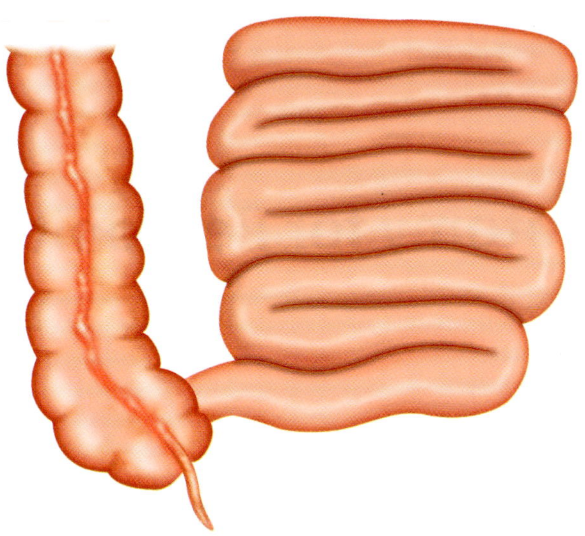

Fig. 37.1 Noble's plication

Strangulated (Nonviable) Small Bowel

Strangulated small bowels should be treated by resection and anastomosis.

Intussusception

Reduction of intussusception should be attempted first, if gut is viable. In most cases, the segment of bowel involved, is nonviable and requires resection-anastomosis.

Volvulus

Sigmoid volvulus is treated by primary resection and anastomosis.

Malignant Obstruction

Resection with primary anastomosis is the preferred option, but for inexperienced surgeon, proximal colostomy for decompression of colon may be right decision. Further surgery is done at a later date.

CLOSURE

- Proximal colostomy or ileostomy may be required in selected cases
- The abdomen is closed en-masse with loop ethilon.

POSTOPERATIVE CARE

- Continue intravenous fluid and electrolytes till flatus is passed
- Nasogastric suction
- Maintain intake-output chart
- Monitor electrolyte balance
- Systemic antibiotic.

POSTOPERATIVE COMPLICATIONS

- Ileus
- Sepsis
- Postoperative chest complications.

CHAPTER

38

Laparotomy for Peritonitis

Dhiraj Choudhury

Peritonitis can nowadays be relatively easily diagnosed and assessed from clinical findings, laboratory investigations and imaging, if presents with typical history and physical signs. But symptoms and signs may vary according to stage of the disease.

INDICATIONS

If an accurate diagnosis can be made, decision is easy to arrive at. But in case of acute abdomen, the old dictum 'it' is better to look and see than to wait and see still holds good. If there is no unanimity between clinical findings and tests, one should be guided by clinical judgement to treat conservatively. But decision may be changed to laparotomy depending on the progress of the patient and new features.

PROCEDURES

1. Abdomen is usually opened by a midline incision.
2. On opening abdomen, rapid evacuation of exudates by suction is the top priority. A sample of the fluid should be preserved for examination.
3. Next step is identification of cause of peritonitis. Start with appendix at the lower abdomen. The operative procedure will depend on the pathology found.

CLOSURE

- Put one or more drains in the abdomen. One drain should be inserted near the site of the procedure and other in the pelvis.
- Close the wound en mass with ethilon.

SECTION

7

Stomach and Duodenum

CHAPTER

39

Pyloromyotomy: Ramstedt's Operation

Dhiraj Choudhury

INDICATION

Infantile pyloric stenosis: Ramstedt's pyloromyotomy is the accepted surgical treatment all over the world.

PREOPERATIVE PREPARATIONS

- Correct dehydration, hypochloremia and hypokalemia with intravenous infusion of half-normal saline adding potassium (10-15 mmol KCl per 500 mL of 0.45% saline).
- Stop feed and perform gastric lavage with normal saline.
- Pass nasogastric tube.

OPERATIVE PROCEDURE

- *Position:* The patient is placed in supine position.
- *Anesthesia:* Usually general anesthesia with endotracheal intubation is used but the operation has been also done under local anesthesia.
- *Incision:* A transverse muscle cutting incision (3–4 cm long) is made in the right hypochondrium overlying the palpable tumor.
- *Exposure:* Deepen the incision through subcutaneous tissue and anterior rectus sheath with cutting diathermy.

  The rectus muscle is split along the lines fibers and peritoneum is opened.

OPERATIVE TECHNIQUE

Retract the inferior margin of the liver upwards. Identify the pyloric tumor and deliver it to wound, and rotate it so that superior surface (least vascular) comes into view.

- A Serosa incision in made antero-superiorly from the pyloro-duodenal junction to gastric antrum (Fig. 39.1).
- The plyoric muscle, which has a gritty consistency, is now separated widely down to sub-mucosa using artery forceps. It results in bulging of intact sub-mucosa from duodenal fornix to gastric antrum (Fig. 39.2).
- Presence of air or bile at the duodenal end of the incision is an indication of perforation. Repair the perforation with interrupted 4–0 chromic catgut sutures, and reenforce by omentum. Bleeding points are dealt with under-running stitches.

CLOSURE

- Close the muscle and sheath en-mas with 3–0 polyglycolic acid sutures.
- Skin is closed with subcuticular stitch.

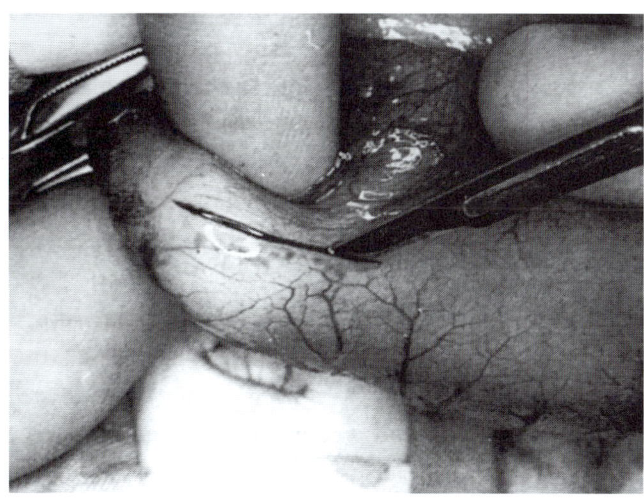

Fig. 39.1 Incision made in the anterior surface of the tumor

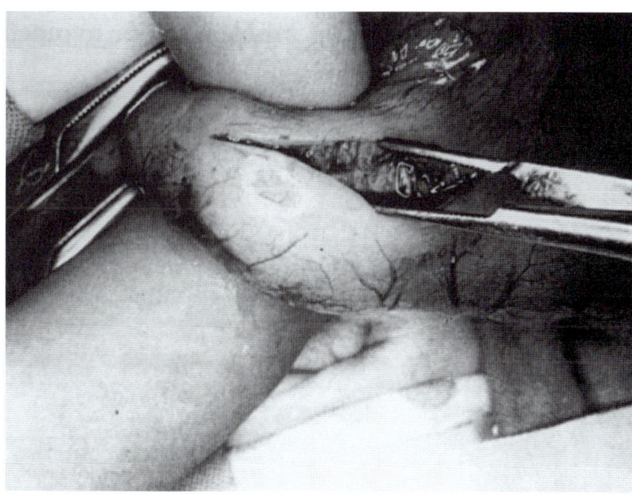

Fig. 39.2 Hypertrophied muscle fibers are split

POSTOPERATIVE CARE

- Intravenous fluid are administered for 2–8 hours
- Oral feeds are started at 2 hours postoperatively and gradually increased
- The child can be discharged on 2nd to 4th postoperative day

Pyloromyotomy can be done laparoscopically with superior cosmesis by experienced laparoscopic surgeon.

CHAPTER 40

Vagotomy

Dhiraj Choudhury

From forties onward, gastric surgery is widely indebted to Dragsted and his associates, who revolutionized the methods, by bringing vagotomy in treatment of duodenal ulcer.

TRUNCAL VAGOTOMY

Division of anterior and posterior trunks of vagus nerve reduces gastric acid secretion by abolishing cephalic phase, but this causes gastric stasis by abolition of antral pump and hence, has to be supplemented by drainage procedure. Moreover, in 7% cases there is fatty diarrhea.

Indications

Truncal vagotomy is nowadays occasionally performed for refractory chronic duodenal or gastric ulcer along with drainage procedure. Gastric outlet obstruction following chronic duodenal ulcer may require gastrojejunostomy and truncal vagotomy.

Preoperative Preparations

- Introduce a nasogastric tube.
- Antibiotic prophylaxis.
- Anti-DVT prophylaxis.

Operative Procedure

- *Position:* The patient is placed in supine position.
- *Anesthesia:* General anesthesia with endotracheal intubation.
- *Incision:* An upper midline incision is preferred (Fig. 40.1).
- *Exposure:* On opening abdomen, a through exploration is done to confirm diagnosis and to exclude other disease. Duodenal ulcer is indicated by presence of cicatrical contracture and petechial hemorrhage when surface of first part of duodenum is rubbed.

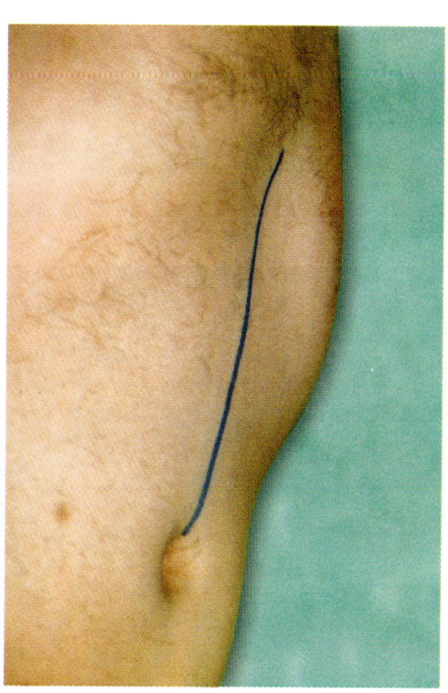

Fig. 40.1 Skin incision

Technique of Truncal Vagotomy

Divide the left triangular ligament with diathermy or scissors and retract left lobe of liver to improve access to esophageal hiatus. Identify abdominal esophagus by palpation of nasogastric tube (Fig. 40.2).

Mobilization of Esophagus

Incise the peritoneum overlying abdominal esophagus transversely and dissect the groove between esophagus and the adjacent crus. Gently insert right index finger behind the esophagus and encircle it. Pass a sling or tape around the esophagus to apply traction (Fig. 40.3).

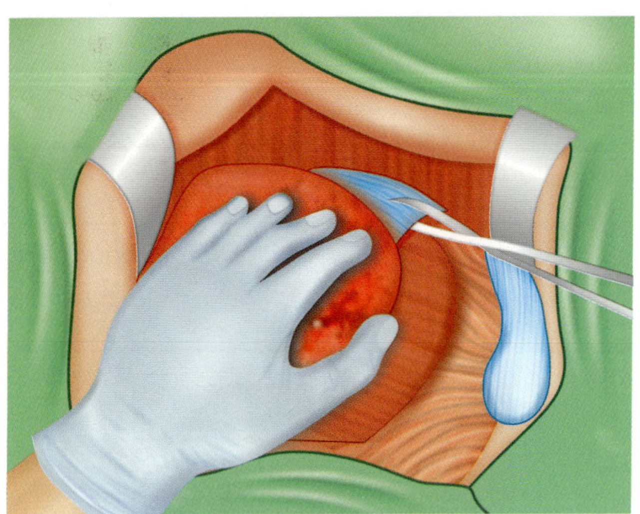

Fig. 40.2 Division of left triangular ligament

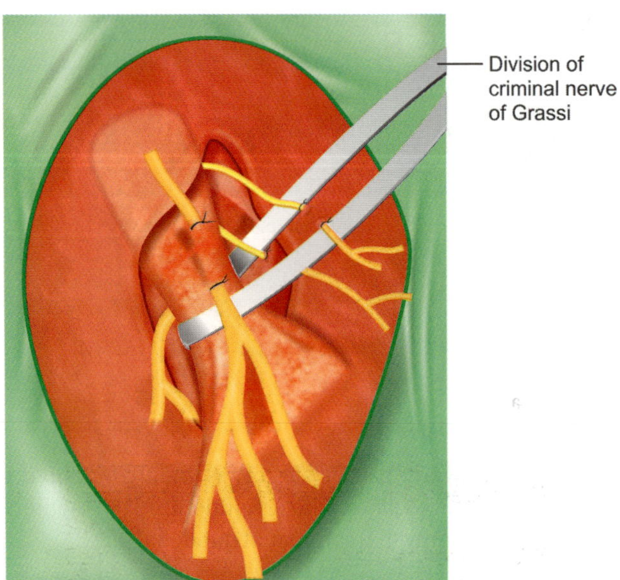

Fig. 40.4 Anterior truncal vagotomy

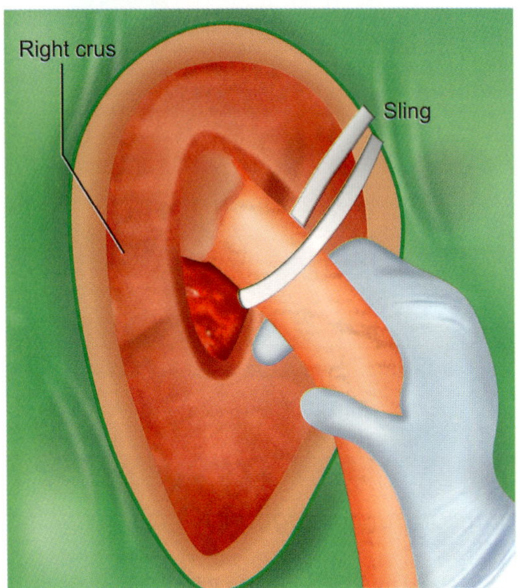

Fig. 40.3 Mobilization of esophagus

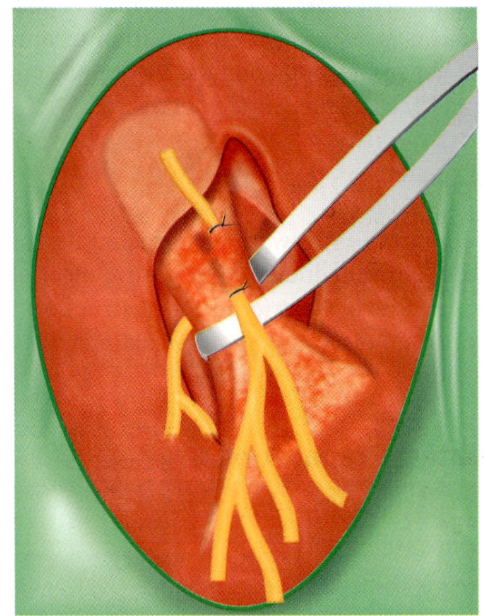

Fig. 40.5 Posterior truncal vagotomy

Anterior (Left) Truncal Vagotomy (Fig. 40.4)

The left or anterior vagal trunk (one or more) lies on the anterior wall of the esophagus. The nerve is separated by a hook or hemostat and divided between long hemostatic forceps. Remove a segment (3–4 cm) of the nerve and tie the ends with catgut to secure hemostasis.

Posterior (Right) Truncal Vagotomy (Fig. 40.5)

The right vagal trunk (usually single) lies on in loose areolar tissue away from the esophagus posteriorly and can be felt as single cord-like structure when the surgeon's index finger encircles the lower most esophagus posterolaterally. Apply hemostats and remove a segment of the trunk. Ligate the cut ends.

Now search for any residual vagal fibers and remove them. It is crucial to divide the criminal nerve branches of Grassi that usually run on the left side of the esophagus. Carry out selected drainage procedure (pyloroplasty or gastrojejunostomy).

Difficulties

- There may be difficulty in exposure of esophagus and vagal trunks particularly in obese patients.

- Esophageal injury should be detected and repaired by all coats sutures with 2/0 proline.

Closure

Close the abdomen en-masse.

PROXIMAL GASTRIC VAGOTOMY: HIGHLY SELECTIVE VAGOTOMY

Highly selective vagotomy aims to denervate only the acid secreting proximal part of the stomach, leaving the alkali secreting antrum with its muscular pumping action still innervated.

Indications and preoperative preparations are same as those described for truncal vagotomy.

Operative Procedure

The abdomen is opened following the steps described under truncal vagotomy.

Exposure

Occasionally division of left triangular ligament and retraction of left lobe of liver may be required for adequate exposure.

Identification of Right and Left Vagal Trunks

Incise the peritoneum over the abdominal esophagus transversely and dissect anterior 2/3rd of circumference of esophagus. The right (posterior) vagal trunk lies posterior-laterally while the left (anterior) trunk lies over the front of esophagus.

Identification of Crow's Foot

The nerve of Latarjet ends at the level of incisura angularis by dividing into several branches resembling a Crow's foot. Unless the patient is obese, the anterior nerve of Latarjet can be seen clearly some 1–2 cm from lesser curvature of stomach. It fans out into several branches as it approaches the antrum.

Dissection of Anterior Nerve of Latarjet (Fig. 40.6)

After identifying Crow's foot, start dissection just proximal to it, on the anterior aspect of stomach by dividing lesser omentum from lesser curvature. Divide and ligate all blood vessels and nerves accompanying them. Continue dissection of the anterior layer of the lesser omentum until main trunk of the left vagus nerve is reached. The left vagus nerve should be completely separated from the wall of the esophagus for a distance of 6–7 cm above esophagogastric junction.

Dissection of Posterior Nerve of Latarjet (Fig. 40.7)

Enter the lesser sac through the greater omentum and identify posterior nerve of Latarjet and Crow's foot. Preserve the Crow's foot and clamp, divide and ligate the terminal branches of posterior nerve of Latarjet. Continue dissection until the right vagal trunk is identified. Now clear the posterior trunk from posterior surface of lower esophagus. Pay particular attention to the nerve of Grassi, which is a branch posterior vagal trunk.

Closure

Close the abdomen en-masse.

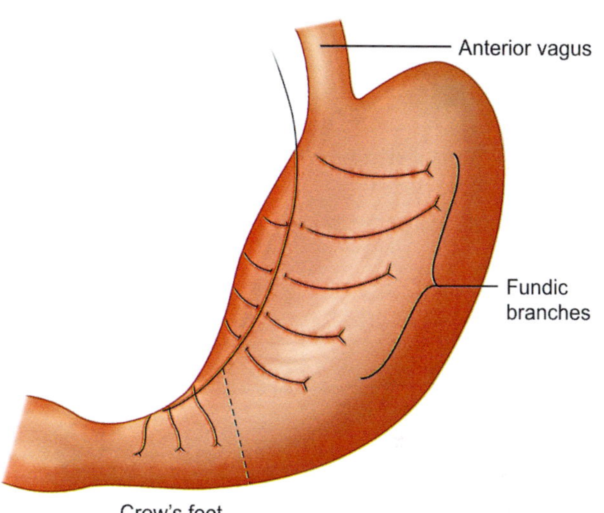

Fig. 40.6 Highly selective vagotomy (anterior)

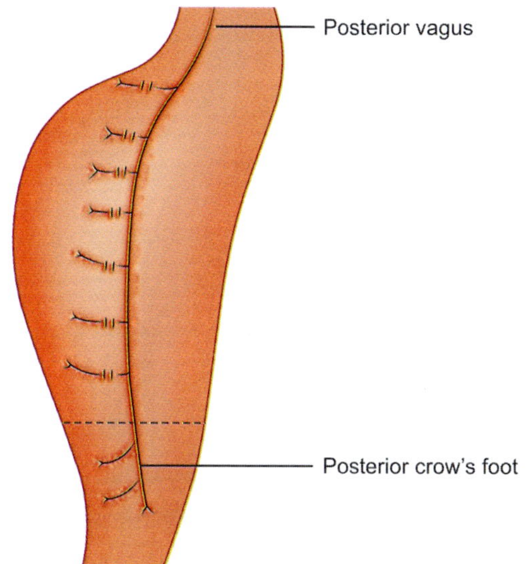

Fig. 40.7 Highly selective vagotomy (posterior)

Postoperative Care

- Intravenous fluid and nasogastric suction is usually continued for 48–72 hours
- Oral liquid is permitted after 48 hours.

Postoperative Complications

- Gastric stasis
- Postvagotomy diarrhea
- Filling of abdominal distensions.

CHAPTER

41

Pyloroplasty: Heineke-Mikulicz Type

Dhiraj Choudhury

Pyloroplasty ensures drainage of gastric antrum following vagotomy.

INDICATIONS

- As a drainage procedure along with truncal vagotomy for duodenal ulcer or gastric ulcer
- Emergency operation for bleeding duodenal ulcer with poor general condition
- The procedure may be used after esophagogastric resection and restoration of esophagogastric continuity.

CONTRAINDICATIONS

Pyloroplasty should be avoided if there is severe scarring and deformity on the duodenal side.

PREOPERATIVE PREPARATIONS

- Nasogastric suction
- Prophylactic antibiotic
- Pyloroplasty carries a low surgical morbidity and mortality rate because of simplicity of procedure.

OPERATIVE PROCEDURE

This procedure is undertaken after completion of truncal vagotomy which has already been described in Chapter 40.

Prepyloric vein of Mayo is the landmark for identification of pylorus.

Kocherization of Duodenum

Mobilize duodenum by Kocher's maneuver by dividing peritoneum lateral to duodenum and carrying finger dissection. This allows good exposure and relaxation of tension on suture line.

Apply two stay sutures one at the upper and one at the lower aspect of pylorus. Prepyloric vein of Mayo helps in identification of pylorus.

Pyloroduodenal Incision

Make a 6–10 cm longitudinal incision across the antrum, pyloric sphincter and proximal duodenum (2.5 duodenal and 3.5 gastric) dividing all coats. Aspirate content: Figure 41.1 shows pyloroduodenal incision, after Kocherization of duodenum. Apply tissue forceps to the wound margins at their centers, and gently draw them apart, so that the wound becomes diamond-shaped (Fig. 41.2). Alternatively, traction on stay sutures draws the longitudinal incision apart until it becomes diamond shaped.

Closure

In original Heineke-Mikulicz pyloroplasty the pyloroduodenotomy was closed transversely in two layers, but in Weinberg's modification, which is favored by the author, closure is done transversely in one layer using interrupted closely placed full thickness sutures using nonabsorbable materials like 2/0 silk or absorbable material like 2/0 vicryl (Fig. 41.3). Palpate the newly formed lumen by invaginating gastric and duodenal walls on each side of the transverse closure with thumb and index finger.

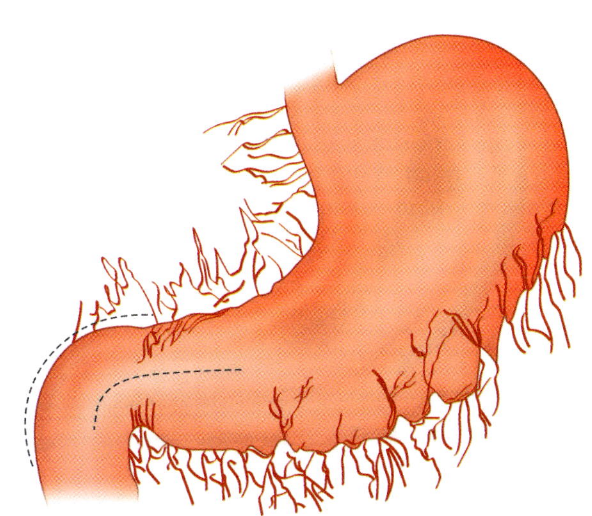

Fig. 41.1 Longitudinal incision

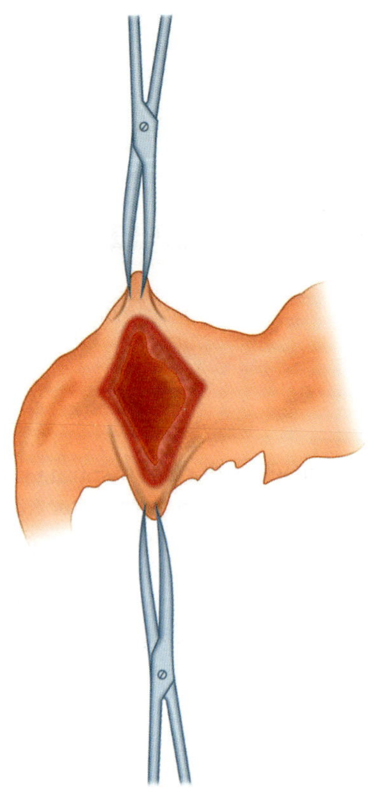

Fig. 41.2 Wound converted to transverse (diamond-shaped one)

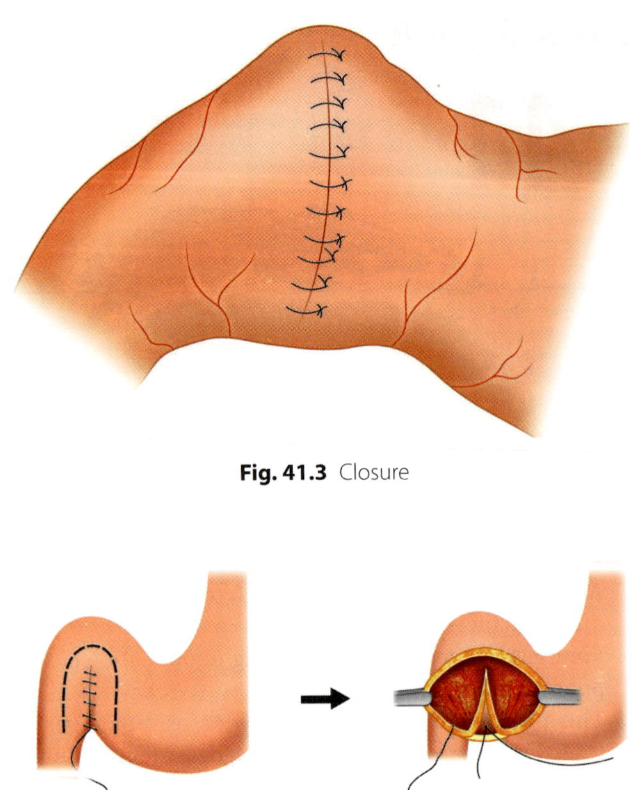

Fig. 41.3 Closure

Fig. 41.4 Pyloroplasty: Finney

FINNEY'S PYLOROPLASTY

This is a gastroduodenostomy done in four layers. In Finney pyloroplasty, gastroduodenal incision is kept close to greater side of stomach.

The pylorus is identified by presence of prepyloric vein. Mobilize pyloric end of stomach first and second part of duodenum by Kocher maneuver. Apply two traction sutures–one on superior margin of midpylorus and other joining pyloric ring on greater curvature of stomach to pyloric ring on duodenal wall.

A U-shaped incision is made into stomach from a point just above the traction suture, through pylorus, down to a similar distance in duodenum. The gastroduodenostomy is done in four layers (Fig. 41.4).

Closure of Abdomen

Abdomen is closed in en-masse.

Postoperative Care

- Nasogastric suction
- Intravenous fluid and electrolytes
- Systemic antibiotic.

Complications

- Hemorrhage
- Afferent loop obstruction.

CHAPTER

42

Gastrojejunostomy

Dhiraj Choudhury

INDICATIONS

- For surgical treatment of chronic duodenal ulcer along with truncal vagotomy
- Pyloric stenosis or gastric outlet obstruction. In elderly patient with low acid value.

PREOPERATIVE PREPARATIONS

In case of gastric outlet obstruction:

- Correction of fluid and electrolyte loss by intravenous administration of fluid and electrolytes
- Nasogastric suction: The stomach should be emptied by gastric lavage, especially if the condition is pyloric stenosis
- Correction of anemia, protein and vitamin deficiency is also important.

OPERATIVE PROCEDURE: POSTERIOR GASTROJEJUNOSTOMY: POSTERIOR, RETROCOLIC, OBLIQUE ISOPERISTALTIC ANASTOMOSIS

Anesthesia—General

The abdomen is opened by midline incision according to steps described under truncal vagotomy in chapter 40.

The transverse colon is turned upwards to expose the transverse mesocolon. A vertical rent is made in the mesocolon with scissors in an avascular area on the left of the middle colic artery.

Bring the dependent part of the posterior wall of stomach to the rent, hold it up by two pairs of Allis tissue forceps. The ligament of Treitz is identified and a loop of jejunum is selected 8–10" from duodenojejunal flexure and hold it by two Allis tissue forceps.

Now, the selected portions of the stomach and jejunum can be placed side-by-side using occlusion clamps, e.g. by twin gastrojejunostomy clamps (Lane) and tissue forceps are removed. The size of the stoma should be 5–6 cm.

The proximal portion of jejunum is anchored to the lesser curvature of the stomach.

To make an anastomosis iso-peristaltic, the afferent loop of jejunum is taken to lie along the distal part of the stomach. By positioning the clamps, the stoma may be made horizontal, vertical or oblique, with very little functional difference, but oblique is generally favored. The clamps and the anastomosis site can be delivered outside the abdomen.

Anastomotic Technique

A side-to-side anastomosis in four layers is carried out:

First Layer

A posterior seromuscular suture (Lembert suture) is made for 6 cm with 2/0 atraumatic catgut, between stomach and jejunum. The short end of the suture is held by a curved forceps (identification) while the long end is preserved for the last layer (Fig. 42.1).

Enterotomy is now made on stomach and jejunum for 5 cm with knife (Fig. 42.2). Cut the bowel wall perpendicular to its surface.

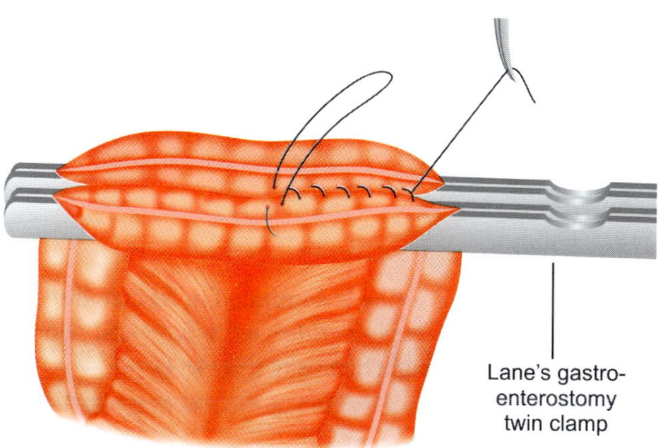

Fig. 42.1 Application of posterior seromuscular suture

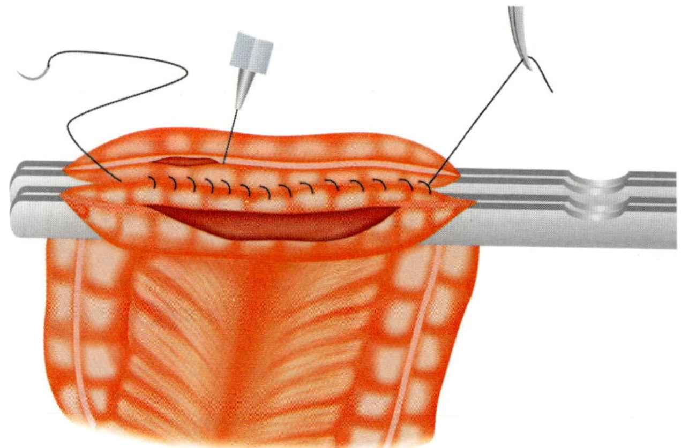

Fig. 42.2 Gastrotomy and enterotomy

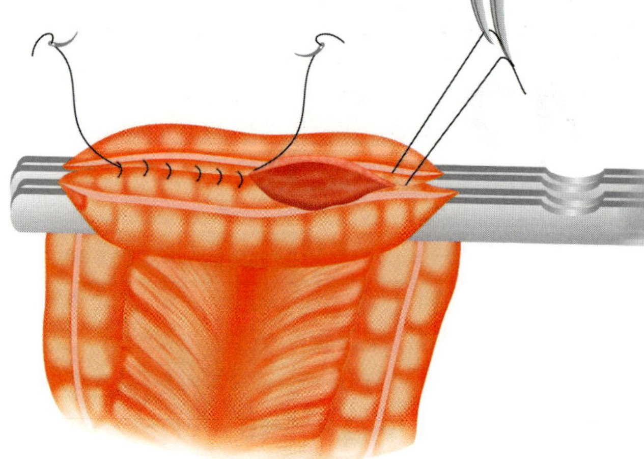

Fig. 42.4 Application of anterior through and through sutures

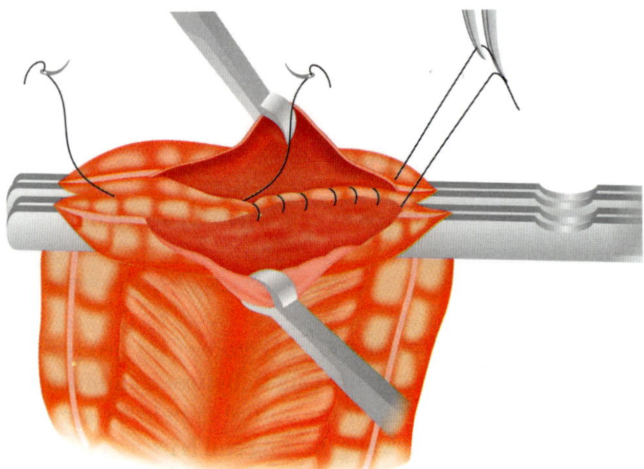

Fig. 42.3 Application of posterior through and through sutures

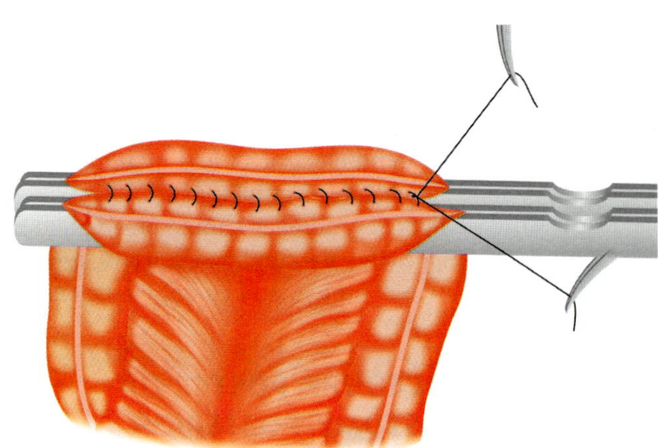

Fig. 42.5 Application of anterior—seromuscular sutures

Second Layer

Posterior through-and-through suture is applied with another 2/0 atraumatic catgut (straight needle is preferred). This is a hemostatic suture and should be locked intermittently and applied with adequate tension. Hold the short end of the suture with a straight hemostat while the long end is used for next layer (Fig. 42.3).

Third Layer

The long end of the suture is continued in reverse direction applying *anterior through-and-through sutures* and tied with short end held by straight hemostat (Fig. 42.4).

Fourth Layer

Apply an *anterior seromuscular suture* with catgut preserved after application of first layer and tie it with short ends of catgut held by curved hemostat (Fig. 42.5).

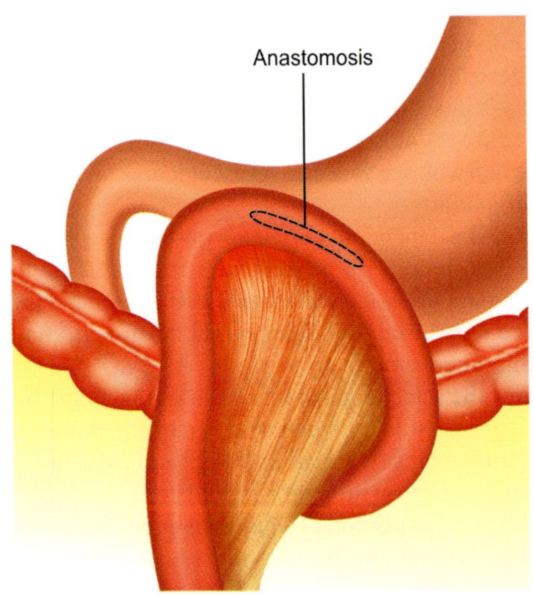

Fig. 42.6 Juxtapyloric anterior gastroenterostomy

Remove clamps and check adequacy of stoma. The jejunum should be anchored to gastric wall for several centimeters on either side of the stoma.

The margins of the rent in mesocolon is stitched to stomach wall by interrupted catgut stitches to prevent internal herniation.

Closure

Transverse colon is put back in its normal position. Abdomen is closed en-masse.

ANTERIOR GASTROJEJUNOSTOMY

This is an anticolic anastomosis which is occasionally indicated for malignant gastric outlet obstruction as a palliative procedure, when posterior gastrojejunostomy is not feasible.

Anterior juxtapylorlic gastrojejunostomy (Fig. 42.6). Recently anterior juxtapyloric gastrojejunostomy is being recommended for benign condition. Choose a fold of anterior wall of the stomach as high as possible when the bypass is done for unresectable distal gastric cancer or as closed to pylorus when the bypass is done for benign pyloric obstruction. A four layers of anastomosis is done.

CHAPTER

43

Partial Gastrectomy

Dhiraj Choudhury

Partial gastrectomy was originally almost accidentally applied to resect a distal gastric carcinoma. Subsequently, it became a popular operative method for treatment of chronic peptic ulcer. But with advent of successful medical treatment, needs of surgery for peptic ulcer has been remarkably gone down.

TYPES

Bilroth I: This was a standard operation for chronic peptic ulcer especially for chronic gastric ulcer until medical treatment became successful. In Bilroth I, duodenum is divided between clamps and distal cut end is kept for anastomosis. The distal stomach is excised and removed (Fig. 43.1A). Part of the cut end of stomach is closed by two layers of sutures to create a lesser curvature. Gastroduodenostomy is done to establish continuity between stomach and duodenum (Fig. 43.1B). It maintains normal pathway for transit of food.

Bilroth II: In this operation, distal two-thirds of the stomach is removed. The duodenal stump is closed. The cut end of the stomach is anastomosed to a loop of jejunum.

Polya gastrectomy: It is closely related to Bilroth II gastrectomy (Fig. 43.2). The standard partial gastrectomy is a polya gastrectomy with valvular anastomosis (small stoma) devised by Finsterer.

STEPS

Anesthesia general with endotracheal intubation.

Position supine

Incision midline incision starting from above umbilicus.

Exploration on opening abdomen examine stomach, duodenum to confirm diagnosis and asses strategy.

Mobilization of stomach and duodenum the gastrocolic ligament is divided along greater curvature of the stomach dividing and ligating the contained blood vessels, extend the dissection on the left up to and including the main left gastroepiploic vessels as they lie near the inferior border of the pylorus. Now, clamp, divide and ligate the right gastric vessels after proper identification. Divide the lesser omentum. Free the first 1–2 cm of duodenum after dividing and ligating small vessels posteriorly.

Section of duodenum: Apply a Payrs clamp across the duodenum just beyond pylorus. A second clamp is applied proximal to this to occlude the stomach. The duodenum is transacted just above the distal Payrs clamp.

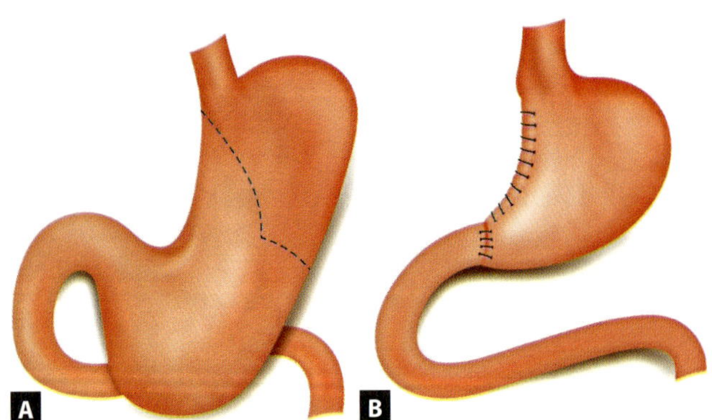

Figs 43.1A and B (A) Billroth I gastrectomy; (B) Gastroduodenostomy

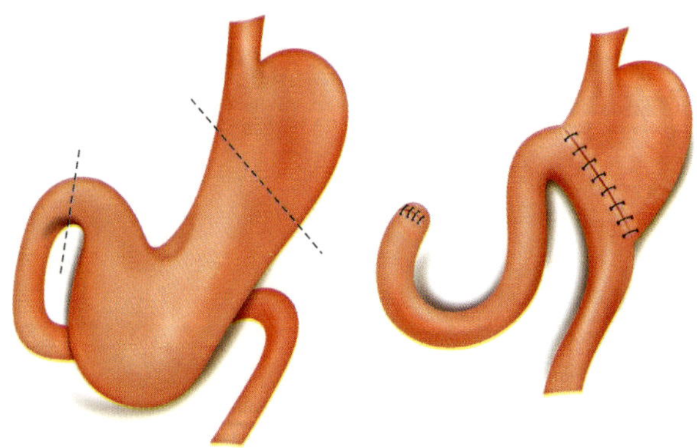

Fig. 43.2 Polya partial gastrectomy

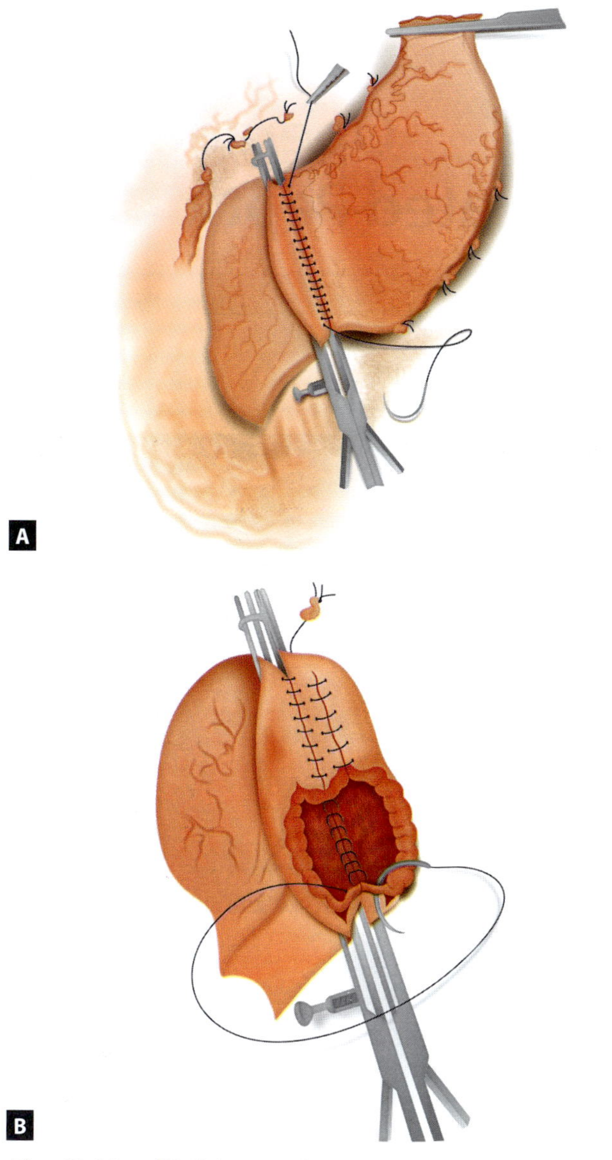

Figs 43.3A and B Polya partial gastrectomy with construction of a retrocolic valvular (short stoma) anastomosis

Closure of duodenum: The duodenal clamp can be closed by a linear stapling device which places a double row of staples across the duodenum. Alternatively, the duodenal stump can be closed with sutures. First apply a running over and over stitch that encircles the clamp and enclosed the crushed duodenum. Gently ease out the clamp and tightening the stitches at the same time. A second invaginating seromuscular suture is now applied.

Transection of stomach and anastomosis: Elevate the pylorus to exert little tension on the left gastric vessels. Identify the vessels, doubly clamp, divide and ligate them.

Select the line of transection of the stomach. Both curvatures of stomach should be free of omentum at the site of anastomosis.

The proximal loop of jejnum is brought through transverse mesocolon and placed along the stomach with afferent loop to lesser curvature. A light occlusion clamp is placed across the stomach proximal to the level of section and a similar clamp is applied to selected length of jejunum. Lock the clamps. A continuous seromuscular stitch is applied to unite the adjacent, surfaces of the two viscera.

A crushing clamp is applied to stomach 1 cm distal to suture line. The stomach is transacted.

Valvular anastomosis: The jejunum is incised for 3–4 cm opposite the lower part of the cut of the stomach. The upper part of the open stomach is closed by through-and-through sutures. The lower 4 cm of the stomach is anastomosed to open jejunum (Figs 43.3A and B).

Staple anastomosis: A long stapling device is placed across the stomach at the proposed line of section and distal stomach is cut off. A proximal loop of jejunum is brought up and sutured to posterior wall of the stomach above the staple line, make a stab wound in the greater curve aspect of the posterior wall of the stomach 2 cm proximal to suture line and make a matching stab wound in the jejunum at the origin of the afferent loop. Two limbs of the stapler are inserted separately into the holes with tips pointing to lesser curve. Lock the two limbs together and actuate the instrument. Four lines of staples will have united stomach and jejunum and knife will have cut the stoma between the center rows of staples.

CHAPTER

44

Operation for Perforated Peptic Ulcer

Dhiraj Choudhury

INDICATION

Perforated gastric or duodenal ulcer is a surgical emergency and better treated by operation. Conservative treatment may be advised if there is improvement of abdominal symptoms and signs (sealed perforation). The choice for closure of perforation versus definitive procedure for ulcer depends on assessment of risk factors by surgeon and experience of the surgeon.

PREOPERATIVE PREPARATIONS

- Nasogastric suction
- Intravenous fluid and electrolytes
- Systemic antibiotic by parental route.

OPERATIVE PROCEDURE

Position: The patient is placed in supine position.

Anesthesia: General anesthesia with endotracheal intubation is used.

Incision: The abdomen is opened by upper midline incision (Figs 44.1 and 44.2).

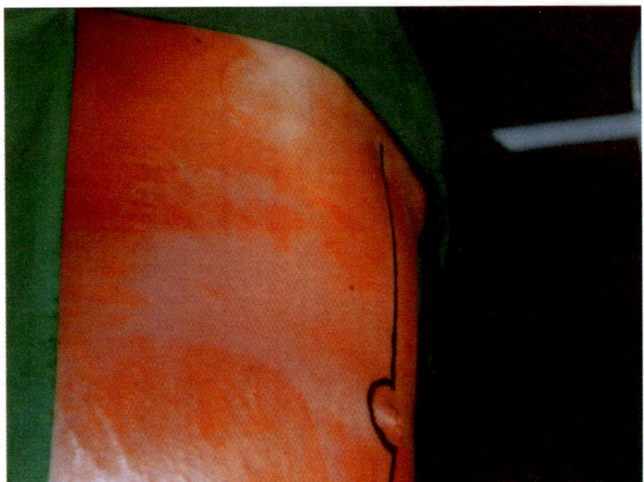

Fig. 44.1 Skin incision (marking)

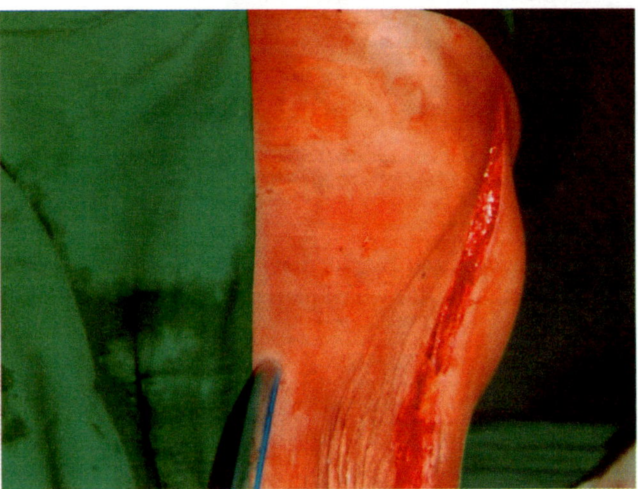

Fig. 44.2 Skin incision applied

Exploration

Escape of gas and bile-stained fluid on opening peritoneum indicates perforated duodenal ulcer. Retraction of liver will expose most frequent sites of perforation. The site may be walled off with omentum.

Peritoneal Toilet

The most important step of operation is thorough peritoneal toilet to remove all the fluid and food debris. A sample of fluid is sent for pathological examination.

Identification of Site of Perforation

Search the first part of duodenum, lesser curvature of stomach for the localization of site of perforation which is commonly anteriorly placed. Posterior perforation which is relatively uncommon can be diagnosed through lesser sac by opening lesser omentum. If searching does not reveal any perforation in stomach and duodenum, explore the whole abdomen particularly gallbladder and colon.

Simple Closure of Perforation

Apply three interrupted stitches with 2/0 vicryl or chromic catgut through the perforated site to close the rent. It is important that the sutures should include sufficient tissue to allow the margins to be approximated without cutting through and should not be tightened too much to prevent tear out. Place each suture in the long axis of the gut to prevent narrowing (Figs 44.3 to 44.5).

Omentoplasty

The closure is reinforced with omentum. Apply a viable segment of omentum over the perforation site and tie the sutures over the plug of omentum (Fig. 44.6). Omentoplasty is presented in Figures 44.7 and 44.8 showing closure of perforation (duodenal and gastric) as schematic diagrams.

Other Procedures

- Vagotomy and pyloroplasty for an early perforated duodenal ulcer in a good risk patient is preferred by some surgeons.
- In case of perforated gastric ulcer, biopsy specimen should be removed before closure of the perforation. Large perforation is better treated by partial gastrectomy if the condition permits and the surgeon is experienced.
- With the advent of effective medical treatment truncal vagotomy and pyloroplasty, is usually not done nowadays.
- In presence of perforation of an obvious cancer, it is safer to close perforation followed by radical surgery after recovery. In good risk patient, an experienced surgeon can undertake immediate resection.

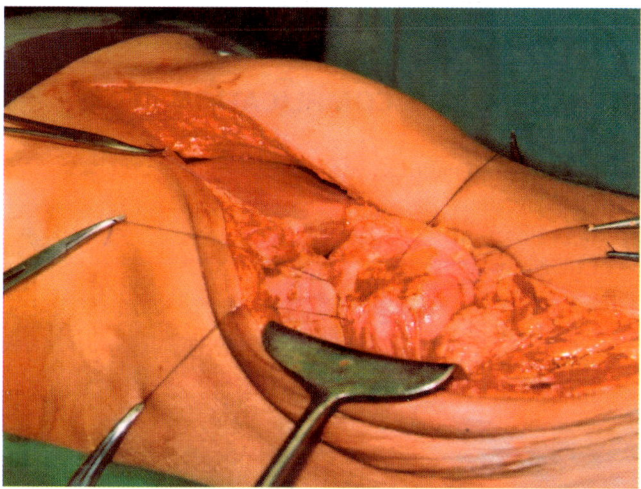

Fig. 44.3 Interrupted sutures applied

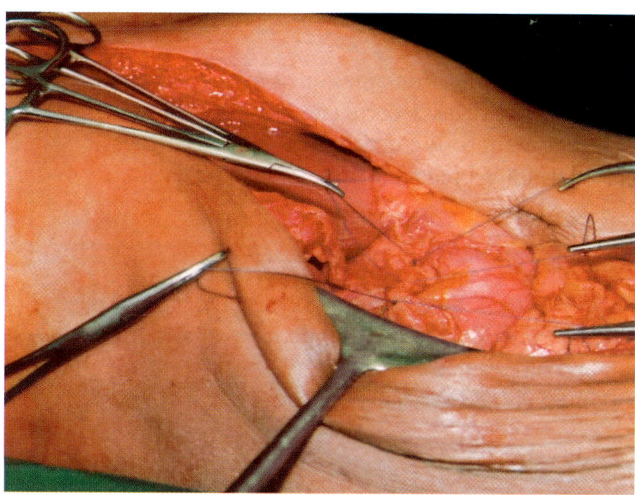

Fig. 44.5 Suture tied

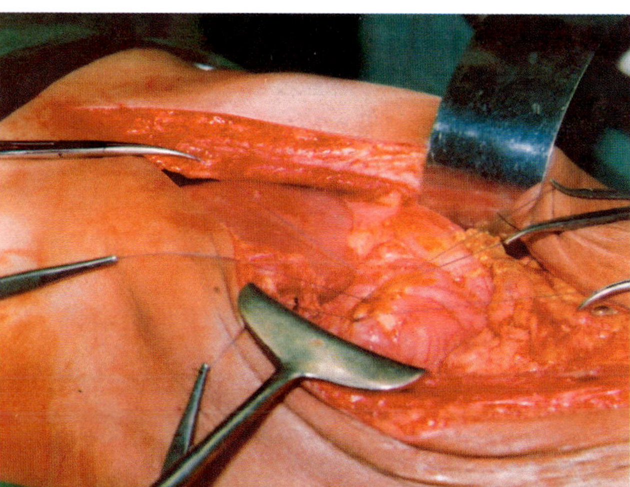

Fig. 44.4 Sutures tied

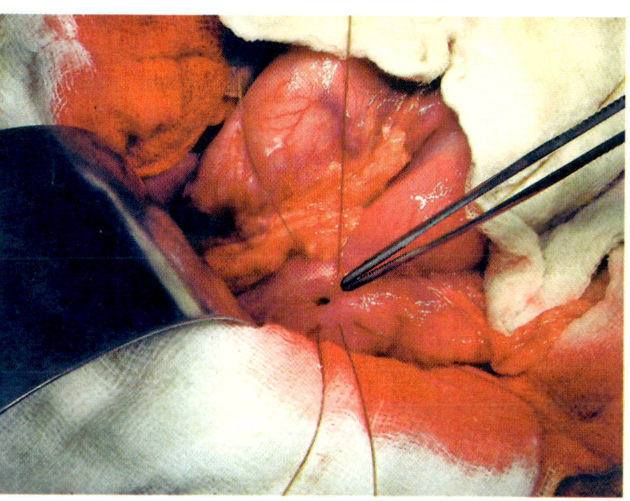

Fig. 44.6 Omentoplasty

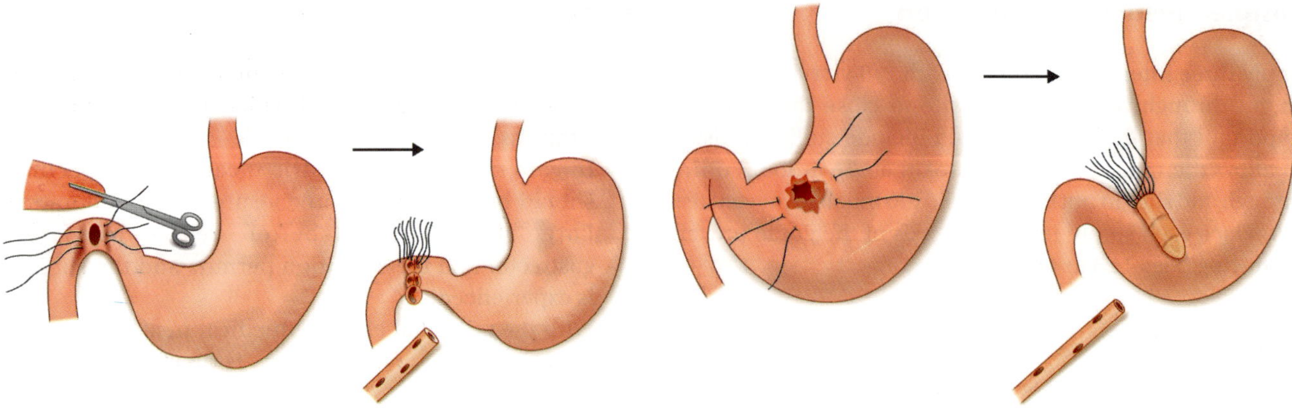

Fig. 44.7 Closure of duodenum perforation (schematic diagram)

Fig. 44.8 Closure of gastric perforation (schematic diagram)

Closure

Aspirate the collection areas once more, particularly above and below the liver. A corrugated rubber drain is inserted in upper abdomen. The abdomen is closed en-masse. Skin is closed by interrupted ethilon stitches.

POSTOPERATIVE CARE

- Continue IV fluid and electrolytes until flatus is passed
- Nasogastric suction, till stomach is emptying satisfactorily
- Systemic antibiotic
- Intravenous H_2 receptor antagonist
- Remove drain after 72 hours
- Chest physiotherapy.

POSTOPERATIVE COMPLICATIONS

Early

- Chest complications
- Paralytic ileus
- Reperforation
- Chest physiotherapy.

Late

- Recurrent ulcer
- Intestinal obstruction adhesive
- Incisional hernia.

CHAPTER

45

Operation for Bleeding Peptic Ulcer

Dhiraj Choudhury

INDICATIONS

- Severe hemorrhage despite adequate conservative measures
- Continued bleeding with loss of one half or more of the estimated blood volume
- Significant rebleed or repeated hospitalization for bleeding
- Endoscopy suggests presence of a visible artery in base of the ulcer
- A patient requiring more than 6 units of blood generally needs operation

The type of operation depends on the age and condition of the patient, size location and bleeding rate of the ulcer.

PREOPERATIVE PREPARATIONS

- Arrange for blood transfusions
- Intravenous omeprazol or proton pump inhibitor
- Endoscopy to assess the cause, site, state and number of lesions.

OPERATIVE PROCEDURE

- *Position:* The patient is placed in supine position.
- *Anesthesis:* General anesthesia with endotracheal intubation is used.
- *Incision:* The abdomen is opened by upper midline incision.

Exposure

Bleeding duodenal ulcer: The most common site of bleeding from peptic ulcer is first part of duodenum, which should be freed from peritoneum by giving incision on its margin (Kocherization) (Fig. 45.1).

Technique

Although suture ligation of the bleeding artery is the mainstay of successful treatment, in most patients truncal vagotomy and pyloroplasty can be done. This is quick, easy and often life-saving.

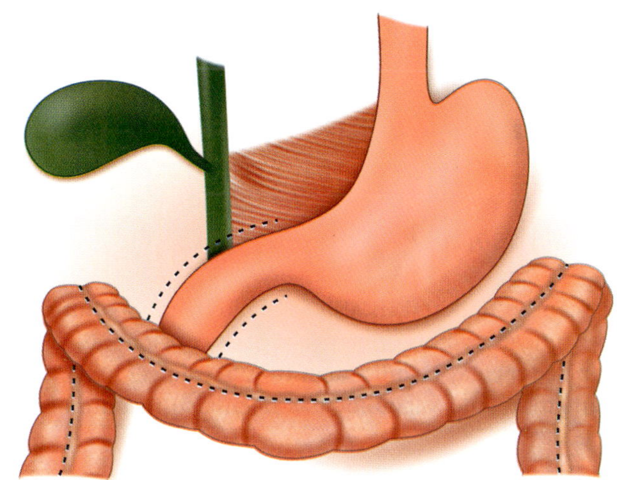

Fig. 45.1 Kocherization

Pyloroduodenotomy

Open the pylorus and duodenum by a longitudinal incision. The bleeding ulcer can be found posteriorly or superiorly. Aspirate the blood to localize the point of bleeding.

Under-running

The bleeding can be controlled by applying well-placed sutures with 0 chromic catgut which underrun the vessel. Carefully insert stitches 0 atraumatic catgut placed transversely to include the artery. Check hemostasis (Fig. 45.2).

Pyloroplasty

The pyloroduodenotomy is closed transversely with interrupted full-thickness sutures using 2/0 atraumatic silk. If pyloroplasty is considered difficult due to scarring then duodenotomy may be closed longitudinally to be followed by gastrojejunostomy.

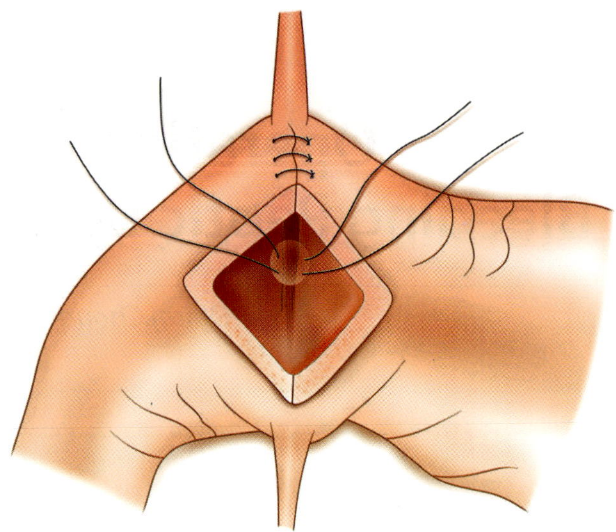

Fig. 45.2 Under-running of bleeding ulcer and pyloroplasty

Truncal Vagotomy

This can be undertaken also in elderly patients but even after truncal vagotomy and pyloroplasty postoperative rate of rebleeding may be more than 10%. In younger fit patients, anterectomy and vagotomy has been also recommended to minimize postoperative rebleeding but this is relatively extensive procedure.

Bleeding Gastric Ulcer

Distal gastrectomy including the ulcer site is the operation of choice if the patient is fit. Underrunning of the bleeding artery with sutures and biopsy from the ulcer may be the minimal procedure but has higher rebleeding rate.

Rarely gastrinoma may be the cause of bleeding peptic ulcer in which case total gastrectomy should be done.

Gastrectomy has high mortality rate.

Closure

Abdomen is closed en-masse.

POSTOPERATIVE CARE

- Continue intravenous fluid and nasogastric suction until the patient is stable
- Administer systemic antibiotic
- Administer intravenous proton pump inhibitor
- Chest physiotherapy.

POSTOPERATIVE COMPLICATIONS

- Hemorrhage
- Pulmonary complications.

CHAPTER

46

Radical Gastrectomy

Parul Shukla

RADICAL TOTAL GASTRECTOMY

Indications

Carcinoma of the proximal body and fundus of the stomach.

Total gastrectomy is also indicated in patients who have tumors, which infiltrate radially into the submucosal planes (linitis plastica).

Anesthesia

General anesthesia with epidural analgesia is preferred.

Position

The patient is placed in a supine position.

Incision

A midline supraumbilical incision provides excellent exposure of the upper abdomen for the surgery. Placement of abdominal self-retaining retractors (Balfour) and use of the Thomson or the Lloyd-Davies retractors will aid in exposure obtained.

Procedure

- Abdomen is opened in the routine manner. An initial inspection and palpation of the liver, parietal and pelvic peritoneum is performed to rule out metastatic disease. Any suspicious nodule should be biopsied and a frozen section diagnosis is obtained.
- Local operability is assessed by opening the lesser sac through a small window made in the gastrocolic omentum. This maneuver enables us to ensure that the major vessels, root of the mesentery, mesocolon and the pancreas are not directly involved by the tumor.
- The greater omentum is now reflected and mobilized from its attachment on the transverse colon and completely separated from the transverse mesocolon till the anterior surface of the pancreas.
- This separation of the anterior leaf of the omentum is continued till the first part of the duodenum on the right side. The right gastroepiploic artery is identified as it arises from the gastroduodenal artery. The right gastroepiploic artery and vein are ligated and divided. Subpyloric lymph nodes are excised along with these vessels.
- The left gastroepiploic artery is now identified and ligated on the left side as it originates from the splenic artery. All the short gastric vessels are serially ligated and divided, taking care to preserve the spleen.
- The gastrohepatic omentum is incised as close to the liver as possible. The right gastric vessels are now ligated and divided.
- Distal division of the stomach is done at the pyloroduodenal junction.
- The stomach is now lifted off the pancreas and the rest of the structures in the stomach bed and the left gastric pedicle can be easily identified. The vessels are skeletonized and all lymphatic tissue around them is dissected and the artery and vein are ligated and divided.
- *Radical lymphadenectomy* is now begun by incising the fascia on the anterior capsule of the pancreas near its superior border. The origin of the splenic artery is identified and all nodal tissue along this vessel is dissected. Lymph nodal tissue surrounding the common hepatic artery is now dissected off by incising the fascia along the superior border of the pancreas and reflecting it upwards over the artery. This dissection begins on the right side exposing the origin of the gastroduodenal artery and continues left-wards till the junction of the hepatic, splenic and left gastric arteries.
- The gastroesophageal junction is cleared on the left side by careful dissection around the hiatus and the crus of the diaphragm.
- The stomach is divided at the cardia end and lifted off its bed.
- Reconstruction (Fig. 46.1).
- Roux-en-Y loop of the jejunum brought up through a window in the transverse mesocolon.

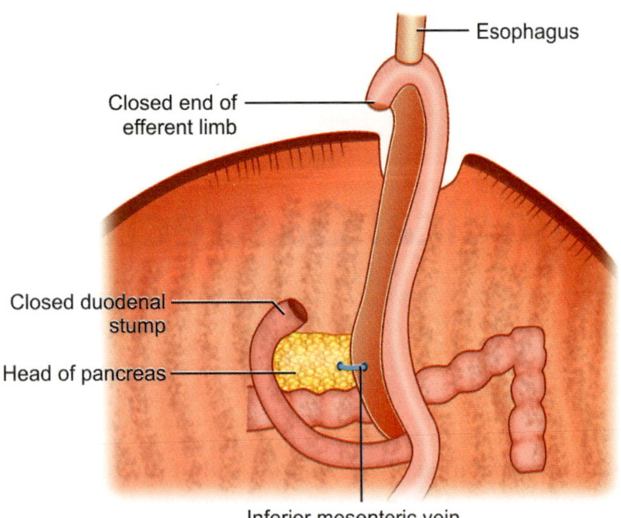

Fig. 46.1 Radical total gastrectomy

- Single layered esophagojejunal anastomosis is performed with absorbable suture material like 3-0 vicryl/*I* PDS to reestablish the continuity of the GI tract. Alternatively, a stapler can be used for the anastomosis.
- Feeding jejunostomy is done to start early enteral feeds.

Two tube drains are placed—one near the duodenal stump and other near the anastomosis.

After confirming complete hemostasis, the abdomen is closed in the usual fashion.

DISTAL RADICAL GASTRECTOMY

Indications

Carcinoma of the gastric pylorus, antrum and the distal third of the body of the stomach.

Anesthesia

General anesthesia with epidural analgesia is preferred.

Position

The patient is placed in a supine position.

Incision

A midline supraumbilical incision provides excellent exposure of the upper abdomen for the surgery. Placement of abdominal self-retaining retractors (Balfour) and use of the Thomson or the Lloyd-Davies retractors will aid in exposure obtained.

Procedure

- The abdomen is opened in layers. The liver is palpated to rule out metastatic disease. A careful examination is made for ascertaining that there are no peritoneal deposits along the parietal walls and in the pelvis. The local operability of the tumor is assessed by making a small opening in the gastrocolic ligament providing access to the posterior wall of the stomach and ensuring that the tumor is free from the pancreas.
- The greater omentum is now reflected from its colonic attachment and lesser sac is completely opened. The omentum is dissected from the transverse measocolon carefully till the anterior surface of the pancreas. This dissection continues till the 1st part of the duodenum. The right gastroepiploic artery is identified here as it takes origin from the gastroduodenal artery. The right gastroepiploic artery and vein are ligated and divided at their origin along with nodes in the subpyloric region.
- The gastrohepatic omentum is now incised as close to the inferior surface of the liver as possible. The whole of the lesser omentum is reflected downwards from the cardiac end of the stomach till the line of division of the stomach. This bares the whole of the lesser curvature of the stomach and ensures complete removal of the right paracardiac and lesser curvature nodes.
- The right gastric leash of vessels is now completely dissected and ligated and divided. The suprapyloric nodes are cleared during this dissection.
- The left gastroepiploic pedicle is ligated and divided, along with nodal tissue on the greater curve.
- By reflecting the stomach upwards and anteriorly, the left gastric pedicle comes into view. The artery and the vein are skeletonized, doubly ligated and divided at the origin.
- Radical lymphadenectomy is now begun by incising the fascia on the anterior capsule of the pancreas near its superior border. The origin of the splenic artery is identified and all nodal tissue along this vessel is dissected. Lymph nodal tissue surrounding the common hepatic artery is now dissected off by incising the fascia along the superior border of the pancreas and reflecting it upwards over the artery. This dissection begins on the right side exposing the origin of the gastroduodenal artery and continues leftwards till the celiac trunk. All nodes along the celiac axis are also excised (Fig. 46.2).
- Stomach is divided distally at the pyloroduodenal junction. This can be easily achieved with the help of a linear cutter stapler. The greater omentum is divided about 5 cm proximal to the proximal limit of the tumor. The proximal division of the stomach proceeds at a distance of 5 cm proximal to tumor.

Reconstruction

A polytype retrocolic loop gastrojejunostomy may be done in 2 layers with 3-0 silk and 3-0 vicryl or PDS to reestablish the continuity of the GI tract. The other option is to perform a Roux-en-Y gastrojejunostomy.

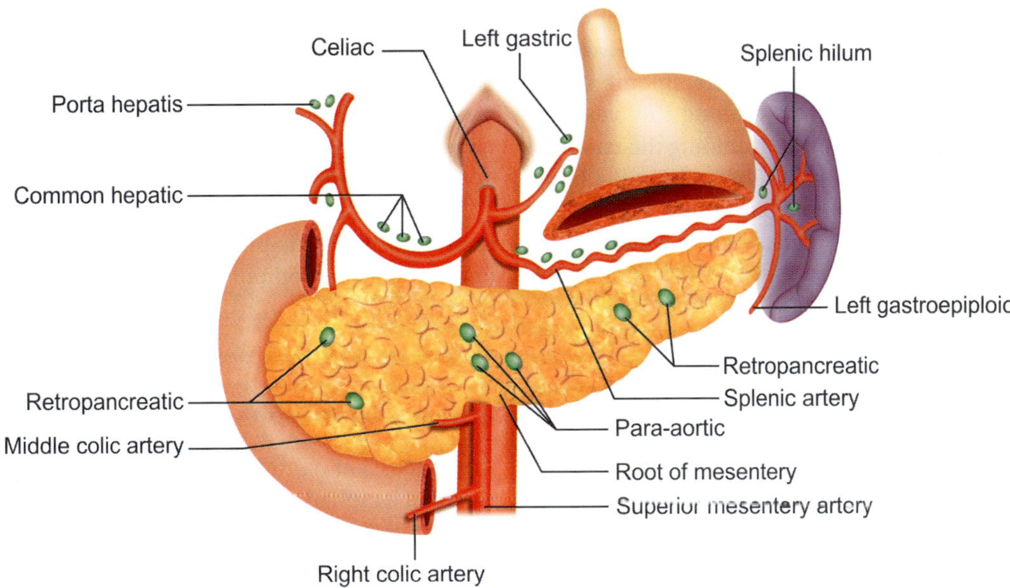

Fig. 46.2 Lymph nodes likely to be involved by gastric carcinoma

A nasojejunal tube (12 fr)/feeding jejunostomy tube may be passed for enteral feeding in the early postoperative period.

Two tube drains of 32 fr are placed. One is positioned at the duodenal stump and the second near the GJ anastomosis.

PROXIMAL RADICAL GASTRECTOMY WITH PARTIAL ESOPHAGECTOMY

Indications

This surgery is performed for adenocarcinoma of the lower end of the esophagus, the CO junction and the proximal part of body and fundus of the stomach.

Anesthesia

General anesthesia with epidural analgesia.

Patient Position

The patient is placed in a semilateral (at about 45° with the horizontal) position with the left side upwards.

Incision

- An oblique left abdominothoracic incision is taken through the 6th or 7th intercostal space depending on the proximal extent of the disease and provides excellent exposure to the lower thoracic esophagus and the stomach.
- Only the abdominal part of the incision is initially taken. This extends from the costal margin to the midpoint between the xiphisternum and the umbilicus. The abdomen is opened and the operability of the tumor is assessed. If the tumor appears to be locally resectable without any obviously palpable liver metastases or peritoneal nodules, the incision is extended into the appropriate intercostal space (usually the 7th) upto the erector spinae muscle with a radial incision to open the diaphragm.

Procedure

- After opening the thorax and the abdomen, self retaining retractors are placed to optimize the exposure. The greater omentum is now reflected completely along its attachment to the transverse colon thereby gaining access to the lesser sac. This dissection proceeds through the avascular fibero-fatty plane along the line of attachment of the greater omentum.
- The stomach is then retracted anteriorly exposing its posterior surface and with careful dissection along the greater curvature all the short gastric arteries are ligated and divided. The left gastroepiploic artery arising from the splenic artery is then doubly ligated and divided. The stomach is thus dissected completely off its bed and away from the pancreas.
- This exposes the left gastric pedicle. The left gastric artery and vein are skeletonized with sharp dissection using either diathermy or scissors and are carefully ligated and divided.

- *Radical lymphadenectomy* is now begun by incising the fascia on the anterior capsule of the pancreas near its superior border. The origin of the splenic artery is identified and all nodal tissue along this vessel is dissected. Lymph nodal tissue surrounding the common hepatic artery is now dissected off by incising the fascia along the superior border of the pancreas and reflecting it upwards over the artery. This dissection begins on the right side exposing the origin of the gastroduodenal artery and continues left-wards till the celiac trunk. All nodes along the celiac axis are also excised. The gastrohepatic omentum is then incised close to the surface of the liver. The lesser omentum is reflected completely onto the lesser curvature.
- The greater omentum is detached 5 cm distal to the tumor.
- The thoracic esophagus is then mobilized and dissected off the aorta and the right pleura. Direct branches from the aorta supplying the esophagus have to be carefully identified and ligated during this part of the dissection. The esophagus is mobilized up to the inferior pulmonary vein and is divided 5 cm proximal to the tumor after securing 2 stay sutures. The stomach is divided 5 cm distal to the tumor along with the whole of the lesser curvature using a linear cutter stapler to prepare a stomach tube.

Reconstruction

Gastroesophageal anastomosis (end-to-side! end-to-end) is completed with the help of either a stapler (usually 25/29 mm*)* or a hand-sewn single layer anastomosis is performed with a absorbable suture material like 3-0 vicryl/PDS.

A *feeding jejunostomy* is performed for early enteral feeds.

A 32 fr tube drain is placed in the thoracic cavity near the anastomosis. The diaphragm is then carefully approximated and sutured. The abdominal and thoracic incisions are closed in a layered fashion, using nonabsorbable monofilament suture.

Editor's Comments

Any discussion on radical gastrectomy invariable starts with extent of lymphatic dissection.

D1 dissection includes removal of N1 group of nodes (1-6) while lymph node stations 7-11 (N2 group), greater and lesser omenta, spleen and distal pancreas is included in D2 gastrectomy. D2 gastrectomy has higher mortality rate than D1 gastrectomy.

For operable gastric cancer, radical gastrectomy remains the initial treatment of choice. Although, there is controversy regarding extent of lymphnode dissection, there is general consensus in performing D2 dissection but with preservation of pancreas and spleen.

CHAPTER

47

Bariatric Surgery

Dhiraj Choudhury

Bariatric or obesity surgery is indicated for certain patients with morbid obesity.

INDICATIONS

The criteria for obesity surgery has been advocated by National Institute for Health and Care Excellence (NICE). It includes:

- BMI (Body mass index) more than 40
- BMI 35–40 with obesity related comorbidity
- Age 18–65 years
- Obesity for more than 5 years
- Failed nonsurgical treatment for weight loss
- Severe obesity where lifestyle measures and medical treatment has not been successful.

CONTRAINDICATIONS

- Presence of inflammatory bowel disease
- Chronic pancreatitis
- Cirrhosis of liver
- Drug or alcohol abuse
- Psychiatric problems.

PREOPERATIVE PREPARATIONS

- Multidisciplinary assessment of patient
- Investigation
- Full blood count (FBC)
- Urea creatinine
- Liver function tests
- Lipid profile estimation of iron, B_{12}, folate.

TYPES OF SURGERY

- *Purely restrictive operations*
  - Vertical banded gastroplasty (VBG)
  - Adjustable gastric banding
  - Sleeve gastrectomy
- *Restriction predominant operations*
  - Roux-en-Y gastric bypass (RYGB)
- *Malabsorption predominant operations*
  - Biliopancreatic diversion.

APPROACHES

- Open conventional method
- *Laparoscopic method:* It is increasingly getting popular.

TECHNIQUE

Vertical banded gastroplasty (VBG): It consists of fashioning of vertical gastric pouch around 20 mL volume with a synthetic band or ring wrapped around the pouch outlet. It forms a 20 mL reservoir above the restriction (Fig. 47.1) This operation is currently favoured. The site of passage of a ring is created using circular stapler through the stomach. The pouch is then fashioned with a vertical staple line from this point to angle of His. This operation has been almost replaced by adjustable gastric banding (AGB).

Adjustable gastric banding (AGB): Adjustable gastric banding involves application of a rigid band with an inflatable silicone ring on the inside which is connected to a reservoir or a port placed on the abdominal wall or sternum. The band is positioned so as to create a small gastric pouch (volume 20 mL) with an adjustable outlet. The stoma is adjusted to the point where food passage is restricted and slows emptying of the pouch. Result is better than VBG (Fig. 47.1).

LAPAROSCOPIC METHODS

Laparoscopic methods are getting increasingly popular. The two most commonly performed procedures are laparoscopic gastric banding (LABG) and gastric bypass.

Laparoscopic gastric banding (LABG): The LABG is composed of three main parts—a silastic inflatable circular 5 mL balloon, 30 cm of silastic tubing and an access port.

The ends of the balloon are connected by means of self locking mechanism around the cardia of the stomach. The tubing is exteriorized on the abdominal wall and attached

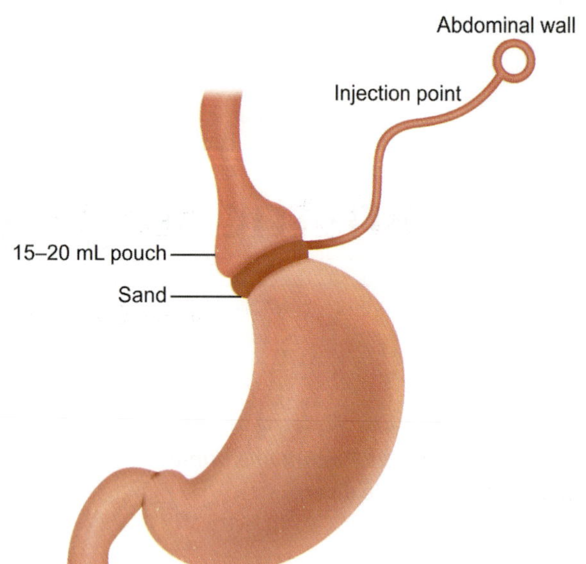

Fig. 47.1 Adjustable gastric band

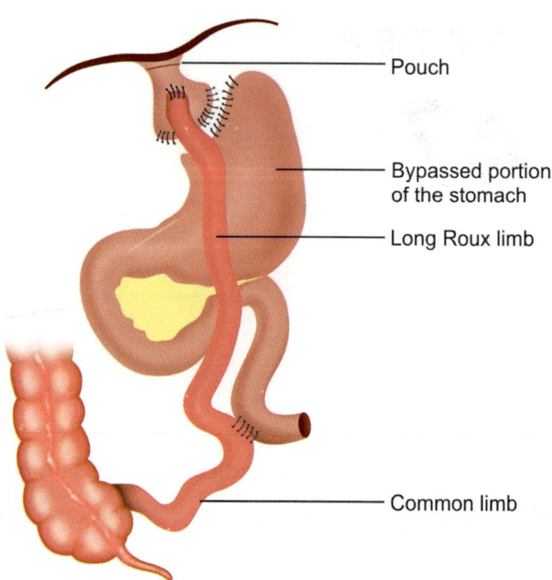

Fig. 47.2 Roux-en-Y gastric bypass

to the access port which is then secured fascia over the left rectus.

The key to successful weight loss after LABG placement is to make periodic adjustments that allow control over the degree of restriction.

Roux-en-Y Gastric Bypass: The operation that has best long-term result is gastric bypass. Using a combination of circular and linear stapler, a gastric pouch is created. The pouch has no connection with rest of the stomach. It is drained by a 70 cm Roux-en-Y loop of jejunum.

Complications: Obesity increase the risk of all types of surgery, particularly chest infection, deep vein thrombosis (DVT) and wound infection.

Gastric bypass involves stapling the stomach, closed a short distance below the esophagogastric junction. A Roux limb is then brought up and anastomosed to the small gastric remnant. Depending on the size of the pouch and calibre of anastomosis there will be a degree restrictive activity. Figure 47.2 shows the Roux-en-Y gastric bypass.

Sleeve gastrectomy: Resect two-thirds of the stomach with the help of a linear cutting stapler. Use of a 56 French bougie passed into stomach by anesthetist as a guide to ensure that the stomach is not too narrow. Figure 47.3 shows sleeve gastrectomy.

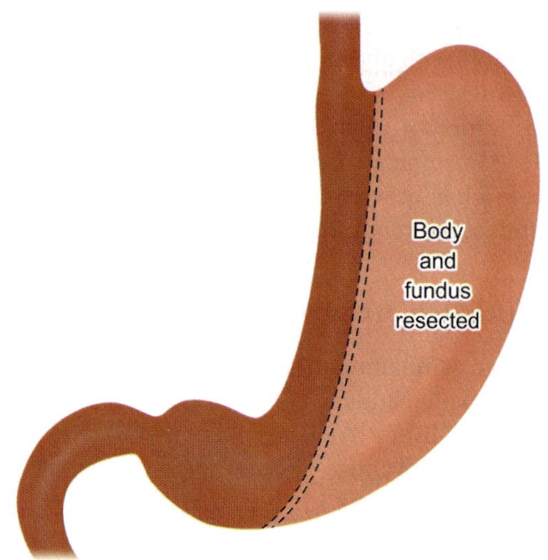

Fig. 47.3 Sleeve gastrectomy

Bilio pancreatic diversion: This consists of significant antrectomy leaving an approximately 200–300 mL gastric pouch. The duodenum is then transacted. Continuity is restored with long alimentary limb which drains the gastric pouch and relatively short common channel through which bile and pancreatic secretion admix with intestinal contents.

SECTION

8

Hepatobiliary Surgery

- **Operative Drainage of Subphrenic Abscess**
  Dhiraj Choudhury
- **Surgery for Liver Infections**
  Dhiraj Choudhury
- **Liver Resection**
  Debasish Banerjee
- **Surgery for Portal Hypertension**
  Debasish Banerjee
- **Cholecystostomy**
  Dhiraj Choudhury
- **Open Cholecystectomy**
  Dhiraj Choudhury
- **Laparoscopic Cholecystectomy**
  Sunanda Roy Mahapatra
- **Surgery of Bile Duct**
  Dipak Kr Ghosh

CHAPTER

48

Operative Drainage of Subphrenic Abscess

Dhiraj Choudhury

ANATOMY OF SUBPHRENIC SPACES (FIG. 48.1)

- Right anterior intraperitoneal space (space of Mitchell) boundary:
  Above—the diaphragm
  Below—opens into right paracolic gutter
  Front—the diaphragm
  Behind—right lobe of liver, gallbladder
  Right—communicated with right posterior space
  Left—falciform ligament
  Source of infection (a) peptic perforation, (b) gallbladder infection.
- Right posterior intraperitoneal space (subhepatic space) boundary:
  Above—the diaphragm, coronary ligament
  Below—opens into paracolic gutter
  Front—inferior surface of right lobe of liver
  Behind—right kidney, right suprarenal
  Right—communicated with right anterior space
  Left—epiploic foramen
  Source of infection (a) duodenal perforation, (b) acute appendicitis.
- Right extraperitoneal space—is a potential space between the diaphragm and bare area of the liver
  Source of infection—liver abscess.
- Left anterior intraperitoneal space:
  Above—the diaphragm
  Below—communicates with general peritoneal cavity
  Front—the diaphragm
  Behind—lesser omentum, stomach
  Right—falciform ligament
  Left—communicates with general peritoneum cavity
  Source of infection—gastric perforation.
- Left posterior intraperitoneal space (lesser sac)
  Above—the diaphragm
  Below—greater omentum
  Front—liver, stomach, lesser omentum
  Behind—diaphragm left kidney, left suprarenal pancreas
  Right—epiploic foramen
  Left—gastrosplenic and lienorenal ligament
  Source of infection—gastric perforation. Collection leads to pseudopancreatic cyst
- Left extraperitoneal space—a potential space containing areolar tissue in the upper posterior part of the liver
  Source of infection—left kidney.

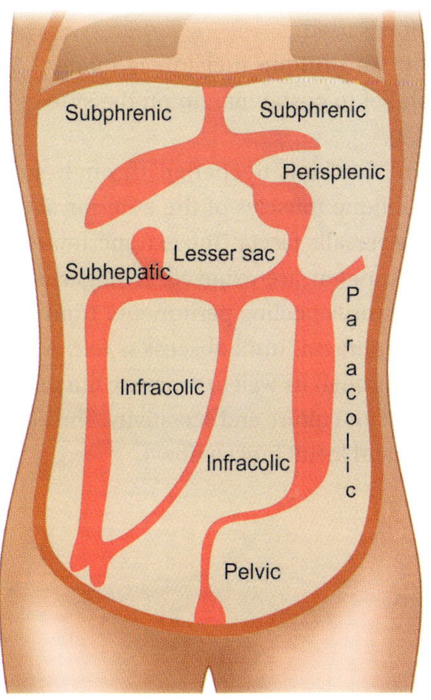

Fig. 48.1 Anatomy of subphrenic spaces

INDICATIONS

Subphrenic abscess is suspected on the basis of a dietum—pus somewhere, pus nowhere, pus under the diaphragm. The most common causes of subphrenic abscess are perforated peptic ulcer, perforation of appendix and acute cholecystitis. Localization of pus can be done by plain X-ray. USG and CT scan, and percutaneous drainage can be attempted under guidance of USG or CT scan. Operative drainage is undertaken when USG or CT-guided percutaneous drainage cannot be safely undertaken or has failed.

OPERATIVE PROCEDURES

Anterior Extraperitoneal Approach for Anterior Abscess

- *Position:* The patient lies in supine position.
- *Anesthesia:* General anesthesia with endotracheal intubation is used.
- *Incision:* An oblique incision is made 2.5 cm below and parallel to costal margin on the side of the abscess (Fig. 48.2).
- *Exposure:* Incision deepened through subcutaneous tissue, oblique muscles of the anterior abdominal wall and transversalis fascia. The extraperitoneal fatty tissue and peritoneum are exposed. A finger is then passed gently upwards peeling peritoneum from under surface of the diaphragm, until abscess is felt. A finger is then inserted through its wall to evacuate the pus. A sample of pus is sent for culture and sensitivity. The opening is then enlarged and loculi broken down.
- *Technique:* When abscess is reached, a finger is inserted through its wall. Pus is evacuated with a sucker. Send a sample of pus for culture and sensitivity. The opening into the abscess is then enlarged and loculi broken (Fig. 48.3).
- *Closure*: Insert a corrugated rubber drain. Close the incision in layers.

Posterior Subpleural Approach for Posterior Abscess

This is suitable for majority of subphrenic abscess locate posteriorly.

- *Position:* The patient is placed in the lateral position.
- *Anesthesia:* General anesthesia with endotracheal intubation is used.
- *Incision:* A transverse incision starting 2.5 cm from midline and extending over or just below 12th rib. An oblique incision is made over the whole length of 12th rib.
- *Exposure:* The incision is deepened through subcutaneous tissue. Divide latissimus dorsi and serratus posterior inferior muscle. The 12th rib is exposed and excised subperiosteally. Its bed is incised transversely at the level of spinous process of the first lumbar vertebra. Divide the fibers of serratus posterior and quadratus lumborum muscles inwards and muscles of 11th intercostal space

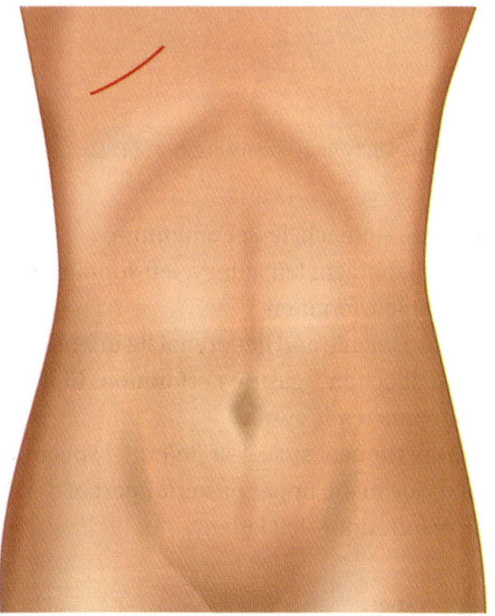

Fig. 48.2 Skin incision for anterior extraperitoneal approach

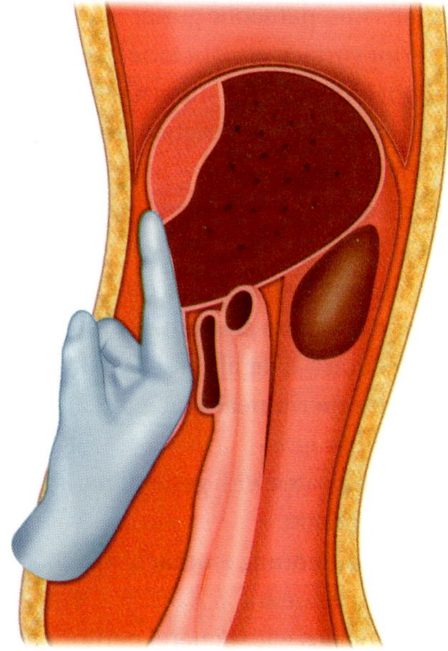

Fig. 48.3 Anterior extraperitoneal approach to site of abscess

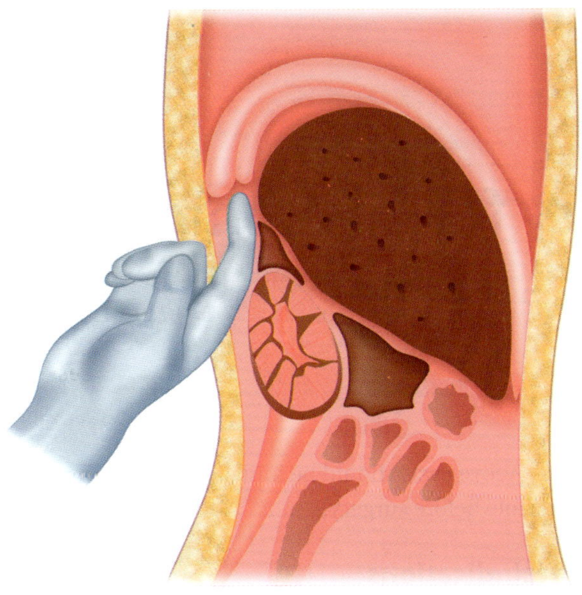

Fig. 48.4 Posterior subpleural approach to site of abscess

outward. This exposes attachment of the diaphragm which is divided.

- *Technique:* The suprahepatic and extraperitoneal spaces on either side are easily explored by passing the fingers upwards under the diaphragm. Any abscess felt is drained (Fig. 48.4).
- *Closure:* Insert a drain and close the incision in layers.

POSTOPERATIVE CARE

- Systemic antibiotic should be administered
- Chest physiotherapy
- Drain is removed if there is no significant drainage.

POSTOPERATIVE COMPLICATIONS

- Pulmonary complications
- Septicemia.

CHAPTER

49

Surgery for Liver Infections

Dhiraj Choudhury

PYOGENIC LIVER ABSCESS

Open surgical drainage may be occasionally required for large pyogenic liver abscess under appropriate antibiotic cover.

Technique

At laparotomy by a subcostal incision, the site of the abscess may be obvious. Sometimes, abscess is located by needle aspiration. The loculi are broken down and a large wide bore drain is inserted and brought out through a separate wound. The pus is sent for culture.

AMEBIC LIVER ABSCESS

Usually abscess can be drained by catheter introduced under CT scan or ultrasound.

Indications for Operative Drainage

Surgical drainage is rarely required for large abscess not suitable for percutaneous needle aspiration, left lobe abscess inaccessible to percutaneous drainage and rupture into peritoneal cavity.

Technique

The abscess is located at laparotomy and drained. The pus resembling anchovy sauce pus is found. A drain is inserted and brought out through a separate wound.

HYDATID CYST OF LIVER

In over 75% of cases, liver is the site of involvement in case of hydatid cyst. Surgery is the curative option. Asymptomatic and inactive cyst may be left alone under USG monitoring of the size. Active cysts should be initially treated by a course of albendazole before surgery.

Contraindications

Surgery is contraindicated at extremes of age, in pregnant women and in patients with extensive or recurrent disease.

TYPES OF OPERATIONS

- *Cystopericystectomy:* Complete excision of the cyst with dissection starting between the pericyst and normal tissue.
- *Ectocystectomy:* The cyst is removed by dissecting between ectocyst and pericyst. It is technically difficult.
- *Endocystectomy:* The plane of dissection is created between endocyst and ectocyst. This is the most commonly performed procedure. Blood loss is considerably less.
- *Liver resection:* This may be indicated for cysts located on the border of liver and for lesions involving left lobe.
- *Liver transplantation*: This may be indicated in extreme cases involving entire liver.

OPERATIVE TECHNIQUE

- *Anesthesia:* General with endotracheal intubation.
- *Incision:* Incision may be right paramedian, upper midline or right thoracoabdominal.
- *Exposure:* On opening abdomen, secure the area around the cyst by any of the following steps:
  - By packing the area around the cyst with packs soaked in silver nitrate (0.5%), or hypertonic saline, or povidone-iodine (1.5%)
  - By use of a plastic drape sutured around the margins of the cyst.
  - The cyst is removed carefully avoiding spillage during surgery.

- *Dealing with residual cavity:* After removal of the hydatid cyst from the liver the residual cavity can be dealt by any of the following methods:
  - Closure of the cavity if the cyst is small
  - Fill the cavity with omental plug. This is the most commonly used method
  - Drainage of the cavity
  - Marsupialization of the cavity.
- *Closure:* Abdomen is closed in layers after securing hemostasis and washing peritoneal cavity with saline.
- Surgical treatment by minimal access therapy consists of puncture, aspiration, injection and reaspiration.

CHAPTER

50

Liver Resection

Debasish Banerjee

INDICATIONS

Malignancy

- *Primary:* Hepatocellular carcinoma, cholangiocarcinoma
- *Secondary:* Colorectal and noncolorectal from any other site.
- *Local invasion:* Gastric, renal, adrenal, colon, gallbladder, hilar cholangiocarcinoma.

Benign

- *Tumors:* Hemangioma, adenoma, cystadenoma, focal nodular hyperplasia
- Trauma
- *Miscellaneous:* Intrahepatic stones, strictures or cysts (polycystic disease, parasitic cysts).

SURGICAL ANATOMY OF THE LIVER

The parenchyma of the liver is divided into 8 segments as described by Couinad, each having independent functional unit. The numbering of the segments starts from caudate lobe (segment 1), proceeds to the right and then turns caudal in a clockwise manner. The left lobe comprises segments 2, 3, 4a and 4b. The right lobe contains segments 5, 6, 7 and 8. American surgeons also describe 4 sectors as follows: Right lateral (segment 6 and 7), Right paramedian (segments 5 and 8), Left paramedian (segments 4a and 4b), left lateral (segment 2 and 3). The attachment of the falciform ligament is between the left lateral and the left paramedian segments (Fig. 50.1).

The hilum of the liver comprises the portal pedicle (common bile duct to the right, hepatic artery to the left and portal vein behind) enclosed in the Glissonian sheath and splitting into right and left branches supplying the corresponding hemilivers (right and left lobes). The two lobes are separated by a sagittal plane corresponding to the cantlie line, which starts in the middle of the gallbladder fossa and extends up to the suprahepatic IVC, slanting to the right. This plane is followed when transecting the liver in a right and left hepatectomy. The right Glissonian pedicle is short (1 to 2 cm) in length. It divides into anterior branch (supplying segments 5 and 8) and inferior branch (supplying segments 6 and 7). The left Glissonian pedicle is longer, runs transversely to the left up to the insertion of the umbilical ligament. Here it turns vertically up and divides into posterolateral branch supplying segment 2, an anterolateral branch supplying segment 3 and a median branch supplying segment 4. The transverse part of the left pedicle, before reaching the umbilical ligament, gives off branches running vertically up to supply the caudate lobe or segment 1.

There are 3 hepatic veins which drain into the IVC just above the liver. The right vein starts between the right lateral and the right paramedian sectors and drains upwards into the suprahepatic inferior vena cava (IVC) after running a short extraparenchymal course. The left hepatic vein runs almost horizontally between the segments 2 and 3 and emerges from

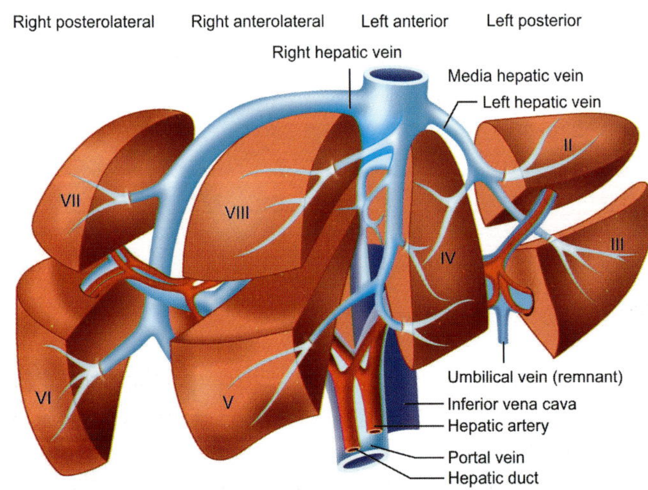

Fig. 50.1 Anatomical segments and sectors of the liver

the parenchyma on the left of the suprahepatic IVC before joining the cava. The middle hepatic vein runs between the right and left paramedian sectors and drains cranially into the left hepatic vein just before it joins the cava.

The double blood supply of the liver by the hepatic artery and portal vein along with the presence of the rich venous network makes the liver highly vascular and the task of resection difficult. However, the resected liver regenerates within weeks of the operation to regain original functional mass.

OPERATIVE APPROACHES TO THE LIVER

Bilateral Subcostal Incision

This is the commonly used approach. The incision is curved, subcostal, convex upwards and usually limited by the mid-axillary lines. The extent of the incision varies according to the portion of the liver planned for removal. A midline vertical extension of the incision from the highest convex point is often employed to excise the xyphoid process. This gives direct and easy access to the suprahepatic IVC and the extrahepatic portions of the hepatic veins. However, the points of meeting for the three divergent incisions in the midline makes it weak and a potential site for leakage of ascites as well as far postoperative hernia. Subcostal incisions also effect respiratory dynamics and associated with atelectasis or pleural effusions.

J Incision

This approach is used for right liver lesions. Incision starts as a midline laparotomy below xiphoid, extends downwards and curves to the right becoming a subcostal incision and finishing below the 10th rib in the posterior axillary line. For left liver resections, a similar incision curving to the left can be used.

Median Laparotomy

This approach is used in emergency trauma. A horizontal T extension can be done, if required. Some surgeons use this approach for left liver lesions.

Thoracoabdominal Approach

With abdominal incisions, exposure, of the subdiaphragmatic region is optimal if table mounted self-retaining retractors (Thompsons system or omnitract) are used for holding the costal margins upwards and outwards. This obviates the need for thoracoabdominal incision which is associated with higher incidence of chest complications.

RIGHT HEPATECTOMY

Resection of right lobe of liver includes segments 5, 6, 7 and 8. This hemiliver is supplied by the right hepatic artery and right branch of portal vein.

A right subcostal incision is used to make an assessment for operability of the tumor. For undertaking liver resection, a full right curved subcostal incision is given starting from right midaxillary line, curving upwards and finishing on the left border of the left rectus muscle. The incision is convex upwards, with the highest point being at midline. From this point a vertically upward midline extension can be used for excising the xiphoid process. The omnitract retractor should be applied for having wide exposure of the subdiaphragmatic region.

Assessment of findings involves noting extent of tumor, diaphragmatic infiltration, peritoneal nodules, hilar lympadenopathy, ascites and any other evidence of extrahepatic disease. Partial infiltration of the diaphragm can be excised en block with the tumor and, therefore, does not indicate inoperability. The gap in the diaphragm can be closed with suture or gortex patch. Ascites, unless proved to be malignant, does not contraindicate resection. Intraoperative ultrasound examination of the liver is essential to rule out left lobe malignancy, if present, makes it inoperable. Ultrasound assessment of the extent of the tumor and its relationship with vascular structures will help plan the resection.

Mobilization of the right liver involves division of the round ligament between silk ties and the falciform ligament with diathermy. The right triangular ligament, enclosing the bare area of the liver is divided with the diathermy from its right border, up to its posterior insertion of the falciform ligament. The inferior ligament is also divided with diathermy (long pencil tip is preferable) helped by elevating and rotating the right lobe to the left by the assistant surgeon. The retroperitoneal bare area of the liver along with the right suprarenal gland is exposed. Tilting the operative table head end up and left side down with additional right and upward traction on the right costal margin will greatly help in undertaking the following steps. Focusing light onto the exposed area is equally important.

The adrenal gland is separated from the liver capsule. Dissection of deeper structures will expose the right adrenal vein and the right edge of the IVC. Further leftward rotation of the right lobe on the IVC along with dissection of tissues on its right border will expose small hepatic veins. These veins drain the liver parenchyma directly into the IVC. These are divided between ligaclips and IVC and transfixed with fine prolene sutures, in order to prevent later slippage. The dorsal ligament of the IVC (avascular connective tissue extending from segment 7 to the caudate lobe and covering the right edge of the IVC) is divided exposing the outlet of the right hepatic vein from the cranial part of the IVC.

Hilar dissection of the liver starts by dissecting the Calot's triangle and dividing the cystic duct. Gallbladder is left in situ. The Glissonian sheath is opened longitudinally. The common bile duct dissected out and looped close to the duodenum. By dissecting out the right border of the common bile duct, the right branch of the hepatic artery is found crossing the common duct either in front or behind, enclosed in lymphatics. Demonstration of pulsation will aid in its identification. The right hepatic artery is followed up to its point of entry into the parenchyma and divided between ties here. This is done to save branches which may arise from it and supply segment 4 or the common bile duct. Next, retraction of the common hepatic duct with the loop interiorly and to the left, combined with division of the posterior layer of the hepatoduodenal ligament will help dissecting out the right portal vein. This is divided between clamps and the ends suture closed with 4-0 prolene. With the division of these structures the right lobe darkens in color and demarcating line appears between the right and the left lobe. The parenchyma is divided along this line. It is not advisable to dissect the right hepatic duct at this stage, as common hepatic duct divides very high up, almost inside the liver parenchyma (Fig. 50.2).

The right hepatic vein is now encircled outside the parenchyma, clamped and divided. Each end is closed with 3-0 prolene sutures. This completes the vascular disconnection of the right hemiliver and, therefore, minimizes blood loss during parenchymal transection. This step may be difficult, especially if the tumor is situated close by. In such cases, division of the right hepatic vein is left till parenchymal transection is completed. The vein is approached intraparenchymally and divided as the last structure.

Transection of the parenchyma is preceded by removing the gallbladder and marking out the demarcating line with cautery. On the inferior surface of the liver, the resection line bisects the bed of the gallbladder. Dissection usually starts at the inferior margin of the liver and proceeds cranially. In the depth of the wound the line of resection should be on the right of the middle hepatic vein, so as not to compromise the venous drainage of segment 4 of the left liver.

Resection of parenchyma is done using different techniques depending on available equipment and expertise. Cavitron Ultrasonic Surgical Aspirator (CUSA) (Fig. 50.3) vaporizes hepatocytes and exposes vascular structures.

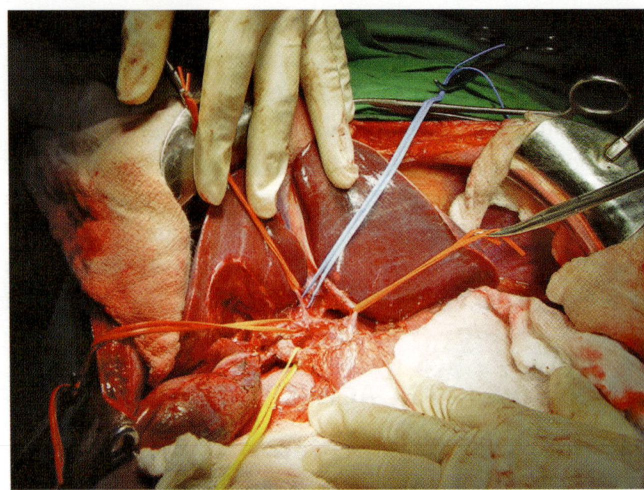

Fig. 50.2 Portal dissection of vascular and biliary structures. Bile duct in yellow, arteries in red and left portal vein in blue sling

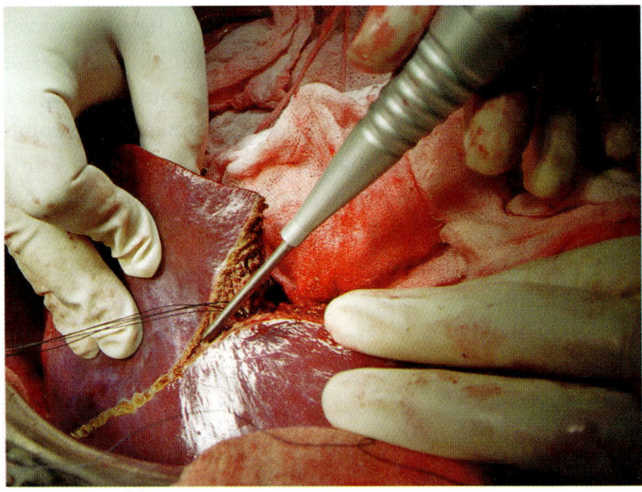

Fig. 50.3 Cavitron ultrasonic surgical aspirator (CUSA) being used to transect the liver

The smaller ones can be coagulated while the bigger ones divided between ligaclips on the right side and silk ligatures on the left. To minimize loss of blood as the parenchyma is being transected the hepatic pedicle (route for the inflow of the blood into the liver may be clamped intermittently up to a maximum total of 60 minutes. Longer clamping times are known to cause postoperative hepatic failure. Very rarely the IVC may need to be clamped (occlusion of outflow of blood) along with occlusion of inflow, to control catastrophic hemorrhage with sutures. Apart from using CUSA, other energy sources like harmonic scalpel, ligasure or water jets can be used for parenchymal transection. Finger fracture technique and pinching followed by crushing small bits of liver tissue using Kelly forceps or Mosquito forceps are used by many surgeons. Bipolar and monopolar spray diathermy or Argon beam coagulating helps in achieving hemostasis while transecting the liver. Two important structures may be divided with care, while transecting the parenchyma. As the resection approaches the hilum, the operator should adjust the dividing line so as to arrive on the right of the bile duct bifurcation. The right hepatic duct is encircled and divided between nonabsorbable sutures. This will avoid any injury to segment 1 or 4 arising from the right duct near the bifurcation of the common hepatic duct. The other important structure to be divided is the right hepatic vein, if it has not been divided already in the extraparenchymal position.

Suture closure of all bile leaking points is essential before closure of the abdomen. Injection of methylene blue into the cystic duct reveals leakage points on the resected surface.

Cholangiograms may be required for large billiary fistula and when the anatomy is unclear. Suturing of bleeders, spray diathermy, application of fibrin glue and abgel; all have been used on the cut surface of the liver achieving hemostasis. The left lobe can be attached to the diaphragm, with sutures through the falciform ligament. Drains are placed and incision closed with nonabsorbable sutures.

LEFT HEPATECTOMY

This operation consists of removing segments 2,3 and 4. This portion is supplied by the left divisions of the hepatic artery and portal vein. This portion is drained by the left and middle hepatic vein. Bile from these segments drains through the left hepatic duct. Segment 1 is not removed in a routine left hepatectomy.

A left subcostal incision is used for initial determination of respectability of the tumor. The incision may be extended to the right and to the xiphoid process, if the surgeon proceeds with resection. Intraoperative ultrasound assessment and application of omnitract retractors for elevation of the costal margins are vital before starting the resection.

Mobilization of the left lobe involves division of the round ligament and the lesser omentum. Care should be taken to prevent splenic upper polar injury by excessive traction while dividing the left triangular ligament. The left phrenic vein transversing the left triangular ligament should be divided between sutures. The lesser omentum should be divided close to carefully looking for an aberrant left hepatic artery, which may be found arising from the left gastric artery and transversing the lesser omentum in 20% cases.

Hilar dissection involves performing cholecystectomy and looping of the common bile duct and retracting it to the right. Then the anterior layer of the hepatoduodenal ligament is opened and the left hepatic artery identified in front of the left portal vein, which runs cranial to the artery. Both the right hepatic artery and the right portal vein should be divided and end suture closed, close to the point of entry into liver parenchyma. This is vital for saving any branches they give off to the caudate lobe (segment 1) of the liver. It is best not to persue the left hepatic duct at this stage as it may be intraparenchymal. The left hepatic vein also runs mostly within the parenchyma and may be difficult to encircle close to the IVC outside the parenchyma.

Parenchymal transection is very similar to as described for right hepatectomy. The difference is that the resection line is on the right of the middle vein. At the lower end of the transection line, the left duct is divided after baring it circumferentially of the parenchymal tissue and saving any aberrant paramedian branch from segments of the right hemiliver or branch from segment 1. Similarly at the upper end of the transection line, the left hepatic vein is divided after it has been joined by the middle hepatic vein. The left liver is detached from the caudate lobe last.

Hemostasis, biliostasis, abdominal drainage and closure of the abdomen is similar to that described for right hepatectomy.

COMPLICATIONS OF LIVER RESECTION

Vascular Complications

Hepatic Vein or IVC Injury

The hepatic veins may be injured while attempting to encircle them in the extraparenchymal position. The inferior vena cava may be torn while mobilizing large posterior tumors. Air embolism should be prevented by using PEEP ventilation and irrigating the area with saline while repair is done with prolene 3-0 sutures. Large IVC tears may require packing followed by application of lateral clamps or cross clamps above and below the liver for proper insertion of stitches under vision. Some tears may require clamping of the hepatic pedicle before repair of the rent can be attempted.

Portal Vein Injury

While mobilizing the left or right portal vein, the operator may injure the vein or a caudate lobe branch. This necessitates clamping and division of the vein after ensuring the patency of the contralateral portal vein. Torn caudate lobe branches should be closed with prolene 5-0 sutures.

Hemorrhage from Resected Liver Surface

Maintenance of low CVP (less than 5) and careful hemostasis while transecting the liver parenchyma avoids excessive blood loss. If hemorrhage is excessive, clamping of the hepatic pedicle is done while suture ligating bleeding points. However, intermittent clamping of the pedicle with intervals of clamp release is usually practiced, with the aim of keeping the total "clamp on" time less than 30 minutes. Longer clamping times may result in postoperative hepatic insufficiency.

Biliary Complications

Biliary Leaks

Bile leakage from the recsected liver surface can cause subphrenic abscess. The fistula may manifest as continuous leak from through a drain given at the time of operation. Injection of methylene blue through the cystic duct into the biliary system can demonstrate a leak point, which can be sutured at the time of resection.

If the caudate lobe ducts are damaged, it is best to remove the caudate lobe as it can cause stricture and recurrent cholangitis.

Postoperative leaks usually closes spontaneously if there is no biliary obstruction. Endoscopic retrograde cholangiopancreatography (ERCP) and papillary stenting may be required for persistent leakage. Reoperation is rarely required.

Bile Duct Injury

Ischemic injury by diathermy, accidental ligation or transection of bile ducts are known complications of liver resection. Roux-en-Y jejunal loop repair is commonly used if detected intraoperatively. Postoperative detection of incomplete stenosis can be treated with ERCP and stenting. Difficult cases will need reoperation.

Hepatic Insufficiency

This is relatively uncommon complications. Ascites, encephalopathy and sepsis (bacterial and fungal) are the usual manifestations seen. Thrombosis of portal or hepatic veins can precipitate hepatic failure. The chance of insufficiency increases with:

a. Removal of more than 60% of functioning liver parenchyma.
b. Presence of cholestasis, obstructive jaundice, chronic liver disease or cirrhosis.
c. Prolonged clamping of hepatic pedicle.
d. Intraoperative hypotension or excessive blood loss.

Infective Complications

Postoperative infections of chest, urinary tract, wound, intra-abdominal collections and biliary system with bacteria or fungus can precede systemic sepsis and multiple organ failure. Close monitoring and aggressive therapy is needed to avoid mortality.

SEGMENT-ORIENTED LIVER RESECTION

Resection of single, two or more segments can be done by dissecting out their individual vascular pedicles. Each segment of the liver is an independent anatomical unit, supplied by branches of the hepatic artery, portal vein and bile duct enclosed in a sheath of connective tissue, from the hilum. So dissection and division of this pedicle will devascularize the segment. The hepatic venous branch draining each segment can be divided as they are encountered while dividing the parenchyma around the devascular segment.

In the liver hilum, on the left side, it is possible to dissect out the triad of branches supplying segment 4 (a and b) and the lateral segments (2 and 3). Dissecting out the right branch, the triad divides into an anterior branch supplying segments 5 and 8 and a posterolateral branch supplying segments 6 and 7. Resection of two segments together will need division of these branches. Dissecting out individual segments requires dissection of parenchyma to isolate and divide individual triads supplying each segment.

LAPAROSCOPIC LIVER RESECTION

Laparoscopic liver surgery requires special equipment like laparoscopic intraoperative ultrasound scanning, energy source like harmonic scalpel, ligasure or CUSA with laparoscopic probe. Surgeons doing advanced laparoscopic surgery in few centers are undertaking such resections.

CHAPTER

51

Surgery for Portal Hypertension

Debasish Banerjee

INDICATIONS FOR SURGERY

Acute or chronic variceal hemorrhage in cirrhosis, noncirrhotic (fibrotic) liver disease and extrahepatic portal obstruction patients are primarily treated with pharmacotherapy and endoscopic variceal ablative therapy. Failure to control hemorrhage with these methods require surgical intervention. Often these patients have splenomegaly with thrombocytopenia and leukopenia due to hypersplenism. Cirrhotic patients may have coagulopathy, intra-abdominal varices, ascites and hypoproteinemia making them high risk for major surgery.

Surgical Options

Direct operation on varices: These are nonshunt procedures, involving devascularization of the gastroesophageal region This involves ligation of the blood vessels supplying the abdominal esophagus and upper half of stomach. Some surgeons combine this procedure with transection and stapled anastomosis of the esophagus or the cardia of stomach to achieve direct disruption of the varices. Splenectomy is performed in most cases for proper devascularization of the greater curvature of stomach and to counter hypersplenism. Operative mortality varies from 15 to 22%, higher in patients being operated for massive bleed.

Morbidity includes: Ascites 11–28%, esophageal stricture: 3–5% and rebleed rate of 15–17%.

Historically several surgeons popularized different procedures having the same aim of controlling variceal bleed.

Crile (1950)—Transthoracic ligation of esophageal varices

Boerema (1949)—Technique of esophageal transection and anastomosis done transabdominally.

Tanner (1961)—Technique of subcardiac portoazygos disconnection with gastric transection and anastomosis.

Hassab (1967)—Transabdominal technique of gastroesophageal devascularization and splenectomy.

Saguira and Futugawa (1973)—Transthoracic extensive esophageal devascularization and esophageal transection combined with transabdominal splenectomy and devascularization of upper stomach, vagotomy with pyloroplasty.

PORTOSYSTEMIC SHUNTS

1. Tips—Minimally invasive procedure
2. Nonselective surgical shunt, e.g. splenectomy with proximal lienorenal shunt, mesocaval shunt, etc.
3. Selective surgical shunt, e.g. distal lienorenal shunt (Warren shunt), coronary caval shunt, etc.

PORTOSYSTEMIC SHUNT: CHOICE OF OPERATION

The portal venous systems do not have valves. Shunts between the low pressure systemic and high pressure portal veins at various points, help to decompress the portal system.

Portosystemic shunts are done mostly in elective situation for patients having hemorrhage from esophagogastric varices or from portal gastropathy. Uncommon indications for this surgery include severe hypersplenism (thrombocytopenia and anemia), intractable ascites and Budd-Chiari syndrome (hepatic venous or inferior venacaval obstruction). Emergency shunt operations are best avoided, because of unacceptably high operative mortality.

Since the portal system has three major veins, portal, mesenteric and splenic vein, these are the usual sites for the different types of shunt. End-to-side or side-to-side portacaval shunts are no longer popular as they involve anastomosis of the portal vein to the inferior vena cava, which precludes any chance of a future liver transplant. Mesenteric caval shunt direct or through a graft and lienorenal shunts between the splenic and renal vein do not have such a disadvantage.

Portosystemic shunts decrease portal pressure and reduce the chance of variceal bleed, hypersplenism and ascites. However, nonselective shunts described above divert blood away from the liver to such a degree that hepatic encephalopathy may occur in cirrhotic patients. These operations can be utilized for patients with portal hypertension due to extrahepatic portal obstruction or intrahepatic presinusoidal obstruction (e.g.) non-cirrhotic portal fibrosis).

Distal lienorenal (between the divided distal end of splenic vein and left renal vein) and coronary-caval shunts (between left gastric vein and inferior vena cava) selectively decompress only the esophagogastric region without reducing the pressure of blood in the portal vein. This reduces the chance of developing postoperative encephalopathy, which makes them ideal for cirrhotic bleeders.

DISTAL SPLENORENAL SHUNT

Distal splenorenal shunt (Warren) involves preserving the spleen while using the splenic vein for creating a portosystemic shunt which selectively decompresses the esophagogastric varices without significantly reducing blood flow to the liver (Fig. 51.1). The chance of developing hepatic encephalopathy in the postoperative period is minimal. The patient is placed supine with a sandbag under the left lower ribs. This helps in exposing the splenic and renal veins. A left subcostal incision is given and ascites aspirated. The greater omentum is bisected between the greater curvature of the stomach and the transverse colon. Division of the gastroepiploeic arcade of vessels between the right gastroepiploeic artery and the first short gastric artery, opens the lesser sac widely. Then the left colonic flexure and transverse colon is mobilized away from the spleen, exposing the upper part of the left kidney. This also exposes the lower border of the pancreas, where the peritoneum is divided to visualize the splenic vein. Small venous branches entering the anterior surface of the splenic vein from the pancreas are divided between transfixing sutures. These veins are delicate and cause bothersome bleed on rupture or slippage. The correct technique is to dissect the pancreas off the splenic vein. The posterior surface of the splenic vein is also dissected out along the veins length. The inferior mesenteric vein, which joins the inferior border of the splenic vein, may be divided if required for proper circumferential exposure of the splenic vein. Before division of the splenic vein, the left renal vein is dissected and exposed over a sufficient length. The retroperitoneum just below the D-J flexure on the left of the superior mesenteric artery in front of the aorta is incised, to expose the anterior surface of the left renal vein. The lymphatic tissue lying in front of the vein is divided between ligatures, to prevent postoperative chylous leakage. The left renal vein is mobilized along its length for about 3 cm, dividing the suprarenal vein, so that it could be caught in a sidebiting vascular clamp and drawn up to the splenic vein for anastomosis. The left gonadal vein is preserved if possible. Next the splenic vein is divided close to the portal vein. The portal vein end of the divided splenic vein is closed with prolene sutures leaving the stump as short as possible, in order to minimize clot formation. The other divided end of the splenic vein is held on a vascular clamp and anastomosed end to side to a venotomy on the left renal vein. Careful alignment of the veins, so as to avoid any kinks on release of the clamps is required. Suturing is usually done with 6-0 prolene. The posterior layer is closed with continuous sutures and anterior with interrupted, in order to prevent purse string narrowing of the anastomosis. The next step of porto-azygos disconnection is achieved by dividing the coronary vein (left gastric vein) close to the upper border of pancreas and the right gastric vein at the lower border of the pylorus. If it is difficult to ligate the coronary vein at the upper border of the pancreas, then it could be divided close to the point where it drains into the portal vein. The transpancreatic collaterals from the splenic vein and collaterals in the splenocolic ligament also forms porto-azygos connections, but these should have already been divided by now, while freeing the splenic vein or mobilizing the left colonic flexure with the transverse colon. Meticulous hemostasis, drainage and closure of the abdomen complete the operation.

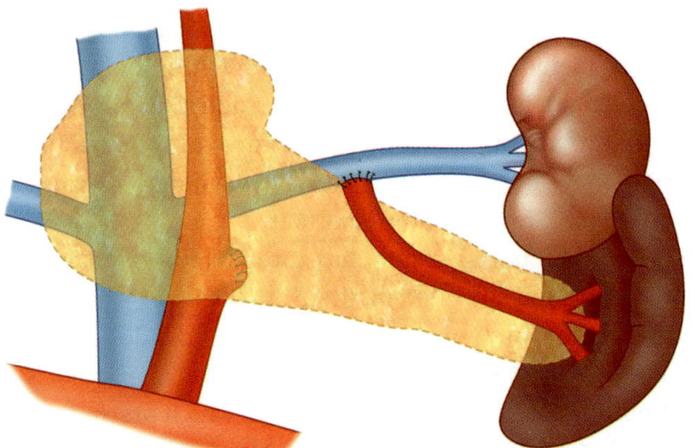

Fig. 51.1 Selective shunt: distal (Warren) splenorenal anastomosis

CHAPTER

52

Cholecystostomy

Dhiraj Choudhury

INDICATIONS

Cholecystostomy may be life-saving procedure in acute cholecystitis with empyema of gallbladder. At present, percutaneous drainage under ultrasonography (USG) or computed tomography (CT) guidance has become the procedure of choice. But operative cholecystostomy may have to be undertaken in elderly critically ill patients with gallbladder lump containing pus.

Preoperative preparations: The patient is prepared with systemic antibiotic, vitamin K injection and intravenous fluids.

PROCEDURE

- *Anesthesia:* This can be carried under local anesthesia if general anesthesia is considered hazardous.
- *Incision:* A small transverse incision is made over maximum pointed tenderness in the right hypochondrium.
- *Steps:* The fundus of the gallbladder is walled off with sterile mops. Two stay sutures are applied and a small incision is made over serosa. The content can be sucked with a sucker introduced through the opening. Material should be sent for culture. An attempt should be made to remove impacted stone with Desjardins forceps. A pursetring suture is applied and a catheter is inserted. (Fig. 52.1) The purse string suture is tightened around the catheter. A corrugated drain is placed around the gallbladder. The gallbladder wall is anchored to peritoneum with absorbable suture.
- *Closure:* A routine closure of abdomen is done.

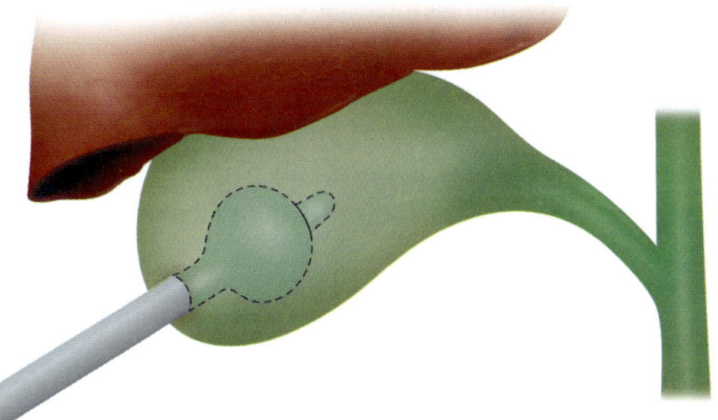

Fig. 52.1 Cholecystostomy. A large Foley catheter is sututred into the gallbladder, taking care not to puncture the balloon when inserting the stitches

CHAPTER

53

Open Cholecystectomy

Dhiraj Choudhury

ANATOMY

The extrahepatic biliary tree consists of gallbladder, cystic duct, right and left hepatic ducts, common hepatic duct and the common bile duct.

The gallbladder is a pyriform-shaped organ about 4" long. It's hepatic surface lies attached to liver by connective tissue containing cystic veins. The other surface is covered by peritoneum.

Anatomically, the gallbladder consists of fundus, body and neck. The *fundus* is dilated blind end which projects little from the liver edge and is related to hepatic flexure. The body passes upwards and backwards and is related to first part of the duodenum. The neck is the narrow part of the gallbladder which may present a small diverticulum called Hartmann's pouch.

The cystic duct (2–4 cm long and 3 mm in diameter) joins the common hepatic duct to form common bile duct (CBD).

The gallbladder receives its blood supply from the cystic artery, a branch of the right hepatic artery. The artery passes through Calot's triangle, bounded by cystic duct inferiorly, liver edge superiorly and common hepatic duct medially. The triangle also contains cystic lymph node.

The most common anomaly of the gallbladder is Phrygians cap where the fundus is constricted and turned back on itself.

INDICATIONS OF OPEN CHOLECYSTECTOMY

- Symptomatic gallstones, biliary colic.
- Mucocele or empyema of gallbladder
- Acalculus cholecystitis
- The presence of contraindications to laparoscopic cholecystectomy
- Failed laparoscopic cholecystectomy/conversion from laparoscopic cholecystectomy
- Carcinoma of gallbladder
- Traumatic rupture of gallbladder.

It should be accepted that, at present, the only indications for open cholecystectomy are failed laparoscopic cholecystectomy or contraindications to laparoscopic cholecystectomy.

PREOPERATIVE STEPS

- Antibiotic prophylaxis.
- Anti-DVT prophylaxis.
- Injection of vit K, if jaundiced.

OPERATIVE PROCEDURE

- *Position:* The patient is placed in supine position on X-ray operating table. Image intensifier is helpful if CBD exploration is planned.
- *Anesthesia:* The patient undergoes general anesthesia with endotracheal intubation.
- *Incision:* The choice of incision lies amongst:
  - Kocher's subcostal incision—good access.
  - Right upper transverse incision—good cosmesis.
  - Right upper paramedian incision.

The author prefers either right transverse incision or Kocher's subcostal incision (Fig. 53.1).

Exposure

The rectus muscle is divided to expose parietal peritoneum which is incised to open peritoneal cavity (Figs 53.2 and 53.3).

A full laparotomy is performed to confirm the diagnosis and exclude other pathology.

The gallbladder is identified and held by sponge holding forceps (Fig. 53.4).

A pack is inserted into right paracolic gutter to displace hepatic flexure and duodenum. A second pack is placed over free border of lesser omentum to apply left oblique and downward traction by assistant's left hand. A Deaver retractor

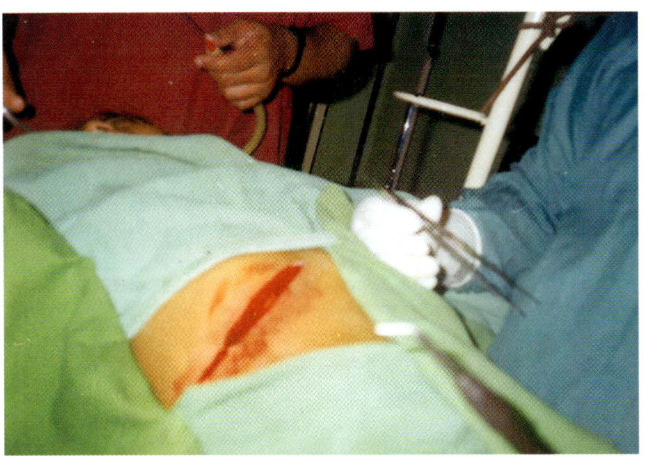

Fig. 53.1 Kocher's subcostal incision

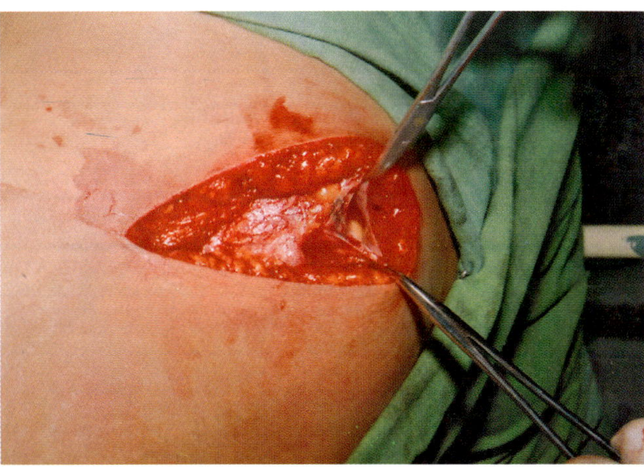

Fig. 53.3 Peritoneal incision

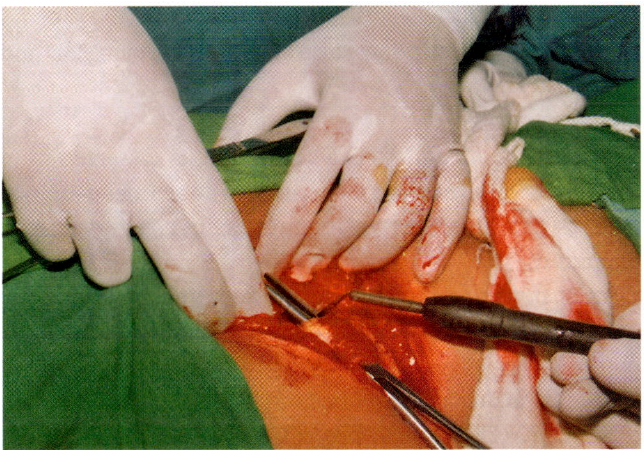

Fig. 53.2 Division of muscles over a straight hemostatic forceps

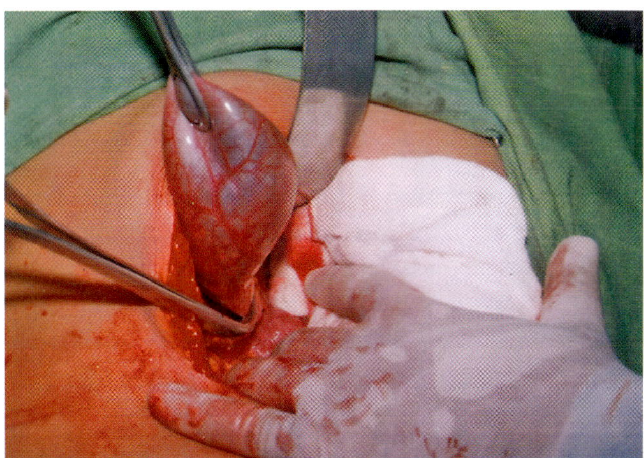

Fig. 53.4 Exposing gallbladder

is used to provide upward traction on left lobe of liver. Hold neck of gallbladder (Hartmann's Pouch) with Moynihan's forceps to apply right oblique traction. This three-way traction fully exposes Calot's triangle (Fig. 53.5). The Deaver retractor is preferably placed over the third mop.

Procedure

Neck-first Method

This is the method of choice.

The peritoneum overlaying the neck of the gallbladder is carefully incised with scissors and dissected free with peanut swab to expose the junction of cystic duct with common bile duct.

The cystic artery is similarly exposed near cystic duct lying above and posterior to duct and followed-up to gallbladder (Fig. 53.6).

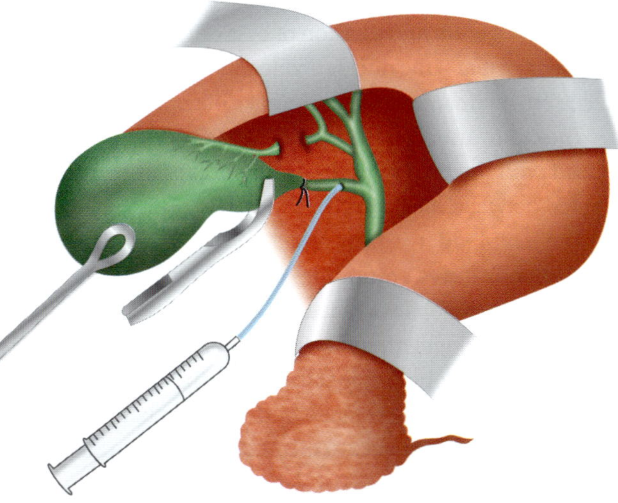

Fig. 53.5 Exposure of Calot's triangle, division and ligation of cystic artery and cannulization of cystic duct, after ligation

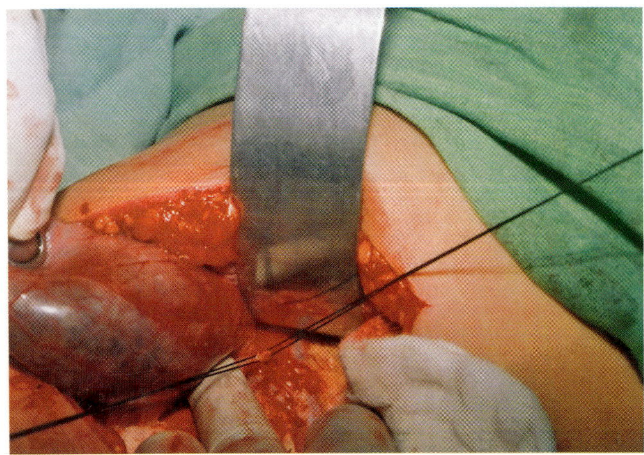

Fig. 53.6 Ligation of cystic artery

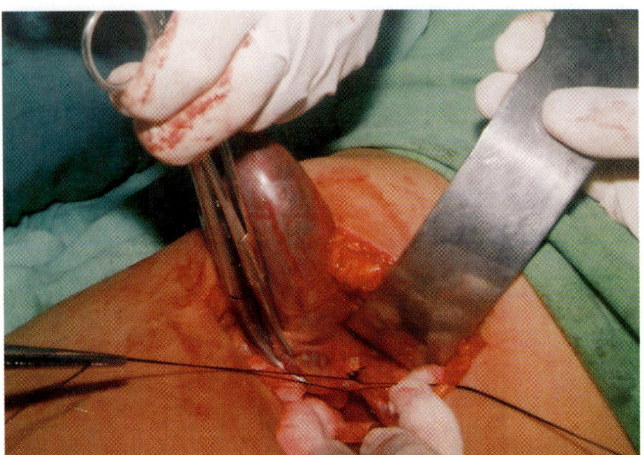

Fig. 53.7 Ligation of cystic duct

It is almost always associated with sizeable lymph node. Preferably ligation and division of cystic artery is done first to avoid risk of tear if the duct is divided first. But in practice, this rule is broken many times for the sake of convenience.

The cystic artery is now ligated with silk or chromic catgut passed with the help of right-angled forceps at two sites and divided between the ligatures.

The gallbladder is now attached to CBD by cystic duct only. Pass ligatures around the cystic duct with the help of right-angled forceps and leave distal ligature untied if *per-operative cholangiography* is planned (Fig. 53.7).

Introduce a cholangiocatheter or infant feeding tube through a small incision made in cystic duct with scissors or by direct puncture. Inject 2–5 mL of contrast billigraffin with a syringe and take a film.

Take another film after injection of 10 mL of contrast. If X-ray shows flow of dye into duodenum and absence of stone, ligate the cystic duct close to its junction with CBD and divide it.

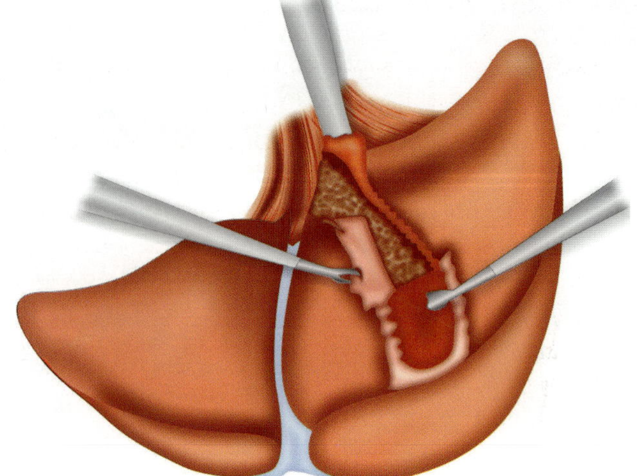

Fig. 53.8 Application of gel foam on liver bed

Removal of gallbladder: The gallbladder is dissected from the liver bed by dividing its peritoneal attachments to liver with scissors. Bleeding from the cut margins can be dealt with diathermy.

It is not imperative to close the peritoneal fringes by suturing with catgut but when done, the needle should not be passed through liver tissues.

Minor oozing from liver bed can be tackled by application of gel foams (Fig. 53.8), or surgical.

Fundus-first Method

Cholecystectomy from the fundus downward is desirable if there is extensive adhesions in Calot's triangle or large stone impacted in the ampulla (Mirizzi syndrome). It is also a method of choice in many cases of acute gangrenous cholecystitis when exposure of cystic duct is difficult and hazardous.

The fundus of the gallbladder is grasped with sponge holding forceps and separation of the gallbladder is commenced at the fundus.

The peritoneal sheath can be divided with scissors on each side and reflected onto liver. A cutting diathermy point may be used to free the gallbladder from liver. The dissection is preferably continued till cystic duct and cystic artery are identified, which are then ligated.

If it is found that any attempt to identify these sutures can cause damage to right hepatic artery or common bile duct, then ligate doubly leaving a part of neck of gallbladder.

Intraoperative Problems

- *Bleeding from cystic artery or an accessory artery:* No attempt should be made in hurry to catch the bleeding point. Apply a hot mop into Calot's triangle under pressure for sometimes. The bleeding point can be caught in a bloodless field after removal of hot mops and ligated properly. If necessary, *Pringle's maneuver* (compressing the hepatic artery in free border of the lesser omentum) may be helpful to reduce bleeding while bleeding point is secured.
- *Bleeding from liver bed:* A hot mop should be applied for 5 to 10 minutes. Bleeding points can be secured either by diathermy or by transfixation sutures.
- *Gallbladder adherent to liver bed:* Partial cholecystectomy or buried in liver or structures in the cystic duct region cannot be safely identified, partial cholecystectomy may be a procedure of choice. This is particularly desirable in patients with cirrhosis of liver and portal hypertension.

  The gallbladder is opened, aspirated and stones removed. The gallbladder wall beyond the liver margin is excised and hemostasis is done by diathermy or interrupted suture. The mucosa in the retained portion of the gallbladder is destroyed with diathermy.

GALLBLADDER CANCER

Operability in Gallbladder Cancer

Operability in gallbladder cancer should be based on several factors. Signs of inoperability include contiguous liver metastasis, ascites, peritoneal nodules and retroperitoneal lymphadenopathy.

Surgery for Operable Gallbladder Cancer

Redical cholecystectomy is the standard operation and should include cholecystectomy, resection of liver in the gallbladder bed and regional lymphadenectomy. The primary aim of liver resection is to achieve tumor-free margins in the liver parenchyma. It can be achieved by performing a wedge resection of liver in the gallbladder bed or a formal resection of segments 4b or 5 of the liver or by extended right hepatectomy. The extent of lymhadenectomy is more or less standardized. Lymph nodes in the hepatoduodenal ligament should be routinely removed. In addition, the lymph nodes behind the pancreatic head and duodenum and those along common hepatic artery and celiac axis should be dissected.

Revision Surgery for Incidental Gallbladder Cancer

Diagnosis of gallbladder cancer on histopathological examination after cholecystectomy is called incidental gallbladder cancer. Controversy exists regarding further management. If the gallbladder cancer is limited only to Mucosa (Tis) or Submucosa (Tia), a simple cholecystectomy is curative. With patients with incidental gallbladder cancer that invades muscularis (Tib) or beyond revision surgery is needed. The revision may include wedge resection of liver in gallbladder bed. Resection of remnant of cystic duct and regional lymphadenectomy.

Palliative Treatment for Gallbladder Cancer

Palliative treatment consists of supportive care or chemotherapy. If the patient is jaundiced, endoscopic biliary stenting may be tried. If not successful, biliary bypass surgery may be required.

Closure

- Check hemostasis.
- Count mops and instruments.
- Place a corrugated drain into Morrison's pouch (most dependent part) and bring it through a stab wound.
- Rectus sheath should be stitched with 2/0 vicryl or proline.
- Skin is closed with interrupted sutures with silk.

Postoperative Care

- In elective operations, oral fluid can be started after 24 hours.
- Systemic antibiotics should be given.

Postoperative Complications

Early
- Biliary leak
- Hemorrhage
- Pancreatitis
- Ileus
- Postoperative chest complications
- Wound infection.

Late
- Biliary stricture.

CHAPTER

54

Laparoscopic Cholecystectomy

Sunanda Roy Mahapatra

INTRODUCTION

Laparoscopic cholecystectomy (LC) is now the gold standard treatment of symptomatic gallstones and is the commonest operation performed laparoscopically worldwide. Laparoscopic cholecystectomy is considered the "Gold Standard" for the surgical treatment of gallstone disease. This procedure results in less postoperative pain, better cosmesis, shorter hospital stays and more disability from work than open cholecystectomy. However, the overall serious complication rate in laparoscopic cholecystectomy remains slightly higher than that seen in open cholecystectomy. In contrast, large retrospective series of LCs from several countries indicate that the overall mortality of cholecystectomy has decreased since the advent of the laparoscopic approach. The overall prevalence of gallstones is about 7% of the population, was higher in women than men (9 versus 5%) and increased with advancing age.

INDICATIONS

The indications for laparoscopic cholecystectomy are the same as for open cholecystectomy:

- Symptomatic cholelithiasis—Billiary colic
- Gallstone pancreatitis
- Acute cholecystitis
- Chronic cholecystitis
- A symptomatic cholelithiasis who are at increased risk for gallbladder carcinoma or gallstone complications
- A calculous cholecystitis
- Gallbladder polyps >0.5 cm and cholesterolosis
- Porcelain gallbladder
- Persons undergoing obesity surgery.

CONTRAINDICATIONS

There are not many absolute surgical contraindication to laparoscopic cholecystectomy. If there is a suspicion of Gallbladder carcinoma then an open cholecystectomy is recommended. Patient suffering from bleeding disorder is a relative contraindication. The other relative contraindications are previous abdominal surgery, pregnancy, cholangitis, severe comorbidities. There are some anesthetic contradictions which are in general for any laparoscopic procedure.

PATIENT PREPARATION

The optimal timing of surgery will depend upon the patient's overall medical condition and underlying diagnosis.

- *Acute cholecystitis*: Patient who presents with acute cholecystitis should be placed on antibiotics and the surgery should be performed within 24 hours or as soon as practical after diagnosis. The previous popular practice was antibiotics and an interval cholecystectomy which is still prevalent. The emergency cholecystectomy is becoming increasingly popular as the rate of conversion for the late approach is greater and there is an increasing number of readmissions while recovering from acute attack.
- *Gallstone pancreatitis*: Patients with gallstone pancreatitis have a high risk of recurrence within 30 days of their attack and, therefore, should undergo cholecystectomy during their hospitalization after their symptoms resolve. The British Society of Gastroenterology guidelines are to do cholecystectomy within two weeks of admission. That include preoperative endoscopic retrograde cholangiopancreatography (ERCP) if needed or laparoscopic bile duct exploration.
- *Obstructive jaundice*: A history of pancreatitis or jaundice raises the likelihood of common bile duct (CBD) stones. Patients with isolated obstructive jaundice with or without cholangitis should either have their CBD cleared with urgent endoscopic retrograde cholangiopancreatography (ERCP) preoperatively or with cholangiography and laparoscopic common duct exploration at the time of

surgery. If ERCP is successful, the patient electively be scheduled for cholecystectomy.

- *Medical comorbidities:* Identification of bleeding diathesis and poor cardiopulmonary reserve will help identify patients who may not tolerate pneumoperitoneum or will have higher likelihood for conversion to open operation. In patients with multiple comorbidities or acute medical problems (such as recent myocardial infarction), a trial of antibiotics with consideration for a percutaneous cholecystostomy tube with delayed laparoscopic cholecytectomy in six to eight weeks may be preferable.

PREOPERATIVE LABORATORY TESTS

Patient should have full blood count and liver function test checked. Additional tests include serum amylase and C-reactive protein (CRP) during acute attacks. May be urea and electrolytes like other operations.

IMAGING

Ultrasonography (US) of upper abdomen establishes the diagnosis of gallstones or abnormalities of the gallbladder wall. The US may also demonstrate CBD dilatation, stones or evidence of acute inflammation of the gallbladder.

Magnetic resonance cholangiopancreatography (MRCP) may be useful to evaluate the common duct in patients with mild elevations of their transaminases or mild CBD dilatation on US.

Isotope scan hepatobiliary iminodiacetic acid (HIDA) may be useful in cases in which the diagnosis remains uncertain after ultrasonography and MRCP.

ERCP is useful in patient presented with CBD.

CT scan has got limited value apart from the acute cases where USS is suboptimal for example in obese patients.

INFORMED CONSENT

Patient should be warned of the risk of conversion usually around 5%, the risk of bile leak 1%, bile duct injury (1 in 400), the risk of injury to bowel and vascular injury. The need for laparoscopic CBD exploration or postoperative ERCP.

STAFF LAYOUT AND POSITIONING OF PATIENT

The patient is operated in the supine position initially and then placed in a steep head-up about 25–35° and left side tilt of 10–15° once the pneumoperitoneum has been established. Some surgeons prefer a nasogastric/orogastric tube is inserted and the stomach aspirated. It is not a mandatory step but nevertheless helpful at times. The surgeon operates from the left side of the patient with the camera person by his side and the assistant and scrub nurse on the other side of the operating table. This is known as North American Technique. In European technique, the patient is placed in either lithotomy or more often modified Lloyd Davises Position and surgeon operates from standing between the legs (Fig. 54.1).

ANESTHESIA

Usually general anesthesia but there are reports of laparoscopic cholecystectomy being performed under high thoracic epidural anesthesia.

CREATION OF PNEUMOPERITONEUM

Before any laparoscopic procedure can begin, access to the peritoneal cavity is performed, first to establish pneumoperitoneum and subsequently to place additional port sites for the laparoscope and various laparoscopic instruments.

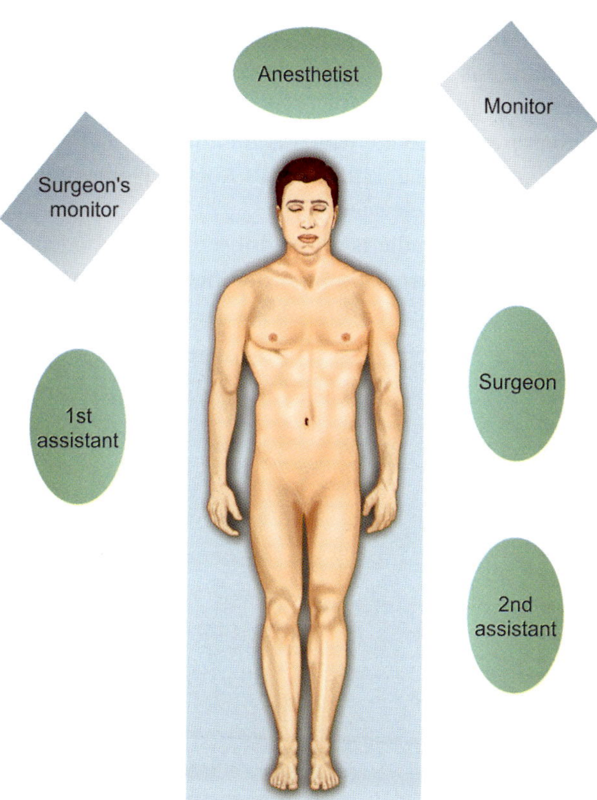

Fig. 54.1 Position of personnel for laparoscopic cholecystectomy

Laparoscopic entry can be performed with an open (i.e. Hasson), or closed (e.g. veress needle, visual entry trocar) technique. Each method has advantages and disadvantages and neither is suitable as an all-purpose method for laparoscopic access. Different approaches can be used for primary and secondary port placement during the same procedure (Fig. 54.2).

Closed Technique

The closed technique is produced by insertion of veress needle through the immediate infraumbilical area. The propensity for visceral and major vascular damage (aorta, iliac vessels and vena cava) is well-documented unless the technique is flawless. It must be remembered that the distance between the anterior abdominal wall and the aorta and its bifurcation into the iliac vessels averages only 2.0 cm.

Palmer's point is located 3 cm below the left costal margin, just lateral to the rectus muscle in the midclavicular line. Like the left ninth intercostal location, Palmer's point can also be used as a site for primary insufflation of the abdomen with a Veress needle when a transumbilical site cannot be used.

Procedure

A small incision is made in the umbilicus and the subcutaneous tissue bluntly dissected to the fascia. The needle is placed to the level of the fascia and the depth marked on the needle, which is then removed. The fascia is then grasped (e.g. Little wood's Kocher clamp) and the abdominal wall is elevated.

The veress needle is grasped just above the measured distance and inserted through the incision at a 45° angle toward the hollow of the pelvis with care not to deviate laterally. Two "pops" should be felt. The first occurs when the needle passes through the abdominal fascia and the second as it passes through the parietal peritoneum.

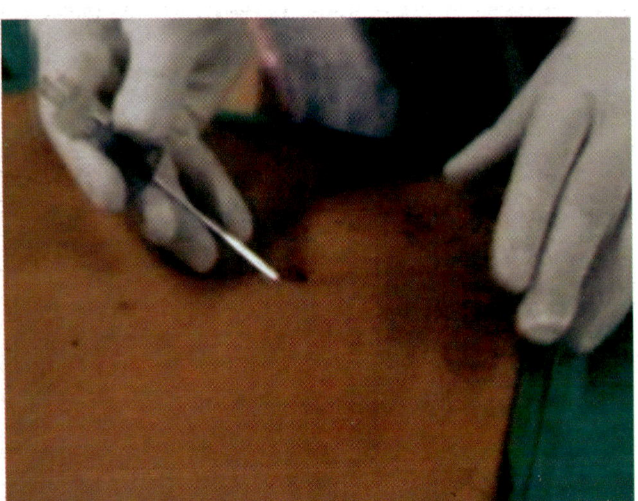

Fig. 54.2 Insertion of veress needle

When the needle passes through the peritoneum and enters the peritoneal space, the displaced hub of the needle will "click" as the protective sheath recoils to cover the end of the needle.

Multiple alternatives are available for confirming veress needle placement. However, no trials are available to suggest the use of one method over another. These include one of the following:

- Saline aspiration and injection. A 10 mL syringe containing 4 mL of normal saline is attached to the veress needle hub. The syringe is aspirated. If nothing returns, saline is injected into the presumed peritoneal space. Intraperitoneal location of the tip of the veress needle is assumed if saline injects freely and the location is confirmed when the water in the veress needle cap droops freely into the peritoneal space by gravity when the syringe is removed.
- If blood or enteric contents are returned upon aspirating the syringe, an inadvertent vascular or visceral injury may have occurred. Under these circumstances, the needle should be left in place and alternative access obtained to assess the potential injury. The needle should be removed under direct visualization.
- Hanging drop method. A drop of saline is placed at the open end of the needle and the abdominal wall is elevated. The suction pressure that is generated should cause the drop of water to be drawn into the abdominal cavity.
- Measurement of intraperitoneal pressure. The intraperitoneal pressure should be ≤ 10 mm Hg. In one large observational study, confirmation of low intraperitoneal pressure method to confirm veress needle placement.

Once the position of the needle is confirmed to be intraperitoneal, carbon dioxide (CO_2) gas insufflation may be initiated. A properly placed needle will allow free flow of the gas. Tympany should be appreciated with percussion of the abdomen in the right upper quadrant.

In the closed method once the abdomen is insufflated, the veress needle is removed and a port placed into the veress needle track. A visual entry port is now most commonly used. Inserting the first trocar under direct vision allows early recognition and immediate management should the vascular or gastrointestinal injury occurs. Care should be taken to avoid a trocar direction (e.g. lateral displacement) or depth that could result in injury to the aorta or iliac arteries. Holding the trocar shaft rather than its top during insertion may help prevent uncontrolled speed and depth of penetration.

Open Technique (Hasson)

The Hasson technique refers to an open method in which an incision (usually periumbilical) is made through the abdominal wall under direct vision. The advantage of the open technique is a low risk for major complications. Some surgeons have abandoned completely the creation of a closed pneumoperitoneum and use the open technique routinely whether or not the patient has had previous surgery. The need for a meticulous technique, even in this situation, is highlighted by the reported incidence of injuries sustained during the creation of an open pneumoperitoneum, although the incidence is undoubtedly lower with this approach.

Procedure

An incision is made in the skin and an instrument used to bluntly dissect the subcutaneous fat. Any vessels that are encountered are cauterized, or ligated and divided. The anterior fascia is incised and stay sutures placed in the fascial edges. These sutures aid with retraction of the abdominal wall and are used to secure the fascia to the port, preventing its displacement during the surgery. At the end of the procedure, these sutures can be removed or alternatively can be used to close the fascial defect.

The peritoneal fat, if present, is bluntly dissected and the peritoneum brought up into the wound with a hemostat. The peritoneum is opened and the index finger is used to sweep the underside of the abdominal wall to clear omentum or bowel, and confirm the absence of adhesions in the region of the incision. A blunt-ended trocar (i.e. Hasson) is then placed through the incision, secured with the stay sutures, and the carbon dioxide (CO_2) gas line is attached to the port to insufflate the abdomen.

Placement of Ports

Four ports are used: One primary (10/11/12 mm), one 5 mm and one 10 mm operating, and one 5.0 mm assisting port. The optical port is at or near the umbilicus and routinely a 0°/30° laparoscope is used (Fig. 54.3).

- The assistant's 5 mm trocar is usually placed at the mid-axillary line halfway between the costal margin and the anterior superior iliac spine. A grasping forceps is placed to grasp the fundus of the gallbladder and retract it and the liver superiorly.
- A second 5 or 10 mm port, which will accommodate the surgeon's right hand instruments is placed in the high epigastric/subxiphoid region just to the right of the falciform ligament. The size of the trocar depends on the size of the clip applier to be used. This trocar is directed toward the gallbladder neck.
- A third trocar for the surgeon's left hand instruments is placed at the right midclavicular line just below the liver edge.

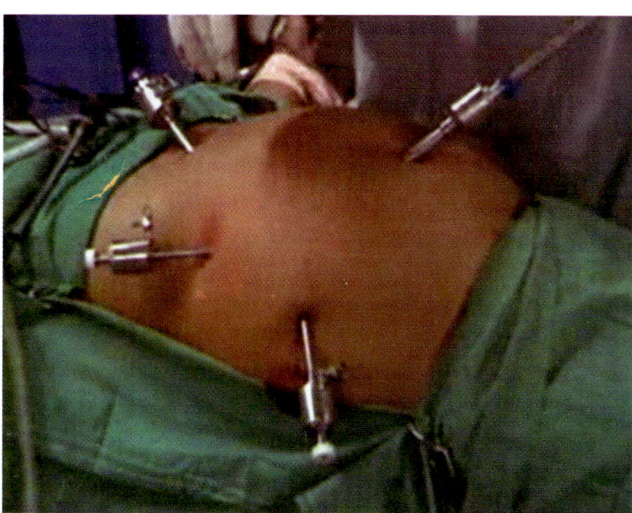

Fig. 54.3 Placement of ports

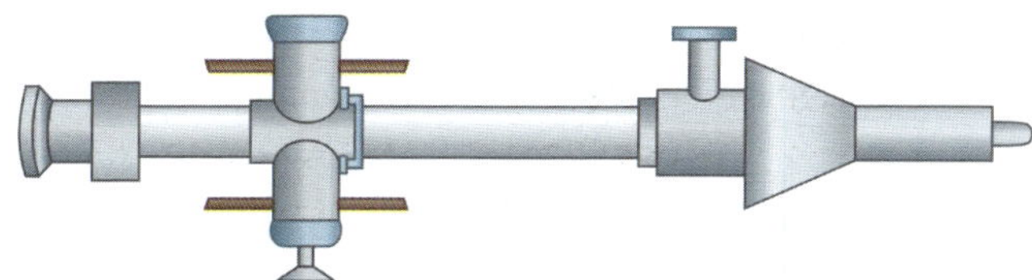

Fig. 54.4 Open (Hasson) cannula, reusable type

An initial 360° scan of the entire abdomen is made primarily to exclude injury/bleeding during the creation of the pneumoperitoneum and secondly to identify any gross macroscopic additional disease. The disposition of the other ports introduced under vision. Feasibility of the laparoscopic operations has been assessed (Fig. 54.4).

GALLBLADDER RETRACTION

Gallbladder Exposure and Dissection

The assistant using the ratcheted toothed grasper pushes the fundus of the gallbladder superiorly and laterally to reveal the infundibulum and porta hepatis. Most commonly, the American gallbladder lift is used to expose the triangle of Calot. The fundus of the gallbladder is grasped by the assistant and flipped upwards and over the superior edge of the right lobe. This maneuver/exposure is not possible in patients with contacted gallbladder or fibrotic/cirrhotic liver. In these cases, the French exposure of the triangle of Calot is used, i.e.

elevation of the gallbladder and segment IV by an atraumatic laparoscopic retractor.

If the gallbladder is very distended, it can be difficult to grasp. Aspirating it with a large bore needle or sharp tipped suction device facilitates purchase by the grasper. The grasper (or stitch or ligating loop) can then be used to close the hole to prevent further spillage of content.

Occasionally, adhesions to the duodenum, omentum, or colon from previous surgery or inflammation may impair this exposure. The surgeon can take down these adhesions safely by grasping the adhesions at their attachment high on the gallbladder and striping them down bluntly towards the infundibulum. Minimal electrocautery should be used in order to reduce the risk of thermal injury to the adjacent bowel.

DISSECTION OF CALOT'S TRIANGLE

The most important consideration in a cholecystectomy is the clear identification of the cystic artery and duct prior to division.

To this end, a thorough dissection of Calot's triangle, bounded by the gallbladder wall, cystic duct, and common hepatic duct, to obtain the anatomical detail is a key step. The surgeon grasps the infundibulum with the left hand forceps and retracts inferiorly and laterally to open the angle between the cystic duct and common duct. This instrument is used to provide retraction in various angles to give anterior and posterior exposure (Fig. 54.5).

Occasionally, a large stone at the gallbladder neck prevents grasping of the infundibulum. This scenario can be managed by dislodging and "milking" the stone back up into the gallbladder body or by placing a stitch into the infundibulum and using that for retraction. The dissection of the junction of the gallbladder and cystic duct begins by the surgeon gently stripping the peritoneum starting high on the gallbladder. Keeping the dissection on a known safe structure (the gallbladder) to develop visualization of the unknown structures is an important principle (Fig. 54.6).

The posterolateral aspect of the gallbladder is the safest area for initial dissection and can be exposed by retracting the infundibulum superior and medical. The surgeon can use minimal cautery or blunt dissection to incise the superficial layer of peritoneum attaching the gallbladder neck to the liver in order to allow further retraction of the infundibulum.

Anterior and posterior dissection continue with alternating inferolateral and superomedial retraction of the neck until the gallbladder is dissected away from the liver, creating a "window" crossed by two structures: the cystic duct and artery. This should be achieved prior to clipping or dividing any tubular structures (Figs 54.7 and 54.8).

There is no need to dissect down to the cystic duct-common bile duct junction unless the cystic duct is very short. The cystic artery should be dissected in a similar fashion. Calot's node or cystic duct lymph node is usually encountered adjacent and anterior to the artery and can be a useful landmark. Electrocautery may be needed for hemostasis before the node can be bluntly swept down (Fig. 54.9).

The surgeon should be aware of certain anatomic variations in order to avoid misidentification of structures. A common anomaly is the right hepatic artery looping onto the infundibulum and being mistaken for the cystic artery. A short cystic duct is also seen quite frequently and could drain

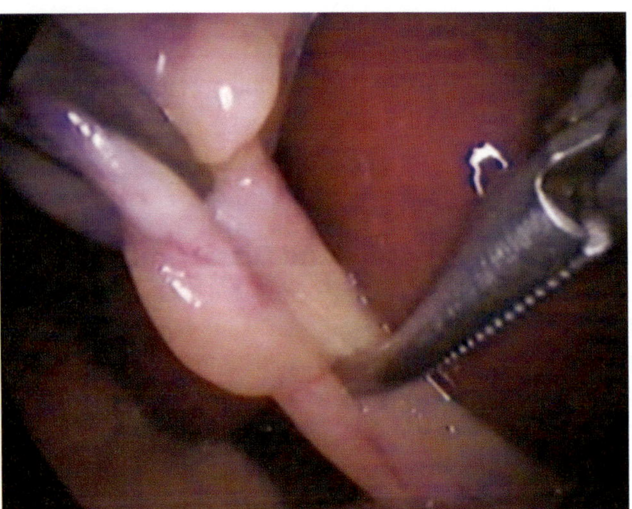

Fig. 54.5 Dissection of Calot's triangle

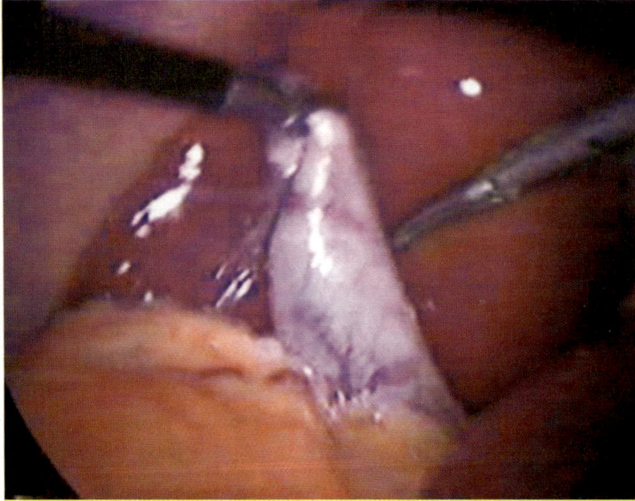

Fig. 54.6 Retraction of gallbladder cephalad, grasping fundus of gallbladder

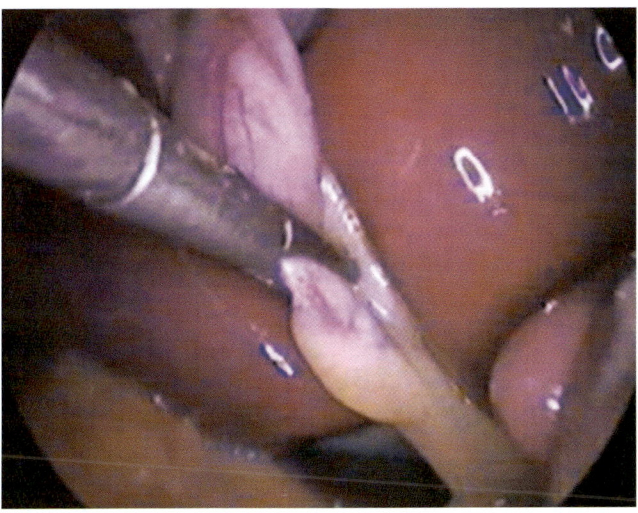

Fig. 54.7 Adhesiolysis

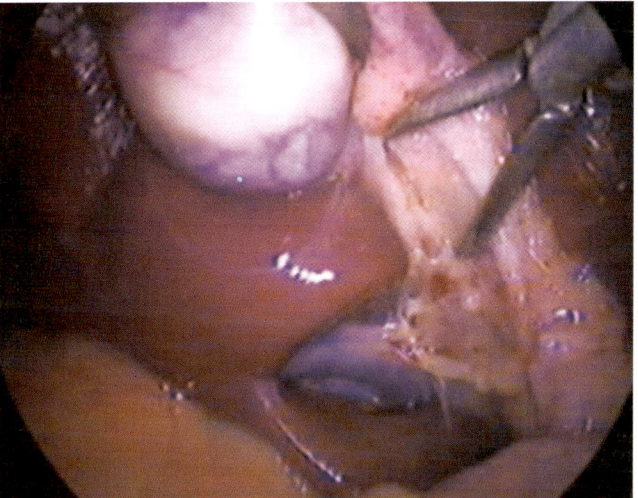

Fig. 54.8 Posterior dissection

into the right hepatic duct, the common duct, or a low-lying aberrant right sectoral duct. In the presence of severe, acute, or chronic inflammation, or with a large stone in the neck of the gallbladder, the infundibulum may be "tethered" to the hepatic duct, which may lead the surgeon to misidentify the common bile duct for the cystic duct.

Division of cystic artery and cystic duct: Once the cystic duct and artery are fully dissected, usually two clips placed medially towards the bile duct and one clip is placed laterally on the cystic duct adjacent to gallbladder.

Both jaws of the clips should be visualized and clearly encompass the duct in order to avoid inadvertent injuries to structures behind the clips and to ensure complete duct closure. Then the duct is fully transected with scissors.

Electrocautery should not be used since the electrical current can be transmitted to the clips and cause delayed necrosis of the stump. The artery is clipped and divided in a similar fashion. The anterior branch of the cystic artery is commonly mistaken for the main cystic artery; therefore, the tissue behind the clipped artery should be dissected to ensure that there is no posterior branch, which can cause troublesome bleeding during the subsequent removal of the gallbladder. The clipped stumps should be inspected for adequacy of closure (Figs 54.10 and 54.11).

MOBILIZATION OF GALLBLADDER

The assistant places continual cephalad traction on the gallbladder fundus while the surgeon alternates medial and lateral anteroposterior traction on the infundibulum with the left hand grasper. This retraction exposes and maintains tension on the plane of tissue attaching the gallbladder to

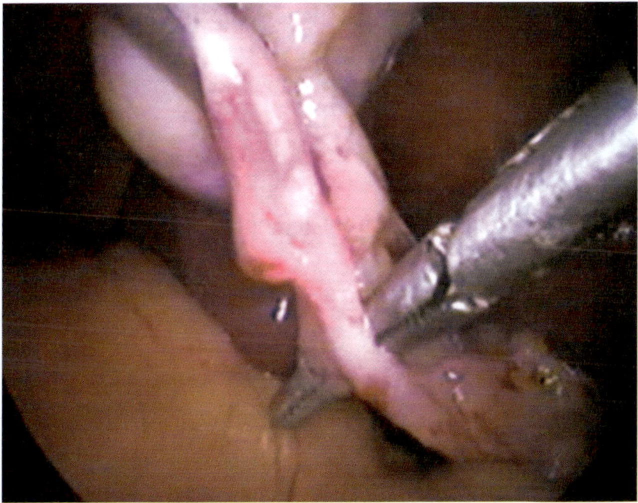

Fig. 54.9 Isolation of cystic duct

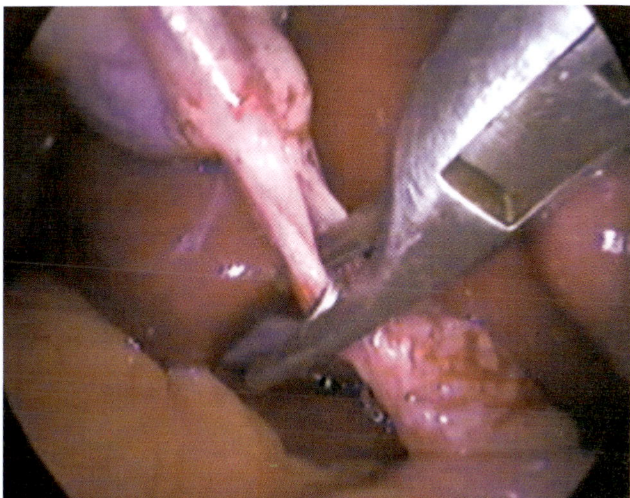

Fig. 54.10 Applications of clip on cystic duct

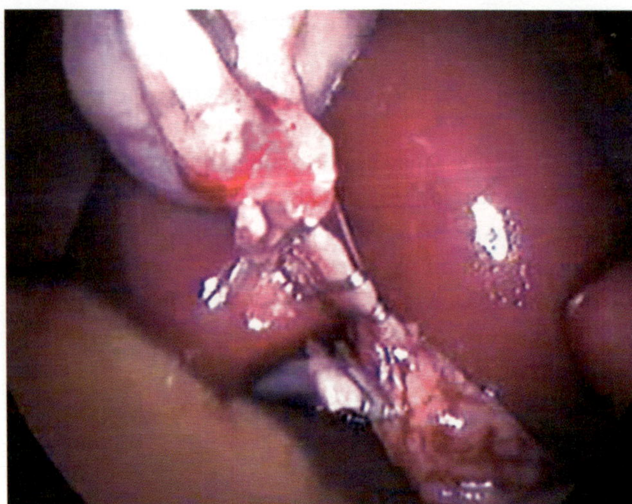

Fig. 54.11 Clipping of cystic artery

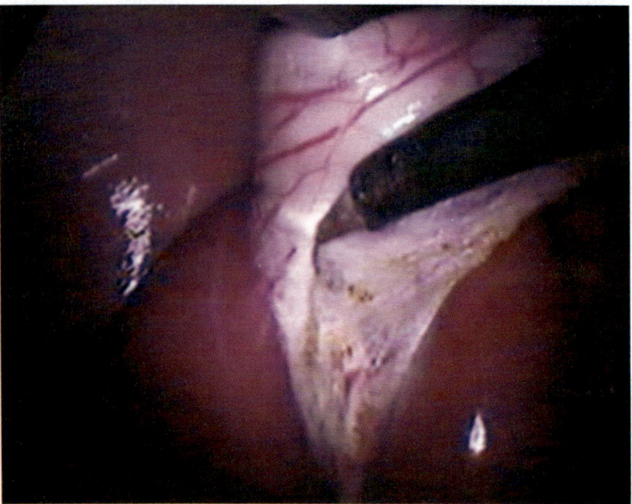

Fig 54.12 Mobilization of gallbladder

the liver. This tissue is gently divided using a hook or spatula cautery in a sweeping motion. This dissection continues from infundibulum to fundus, and bleeding should be minimal if dissection is performed in the correct plane. Prior to completely detaching the gallbladder, the liver should be inspected for areas of bleeding or bile leakage. The right upper quadrant is irrigated, and then the gallbladder is fully released (Fig. 54.12).

Occasionally, persistent minimal bile leakage occurs from the liver bed. This leak may be from a transected duct of Luschka or, more likely, from a superficial duct within the liver that was unroofed during the dissection. If the end of the duct can be grasped then the duct should be clipped. Otherwise, one may perform intracorporeal suturing of the opening of the duct, or simply leave a closed suction/Robinsons drain to control the leak.

INSERTION OF DRAIN

This is not a mandatory step. It is usually advised if the dissection was difficult or there is bile spillage. Usually size 12/14 drain is inserted through one of the 5 mm port. Most people use the lateral most port for this.

REMOVAL OF GALLBLADDER AND PORT CLOSURE

The umbilical incision is the ideal location for extracting the gallbladder. The umbilical incision has no muscle layers and is easy to extend with the minimal pain and cosmetic sequelae. To limit bile contamination of the abdomen and wound, an extraction bag is used when the gallbladder is acutely inflamed and friable or when there was inadvertent perforation of the gallbladder. Any remaining loose stones can be placed in the bag as well. The laparoscope is transferred to the subxiphoid position, and the bag or a large toothed grasper is positioned within the umbilical trocar (Fig. 54.13).

The gallbladder is placed into the bag or the infundibulum is grasped with the forceps. The trocar is removed, and the gallbladder is withdrawn through this incision under laparoscopic vision. If the gallbladder is very large or contains large stones, the fascial incision may need to be stretched or enlarged. Once the gallbladder is removed the right upper quadrant can be irrigated if necessary, and the other trocars can be removed under direct vision while allowing escape of CO_2. The umbilical fascia is then closed with the stay sutures originally placed or with sutures taken under direct vision.

The specimen can also be retrieved through the subxiphoid port site. Some surgeons feel that the subxiphoid site may be better for specimen extraction as the subxiphoid site has a lower likelihood or hernia formation; however, formal study of this has not been performed.

The skin is closed with subcuticular absorbable stitches and with steri-strips or with surgical glue. The incisions are infused with bupivacaine/lignocaine for postoperative analgesia (Fig. 54.14).

CONVERSION TO AN OPEN OPERATION IS INDICATED

- Hemorrhage
- Unusual or confusing anatomy
- Failure to progress laparoscopically in a timely fashion

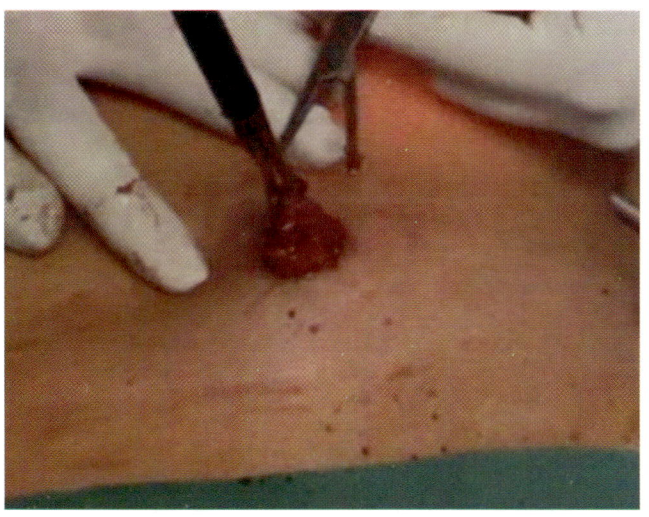

Fig 54.13 Removal of gallbladder through umbilical port

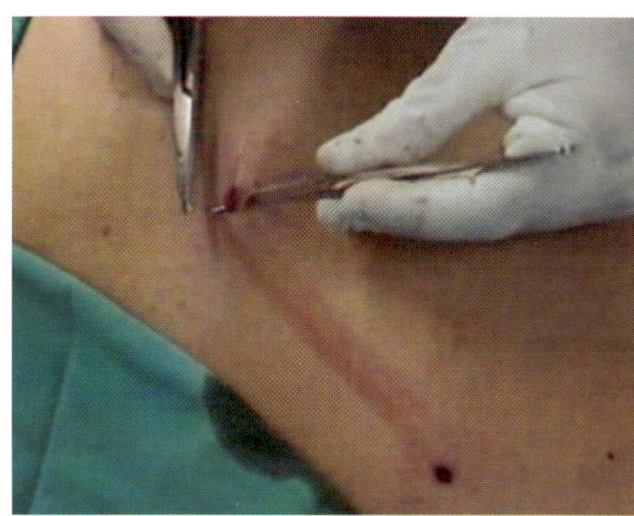

Fig 54.14 Closure of wound

- Bowel perforation or major injury to the bile ducts
- Mirizzi's syndrome
- Potentially resectable gallbladder cancer
- Dense adhesions distorting anatomy at Calot's triangle
- Common bile duct stones that cannot be removed laparoscopically or endoscopically (due to Billroth II anatomy, previously failed ERCP, or lack of an experienced endoscopist).

POSTOPERATIVE COMPLICATIONS

- Bile leak, the risk is around 1%
- Bile duct injury (1 in 400 cases)
- Postoperative hemorrhage both from liver bed and also can be from port site
- Hollow viscous injury
- Vascular injury.

CHAPTER

55

Surgery of Bile Duct

Dipak Kr Ghosh

ANATOMY

Bile from each segment of the liver is drained by a separate duct. Ducts from segment II, III and IV form the left hepatic duct which runs close to the base of the segment IV. It has an extrahepatic course of 2 cm approximately and can be made available for surgical procedures by incision of the Glisson's capsule to obtain an appropriate length. Ducts of segment VI and VII unite to form the right posterior sectorial duct which unite with the right anterior sectorial duct formed by union of segmental ducts V and VIII. The sectorial ducts unite inside the liver to form the right hepatic duct which has a short extrahepatic course and unite with the left hepatic duct to form the common hepatic duct which, in turn, receives the cystic duct from the gallbladder to from the common bile duct (CBD).

The CBD runs in the free margin of the gastrohepatic omentum flanked by the hepatic artery medially with portal vein lying posterior to it. All these together form the anterior boundary of the aditus to the lesser sac (Foramen of Winslow). The CBD has a variable length (5–9 cm) and drains into the duodenal ampulla surrounded at its termination by sphincter of oddi.

The main pancreatic duct may join it before its termination or separately drain within or outside the sphincter. The CBD is divided into supraduodenal, retroduodenal and intrapancreatic parts. Blood supply of the bile duct is derived from cystic artery with its known variations, ascending branch of the gastroduodenal and posterior superior pancreaticoduodenal arteries.

The main vessels run along the 3 and 9 o' clock positions of the duct which then shoot off subserols transverse branches to form subserous and submucous circular plexuses. This knowledge may help in prevention of ischemia and consequent fibrosis of the duct during surgical interventions.

DUCTAL ANOMALIES

The right posterior sectorial duct may join the duct formed by union of right anterior sectorial duct and left hepatic duct to form the common hepatic duct in 12% of cases. In 16% of cases, the right anterior sectorial duct joins the duct formed by right posterior sectorial duct and left hepatic duct.

A cholecystohepatic duct may enter the gallbladder from the liver. Other anomalies like cystic duct draining into right hepatic or a sectorial duct may also exist.

SURGERY OF BILE DUCT STONES

Presence of calculi in the bile duct (Choledocholithiasis) is to be suspected in patients with cholelithiasis if there is history of recurrent biliary colic followed by jaundice and presence of a dilated CBD on ultrasonography (USG). Sometimes magnetic resonance cholangiopancreatography (MRCP) or endoscopic retrograde cholangiopancreatography (ERCP) demonstrated their presence. Stones are also palpated and revealed by operative cholangiogram and/or choledochoscopy at laparotomy. Several techniques are available for treatment which are sometimes used in combination. These are: (1) Endoscopic sphincterotomy and transduodenal clearance of the ducts—suitable for calculi <2 cm in diameter, (2) Extracorporeal shock wave lithotripsy (ESWL)—may be used to break calculi into smaller fragments, (3) Laparoscopic choledocholithotomy and (4) Open technique of choledocholithotomy.

Choledocholithotomy

This means opening the bile duct and cleansing the duct of calculi. An on-table operative cholangiogram may be performed to decide on the step when one is in doubt about the necessity of opening the duct.

Steps of Choledocholithotomy

The peritoneum at the free margin of gastrohepatic omentum is incised and a length of common duct is exposed. The structure is punctured with a fine needle on syringe to aspirate it and confirm its identity. A vertical incision is then made on the anterior wall of the CBD. This should be of sufficient length to deliver the calculi and should not extend long enough inferiorly to avoid damage to transverse blood vessels running over the duct at its lower end. The incision may be made directly over the impacted calculus steadying it with thumb and index finger of the left hand or at a site where calculi can be conveniently brought by manipulation. Stay sutures are applied to the edges of the incision for control.

Pressure on the duct at appropriate points may deliver the calculi out through the opening. A rubber catheter may be attached to the tip of the sucker and introduced upwards and downwards into the duct. Suction applied to the catheter may help in bringing the calculi into the area of the opening in the duct. The specially designed Desjardins forceps which holds the stone without crushing may be gently passed into the common duct, right hepatic duct, left hepatic duct systemically keeping the head-end of the operating table lowered.

Calculi held at its fenestrated end are extracted out one after another. The same maneuver is followed for the lower end after reversing the head raised position. Balloon tipped soft catheter may also be used for this extraction. The duct in its entire length has also the right and left hepatic ducts is next washed thoroughly with water or normal saline to flush out residual calculi or fragments. The whole procedure of clearance is repeated once again. If available, a choledochoscope is passed to inspect the lumen of the duct to look for residual calculi or fragment at this stage.

As a simple technique, a lubricated rubber catheter of appropriate size and stiffness may also be gently passed downwards to the duodenal lumen where it can be detected by palpating through the duodenal wall. The sphincter of oddi may be palpated around it to exclude residual calculus at lower end of the duct.

After being satisfied about the adequate clearance of the duct the horizontal limb of T-tube preferably made of India rubber or latex is introduced through the incision so that the end of the limb extends both above and below the incision. The limb and its ends should lie freely inside the duct and should not extend so far below as to declude the opening of the pancreatic duct which may predispose to postoperative pancreatitis.

It is a good practice to cut out a strip from the entire ventral aspect of the horizontal limb of T-tube to assure uninterrupted flow of bile. The junction of the T-tube is placed in the lower end of the incision which is closed by interrupted 3/0 chromic catgut sutures. Some surgeons feel that it is important to exclude the mucosa from the bites. A completion cholangiogram is performed through the T-tube (taking care not to introduce air bubbles) to confirm clearance of calculi from the duct system. The T-tube is next brought out through a stab wound in the lateral abdominal wall making sure that it lies laterally without tension and is fixed securely to the skin by a silk stitch encircling the tube. A corrugated rubber sheet or tube drain is next placed in the hepatorenal pouch to drain out any leakage postoperatively and brought out through lateral abdominal wall where it is secured with a stitch.

For calculus impacted or lodged in diverticulum in the inaccessible retroduodenal part of CBD, duodenum is kocherized and the CBD is incised directly over stone to deliver it out and the incision is closed by interrupted sutures over a T-tube splint. If the calculus cannot be removed through the bile duct by choledochotomy, the duodenum is incised longitudinally over the papilla, sphincterotomy performed and the duct explored in retrograde manner. Postoperatively, bile drains into a bedside receptacle through a sterile connection. The T-tube is clamped intermittently from the end of the first week for increasing periods. One should keep watch for onset of colic pain, fever with chill, yellow discoloration of urine, white stool or leakage of bile around the exit of the T-tube. In such a case, T-tube should be unclamped and again allowed to drain freely. In any case, a postoperative T-tube cholangiogram is performed around the seventh day which should demonstrate free flow of dye into the duodenum and no filling defect should be apparent in the dye-outlined bile duct from the tapered lower end to the right and left hepatic ducts. On being satisfied, the T-tube is removed by gentle and steady pull around the tube.

Residual calculi in the duct may be treated successfully in most cases through endoscopic sphincterotomy and extraction using a Dormia basket or similar instrument. For stones larger than 2 cm, it may need removal by surgery involving re-exploration of CBD. Stones can also be dealt with through the transhepatic route for calculi in the left region of the duct system. Ursodeoxycholic acid (Udiliv) or analogue has been used to prevent recurrence or for preventing the calculi from getting larger.

Note on Operative Cholangiogram

This is performed to ascertain presence of calculi in the bile ducts prior to deciding on choledocholithotomy in cases where there is no clear evidence in its favor and also as a completion cholangiogram through T-tube to rule out residual calculi or fragments.

Technique

After dissection of Calot's triangle and prior to cholecystectomy, the cystic duct is dissected clean (Skeletonized) and held with a sling of silk or other suture material. The cystic duct is tied off close to the gallbladder. A fine plastic tube, usually a pediatric Ryle's tube of suitable caliber, is attached to a saline-filled syringe and the whole is made air free by pushing out the fluid. A syringe filled with radiopaque dye (Urograffin may be used) is kept ready and air-free. The cystic duct is incised at a convenient point and the plastic tube introduced through it across the valve of the cystic duct into the CBD. Withdrawal of bile into the syringe on negative suction confirms the presence of the tip of the tube in the lumen of the CBD. The tube is fixed in position by tying the suture used as a sling and the saline-filled syringe is replaced by the dye-filled one taking care not to let air bubbles in doing this change over. The amount of dye to be pushed depends on the caliber of the CBD and varies from 4–10 mL. The dye is first pushed in the headward position to fill the upper segment of the common duct and the right and left hepatic ducts and pictures taken.

The position is then reversed and further amount of dye is pushed to outline the lower end of the CBD. The dye should enter the duodenal lumen and outline its mucosa. Any negative shadow is interpreted as a calculus. An air bubble which has a characteristic rounded shape with smooth outline should not be mistaken for a calculus.

Biliary Drainage Procedure

Surgery for choledocholithiasis may be complicated by inadequate clearance of the ducts leaving behind residual calculi or fragment. Also certain conditions may predispose to formation of recurrent calculi. It is important to assure adequate drainage of bile into the intestine in these cases. Two surgical maneuvers are used for this purpose and need to be considered here. These are: (1) Transduodenal sphincterotomy/sphincteroplasty and (2) Choledochoduodenostomy.

Transduodenal Sphincterotomy/ Sphincteroplasty

This entails opening the duodenal lumen, identification of the sphincter of oddi and incision of the sphincter to widen it. It is specifically indicated in condition, like multiple small calculi and sludge present in the ducts including the intrahepatic portion and stones lodged at the lower end of CBD.

Choledochoduodenostomy is indicated in above condition and also in condition like Bismuth type 1 bile duct stricture, some patients with choledochal cyst and as a palliative procedure in malignant conditions obstructing the CBD at its lower end. For example, carcinoma head of the pancreas, cholangiocarcinoma, etc. when it may be wise to transect the CBD and perform an end to side choledochoduodenostomy. The choice between transduodenal sphincterotomy and choledochoduodenostomy in conditions where both are indicated is basically indicated by the size of the CBD. It should be 2 cm or more in diameter (1.5 cm according to some) to justify choledochoduodenostomy.

Technique of Sphincterotomy/Sphincteroplasty (Figs 55.1 to 55.3)

The duodenum is kocherized. An adequate incision is made on the posterior peritoneum lateral to the lateral border of the duodenum which is then mobilized medially by gentle dissection taking care not to injure the spermatic and other retroduodenal veins. The duodenum is then incised longitudinally in its long axis, the center of the incision should correspond with the position of the duodenal papilla. Through the already opened CBD (choledochotomy) a rubber catheter with a stiff tip or a Bake's dilator is passed into the duodenal lumen or pushed to project the mucosa or its tip. The sphincter of oddi is identified and incised at 11 o'clock position to protect the pancreatic duct (Sphincterotomy). A specially designed grooved dilator is employed by some. In sphincterotomy, the muscle layer at the sphincter of oddi is partially incised, while in sphincteroplasty the muscles in the sphincter is divided totally. The incision may be extended for adequate length to match the diameter of the supraduodenal duct taking care that this does not go so far as to open up the

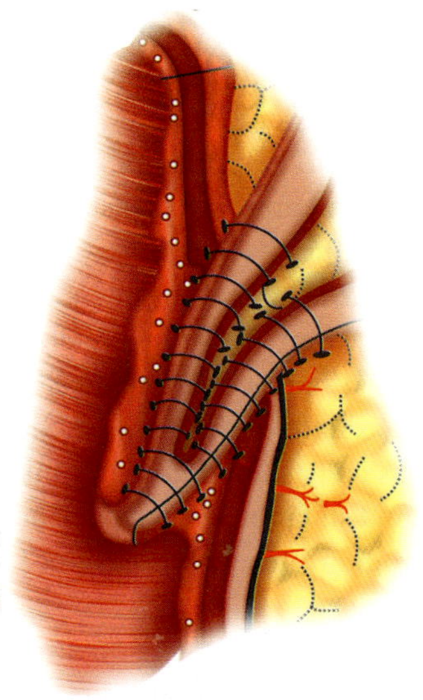

Fig. 55.1 Normal

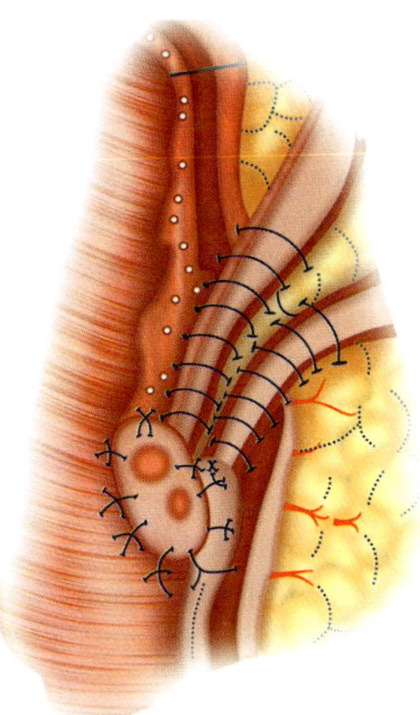

Fig. 55.2 Sphincterotomy

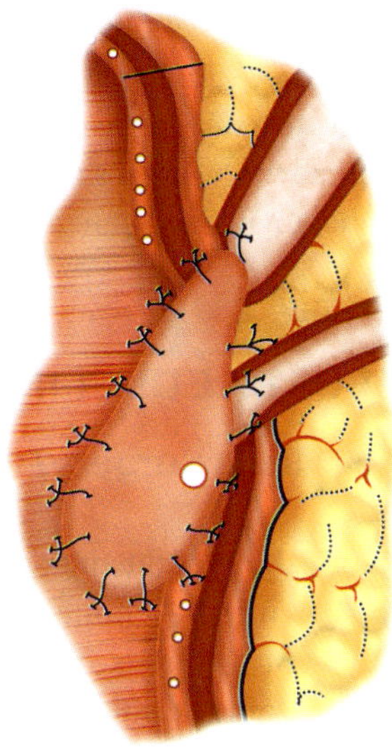

Fig. 55.3 Sphincteroplasty

duodenal lumen. The mucosa of the bile duct and that of the duodenum are then sutured by interrupted 3/0 chromic catgut sutures, progressively incising and suturing bit by bit. The duodenum is then closed vertically in two layers, 3/0 chromic catgut or vicryl through and through and then outer 3/0 or 2/0 atraumatic silk. One may close the duodenum longitudinally also or use continuous or interrupted sutures for the two layers provided the adequacy of its lumen and integrity of anastomosis is maintained.

Complications

Complications of the procedure include hemorrhage evidenced by malena and hypotension if bleeding is severe, and duodenal perforation.

Choledochoduodenostomy (Figs 55.4 to 55.6)

A dilated common bile duct with recurrent bones of cholangitis with or without stone is an indication for choledochoduodenostomy. The common should be preferably 2.5 cm in diameter. O is just below the entrance of cystic duct.

Steps: The CBD is aspirated through a syringe and fine needle to draw bile and confirm its identity. The CBD is then incised vertically (some use an oblique cut) for an adequate length (2–2.5 cm). The duodenum is kocherized and incised longitudinally, the length of the incision is kept to about half of that of CBD incision.

The CBD and duodenum are then anastomosed by full thickness interrupted 3/0 or 2/0 vicryl sutures. The cut edges of the two incisions are approximated in the form of an isosceles triangle. The ends of the duodenal incision are approximated to the middle of the two sides of the CBD incision and the center of the posterior edge of the duodenal incision to the lowest part of CBD incision. The anastomosis is completed by interrupted sutures of the posterior margins. The center of the anterior margin of the duodenal incision is then approximated to the upper most point of the CBD incision and the two halves of the anterior margin of the duodenum thus created is approximated to the two sides of the CBD incision to complete the isosceles triangle. The anastomosis should be tension free. A rubber tube or a sheet drain is placed beneath the anastomosis and abdomen closed in layers.

Complications

1. Leakage, peritonitis and fistulae.
2. Postoperative pancreatitis (Usually when anastomois is done in a narrow duct).
3. The controversial sump syndrome. This is believed to be caused by stasis of vegetable debris, calculi or fragments and infected in the bypassed segment of the bile duct. A narrow stoma may also be a factor. The patient suffers from digestive disturbance and cholangitis with chill and fever.

BILE DUCT INJURIES

Majority of bile duct injuries occur during operation of cholecystectomy. The bile duct may also be injured during other surgical procedures, like gastrectomy or operation on the pancreas. Rarely, blunt injuries produce disruption of bile ducts.

Operative bile duct injuries may be categorized as (1) Ligation (2) Ligation-excision of a segment (3) Complete

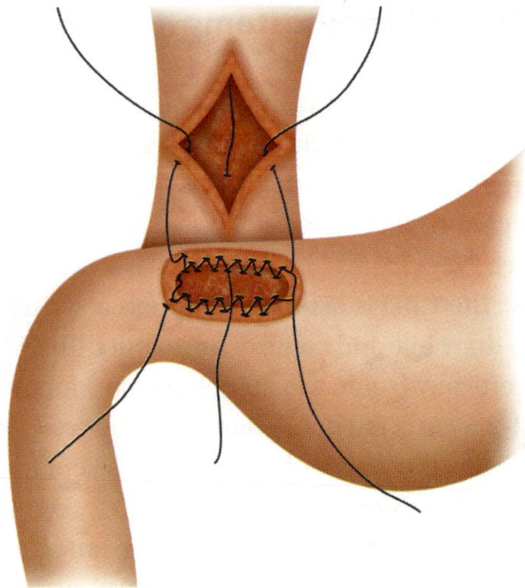

Fig. 55.4 Application of posterior sutures

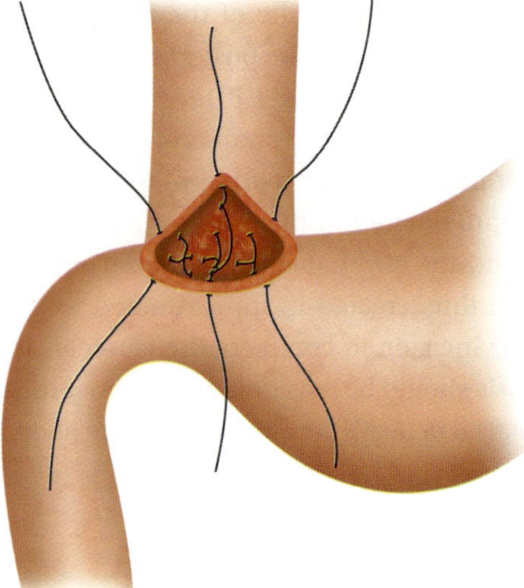

Fig. 55.5 Application of anterior sutures

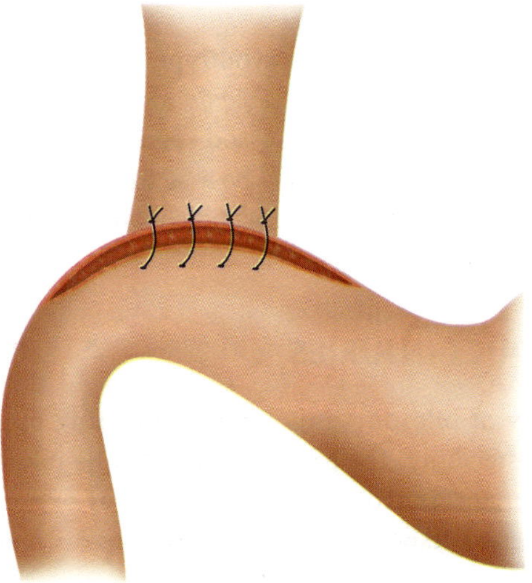

Fig. 55.6 Completion of anterior sutures

transection (4) Lateral and incomplete injuries or cystic duct leaks (5) Crushing trauma, e.g. clamping injuries following panic reaction to hemorrhage (6) Thermal injuries as encountered at laparoscopic cholecystectomy.

The injury may be detected on table or becomes apparent in the postoperative period with *Obstructive jaundice* (usually within 48 hrs) or features of *Excessive bile leakage* (2nd to 7th day). Bile leakage may be manifested as *bile peritonitis* or *external biliary fistula.* A fistula occurs when drainage had been provided at the primary operation or instituted following postoperative intraperitoneal bile collection and peritonitis. Massive intraperitoneal bile collections may lead to a serious situation presenting with hypotension, dyspnea, fever and complicated by features of septicemia and resultant organ failure *(Waltman-Walters syndrome/*demanding prompt surgical intervention to achieve adequate drainage and toilet.

A ligated or crushed duct stimulates fibrosis leading to a complete or incomplete *biliary stricture.* An external biliary fistula may heal by fibrosis to culminate in a *biliary stricture.* A hepaticojejunostomy or fistulojejunostomy (see later) may also be complicated by stricture formation.

Acute cholecystitis with Mirizzi's syndrome, prolonged T-tube *in situ* with cholangitis and pancreatitis may also lead to biliary strictures.

MANAGEMENT OF BILE DUCT INJURIES

When Detected during Surgery?

Simple ligature and crushing of the duct should be undone immediately and this may be enough for short period occlusion. If in doubt, a T-tube is introduced through a choledochotomy away from the site and passed across the area to act as a stent.

Lateral injuries or incomplete cuts may be sutured by interrupted 3/0 vicryl eversion sutures in single layer over a T-tube introduced similarly.

Complete transection or ligature-excision of a segment, after undoing the ligature and trimming the margins, may be reconstructed by end-to-end anastomosis with one layer interrupted 3/0 vicryl eversion sutures over a T-tube stent introduced remotely. If the duct is wide enough at the site, hepaticojejunostomy into a Roux jejunal loop (see later) after tying off the distal end of duct is recommended.

The duodenum is kocherized and soft tissue dissection performed without compromising the blood supply of the ducts to achieve a tension-free anastomosis. Adequate drainage through a multi-holed tube or rubber sheet is provided to cover leak from the anastomosis and abdomen closed in layers.

Divided sectorial ducts may be ligated off. A large caliber duct is anastomosed end to side to a Roux loop of jejunum.

It is, however, important to realize that reconstructive surgery of bile ducts demands a certain degree of expertise and experience. There should be no hesitation to seek help from an experienced surgeon, when one encounters a problem caused by iatrogenic injury of bile duct during surgery and such help is available. It is prudent to provide adequate drainage only through tube or rubbersheet drains to hepatorenal and subphrenic spaces as also to dependent area in pelvis, e.g. pouch of Douglas and close the abdomen. The patient may be subsequently referred to a proper center for specialized treatment. One should not tamper with the bile ducts roughly in a casual manner to interfere with their vascularity and integrity which will predispose to the formation of a stricture due to ischemia.

Treatment of Complications Detected During Postoperative Period

Bile Collections and Peritonitis

Bile leaks have been classified as minor and major leaks. While the former is treated expectantly or by guided aspirations, the latter demands aggressive intervention.

Broad spectrum antibiotics with adequate cover for Gram-positive, Gram-negative and anaerobic infections are instituted and attention given to adequate fluid and electrolyte replacements. Localized collections may be drained by guided aspirations under USG or CT. Pigtail catheters, sometimes in pairs, are used for continued drainage. Surgery is indicated for large collections as also those which are septate or situated in between loops of intestines. An adequate incision is made—midline, right paramedian, subcostal or transverse depending as found, in USG/CT on disposition of the intraperitoneal collections. All collections are drained and septi broken up.

A leaking sectorial duct is ligated off or anastomosed to a Roux loop of jejunum as mentioned earlier.

External Biliary Fistula

Following evacuation of collections, continued drainage is maintained through tube or rubbersheet drains placed in dependent areas including subphrenic space, hepatorenal pouch and pouch of Douglas. The expectation is to establish an *external biliary fistula* which may eventually dry up as in a sectorial duct fistula, or heal by fibrosis to form a biliary stricture. An external biliary fistula may continue to persist without signs of drying up or may coexist with an incomplete stricture in which cases surgery is indicated. The fistulous tract is cored out starting from the parietes to the origin in the biliary tract. The dissected fistulous tract is opened up. The incision is extended to the bile duct and the opening anastomosed to a Roux loop of jejunum (Fistulojejunostomy) with interrupted eversion sutures using 3/0 vicryl and adequate drainage is provided by tube or rubbersheet drains before closing the abdomen. The risk of stricture formation in the future is high following fistulojejunostomy. However, this is an acceptable temporising measure.

External fistula from incomplete cut in the bile duct, a lateral injury or a cystic duct leak is successfully dealt with by endoscopic stenting in the large majority.

Biliary Stricture (Fig. 55.7)

The type of reconstruction depends on the level and length of the stricture. Bismuth's classification remains the most acceptable-Type 1 when the upper limit of the stricture is more than 2 cm away from carina, type 2 when this distance is less than 2 cm, type 3 when this is at the carina and communication between the right and left hepatic ducts is maintained, type 4 when strictures involve carina with loss of communication between the right and left hepatic ducts, type 5 when strictures are higher up and include those that involve sectoral ducts.

Endoscopic or transhepatic dilatations and stenting or ballooning have been practiced for accessible biliary strictures but is unlikely to be of permanent benefit for established biliary strictures.

The available surgical techniques are:

Excision of stricture and end-to-end anastomosis over a T-tube stent: This is a procedure which is difficult to perform satisfactorily without tension and although once practiced widely, has become an almost obsolete procedure.

Choledochoduodenostomy: This is suitable for Bismuth type 1, and also some selected type 2 strictures provided that the anastomosis can be achieved without tension and adequate blood supply is preserved after mobilization of ducts and kocherization of duodenum.

Hepaticojejunostomy: While the hepaticojejunostomy can be performed utilizing a portion of the bile duct which is proximal to the stricture, it may be observed that for best results, one should try to achieve an accurate mucosa to mucosa anastomosis for which the ductal side of the anastomosis should be adequately dilated. Also, the lining mucosa should be healthy and free from inflammatory changes as far as practicable. These requirements are best satisfied if the

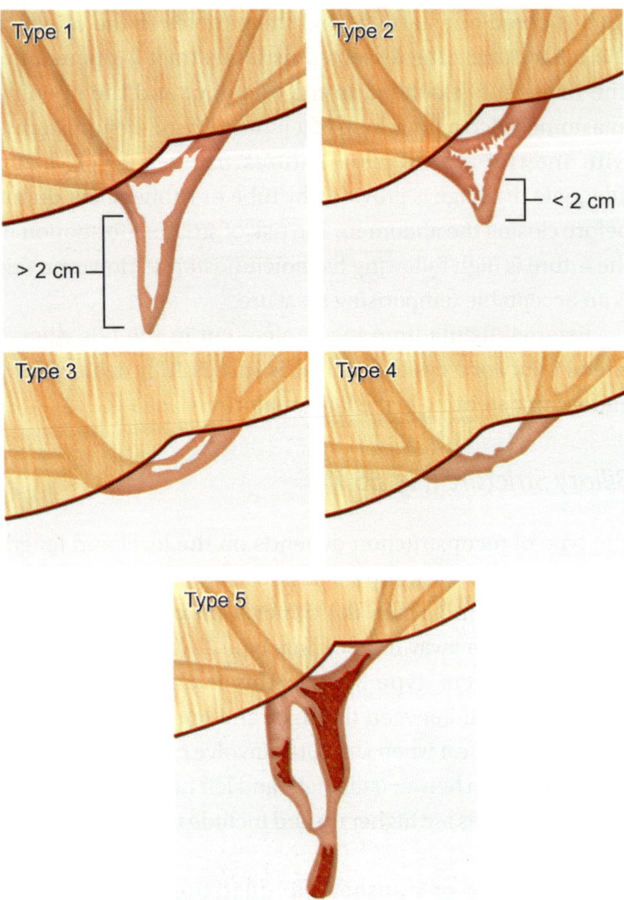

Fig. 55.7 Types of biliary strictures

anastomosis is performed at an area remote from the stricture. This consideration has made the left hepatic duct approach, as popularized by Hepp and Coninaud, a very acceptable one and is preferred whenever it is possible to use it for a bypass of the ductal system.

Steps of the operation: Abdomen is opened by an extended subcostal, Chevron (Roof top) with a vertical limb from the convexity in the midline; a long midline or right paramedian incision may be made in a thin person with a narrow subcostal angle. Bands and adhesions stretching from the interior to the parietal peritoneum are divided to obtain a more clear view. The ligamentum teres is divided and traction on the end attached to liver in upward direction helps in identification of the stricture and subsequent steps. The colon which is adherent to the undersurface of the parietal peritoneum and inferior surface of liver is mobilized through combination of blunt and sharp dissections and displaced medially and downwards. The convex surface of duodenum now comes into view. The duodenum is dissected free and reatracted medially and to the left. The stricture becomes apparent as a firm fibrous nodule. The dilated duct above the nodule is dissected and pricked with a fine needle on syringe to draw out bile and confirm its identity. An anastomosis between upper stump of the duct and Roux loop of jejunum is shown in Figures 55.8 to 55.10.

Left duct approach— (Hepp and Coninaud): An incision is made along the Glisson's capsule of liver below the quadrate lobe and the so-called 'hilar plate' is displaced down to expose a length of the left hepatic duct. An incision is made between two stay sutures to open the duct which allows for copious flow of bile (Figs 55.11 and 55.12).

The jejunum is then traced onwards from the duodenojejunal flexure up to 25 cm approximately and divided through and through along with the mesentery. The distal jejunum is closed in two layers. A hole is created in a convenient and avascular part of the transverse mesocolon and the closed distal jejunal loop transported through this so that its anterior mesenteric surface is made to lie without tension alongside the opened part of left hepatic duct. An incision measuring about half of that in left hepatic duct is made on the anterior mesenteric surface of the jejunal loop 5 to 10 cm away from the closed end. The duct to jejunum anastomosis is then performed using single-layer full-thickness interrupted 3/0 vicryl eversion sutures. It is advisable to place the suture through the jejunum in such a way so that the mucosa of the jejunum rides up the lumen of the duct. This is achieved by taking an extra bite through the mucosa only, apart from the full-thickness bite. The jejunal wall is sutured to the Glisson's capsule by seromuscular bites immediately proximal and distal to the anastomosis to reduce the tension. The jejunal loop is then fixed to the hole in the transverse mesocolon by a few interrupted sutures taking care that the length of the loop from the anastomosis lies relaxed without any tension. The proximal end of the jejunum is then anastomosed end-to-side with distal jejunum about 30 to 40 cm away from the hepaticojejunostomy in two continous layers using 3/0 or 2/0 vicryl for the full-thickness and the same suture or 3/0 atraumatic silk for the seromuscular layer. After peritoneal toilet, the abdomen is closed in layers. A tube or rubbersheet drain is laid below the hepaticojejunal anastomosis before closure and brought out through a stab wound in the lateral abdominal wall. A fine plastic tube can be introduced through an incision in the Roux loop and laid across the anastomosis to act as a stent—this is brought out through a stab wound in the lateral abdominal wall. Some surgeons including the author close both jejunal loops and construct a side to side

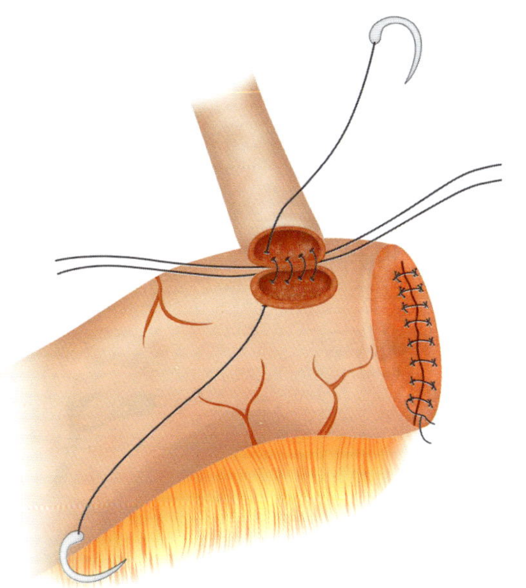
Fig. 55.8 Hepaticojejunostomy Roux-en-Y (Posterior sutures)

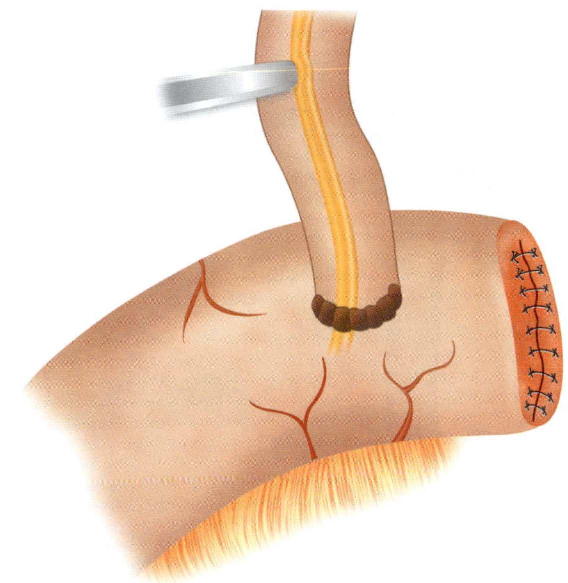
Fig. 55.10 Hepaticojejunostomy completed

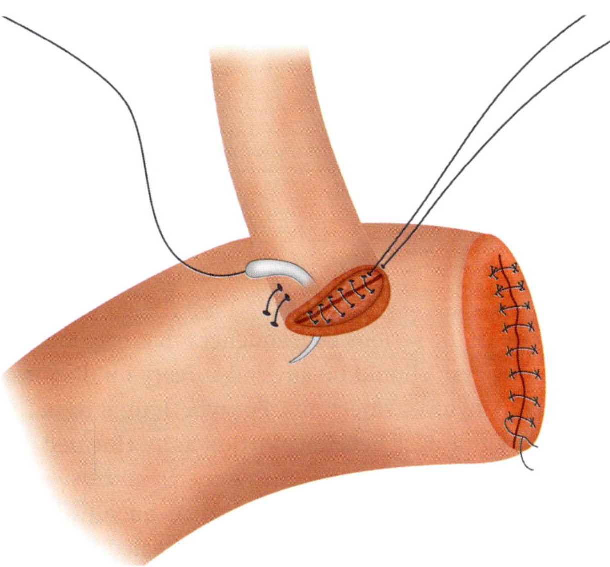
Fig. 55.9 Hepaticojejunostomy (anterior sutures)

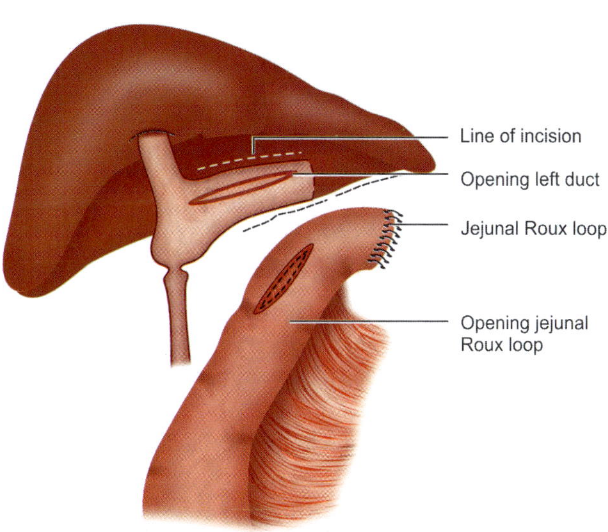

Fig. 55.11 Left hepaticojejunostomy

jejunojejunostomy. For Bismuth type 4 or 5 stricture, it may be necessary to perform multiple anastomoses between the biliary tract and the Roux loop of jejunum. The same thing holds true for multiple-origin high up biliary fistulae also.

Results of Biliary Reconstruction Procedures

All these procedures are liable to be complicated by sepsis and stenosis of the anastomosis leading to episodes of cholangitis, obstructive jaundice and formation of calculi proximal to the anastomosis. While most of these complications are related ultimately to narrowing or stenosis of the anastomosis and become manifest within one year, a few continue to occur up to 3 years and rarely even later.

Surgery of Choledochal Cysts in Adults

Choledochal cyst (Syn. Congenital bile duct cyst) is a congenital condition of cystic dilatation of biliary tract which is usually extrahepatic and may be isolated or found combined

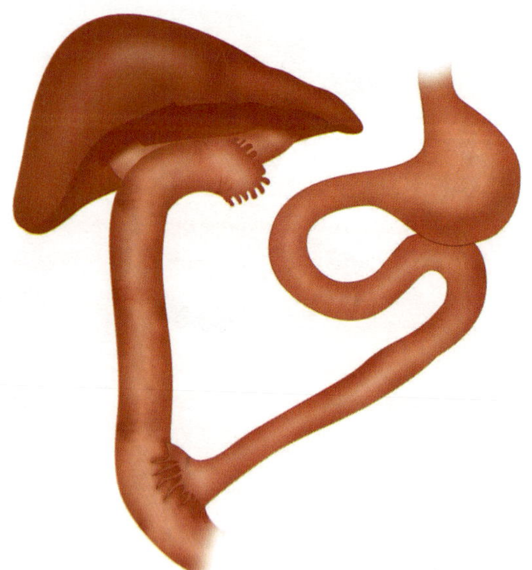

Fig. 55.12 Completion of anastomosis between left duct and Roux loop of jejunum

with intrahepatic dilatation also. Much more common in females, this is diagnosed usually before age of 10 years but about 25% may present after 20 years of age. The "Classical Triad" of presentation include jaundice, pain abdomen and a palpable mass.

In the common form, it is extrahepatic starting from just below the carina and extends down to the lower end within duodenum and may extend to the pancreas also.

Alonso-Hej et al's (1959) classification modified by Todani (1977) divides the cysts into (Fig. 55.13).

Type-I: Cystic dilatation, focal dilatation, fusiform dilatation.

Type-II: Cystic diverticulation from the bile duct.

Type-III: Cystic dilatation at lower end within duodenum—'Choledochocele'

Type-IV: IVa, extrahepatic as well as intrahepatic dilatations.

IVb: Multiple extrahepatic cysts.

Type-V: Intrahepatic dilatations only (Caroli's disease).

The condition is liable to be affected by complications-cholecystitis with cholelithiasis, cholangitis, intracystic calculi formation, recurrent pancreatitis and the more serious conditions like carcinomatous change and rupture of the cyst. Recurrent infection may lead to cirrhotic changes in liver and portal hypertension.

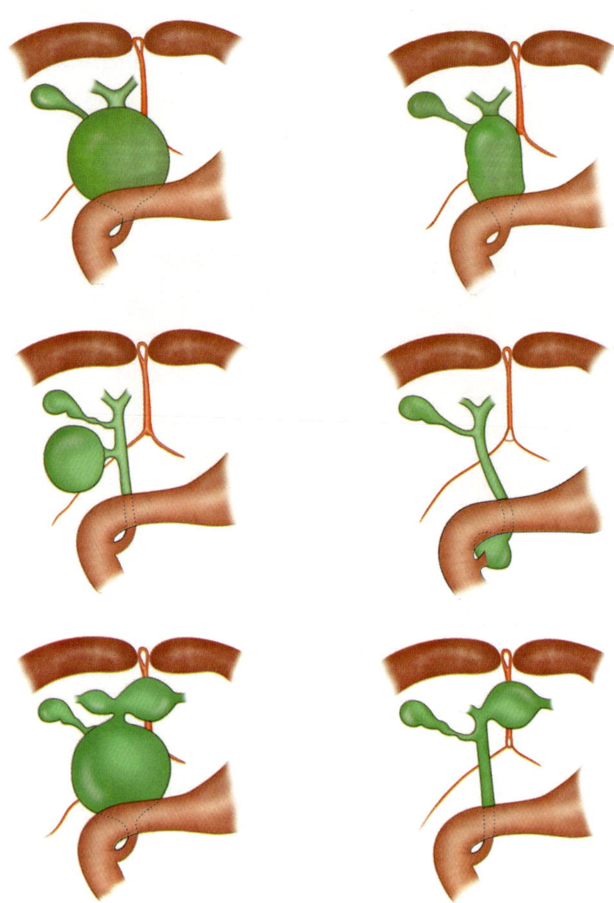

Fig. 55.13 Types of choledochal cysts

Because of the serious consequences that may follow, a choledochal cyst, should be advised surgery on diagnosis. This usually involves resections. For type-I, total or radical excision of the cyst bearing portion is performed and followed by Roux hepaticojejunostomy. In short-segment type-Ib, it may be possible to perform an end-to-end anastomosis over a stent. Type-II may be treated by ligation or closure of the connection with the bile duct but may need Roux; hepaticojejunostomy if narrowing of the bile duct is apprehended in the former technique. Type-III is treated by transduodenal sphincteroplasty/sphincterotomy, which may have to be added to resection in some cases of type-IC, type-IVb/and extrahepatic component of type-IVa have to be treated by multiple excisions and anastomoses into Roux loop of jejunum. Type-V and intrahepatic component of type-IVb may be treated by stenting or subjected to segmental resections of liver, right or left lobectomy or even hepatic resection followed by liver transplantation.

Only drainage may have to be resorted to in the unfit and ill patients and patients with severe cholangitis or ruptured cysts. This can be achieved by (i) endoscopic drainage through nasobiliary drain or stent, (ii) Percutaneous transhepatic biliary drainage (PTBD), (iii) T-tube drainage, e.g. in rupture, (iv) Choledochoduodenostomy or (v) Roux hepaticojejunostomy.

Resection of Choledochal Cyst

A subcostal or right paramedian incision is made. The gallbladder and cystic duct is subjected to careful dissection which extends to the choledochal cyst-one should be careful not to damage the right hepatic artery which may be adherent to the cyst wall. The anterior, medial, lateral, and posterior cyst walls are dissected carefully in a caudal direction. The cyst is dissected posteriorly of the portal vein and hepatic artery encircled in a sling of cotton tape or rubber catheter. The cyst may have to be opened longitudinally to facilitate the dissection by pulling on the edges. If present, intracystic calculi may be removed at this stage. The lower end of the cyst extends into the intraduodenal part of the bile duct. The duodenum is mobilized by kocherization (incision of posterior parietal peritoneum lateral to duodenum) and the lower end of the cyst is dissected with care. The high anomalous pancreatic duct-biliary junction needs to be protected. The cyst-bearing bile duct is divided proximal to this junction ligating off the lower end. Accidental ligation or injury to the pancreatic duct at this juncture may lead to serious complications like pancreatitis or postoperative pancreatic fistula. Applying traction on the divided cyst, dissection is made to proceed cranialwards. The anterior, lateral and medial walls can be dissected without much problem, but the posterior wall needs to be separated from the portal vein and hepatic artery. Adhesions resultant from repeated episodes of cholangitis may render this a difficult procedure and if so needed, the posterior wall of the cyst may be incised and divided into inner and outer layers, the latter is left adherent to the blood vessels and the inner layer dissected or stripped out and removed with the cysts, accepting whatever small risk is there in respect of malignant change. Injury to the portal vein or hepatic artery is thus avoided. The cyst along with cystic duct and gallbladder attached to it is dissected upto its upper limit just below the carina where it is divided, to remove the cyst along with the gallbladder. Reconstruction is achieved by hepaticojejunostomy to a Roux loop of jejunum. If the cystic change extends to right and/or left hepatic duct, these have to be divided to achieve complete removal and reconstruction accomplished by two separate anastomoses to the Roux loop of jejunum. After hemostasis, the abdomen is closed in layers with provision to draining through tube or rubbersheet drain.

Complications of the Operation

1. Anastomotic leak which is not common—the resultant fistula usually dries up with expectant treatment,
2. Pancreatitis,
3. Pancreatic fistula, etc.

SECTION

9

Pancreas

CHAPTER

56

Surgery of Pancreas

Dipankar Sen Gupta

SURGERY FOR ACUTE PANCREATITIS

Introduction

Acute pancreatitis is an acute inflammatory condition of the exocrine pancreas. It is diagnosed by a typical clinical presentation of upper abdominal pain associated with or without organ failure, together with significantly raised levels of the pancreatic enzymes: amylase and lipase. Confirmation of the diagnosis is made by using a contrast-enhanced CT imaging.

Acute pancreatitis can be mild or severe. Mild pancreatitis is treated by conservative measures. Severe pancreatitis is also managed medically to begin with, but may require surgery for the following indications.

Indications of Surgery

Infected Pancreatic Necrosis

This is established by a combination of contrast CT to demonstrate necrosis and a fine needle aspiration culture of the necrosis to demonstrate infection. The patient should also show evidence of non-improvement of clinical status after using appropriate antibiotic together with other routine intensive care support. The following points need mentioning: (i) fever (ii) persistent high white cell count (iii) high CRP > 150 mg/dL.

Pancreatic Abscess

This is a circumscribed intra-abdominal collection of pus in the peri-pancreatic area in the absence of any pancreatic necrosis and characterized by the typical clinical manifestation of fever with raised white cell count.

Preoperative Preparations

- General preparations.
- *Establishment of antibiotic policy:* Assessing what antibiotic group has already been used and what antibiotic to use perioperatively.
- Perioperative use of octreotide (dosage 0.1 mg subcutaneously × 8 hrly) and to start 20 minutes before surgery.
- Assessment of urinary output and renal status prior to surgery and fluid/diuresis corrections as required.
- Correction of prothrombin time by using vitamin K, fresh frozen plasma (FFP) transfusions and arrangement of fresh donors during surgery.
- Assessment of serum albumin level and an attempted correction of albumin as far as possible.
- *Timing of operation*: Three weeks or later, after the onset of disease.

Operating Procedure

- Position of the patient: Supine
- General anesthesia and introduction of a Ryle's tube into the stomach and a Foley's catheter into the urinary bladder (if not in place already).

Incision

Choice: i. Midline
ii. Rooftop
iii. Upper transverse abdominal.

In surgery for acute pancreatitis, a mid-line incision is preferable as the extent of the disease is variable inspite of preoperative CT localizations.

Exposure

Difficult in surgery of acute pancreatitis as clear visceral landmarks are not always evident due to inflammation and edema of all tissues.

Operative Technique

Once the peritoneal cavity has been reached, gentle finger dissection is the only method that can be used to locate and open up the area of necrosis/abscess. Thorough study of the preoperative CT imaging is done to identify the location of the necrosis/abscess. Great caution is to be exercised as there is a definite risk of entering the bowel lumen or causing hemorrhage.

The transverse colon is situated anatomically on the pancreas and is greatly involved in the inflammatory process. The first few loops of the jejunum get adherent to the transverse mesocolon (which is also on the pancreas because of the spread of peripancreatic inflammation. In addition to that, the transverse colon can develope fistulous connection with the pancreatic bed or its vascular supply may be compromised due to inflammatory infarction of its supplying blood vessels. Separation of these involved/adherent bowel is not easy and the lumen can be opened inadvertently. If that happens, it is a disaster and is best avoided.

Once the area of necrosis has been reached, the dead tissues have to be teased away gently from the viable structures by finger dissection alone. There is always a great risk of bleeding from the pancreatic bed area during separation of necrosis. The aim here is to remove all necrotic tissues avoiding significant hemorrhage. Inadequate removal of necrosis would require a second hazardous surgery at a later date.

Summary of Problems Faced during Necrosectomy

- Inadequate necrosectomy—to be avoided by careful intelligent digital probing.
- *Hemorrhage from pancreatic bed:* This is partly avoided by planning the timing of the surgery. Hemorrhage is significant if any surgical interference is made earlier than 3 weeks from the onset of disease. The risk of hemorrhage precedes as time passes by and later the surgery, lesser the chance of significant blood loss.
  Some bleeding is inevitable and this is controlled by pressure packs. Usually, a little bleeding continues even after removing the packs and if this is at an acceptable level, it is managed by irrigation of the pancreatic bed and transfusion of fresh blood.
  Sometimes, though rarely, significant bleeding can continue. In that case, it has to be controlled by pressure packing again which may have to be removed/changed after a day or two.
- Entry into the colon or the presence of an existing colonic fistula is a life-threatening situation. A proximal loop ileostomy must be established and the diseased colon may either be exteriorized or resected and then exteriorized. Simple repair will be unwise.
- A vascularly compromised colon due to inflammatory infarction of its blood supply has to be treated similarly, leg, proximal ileostomy, resection and exteriorization of viable bowel as mucocutaneous fistula.
- Injury to proximal jejunal loop is again best avoided. However, in the case of such an accidental event a simple repair is advised, after having established that there is no partial distal obstruction due to adhesions or kink. Alternatively, the injury site can be used for placing—feeding jejunostomy tube.

Closure

Several methods are available and the choice of a particular method will depend on the nature of the problems faced during surgery.

- Simple anatomical closure as in any laparotomy with drainage tubes in the operated bed—this method can only be used when the surgery has been necessitated at a later date from the onset of the disease. This delay firstly indicates a disease score of lesser virulence and secondly allows the inflammatory process to settle, thereby reducing the risks of hemorrhage and bowel damage.
- Anatomical closure with irrigation set up, i.e. size 18 Ryle's tube to introduce normal saline for irrigation and wide bored chest drainage tubes to wash out hemorrhage necrotic remnants. The number of such strategically placed tubes will depend on the extent of the operated pancreatic bed.
- Closure with pressure packs to stop significant bleeding. In this situation, it will be necessary to re-explore and review the position after 1 or 2 days.
- Partial closure with laparostomy formation (i) to control significant hemorrhage with pressure packs, and (ii) to irrigate grossly infected necrotic area.
- Terminal ileostomy and exteriorization of colon (damaged/fistulating/vascularly compromized) as mucocutaneous fistula.

Postoperative Care

- Cardiorespiratory and ventilator support may or may not be required depending on the general and multiorgan status of the patient.
- Fluid/nutrition/antibiotics as per requirement.
- Renal support may be required when necessary.
- Octreotide is given 8 hrly for 7 days/Irrigation of the pancreatic bed by saline with a close monitoring of input and output and culture/sensitivity study of the output material to detect sepsis.
- Routine monitoring of Hb, PCV, white cell count, electrolytes and urea-creatinine.
- Monitoring of fever, pulse rate and blood pressure and care of ileostomy or colostomy areas when present.
- Oral/jejunostomy feed can be started 3–4 days after surgery.
- Irrigation to continue till returning fluid clears up and is sterile. The drain tubes can be removed later.
- Once fever subsides and general condition improves, the patient can be shifted out of the intensive care unit.

Postoperative Complications

- Hemorrhage from the pancreatic bed is life-threatening. Packing of the pancreatic bed is one option of treatment. Angiographic embolization is also a good option.
- Infection and sepsis of the pancreatic bed may require a second surgery. Inadequate necrosectomy could be a cause.
- Development of an intestinal fistulae (colon or small bowel) is probably caused by compromised bowel not detected or judged during the surgery. A second surgery will be required but the outlook is very poor.
- General deterioration of condition, inability to be weaned from cardiorespiratory and ventilator support indicates a multiorgan system failure. The underlying cause is probably sepsis due to severe grade acute pancreatitis. Acute respiratory distress syndrome (ARDS), renal failure, hypotension, encephalopathy, disseminated intravascular coagulation (DIC) are the eventual manifestations leading to death.

PANCREATICOJEJUNOSTOMY

Introduction

Pancreaticojejunostomy or drainage of the pancreatic duct is an operation done in patients with recurrent severe or moderate abdominal pain arising due to chronic pancreatitis with dilated pancreatic duct. Most of them have pancreatic ductal stones. A USG of upper abdomen initially suggests the presence of pancreatic stones. An MRCP or an ERCP is required to show the degree of ductal dilation, as also the disposition and lie of the pancreatic duct stones. Since most of the pancreatic duct stones are radiopaque, a straight X-ray of the abdomen is also required to see the stones. This X-ray abdomen will be of immense value in judging the clearance of all stones during the operation.

Indications

Drainage of the pancreatic duct by anastomosis to jejunum may be indicated for symptomatic chronic recurrent pancreatitis. Ductal dilatation of the pancreatic duct of at least 6 mm. Mostly, stones are found in the dilated ducts. However, a calculus ductal dilatation of the pancreatic duct is also possible (in a smaller percentage of cases), and they are also candidates for surgical drainage, provided the duct is sufficiently dilated.

Preparations

Routine preparation as in any abdominal surgery. Diabetes due to chronic pancreatic disease may be an associated factor, and sugar control is essential.

Octreotide is to be given in the perioperative and postoperative period.

Operative Procedures

- *Position of patient:* Supine.
- *Anesthesia:* General with a nasogastric tube positioned in the stomach.
- *Incision:* Rooftop or midline.
- *Exposure:* The stomach, transverse colon with mesocolon are exposed. The rest are packed for good exposure of the pancreatic body.

Technique: First Part–Exposure of Duct and Lithotomy (Fig. 56.1)

- The lesser sac is entered, through the greater omentum.
- The anterior surface of the pancreas is reached, and any vein encountered is dissected away or tied and cut to give a good exposure. The transverse mesocolon with the colonic vessels are dissected downwards and away from the pancreatic surface.
- The pancreatic duct with stones, is felt in the mid-body area by the finger. A needle is inserted into the pancreatic

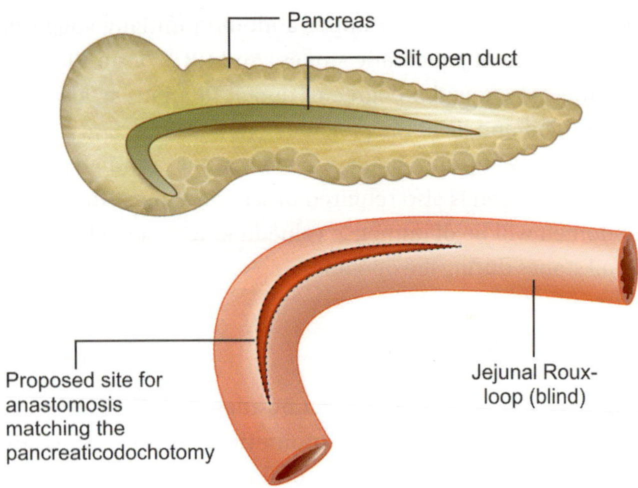

Fig. 56.1 Slit open main pancreatic duct and proposed site in Roux-loop of jejunum for anastomosis

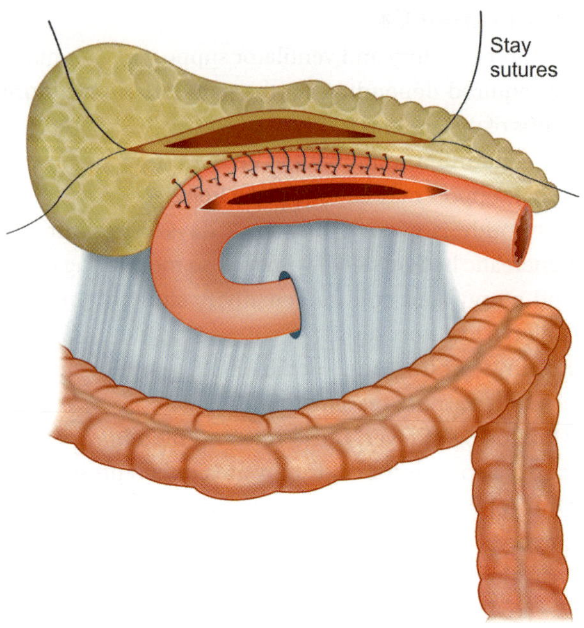

Fig. 56.2 Application of first layer of sutures

duct and aspirated. A clear transparent fluid confirms the presence of the needle into the pancreatic duct.

- The pancreatic duct is incised and opened transversely in between stay sutures. Once the lumen has been reached, the duct opening is extended by scissors firstly towards the tail, till the last of the stone lying in the tail is reached. Using a Desjardines or similar type stone holding forceps, all stones are removed, although a few granules may be found to be adherent to the pancreatic acini tissues and unremovable.
- The same method of extension of incision by scissors is made transversely towards the head region, and stones removed. Once again small bits of stones adhere to the main substance of the pancreas which are difficult, sometimes, impossible to remove. These are left behind. Great care is taken as the head region is approached and the pancreaticodochotomy is made bit by bit, for fear of hemorrhage. Eventually, the whole duct is laid open, and a point is reached very near the ampulla. All stones are removed.
- It is now necessary to cut back in the direction of the accessory duct, that is to the right and below. This is done after careful probing to find the lie of the duct. Once again, the incision is extended bit by bit for fear of hemorrhaging. Again all stones are removed.
- After completion of laying open of the main pancreatic duct as mentioned above and removal of all visible stones, it is quite common to realize that there are one or two stones left behind. This is established by sounding technique using metal dilators. Where facilities are available, a choledochoscope can be used to try and note their presence. The difficult part is to negotiate and remove all these stones. Sometimes, sounding can give a false impression, as the grate made by small adherent granules can mimic the presence of a larger stone. This is where a check X-ray of a previously noted radiopaque stone can be very useful for comparison. Anyhow, most of the stones are removed, and an accurate assessment is made by check X-ray as to how many, if any, have been left behind.
- When the dilated pancreatic duct did not contain any stone, a smaller (and less hazardous) incision in the body and head suffices for anastomosis.

Technique: Second Part–Anastomosis

The operation choice is of longitudinal pancreatico-jejunostomy, which creates a long side-to-side anastomosis between the incised duct and a Roux-loop of jejunum.

- A Roux-loop of jejunum is prepared. The blind limb of the Roux-loop is brought to the lesser sac preferably by the retrocolic route.
- The end of the blind loop stump is closed in 2 layers by continuous 3-0 vicryl and 3-0 silk.
- The blind loop is placed like an inverted J, with the transverse limb pointing to the left. The stump should be located 3 cm distal to the tail-end of the pancreaticodochotomy. The seromuscular coat of the transverse limb is then fixed to the tissue of the pancreas just below the ductal opening, using 00 interrupted silk at suitable interval (First layer) (Fig. 56.2).

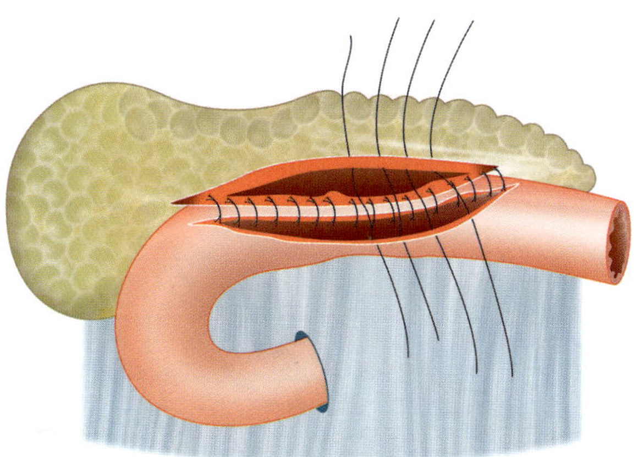

Fig. 56.3 Application of second and third layers of sutures

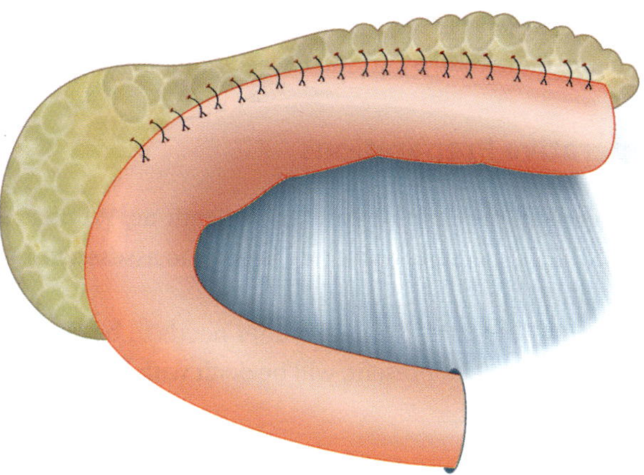

Fig. 56.4 Completion of anastomosis

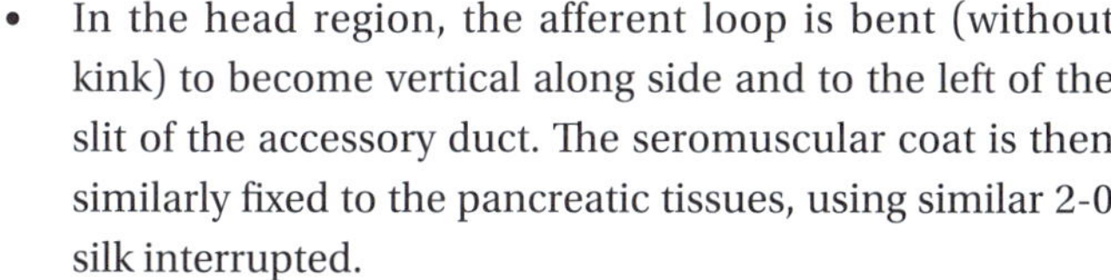

- In the head region, the afferent loop is bent (without kink) to become vertical along side and to the left of the slit of the accessory duct. The seromuscular coat is then similarly fixed to the pancreatic tissues, using similar 2-0 silk interrupted.
- The jejunal loop is then opened by a knife to expose the lumen extending from the tail end of the pancreatico-dochotomy site along the whole length of the transverse limb and down a little bit in the longitudinal limb, till the point where the accessory pancreaticodochotomy ends.
- An anastomosis between the cut open pancreatic duct and jejunal limb is made using through and through interrupted sutures of 2-0 vicryl which are properly spaced and placed posteriorly and then anteriorly to complete the anastomoses (second and third layers) (Fig. 56.3).
- A reinforcing interrupted 2-0 silk suture is given to hold the anterior seromuscular jejunum and the tissues of pancreas (fourth layer) (Fig. 56.4).
- The retrocolic rent in transverse mesocolon is fixed to the jejunal limb.
- The Roux-en-Y jejunojejunostomy is completed.
- The lesser sac is closed and a drain is placed here.

Closure

Anatomical routine closure with drain.

Postoperative Care

The patient is maintained with IV fluids/antibiotic/nasogastric tube and monitoring of pulse, blood pressure, renal flow, intake/output and electrolytes.

About 3 days later, when bowel sounds return, oral feed is restarted and IV omitted. Drain is removed after 5–6 days when dry.

Postoperative Complications

- General complications of abdominal surgery.
- Chance of leak of pancreatic juice is there, but this is an uncommon happening.
- Problem is actually of inadequate removal of stones and recurrence of pain. Therefore, a careful documentation of amount and number of stones left back is very essential for future follow-up.

PSEUDOCYST OF PANCREAS

Acute pancreatic fluid collections occur in 40% of patients with acute pancreatitis. 50% of this collection will resolve spontaneously and 50% will persist as a pseudocyst which may cause symptoms necessitating surgery.

It takes 4–6 weeks for the fluid collection to resolve. If after 6 weeks there is a residual collection of more than 6 cm in diameter, it merits consideration of surgery.

The assessment may primarily have been CT imaging, but study of regression of cysts at a regular interval is done satisfactorily by ultrasonography. Cysts more than 6 cm diameter that persist for more than 6 weeks is a condition that may give rise to symptoms, which include gastric or duodenal compression or compression of the CBD. Less frequently, the cyst may point downwards and require a different approach in surgery, although percutaneous aspiration or endoscopic/laparoscopic drainage have also been described. Conventional open transgastric internal drainage (Jurash) has always given satisfactory results.

Indications

- Symptoms as vomiting/pain upper abdomen/fullness after a small meal

- Evidence of sepsis
- Cyst size more than 6 cm, and 6 weeks after acute attack.

Preoperative Preparations

Routine general preparations and investigations. White cell count/CRP/P. Time/serum albumin is done to assess settling of pancreatitis.

During USG studies, the gallbladder needs to be studied for gallstones which, if present, will be dealt with in the same setting.

Operative Procedure: Transgastric Cystogastrostomy or Roux-en-Y (Cystojejunostomy)

- *Position of patient:* Supine
- *Anesthesia:* General
- *Incision:* Rooftop or midline incision

Transverse upper abdominal incision may also be given:

Unless the cyst is pointing below the stomach, a rooftop or transverse incision will give excellent approach.

A lower pointing cyst will be better tackled by a midline incision.

Exposure

The stomach and the cyst walls are identified. It is established:

- The cyst is truly retrogastric (as in majority of cases).
- The cyst wall is well-formed and capsulated.
- The cyst wall is densely adherent to the posterior wall of the stomach.

The transverse colon and the small intestines are packed aside using mops to give a clear view of the stomach with the protruding retrogastric cyst.

Techniques (Fig. 56.5)

- Anterior wall of the stomach is picked-up in between two stay sutures. In the region of the body and antrum that is accessible to the surgeon and also is anterior to the maximum bulge produced by the cyst.
- A longitudinal anterior gastrotomy is made.
- A needle (with attached syringe) is introduced into the cyst through the posterior stomach wall and clear fluid is aspirated.
- Two deep non-absorbable stay sutures are placed to pullup the posterior wall of the stomach with the adherent cyst wall at an appropriate place easily accessible and at the site of the maximum bulge.

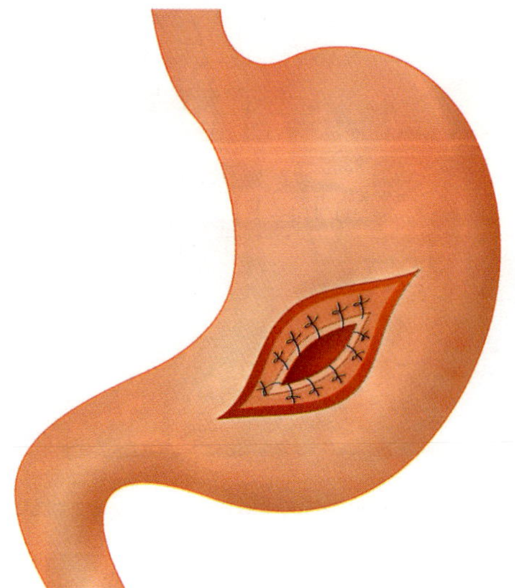

Fig. 56.5 Cystogastrostomy

- A stab knife longitudinal cut is made (about 1 cm wide) and deep enough to cut into the cyst.
- An index finger is immediately introduced into the cyst wall to stop the hemorrhage from the cut cyst and stomach wall.
- Two through and through 2-0 vicryl sutures are placed on two sides of the linear cut and the two edges are both pulled and lifted.
- The initial 1 cm cut is then increased longitudinally using scissors, so that 2–3 fingers can be introduced and a satisfactory stoma is made.
- As there is significant hemorrhage from the cut edges of the stomach and cyst wall—a rapid series of about 10–12 through and through interrupted 2-0 vicryl sutures are placed all around the stoma, and then individually tied (Fig. 56.5).
- If there are any more bleeding from the cut edges of the stomach and cyst wall, extra-interrupted sutures are placed to achieve complete hemostasis.
- The cyst is completely evacuated of all fluid contents using gentle suction.
- Digital feel of the cyst cavity and wall is made and residual sterile necrotic tissues are looked for and gently evacuated.
- The cyst wall is irrigated with saline and a clear returning fluid is seen.
- An edge biopsy of the cyst wall is taken.
- The anterior stomach wall is closed in 2 layers—continuous - 2-0 vicryl and 2-0 silk.
- Abdomen is closed in layers.
- If the cyst was found to be pointing at a site inferior to the stomach, the maximum protruding point is identified,

aspirated to make sure and then cut opened for a diameter of about 2 cm. The occurrence of hemorrhage from the cyst wall in this case is minimum. Once again, an edge biopsy of the cyst wall is taken.

A Roux-en-Y end-to-side cystojejunostomy is established using one layer interrupted 2-0 vicryl sutures (Fig. 56.6).

Closure

Routine anatomical closure. A drain is given.

Postoperative Care

Routine postoperative management with nasogastric aspiration/IV fluid/monitoring of pulse/BP/intake-output/ renal parameters/electrolytes/white cell count/Hb.

After about 3 days, the nasogastric tube is withdrawn and oral feed commenced—water first, then liquids and then solid.

Postoperative Complications

- Usually recovery is satisfactory and uncomplicated.
- There may be bleeding from inside the cyst wall. This should respond to conservative measures and blood transfusion.
- Risk of infection to be combated with antibiotics.
- Leaks/gastric fistula-very rare and usually underlines residual unresolved pancreatic inflammation—to be treated conservatively with initial parenteral nutrition and later establishment of a feeding jejunostomy.

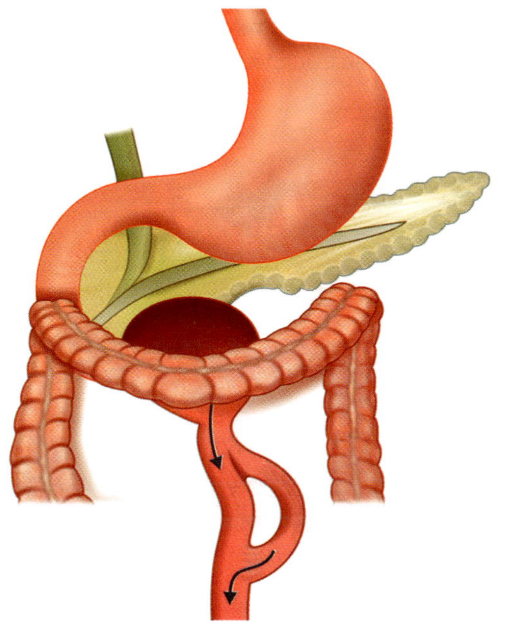

Fig. 56.6 Cystojejunostomy (Roux-en-Y)

SURGERY OF PANCREATIC CANCER

Pancreatic ductal adenocarcinoma remains a leading cause of death with survival rate less than 5% all over the world. Surgical resection with negative resection margin remains the gold standard of treatment but can be achieved in small number of patients.

PANCREATICODUODENECTOMY/ WHIPPLE'S PROCEDURE

Introduction

Neoplasm at the lower end of the common bile duct requires a radical excision policy. Four types of neoplasm are encountered in that critical zone.

1. Papillary tumor of the ampulla of vater, which results in the blockage of both the CBD and pancreatic duct (PD) at the very tip of the ampulla. (This results in ductal dilatation of both the CBD and PD for the entire length and can be imaged and assessed accordingly).
2. Carcinoma of the head of pancreas, which results in the blockage of both CBD and PD at the head region, thereby, sparing the last 1 cm of the CBD and PD (the ductal dilatation of the CBD and PD on imaging can be seen to end about 1 cm away from the ampulla), with a small length of normal CBD and PD left at the tip, which actually represents the intra-duodenal length of the ducts.
3. Cholangiocarcinoma of the lower end of CBD, which results in blockage of the CBD only (On imaging the CBD is wholly dilated but the PD appears normal).
4. Carcinoma duodenum at the ampullary area (imaging pictures will depend on whether the ampullary opening is involved or not).

The extent of excisional surgery required for all these four conditions is the same and was described in details by Whipple. Recent analysis suggests that a more radicle approach is required. This involves routine cholecystectomy and radical excision of adjacent lymph nodes, and should give longer survival.

Indications

- Papillary carcinoma of the ampulla of vater.
- Carcinoma head pancreas.
- Cholangiocarcinoma lower end of CBD.
- Carcinoma duodenum at the ampullary area.

Preparations

Judging Operability

- USG/CT identifies the obvious advanced stages, i.e. presence of liver metastases, obvious ascites with presence of malignant cells.
- In the absence of obvious metastatic disease, the next judgement is assessing the clearance of the tumor in relation to the portal vein. This judgement is especially necessary in the case of carcinoma head pancreas. CT/MRI imaging should identify the proximity or invasion of the portal vein. When the portal vein is involved or invaded, the neoplasia is locally advanced and a radical approach may not succeed.
- Local involvement of the uncinate process of the pancreas is another thing to look for. As the uncinate process hooks back behind the superior mesenteric vessels, tumors involving the uncinate process are not ideal for attempting a radical clearance.
  In general, <20% patients have resectable disease.

Minimizing Jaundice

Neoplastic obstruction of the lower end CBD results in jaundice. This needs to be addressed at the very beginning, especially when the bilirubin >10 mg and there is associated coagulopathy. There are several options available.

- The first option is preoperative ERCP stenting. Jaundice will take 2–3 weeks to subside, when surgery can be attempted. The patient can go home during the waiting period.
- A percutaneous transhepatic biliary drainage (PTBD) is the next option when ERCP stenting has failed. A PTBD catheter is left in position to drain bile. The patient needs to be hospitalized during the waiting period, which demands a lengthy hospital stay.
- A percutaneous transcholecystic drainage is an option, when the gallbladder is grossly distended and palpable (not commonly done).
- When icterus is mild (or when the above have failed), surgery can be attempted after taking the special preparations for jaundice.

Preparations for Jaundice

- Injection Vitamin K 10 mg × IM × daily x 5 days to correct the P. time.
- Preoperative antibiotics for 2–3 days at least to prevent sepsis.
- Proper hydration is an absolute requirement using IV fluids. Diuresis with mannitol is done to establish a good renal flow with an aim to prevent the development of hepatorenal syndrome. Patient needs to be catheterized to monitor the urinary output.
- Arrangements for FFP to correct P. time, if necessary, prior to and during surgery.
- Arrangements of fresh donors (not old blood) to be used during surgery. It is best to have at least 3–5 fresh donors ready.
- A perioperative antibiotic policy to supplement the preoperative antibiotic used.
- Octreotide to be started 1/2 hour prior to surgery. However, some studies disagree to the benefits of using routine octreotide.

Operative Procedures

- *Position of patient:* Supine.
- *Anesthesia:* General with nasogastric tube and Foley's urinary catheter in position.
- *Incision:* Preferably rooftop. Midline can also be used. Some prefer transverse upper abdominal incision.

Exposure

- The falciform ligament is cut and retracted.
- Loops of small bowel are packed and pushed below.
- The liver, gallbladder, stomach, duodenum and transverse colon are exposed with the pancreas.

Technique: First Part–Resection (Fig. 56.7)

- *Operability is judged:* Liver, omentum, peritoneum has to be clear, with no evidence of malignant ascites. The tumor

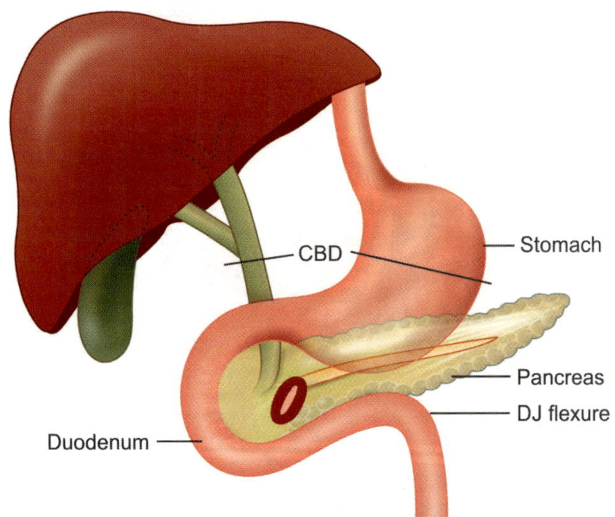

Fig. 56.7 Resection lines for pancreaticoduodenectomy

is not locally advanced. The transverse mesocolon and the unicate process area and the beginning of the root of mesentery are clear.

- If facilities are available an attempt may be made to confirm malignancy. A transduodenal fine needle aspiration is done after kocherization of the duodenum and fixing the tumor area between two fingers. The material is sent for cytology/frozen section study and the report is expected before the actual beginning of the radical excision.
- The kocherized duodenum is further mobilized and the superior mesenteric vessel site is reached. A finger is insinuated gently in front of the superior mesenteric vein and behind the neck of the pancreas. The finger is very gently used to probe the clearance of the neck of the pancreas from the superior mesenteric vein and the portal vein. Once this has been achieved, surgery can begin.
- The lesser sac is opened, separating the transverse colon and mesocolon from the stomach. The transverse mesocolon is carefully separated from the anterior pancreas. This is a very tedious dissection where an extra careful approach is required as one or two veins can be draining directly into the portal vein. If a vein is torn (and they are prone to tear easily), immediate attention is essential to control the hemorrhage.
- The gastroduodenal artery is the next thing to approach. A palpation/dissection of the supraduodenal area shows the line of the lie of the hepatic artery. On retracing that line back carefully, the origin of the common hepatic artery is identified, together with the downward course of the gastroduodenal artery. The gastroduodenal artery is securely tied in two places and cut in-between.
- The stomach is transected next, proximal to the antrum. This is done in-between intestinal clamps. Using staples is another option. The stump is then turned back to the right, tying and dividing its supplying vessels, thereby folding it on the first part of the duodenum and exposing the neck of the pancreas. In pylorus-preserving procedure, the duodenum is divided 2 cm distal to pylorus (First portion of duodenum).
- The CBD/CHD is then identified and the gallbladder mobilized. The cystic artery is tied and cut, and the gallbladder dissected free from the liver bed, so that it is brought downwards and left hanging by the cystic duct. The Callot's triangle is dissected clean and all tissues, lymph nodes are pushed downwards.
- The CHD/CBD is then dissected free very carefully and judiciously from the portal vein, and a loop or sling is applied on it and drawn outwards. The portal vein is then identified on the supraduodenal part and dissected free.
- The neck of the pancreas is inspected once again and a finger is passed gently between the neck and portal vein from below upwards (or from above blow). A sling or loop is then passed through this plane and the neck of the pancreas is pulled anteriorly.
- An occlusion clamp is placed on the body side and a crushing clamp (large straight artery forceps) on the head side of the neck of the pancreas. The neck is then divided by a knife, by using the sharp blade posteroanteriorly to prevent any accidental injury to the portal vein lying behind. Hemorrhage from the body of the pancreas is controlled by stitches using 4-0 or 5-0 silk. The cut pancreatic duct is inspected, gently probed and a suitable tube (e.g., size 5 or 6 infant feeding tube) is introduced as a pancreatic stent into the pancreatic duct, fixed to the edge of the duct with 4-0 catgut and cut at a level so that about 3 cm is left sticking out.
- The CHD is then transected above the cystic duct junction at a suitable point. All tissues/gallbladder/CBD/L nodes are dissected down from that area taking care to protect the portal vein which is lying just posteromedially.
- Attention is now given to the D-J flexure, which is then dissected free from the surrounding peritoneal reflections. The inferior mesenteric vein is noted and preserved. A suitable site is identified in the proximal jejunum about 6-10" from the D-J flexure and transected. The cut end of the proximal jejunum is tied or stapled and is negotiated around the duodenal side to be pulled out laterally. Outward traction is given at the D-Jejunal flexure and more adhesions are cut with sharp scissors. A band of tissue (ligament Treitz) will be found to be holding onto the D-J flexure, and this has to be clamped and cut for the D-J flexure to be fully released. The proximal cut jejunum, the D-J flexure and by continuity the 4th part of the duodenum is pulled in continuity toward the lateral aspect, and the supplying mesenteric vessels to the proximal cut jejunum are tied and cut till the lower edge of the head pancreas is reached.
- The duodenum and pancreatic head is now attached only at the uncinate process area and above that to tissues going medially towards the portal vein. There is a definite risk of hemorrhaging in this area and utmost caution is necessary. The uncinate process is carefully dissected and all tissues coming or going to it are clamped, cut and tied one bit at a time. The remaining tissues are also clamped bit by bit using a Kocher's forceps, and cut and transfixed to prevent slippage of ligature. A slow progress is made in this area, and eventually the pancreatic head with the duodenum together with the lower end CBD, antral stump, en bloc adjacent lymph nodes and proximal

jejunal stump is completely free to be removed as a specimen. The first part of the surgery is complete.

Technique: Second Part–Reconstruction (Fig. 56.8)

- The resected bed is carefully inspected and hemostasis in meticulously performed.
- The cut jejunal end lying distally is picked up and the stump is closed in 2 layers—continuous 000 vicryl and 3-0 silk.
- The closed stump end is then brought to the supracolic compartment preferably by the retrocolic route or by the anticolic route, without any twisting of its vascular pedicle, which may happen during the maneuver of pulling out and dissection at the D-J flexure.
- An end-to-side anastomoses is then done between the cut end of the CHD and the antimesenteric border of the jejunal stump, about 3–4 cm, from the closed stump end. Anastomosis is done using one layer 4-0 vicryl interrupted sutures.
- The jejunal limb is then placed alongside the cut end of the pancreas so that the alignment has no kink or twist and is about 3–5 cm distal to the hepaticodochojejunostomy. The aligned jejunal limb is then held at the superior and inferior end of the cut pancreas using 2-0 silk sutures. A seromyotomy is then made on the jejunal limb between these stay sutures.
- A small opening is made on the mucosa of the jejunum (thereby entering the lumen) opposite to the point where the pancreatic duct is opening. The cut end of the pancreatic stent whose other end has already been placed inside the pancreatic duct is now pushed into the jejunal lumen through the mucosal opening. Careful inspection is made to ensure that the cut end is pointing towards the distal jejunum. 6–8 interrupted 4-0 vicryl sutures are then placed, 3–4 of them anteriorly and 3–4 of them posteriorly, taking the full thickness of the pancreas and one wall of the duct (anteriorly or posteriorly) on one side and through and through full thickness jejunum (mucous membrane and seromuscular coat) anteriorly or posteriorly on the opposite side. All 6-8 sutures (3–4 anterior and 3–4 posterior) are carefully inspected to note that they have been spaced and placed properly. The extremely important sutures are then tied carefully around the pancreatic stent. Once these sutures have been placed, the cut end of the pancreas is now impinging into the seromyotomied portion of jejunum. Overlapping interrupted 2-0 or 3-0 silk sutures are then placed taking the seromuscular coat of the jejunum on one side and the pancreatic tissue and fascia on the other side. Such sutures are placed circumferentially (anteriorly and posteriorly at a regular interval) to complete the anastomosis.
- An end-to-side gastrojejunostomy is done in 2 layers, using continuous 2-0 vicryl and 2-0 silk. If the antral end had been previously closed and stapled, then a side-to-side gastrojejunostomy is performed. The gastrojejunostomy is obviously sited distal to the pancreaticojejunostomy (Fig. 56.9).
- A feeding jejunostomy is then done distal to the gastrojejunostomy.
- The operated site, pancreatic and portal vein areas, anastomotic sites are all inspected for any hemorrhage or bile leak, and a drain is then placed on the high upper flank, just below and behind the CHD and pancreatic anastomosis.

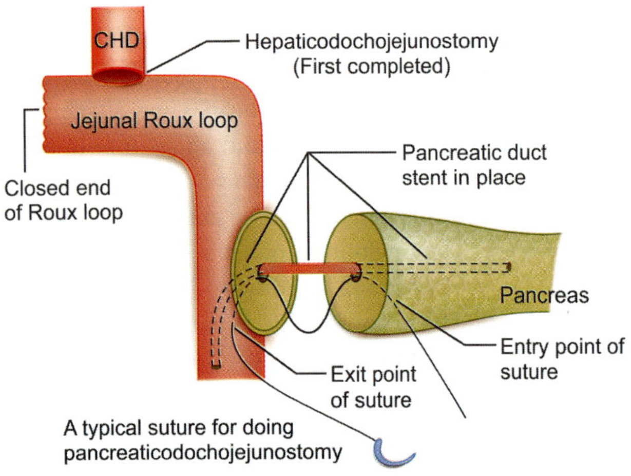

Fig. 56.8 Schematic diagram showing reconstruction

Closure

Anatomical closure is done in layers, with a drain as mentioned.

Postoperative Care

The patient is preferably kept in the intensive care and monitoring is done for pulse, BP, and urine outflow/hour. Intake-output is recorded and about 3 days is given for the abdomen to settle, when jejunostomy feeding is started. Once jejunostomy feed is tolerated and the patient is stable, his IV fluids can be omitted and he can be shifted out of the intensive care. Octreotide is given for 7 days.

About 8–10 days time is given from the date of the operation, when oral intake is allowed. Prior to this, a check USG is made to ensure there is no intra-abdominal collection; and white cell count/electrolytes and renal parameters are satisfactory.

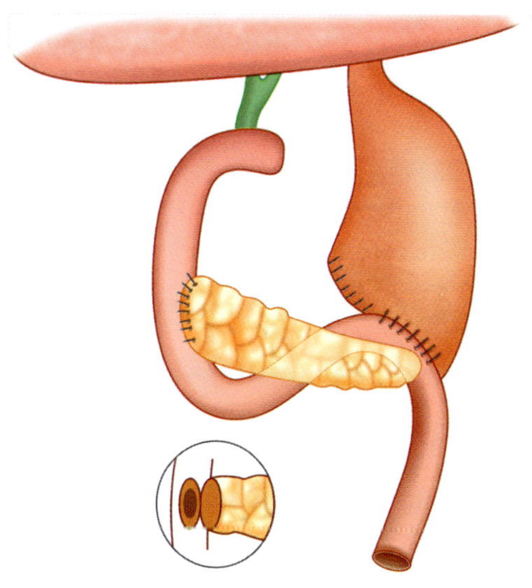

Fig. 56.9 Reconstruction after conventional pancreato-duodenectomy with end-to-side pancreaticojejunostomy

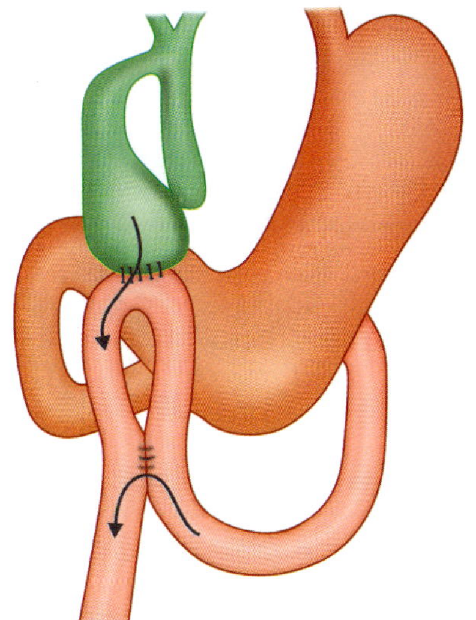

Fig. 56.10 Cholecystojejunostomy with entero-anastomosis

Once oral intake is tolerated, it is gently built up to liquids, semisolids and soft diet. There is a likely increase in drainage during this period, which should settle down in 3-4 days. The drainage tube is removed after it becomes dry and the jejunostomy is removed at a subsequent suitable date.

Postoperative Complications

Morbidity is high (40%)

- Bleeding
- Anastomotic leak
- Biliary leak
- Ileus
- Diabetes
- Sepsis - wound
- Delayed gastric emptying
- Pancreatic fistula
- Pancreatic insufficiency
- Weight loss
- Dumping
- Reflux

Palliative procedure, surgical bypass can be done to provides drainage of biliary system. Cholecystojejunostomy with enteroanastomosis is preferred in carcinoma head of the pancreas, when radical operation is not possible (Fig. 56.10).

SECTION

10

Spleen

CHAPTER

57

Surgery of Spleen

Dhiraj Choudhury

ANATOMY OF SPLEEN

The spleen, the largest lymphoid organ in the body, is located in the left upper quadrant of the abdomen. It is held in position by ligaments, namely lienorenal, splenophrenic, gastrosplenic and splenocolic. These ligaments are avascular except gastrosplenic which contains short gastric vessels.

The convex superior surface of the spleen is related to the diaphragm, while the concave inferior surface is related to stomach, tail of the pancreas, splenic flexure of the colon and left kidney.

The splenic artery, a branch of the celiac artery, runs along the upper border of the pancreas and enters through the hilum. The splenic vein emerges from the hilum.

Accessory spleen is a common occurrence and may be found in the hilum of the spleen, gastrosplenic ligament, lienorenal ligament and in any site of the abdomen.

SPLENECTOMY

Indications

- *Irreparable:* Splenic trauma. Splenic injury causing hemodynamic instability in spite of adequate resuscitation requires immediate operation. Conservative treatment may be tried if the patients are stable with no other intra-abdominal injury and if extent of splenic damage is minimal on CT scan or laparoscopy. Other traumatic conditions include:
- Iatrogenic injuries.
- Delayed rupture of spleen.
- Spontaneous rupture of pathological spleen.
- Hematological disorders—
  - Idiopathic thrombocytopenic purpura
  - Thrombotic thrombocytopenic purpura
  - Hereditary spherocytosis.
- Primary tumors.
- Splenic cysts
- Splenic abscess
- As a part of radical upper abdominal surgery, e.g. total gastrectomy.

Preoperative Preparations

- For emergency splenectomy follow ALTS protocol consisting of control of airway, breathing and circulation.
- Administer pneumococcal vaccine.
- Antibiotic prophylaxis.

Operative Procedure

Emergency Splenectomy

Anesthesia: General.

Incision: A long midline incision provides quick wider exposure. A left oblique sub-costal incision is an alternative (Fig. 57.1).

Exposure: Once in abdominal cavity, remove blood and clots by mopping, scopping and suction.

Technique—Mobilization of spleen: The surgeon standing to the right of the patient introduces his left hand round the spleen while the assistant retraces the skin wound for better exposure. Assess the nature of injury (Fig. 57.2).

Temporary control of bleeding: In case of massive hemorrhage temporary hemostasis can be achieved by compressing the splenic vessels in the hilum between thumb and finger of surgeon's right hand.

Now divide the posterior layer of lienorenal ligament under direct vision (Fig. 57.3). Now the spleen is rotated medially and delivered through the incision while a large pack is inserted.

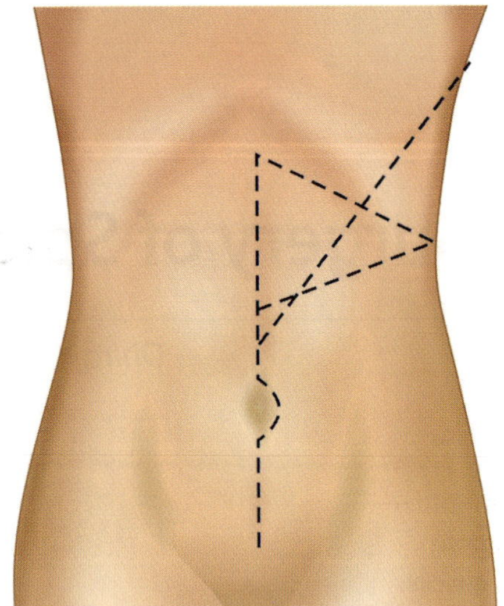

Fig. 57.1 Skin incisions for splenectomy

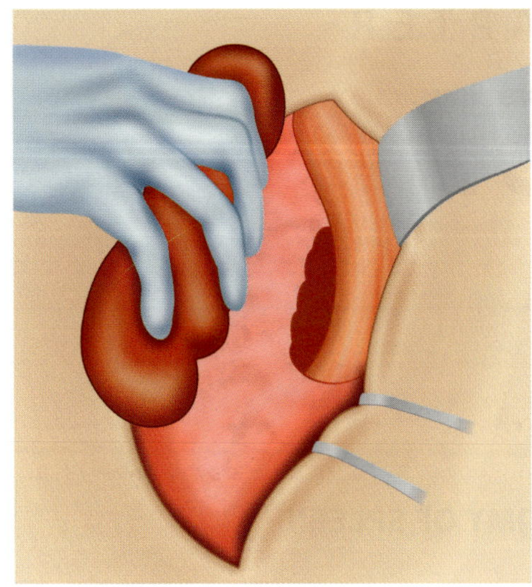

Fig. 57.3 Dividing the posterior layer of lienorenal ligament

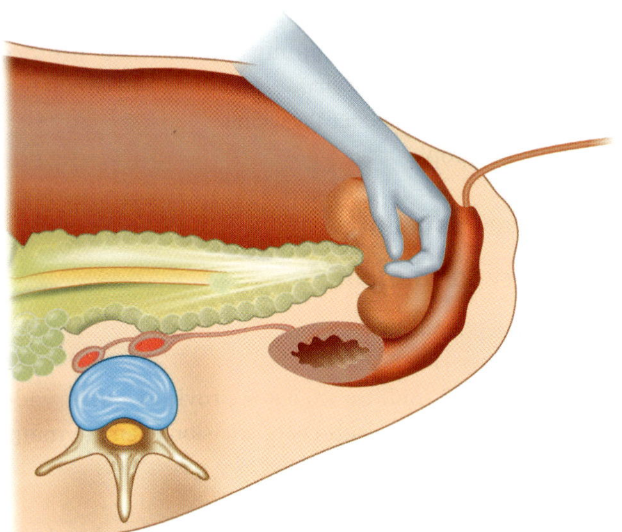

Fig. 57.2 Mobilization of spleen schematic diagram

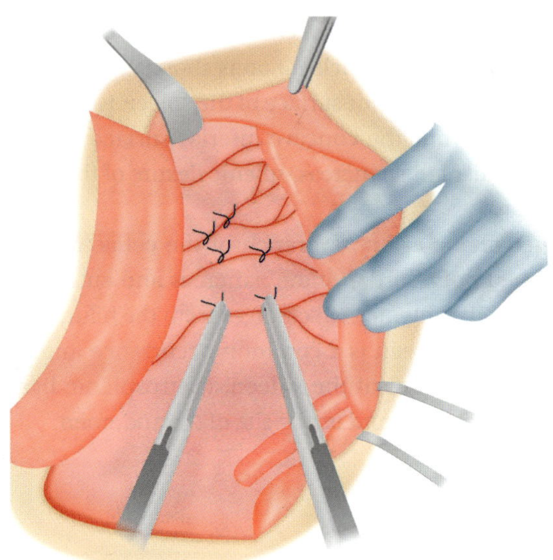

Fig. 57.4 Ligation of short gastric vessel

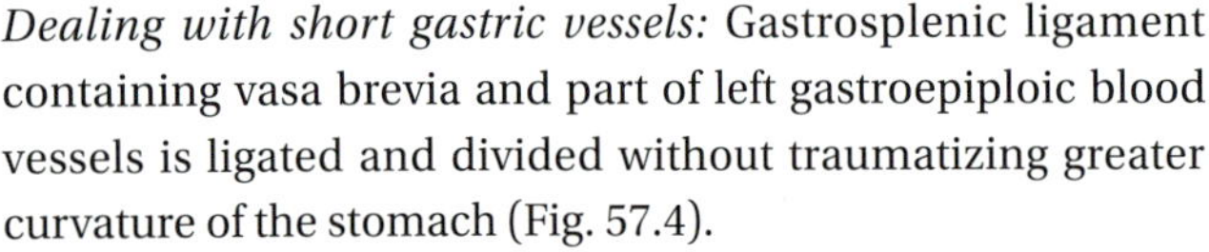

Dealing with short gastric vessels: Gastrosplenic ligament containing vasa brevia and part of left gastroepiploic blood vessels is ligated and divided without traumatizing greater curvature of the stomach (Fig. 57.4).

Dealing with splenic vessels: The tail of the pancreas is carefully separated from the hilum of the spleen. Now doubly ligate the splenic artery and vein individually with silk and divide them (Fig. 57.5). However in case of difficulty, the tissues can be clamped, transfixed and ligated with silk. The spleen can now be removed after division of the remaining avascular attachments.

Surgical alternatives to splenectomy (Fig. 57.6) salvage operations.

- *Splenorrhaphy:* Minor splenic laceration can be sutured with 0 vicryl.
- *Partial splenectomy:* In case of partial or complete avulsion at the upper or lower pole, partial splenectomy can be carried out.
- *Splenic wrapping:* In case of major de-capsulation injuries, spleen may be wrapped in the mesh to secure hemostasis. Splenic artery ligation is valuable in case of multiple tears.

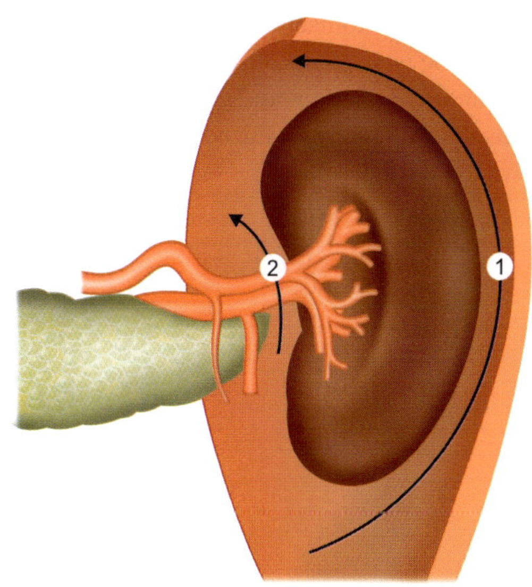

Fig. 57.5 Splenic vessels at hilum

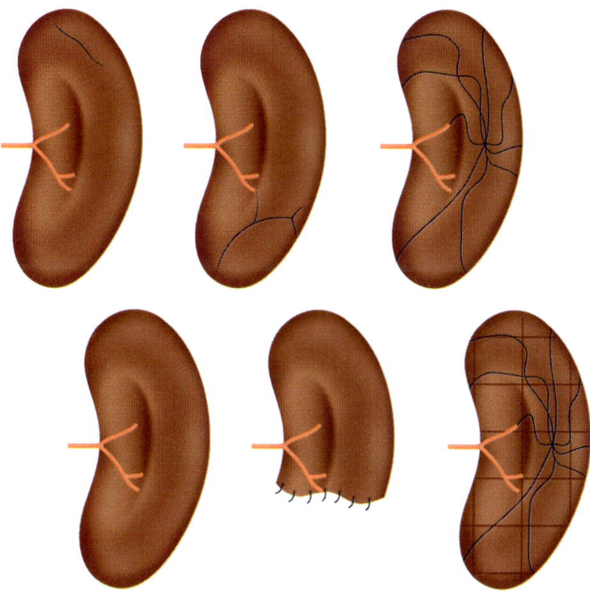

Fig. 57.6 Shows various salvage operations

Elective Splenectomy

Incision: A midline incision with a T-shaped extension or left subcostal incision is suitable, for moderately enlarged spleen. A thoracoabdominal incision in the line of the left 9th rib may be desirable for hugely enlarged spleen.

Exploration: A general exploration of the abdomen should be done particularly with examination of the spleen, liver and lymph nodes.

Technique: In case of huge splenomegaly, early control of splenic artery at the upper border of the pancreas is desirable. Enter the lesser sac by dividing the gastrosplenic ligament and ligate the splenic artery in continuity at the upper border of the pancreas.

Mobilization of spleen: The surgeon introduces left hand over the spleen in order to deliver it into the wound. Dense adhesion may be present between spleen and left diaphragm which are divided, gastrosplenic ligament is divided and short gastric vessels ligated. As spleens mobilized, the splenorenal ligament is exposed and carefully incised. Now, the spleen may be mobilized outside the wound and splenocolic ligament can be divided between curved clamps. The spleen is non retracted medially, while tail of the pancreas is separated by blunt dissection from splenic vessels.

Now, attention is paid to the splenic hilum. Gently separate the tail of the pancreas from the hilum by gauze dissection. The splenic artery and vein are identified and individually ligated and divided. The artery is doubly ligated with silk before the vein.

Removal of spleen: Divide the residual peritoneal attachment (avascular) between the spleen, stomach and colon and remove spleen.

Search for accessory spleen: When splenectomy is performed for blood dyscrasias (hypersplenism), search should be made for accessory spleen and it should be removed if found. The search should be made in hilar region, splenorenal ligament, greater omentum retroperitoneal region surrounding tail of pancreas, mesentery of large and small intestine, pelvis.

Closure

- Check hemostasis in splenic bed and vascular pedicle.
- Insert a drain to splenic bed.
- Close abdomen en-mass with loop ethilon or in layers.

Postoperative Care

- Continue intravenous fluid and nasogastric suction for 48–72 hours.
- Administer systemic antibiotic.
- Immunization with antipneumococcal vaccine.
- Remove drain when it stops draining.
- Chest physiotherapy.
- Skin sutures are removed after 7th day.

Postoperative Complications

- Respiratory—particularly basal atelectasis, pneumonia.
- Reactionary—hemorrhage.
- Subphrenic abscess.
- Gastric or pancreatic fistula (rare).
- Acute dilatation of stomach.
- Overwhelming postsplenectomy infection (OPSI). This is more common in children and elderly people. OPSI may cause death in 5% splenectomized patients.
- Portal vein thrombosis.

SECTION

11

Small Bowel

CHAPTER

58

Operations on Small Bowel

Dhiraj Choudhury

SMALL BOWEL RESECTION AND ANASTOMOSIS

Indications

- Intestinal obstruction with critical ischemia: Non-viable gut.
- Congenital atresia
- Small bowel trauma
- Strictures-tubercular or Crohn's
- Tumors of bowel or mesentery.

Operative Procedure

- *Position of the patient:* The patient lies in supine position.
- *Anesthesia:* General anesthesia with endotracheal intubation is used.
- *Incision:* Abdomen is usually opened by midline incision.
- *Exploration:* On opening abdomen a thorough diagnostic exploration is carried out. Deliver the diseased segment into the wound and apply packs to protect peritoneal cavity.

Technique

Apply two occlusion clamps in healthy bowel to occlude the bowel on either side of proposed lines of resection. Carefully incise the peritoneum of the mesentery superficially along the line chosen for division of vessels. This will expose mesenteric vessels.

Divide the mesenteric vessels under direct vision between artery forceps and ligate them with absorbable or non-absorbable sutures. The lines of division of mesentery is in the line of shallow V. Apply crushing clamps at a 30° angle to the bowel. This allows better perfusion of the antimesenteric border (Fig. 58.1).

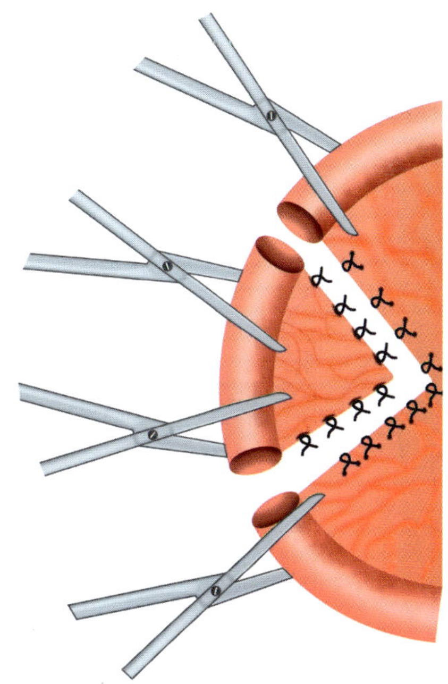

Fig. 58.1 Resection of bowel

Cut across the bowel with a knife and remove diseased segment of bowel. Cover the cut ends of remaining bowel with betadine soaked swabs.

Anastomosis: Perform end-to-end anastomosis by hand sewn methods or with the help of stapler which has already been discussed in Chapter Intestinal anastomosis (Figs 58.2A to D) demonstrates two layers end-to-end anastomosis between two loops of small bowel.

STRICTUREPLASTY

Indications

Tubercular strictures or stricture due to Crohn's disease.

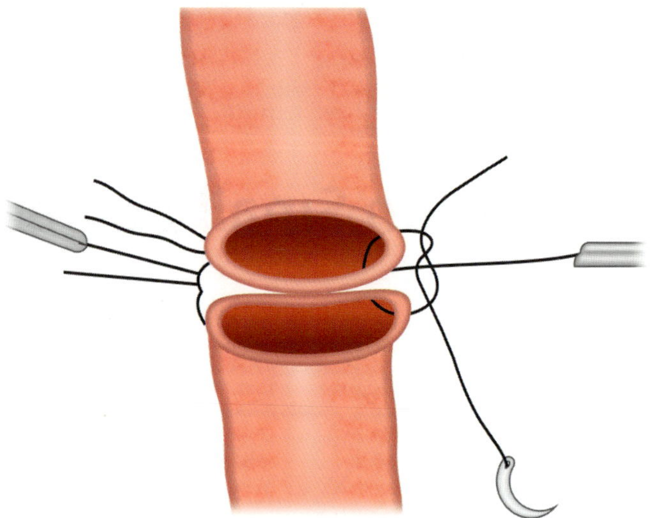

Fig. 58.2A Posterior seromuscular sutures

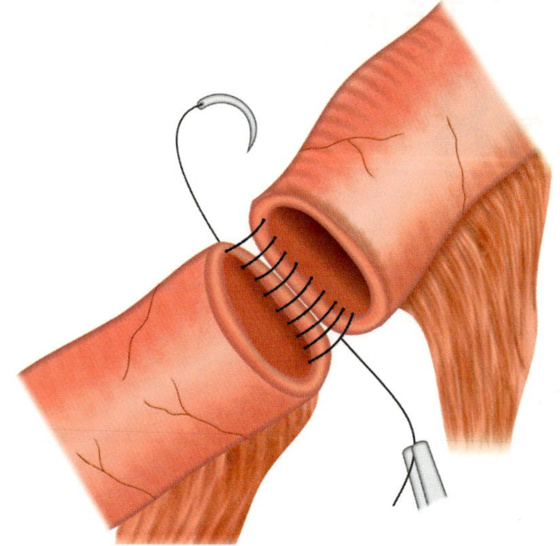

Fig. 58.2B Posterior through and through sutures

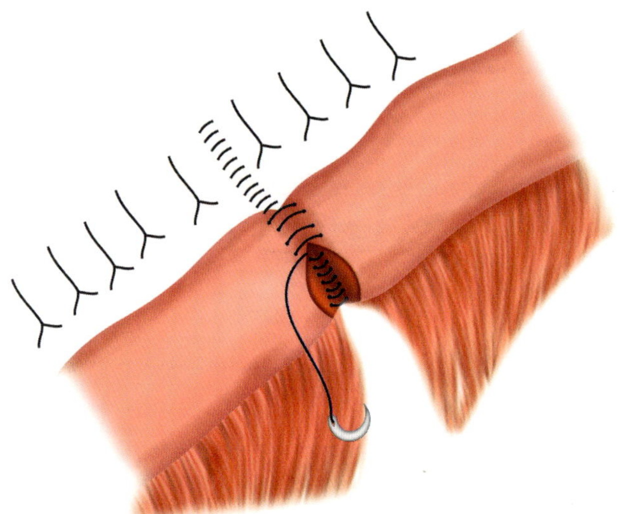

Fig. 58.2C Anterior through and through sutures

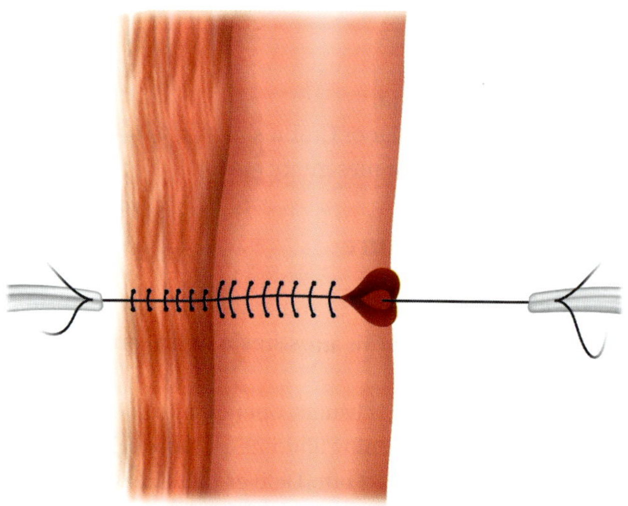

Fig. 58.2D Anterior seromuscular sutures

Technique: A longitudinal full-thickness incision is made across the stenotic area extending into normal bowel on either side for 1 cm (Fig. 58.3).

The incision is closed transversely using either interrupted single layer full thickness sutures using 2/0 vicryl or two layers of sutures (Fig. 58.4).

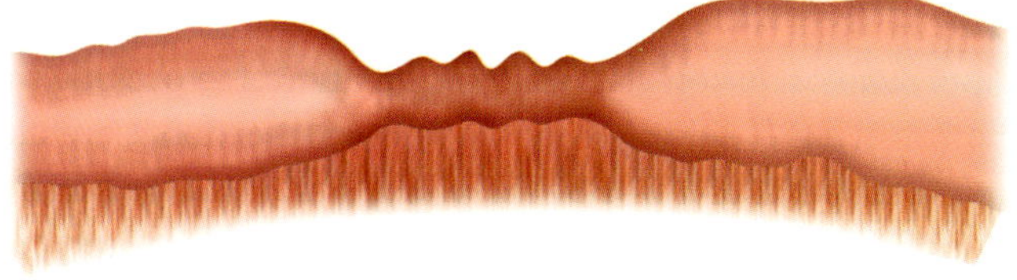

Fig. 58.3 Longitudinal incision

THE ROUX-EN-Y LOOP

A defunctioning loop of jejunum (The Roux-en-Y loop) provides a useful conduit for connecting upper alimentary tract or biliary tree to small bowel.

Indications

- Biliary drainage and bile duct reconstruction.
- Reconstruction after total gastrectomy or esophago-gastrectomy.

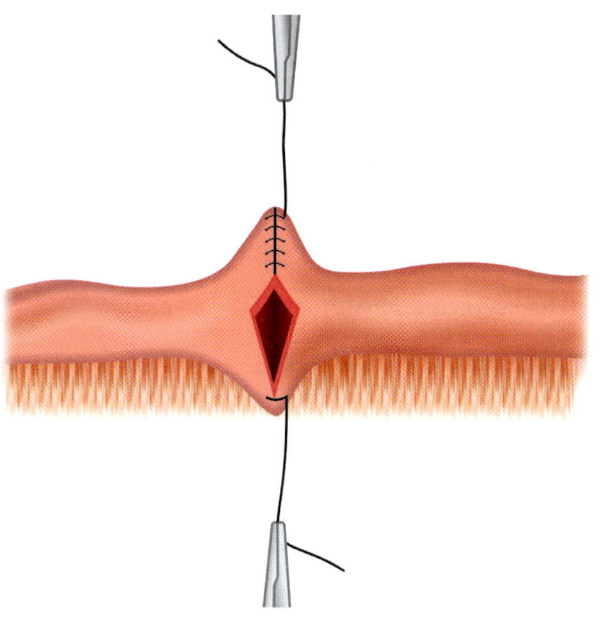

Fig. 58.4 Strictureplasty—transverse closure single layer

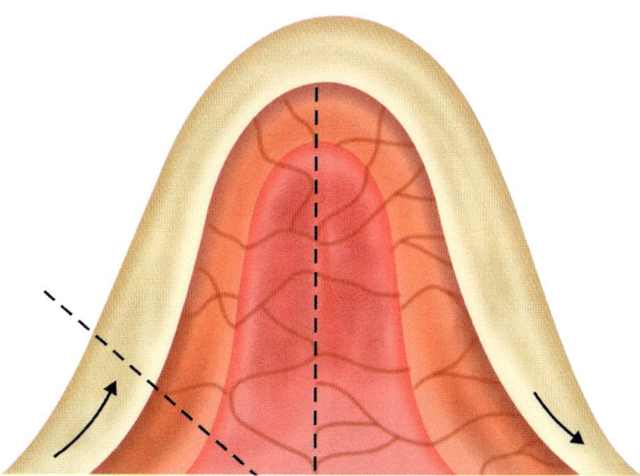

Fig. 58.5 Line of transection of bowel and division of vascular arcade

Technique: Select a loop of jejunum 10–15 cm distal to duodenojejunal flexure. The number of vessels requiring division depends on the length of the conduit. From the point chosen for intestinal transection, incise the peritoneal leaves of the mesentery and divide at least one vascular arcade. Ligate the vessels (Fig. 58.5).

Divide the bowel between clamps. Straighten the limb and take it by shortest route to the site of anastomosis. Close the cut end. Restore the intestinal continuity by anastomosing short efferent loop to the base of the long loop (end-to-side) (Fig. 58.6).

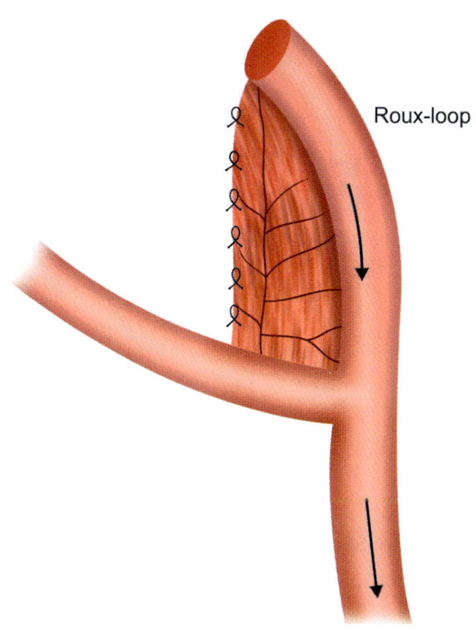

Fig. 58.6 Construction of a Roux loop

Advantages

- It can stretch further and it is empty of intestinal contents, thus preventing contamination of organ (bile duct) to be drained.
- Active peristalsis down the loop encourages drainage.

MECKEL'S DIVERTICULECTOMY

Indications

- Meckel's diverticulum causing acute abdominal conditions, like diverticulitis. Internal obstruction due to band intussusception
- Incidental finding during laparotomy for other cause. The conditions are usually diagnosed during laparotomy.

Operative Procedure

- *Anesthesia:* General
- *Incision:* A midline is preferred because of greater flexibility.

Technique

- The loop of the terminal ileum bearing Meckel's diverticulum is delivered into the wound. If mesodiverticulum is present, it should be freed divided and ligated.

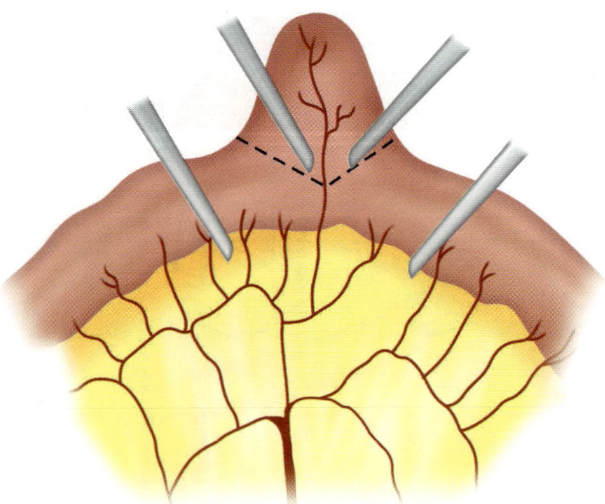

Fig. 58.7 Meckel's diverticulectomy

- The diverticulum can be excised by wedge or V-shaped excision of the base after application of clamp obliquely (Fig. 58.7)
- Sometimes segmental resection of the involved ileum with end-to-end anastomosis has to be undertaken.

ILEOSTOMY

See chapter on Intestinal Stomas (Chapter 35).

SECTION

12

Appendix

CHAPTER

59

Appendectomy: Open Method

Dhiraj Choudhury

INDICATIONS

- **Emergency operation** is indicated for acute appendicitis.
- **Elective operation** is required for appendicular lump after initial conservative treatment (interval appendicectomy) or for chronic or recurrent sub-acute appendicitis.

PREOPERATIVE PREPARATIONS

- Intervenous fluid is started in case of acute appendicitis.
- Systemic antibiotic.
- Nasogastric suction.

OPERATIVE PROCEDURE

- *Position:* The patient is placed on supine position.
- *Anesthesia:* General anesthesia with endotracheal intubation, is used.
- *Incision:* The choice lies between, Lanz transverse skin crease incision (cosmetically best), McBurny's Gridiron incision, and lower mid-line incision (if diagnosis is not certain). These have been described in Chapter 33. Author prefers Lanz transverse incision. Make a 4 cm long transverse incision starting above and just medial to anterior superior iliac spine (Fig. 59.1).
- *Exposure:* The incision is deepened through subcutaneous fat and fascia scarpa until external oblique aponeurosis is exposed. Secure hemostasis with diathermy.

  Incise the external oblique aponeurosis in the line of fibers. Make a small incision with scalpel and enlarge with scissors. Hold the two leaves with hemostats (Fig. 59.2), retracting the edges.

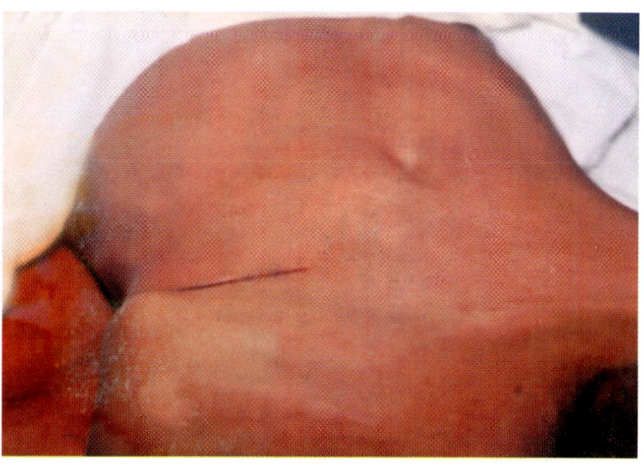

Fig. 59.1 Lanz incision (transverse)

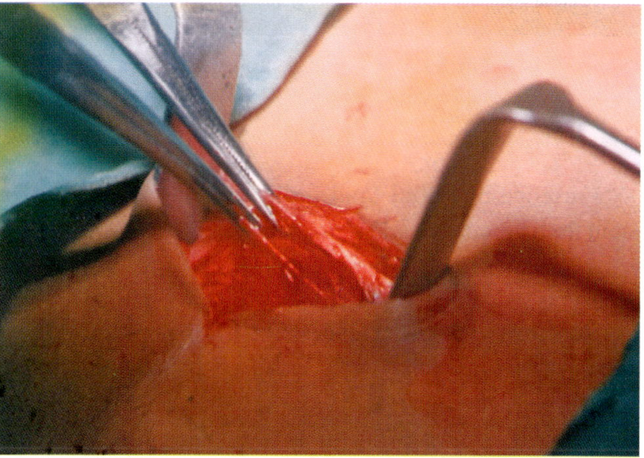

Fig. 59.2 Incision of external oblique aponeurosis

The underlying internal oblique and transversus is split in the line of fibers. Insert Langenbach's retractor (Fig. 59.3) to enlarge the opening. Lateral wound extension, by extending skin incision, dividing the internal oblique, transversus abdominus, may be required for high retrocecal or sub-hepatic appendix. Sometimes, medial wound extension may be necessary.

Hold the peritoneum with two hemostats and rule out holding of any internal structure, before making an incision. Enlarge the incision with scissors (Fig. 59.4).

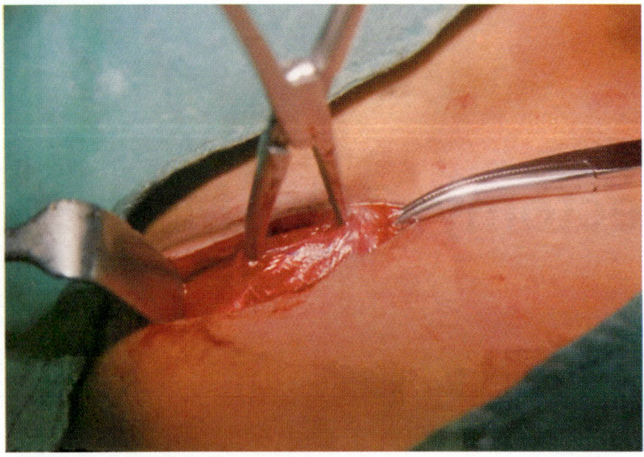

Fig. 59.3 Splitting of internal oblique and transversus abdominis

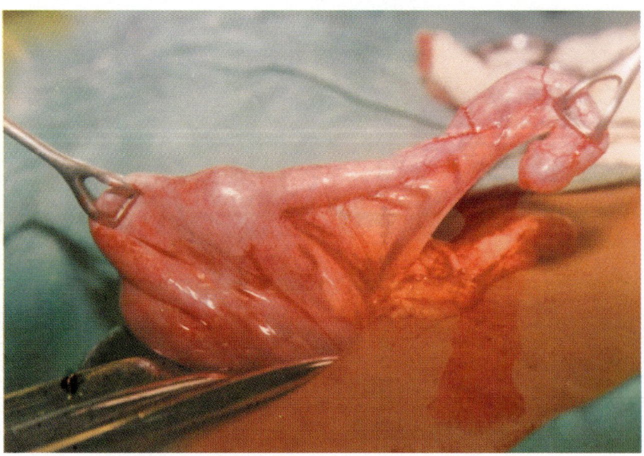

Fig. 59.5 Exposure of appendix

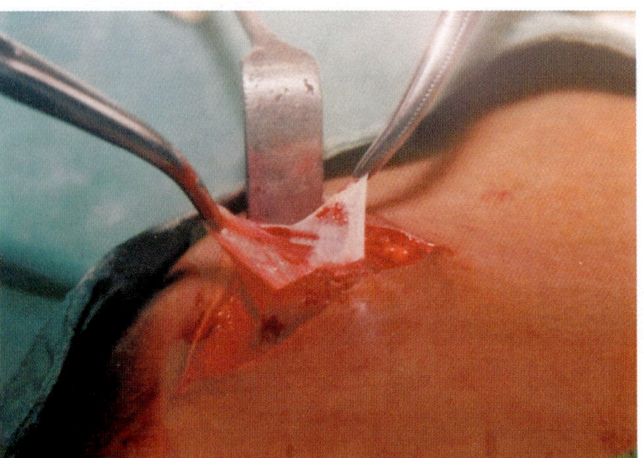

Fig. 59.4 Opening peritoneal cavity

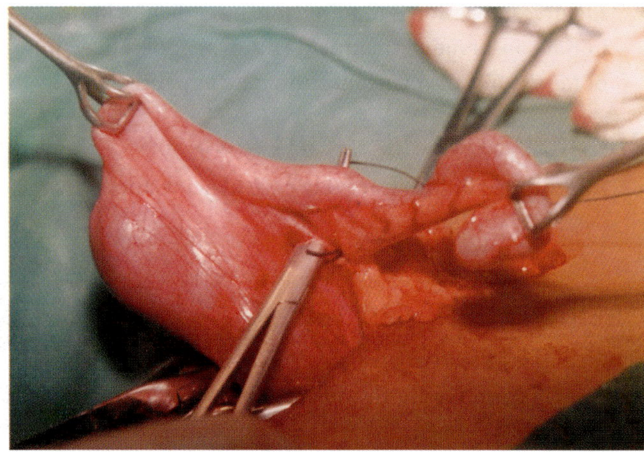

Fig. 59.6 Ligation of appendicular artery by passing ligature through a hole in mesoappendix

Presence of turbid fluid indicates acute appendicitis. Send fluid for culture and sensitivity test.

Identification and Delivery of Appendix

Often cecum is the first structure seen. Once the fascia transversalis and peritoneum are exposed, these are gently picked up with hemostat. A second hemostat is then placed and the first hemostat repositioned. Palpate to ensure there is no bowel can get between hemostats before a small cut is made and then extended under direct vision.

Identify cecum from its taenia and deliver it into the wound. When the cecum does not present, insert an index finger into right iliac fossa laterally and move it medially until cecum is located.

Follow the anterior taenia coli downwards to the base of appendix. If the appendix is retrocecal or pelvic in position, deliver it with index finger of working hand. Sometimes the appendix may be delivered directly. If it is not possible to deliver appendix into wound, enlarge the incision by dividing the fibers of internal oblique and transversus abdominis laterally and medially (Rutherford Morrison's muscle-cutting incision). Steady the cecum and appendix with Babcock's forceps (Fig. 59.5). The cecum may be returned to abdominal cavity.

Dealing with Appendicular Artery

The mesoappendix containing appendicular artery can be clamped, divided and ligated with chromic catgut or silk. Alternatively, mesoappendix can be ligated first with catgut

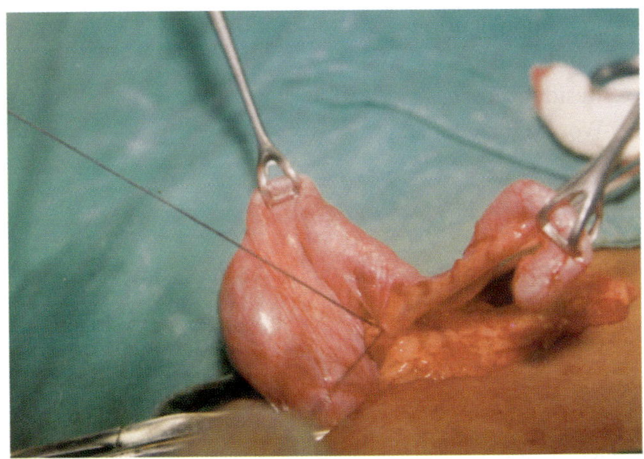

Fig. 59.7 Ligation of appendicular artery

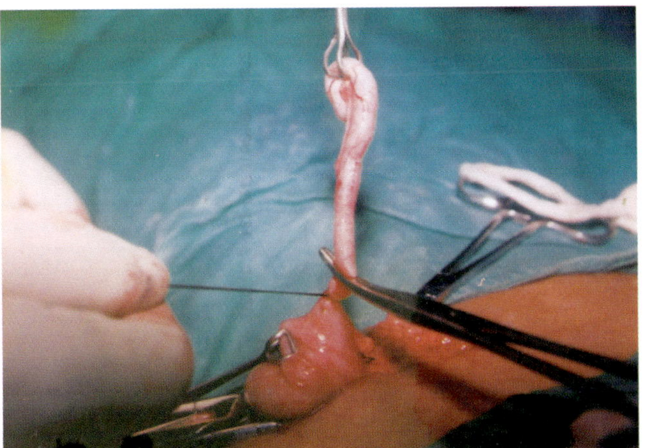

Fig. 59.8 Ligation of appendicular stump

or silk, passed through a hole near the base and then divided (Figs 59.6 and 59.7).

Ligations of Appendicular Stump

- Crush the base of appendix with Kocher's artery forceps and then re-apply it distally. Ligate the base of appendix with 2/0 chromic catgut (Fig. 59.8)
- Transect the appendix with scalpel 5 cm distal to ligature and remove it. Apply povidine iodine to appendicular stump.
- *Burrying appendicular stump:* Burrying appendicular stump with purse string suture is optional and depends on surgeon's choice.
- Apply a circular seromuscular suture with 2/0 chromic catgut around the base of appendix and tighten the suture while invaginating appendicular stump (Fig. 59.9).

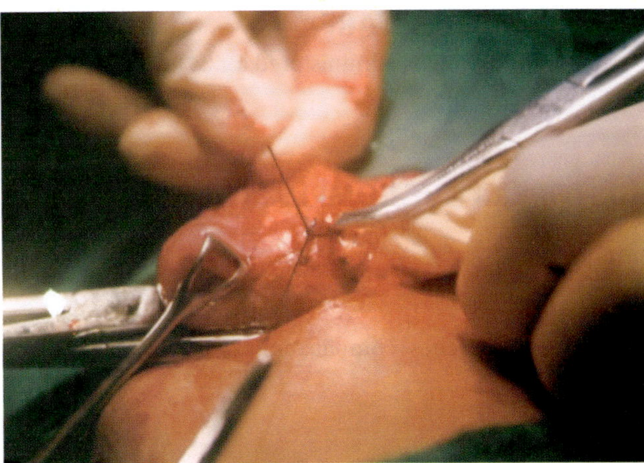

Fig. 59.9 Burrying of appendicular stump

Saline lavage is undertaken if there is significant contamination.

Closure

- Check hemostasis.
- Examine terminal ileum for Meckle's diverticulum.
- Close the incision in layers; peritoneum with continuous catgut sutures, muscles with interrupted catgut, external oblique aponeurosis with continuous catgut stitches. Skin is closed with interrupted ethilon suture.

SPECIAL PROBLEMS

- An adherent retrocecal appendix is best removed by retrograde method.
  The base of the appendix is clamped, divided and ligated. Starting at the base, the mesoappendix is clamped, divided in small pieces until the whole organ is removed. Ligate the mesoappendix now.
- Appendicular abscess is treated by placing a corrugated rubber drain and closing the abdomen around the drain.
- If the appendix looks normal, search terminal ileum for Meckel's diverticulum or Crohn's disease and in children ileal mesentery for lymphadenitis. Diverticulectomy is usually carried out for Meckel's diverticulum along with appendicectomy but in Crohn's disease appendix should not be removed.
- A carcinoma cecum requires right hemicolectomy.
- An appendicular tumor (carcinoid) if less than 2 cm in diameter situated near tip, can be removed by appendicectomy, which should include as much mesoappendix as possible. If the tumor is greater than 2 cm subsequent, right hemicolectomy is required.

POSTOPERATIVE CARE

- Intravenous fluid is administered for 24 hours.
- Systemic antibiotic.

POSTOPERATIVE COMPLICATIONS

Early

- Hemorrhage
- Postoperative chest complications
- Retention of urine
- Paralytic ileus
- Residual abscess
- Wound infection.

Late

- Intestinal obstruction-bands and adhesion
- Intestinal fistula
- Incisional hernia.

CHAPTER

60

Laparoscopic Appendectomy

Om Tantia, Samik Kumar Bandyopadhyay

HISTORY

Laparoscopic appendectomy was first performed in Kiel by Kurt Semm in 1980—5 years earlier than laparoscopic cholecystectomy. The credit for the first series of laparoscopic appendectomies goes to Schreiber but it was the report form Pier et al. in 1991, analysis of the results of 625 patients undergoing the procedure was described, that drew popular attention. Day case laparoscopic appendectomies are also being performed.

INDICATIONS

The indication for performing a laparoscopic appendectomy should be the same as that of open appendectomy. The most common indication is acute appendicitis. However, it may also be performed for dense appendicular adhesions, appendicular endometriosis and periappendicular peritoneal endometriosis. Apart from usual advantage of laparoscopic surgery, another advantage is opportunity to diagnose other conditions responsible for pain.

CONTRAINDICATIONS

- Patient not fit, i.e. not fit for general anesthesia
  - Hemodynamically not stable
  - Uncorrected coagulopathy
  - Severe chronic obstructive pulmonary disease precluding general anesthesia
- Surgeon not fit—An untrained surgeon is possibly the most important contraindication
- Place not fit—An institution with proper equipment is the place where the operation should be attempted.

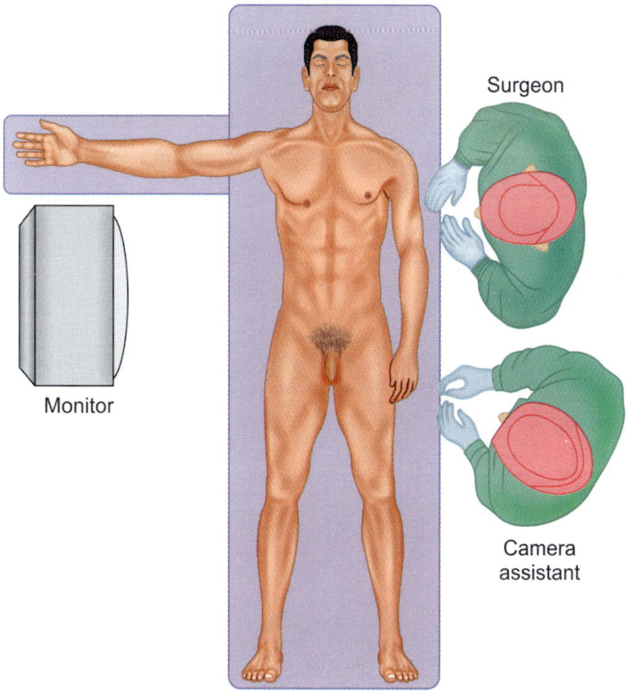

Fig. 60.1 Operating room layout

STEPS OF OPERATION

- The operation is performed under general anesthesia with endotracheal intubation.
- The patient is asked to empty the bladder before being sent to the operating room. Catheterization of the patient is optional.
- An angled scope, however, allows the surgeon to scrutinize all the nooks and corners thoroughly. We prefer using a 5 mm 30° telescope (Fig. 60.1).

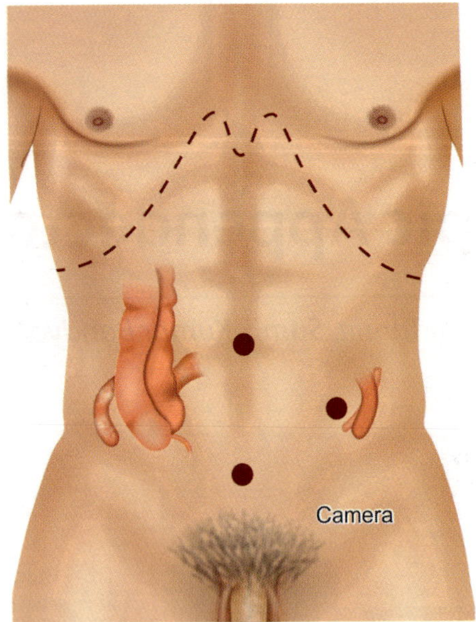

Fig. 60.2A Port placement—option 1

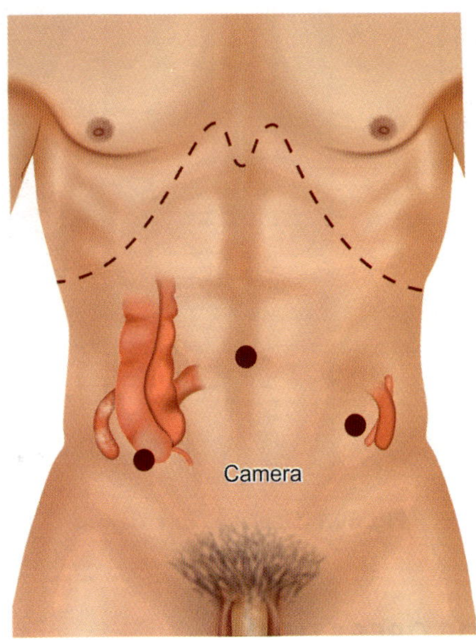

Fig. 60.2B Port placement—option 2

- *Position:* A steep Trendelenburg's position is helpful as it allows the small intestine to drop off into the upper abdomen. Elevation of the right side of the abdomen allows better visualization.
- *Port positions:* An array of options exists regarding the positioning of the port. Pneumoperitoneum is usually created through umbilicus (open access or Veress needle ascess depends on the surgeon's preference). The initial 10 mm port is made at the umbilicus and the accessory ports are then made under direct vision.

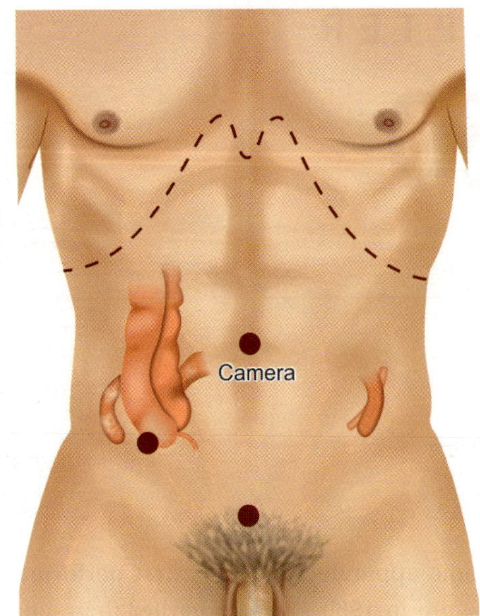

Fig. 60.2C Port placement—option 3

We prefer to introduce a 10 mm port at the umbilicus as the 1st port. Once the accessory ports are introduced, the telescope is shifted to the 5 mm port in left iliac fossa. This arrangement satisfies the principle of triangulation and allows easy access to the sub-hepatic region, if found necessary (Figs 60.2A to C), shows various options for port placement.

Steps

Identification of Cecum and Diagnostic Laparoscopy

- Cecum is identified and the taenia are followed to identify the appendix.
- Lysis of the lateral avascular cecal fold may be necessary in some patients with a retrocecal appendix.
- Inspection of the pelvic organs in female patients and examination of terminal ileum is performed in all patients. This step assures greater significance if the appendix appears non-inflamed.

Displaying the Whole Appendix (Fig. 60.3)

- Mobilization of the cecum if required.
- Lysis of periappendicular adhesions if straightening out of the appendix is necessary.

Lysis of Mesoappendix

This can be performed by a variety of energy sources—ultrasonic shears, bipolar cautery or monopolar cautery.

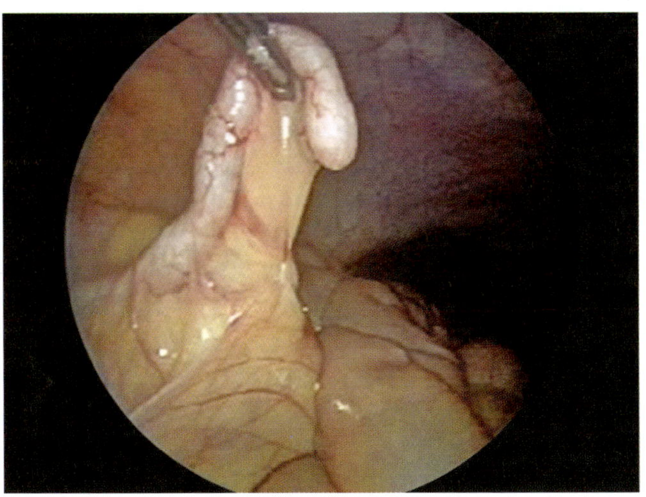

Fig. 60.3 Displaying the appendix

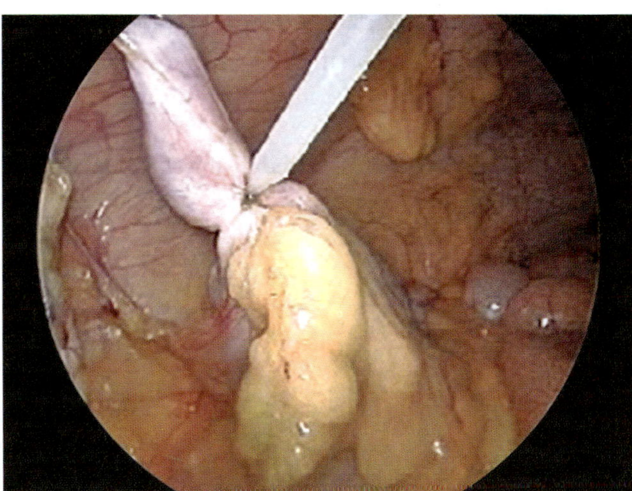

Fig. 60.4 Base ligated by endoloop

The appendicular vessel can be dissected out and may be controlled by ligature clip or energy sources. Alternatively, vascular staplers have been used for this purpose.

Amputation of the Appendix

The base of the appendix may be ligated by intracorporeal sutures or pretied endoloop ligatures may be used for the same purpose (Fig. 60.4). Clips or ligatures may also be placed proximal to the proposed level of transection. The appendix is then cut with scissors.

Extraction of the Appendix

- It is preferable to place the appendix in an endobag before taking it out through the umbilical port—this serves to prevent port contamination and lessens the risk of port infection.
- Alternatively, the appendix may be grasped by a 5 mm grasper in a sleeve reducer passing through the 10 mm umbilical port and withdrawn into the sleeve reducer following which the reducer and appendix grasped by the instrument are removed simultaneously.

The Final Look (Fig. 60.5)

The appendicular stump and the mesoappendix are examined for any sign of bleeding. The ports are then removed under direct vision and the pneumoperitoneum is released.

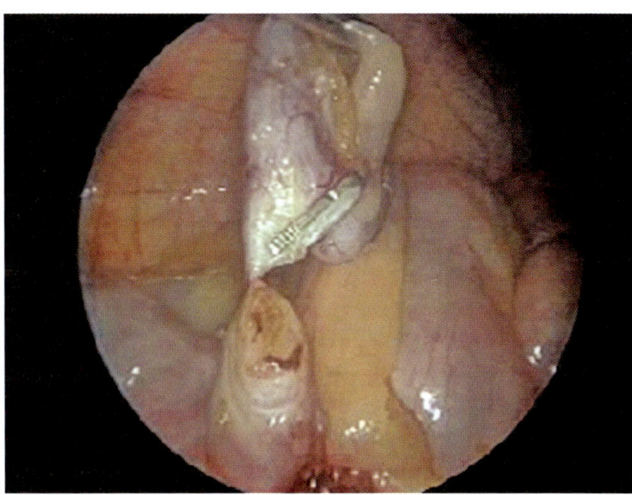

Fig. 60.5 Inspection of appendicular stump

Optional Extra Maneuvers

- A small gauge piece soaked in povidone iodine may be used to gently cleanse the appendicular stump after partial transection of the appendix following which the gauge piece is removed and the appendicular transection is completed. Alternatively, the mucosa of the stump may be carefully cauterized.
- Closure of 10 mm port by port closure needle is a safe and important step.
- Suction of purulent exudates or debris from the variety of the appendix is preferable. If necessary, a local lavage may also be performed.

Before starting dissection, an extremely inflamed appendix may be secured with a pretied suture ligature which may be used to elevate or move the appendix with minimal trauma.
- Placement of a drain is dictated by the situation and the surgeon's preference.

POTENTIAL ADVANTAGES OF LAPAROSCOPIC APPENDECTOMY

- Thorough exploration of peritoneal cavity.
- Definitive treatment for nonappendiceal lesions
- Negative or unnecessary laparotomy avoided.
- No need for extension of incision for abnormal location of appendix.
- Thorough peritoneal toilet in case of appendicular perforation possible.
- Reduced incidence of complications—wound infection, postoperative adhesions, incisional hernia, infertility.
- Excellent cosmesis.
- Less postoperative adhesion.
- No postoperative discomfort and narcotic requirement.
- Reduced hospital stay.
- Early return to routine work.

LAPAROSCOPIC APPENDECTOMY IN PREGNANCY

Acute appendicitis in pregnancy is a common problem occurring with an incidence of 1 in every 1500 pregnancies. The diagnosis becomes more difficult with advanced pregnancy because abdominal pain with associated gastrointestinal symptoms and leukocytosis may be present in the 3rd trimester of pregnancy.

The delay in diagnosis and treatment results in a 10–15% perforation rate. There is an increase in fetal mortality in 5–28% in this situation while premature delivery can go up to 40%. Therefore, a high index of suspicion and early action is warranted.

SUGGESTED PRINCIPLES

- A left lateral position helps to prevent inferior vena cava (IVC) compression.
- Minimizing the reverse Trendelenburg's tilt also helps in preventing IVC compression.
- An intra-abdominal pressure of around 10 mm Hg is safe for the fetus.
- An open Hasson technique may be performed especially in advanced pregnancies—the entry is usually subxiphoid
- Antiembolic devices are preferred.
- End tidal CO_2 monitoring is vital (25–30 mm is the preferred range).
- Fetal monitoring and use of tocolytic agents are necessary.
- A low operative time is preferred.
- Fetus needs protection, if cholangiography is required.
- An informed consent explaining all eventualities must be obtained beforehand.

WHAT TO DO IF THE APPENDIX APPEARS NORMAL?

Some surgeons have advocated leaving the appendix *in situ* to prevent unnecessary appendectomies. However, to avoid postoperative confusion, most surgeons now remove a normal-looking appendix. The usual reasons for such a decision are:
- The situation may represent mucosal appendicitis or neurogenic appendicopathy—leaving such an appendix may be dangerous.
- The patient may continue to have chronic abdominal pain if the appendix is left behind as the organ can be a site of chronic pain.
- Missed and future appendicitis are prevented.
- There is no added morbidity or cost of hospitalization.

SPECIAL SITUATIONS

Retrograde Laparoscopic Appendectomy

The appendix in some patients may be embedded in a dense phlegmon, where, it cannot be dissected off properly. Also, the distal part of a long appendix cannot be dissected off easily in some patients. The appendicular base may, in these patients, be mobilized, dissected and transected. The transected end of the appendix may be then manipulated to separate and remove the organ.

Submucosal Appendectomy

In rare situations, where the mesoappendix is densely fibrotic and contracted resulting in dense adhesions between appendix and any part of the bowel, this technique may be used. In some patients where attempts at dissection may result in a bowel injury, a longitudinal incision may be made on the lateral part of the appendix down to the muscle and the entire appendicular mucosa may be dissected off, ligated and removed.

Two-Port Appendectomy

This is actually a lap-assisted approach where the appendix can be exteriorized through a 10 mm right iliac fossa port in thin individuals with a mobile cecum and long appendix.

Single Port Appendectomy

This was described by Pelosi where a 10 mm trocar with a 5 mm working channel is used. Adhesiolysis is done by the working channel and the appendix is exteriorized after desufflation and amputated.

CURRENT STATUS OF LAPAROSCOPIC APPENDECTOMY

Laparoscopic appendectomy has been found to be a technically feasible and safe procedure. Multiple randomized controlled trials and meta-analysis have demonstrated this.

The cost of treatment is, no doubt, higher than conventional operative therapy but the difference may be more than offset if the lesser hospitalization, lesser use of parenteral activities, earlier ambulation and earlier return to work is considered. Cosmesis, of course, is excellent, especially if smaller trocars are used and perioperative pain is negligible. Wound infection is much less.

The laparoscopic treatment assumes more importance while considering surgery in women of reproductive age group and obese patients. A comprehensive diagnosis is possible in the first group where a long incision with a risk of infection is avoided in the second. Furthermore, anomalous position of the appendix, e.g. in subhepatic area needs only a minor alteration in the position of accessory ports and avoids a morbid muscle cutting incision which is required in open surgery is avoided. Additional therapeutic procedures, e.g. adhesiolysis or lysis of a band capable of causing obstruction in future may be performed without altering the postoperative recovery or without adding any separate incision.

COMPLICATIONS OF LAPAROSCOPIC APPENDECTOMY

These can be considered under the following headings:
- Complication of access, e.g.
  - Visceral injury, e.g. to bowel or urinary bladder
  - Hemorrhage—from vascular injury or port sites
- Complications of carboperitoneum, e.g.
  - Accidental embolism
  - Acidemia
  - Inferior vena cava compression
- Complications specific to laparoscopic appendectomy.
  - Thermal injury to cecum, small bowel, etc. or stump ischemia must be avoided by a careful use of electrosurgery.
  - Hemorrhage from an aberrant appendicular artery may occur due to a slipped clip or ligature. This may result in few intraperitoneal bleeding or retroperitoneal hematoma. A low threshold for conversion is warranted.
  - Port infection—this is usually avoided if the correct steps are followed.
  - Intra-abdominal abscesses may occur in patients with a perforated appendix. Careful cleansing of the peritoneal cavity as per principles of surgery and judicial use of drains is, therefore, advised.
  - Stump appendicitis—a long stump left behind at laparoscopic appendectomy results in this problem. Therefore, it is advisable that only 5 mm of appendix should be left behind from the last ligature at the appendicular base.

In conclusion, it may be said that laparoscopic surgery is an attractive option for treating patients suspected to be suffering from appendicitis and for assessment of patients presenting with right iliac fossa pain.

SECTION

13

Large Bowel

CHAPTER

61

Colectomy

Subhayan Bera

INTRODUCTION

Colon is a hollow organ. It is long and tubular in shape. In this chapter we will discuss the surgical principle involving resection of colon from ileocecal junction to rectosigmoid junction in segments or as a whole. Different parts of this organ may be involved in different surgical diseases. It is not possible to describe all the possible surgical situations which are encountered in day-to-day surgical practice. The necessary modification will come with experience.

SURGICAL ANATOMY

The most important consideration in colonic resection is its pattern of blood supply. The basic principle is to include the territory of an arterial supply in resection. Otherwise avascularity might cause significant and serious complications. In case of malignant disease, the other principle, which is considered very often is to include one arterial areas proximal and distal to the lesion. In this regard the right and left branches middle colic artery are considered as two territories (Figs 61.1 A to D).

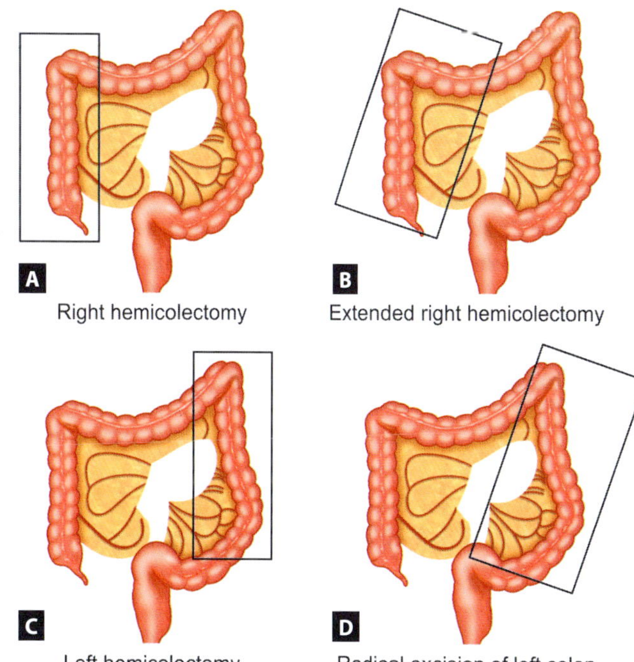

Figs 61.1A to D Anatomical basis of different types of colectomy

INDICATIONS

Indications for colonic resection may be elective, urgent or emergency. Common indications are colonic tumors (both benign and malignant) and inflammatory bowel disease. Less common indications are advanced ileocecal intussusception, injury, vascular disease, diverticular disease, volvulus, etc. All these conditions usually produce obstruction, visible bleeding, anemia, pain, mass or chronic ill health.

SPECIAL PREPARATION

Colon contains stool. This is a potential source of infection. Though it was tried previously, it is not possible to make stool completely sterile with non-absorbable oral antibiotics. Also if the colon contains some stool, the chances of spillage during operation will always be there.

Nowadays in elective situations, colon is made empty as far as practicable. Only clear fluids are given orally for the last 24–48 hours to reduce the formation of stool. Colon is mechanically emptied with special methods. Colonic lavage powder or sodium picosulphate preparations are commonly used for this purpose. Preoperative non-absorbable oral antibiotics are of little help. Prophylactic systemic antibiotics are necessary to reduce the chances of infective complications further.

In emergency situations or due to obstruction, where colonic preparation is not possible, on-table lavage may be done after laparotomy before actual resection. Very often protective colostomy is done and primary anastomosis is avoided.

For right-sided colonic lesions, strict bowel preparation is not always necessary.

Using general criteria DVT prophylaxis should be used.

Right Hemicolectomy

In this procedure, the ascending colon with adjoining part of terminal ileum and right side of the transverse colon are excised in continuity. The territory of ileocolic, right colic and right branch of middle colic vessels is excised. The actual length varies from patient to patient due to the location of pathology and other factors.

Indications

Elective:

- Most commonly carcinoma cecum, ascending colon, hepatic flexure
- Appendicular neoplasms—carcinoid >2 cm
- Crohn's disease
- Ileocecal tuberculosis.

Emergency:

- Indicated for right colonic obstructing lesions, perforation, hemorrhage e.g. cecal volvulus, diverticulitis.

Anesthesia—Usually general anesthesia.

Position—The patient is placed in supine position.

Incision

Almost any colonic operation can be performed through the midline incision skirting the umbilicus on either side. The supine position is the position of choice. The length and placement of the incision will depend on the site of the pathology and constitutional factors. Paramedian, left or right and transverse incisions are also favored by some surgeons. In emergency condition, incision is planned in such a way that it can be extended if needed (Fig. 61.2).

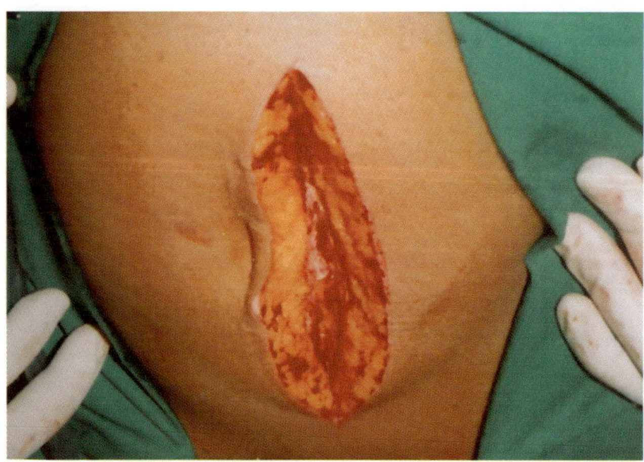

Fig. 61.2 Midline incision

Exposure and Assessment

On entering the abdomen it is necessary to assess the lesion carefully. Full laparotomy is necessary in a systematic manner. Particularly in case of malignant lesions, involvement and infiltration of the adjoining organs, lymph node involvement, spread inside peritoneal cavity and any involvement of liver are assessed carefully. Another, often forgotten, aspect is to check for metachronous and synchronous lesions in the colon. In case of distal obstructive lesions check the state of distended cecum for impending gangrene or perforation.

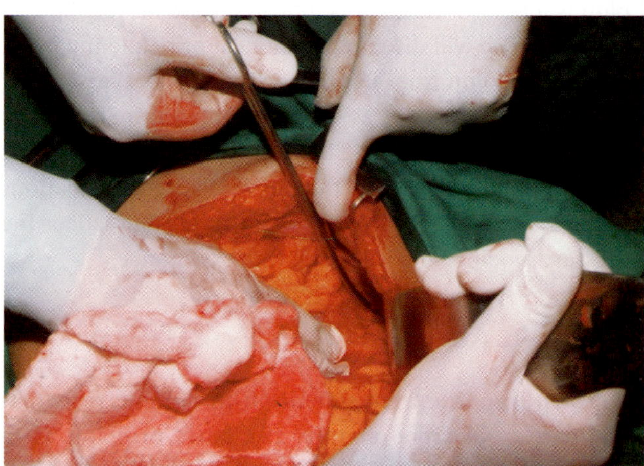

Fig. 61.3 Mobilization of right colon

This assessment is an extremely important step before starting the actual resection. Surgeon should decide whether radical surgery would be possible and would radical surgery alter the prognosis at all without increasing the risks.

Procedure

Mobilization of Right Colon (Fig. 61.3) (Lateral to Medial)

The lateral peritoneal attachments of the right colon (White line of Toldt) are incised, after gently retracting cecum and terminal ileum anteromedially. Peritoneum in the right paracolic gutter is incised. The lower and upper ends are curved and extended medially below the cecum and hepatic flexure respectively; the length of this extension depends on the nature and location of the lesion. Near the hepatic flexure, some parts of the greater omentum need to be divided

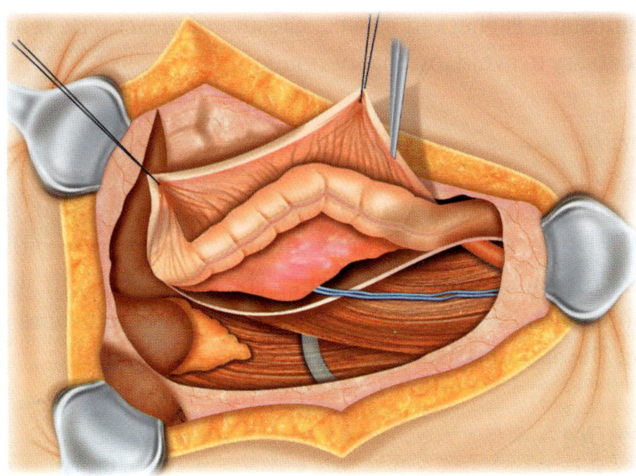

Fig. 61.4 Display of right ureter (schematic diagram)

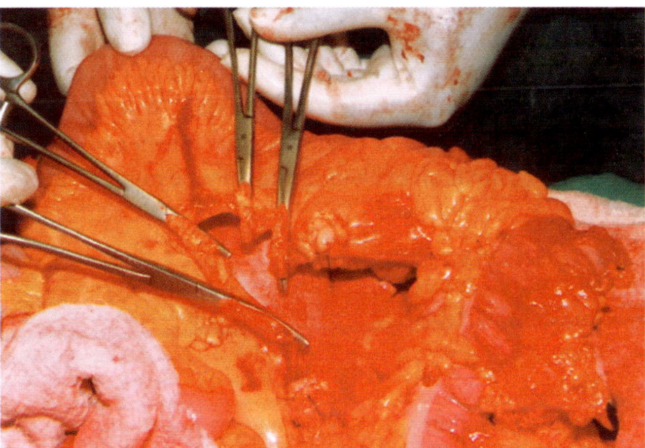

Fig. 61.5 Division of vessels

The hepatic flexure is mobilized by division of the hepatocolic ligament. In malignant disease, this line goes near the greater curvature of stomach. In case of malignant disease attached greater omentum included with resected part of transverse colon. Near the cecum, the incision will go to the lower lip of the mesentery to some extent.

The right colon is gradually lifted off medially from the retroperitoneum up to the superior mesenteric vessels with blunt dissection. Usually no significant blood vessels are encountered during this maneuver. Care needs to be taken so that duodenum, right ureter and gonadal vessels are identified and not injured (Fig. 61.4).

Division and Ligation of the Vessels (Fig. 61.5)

Once the right colon is mobilized the ileocolic, right colic and right division of middle colic vessels can be seen and palpated easily. These are divided individually close to the origin from superior mesenteric vessels. This should devascularize whole of the ascending colon, about right part of transverse colon and few inches of terminal ileum. Division of mesentery with vascular arcade should proceed gradually close to the mesenteric side of ileum. The terminal ileum is prepared for resection some distance away from ileocecal valve. After small intestine has been prepared at its mesenteric border, a fan-shaped excision of the mesentery to right colon is carried out. This includes part of right branches of middle colic artery. Similarly, transverse mesocolon with vascular arcade should be divided gradually close to the mesenteric side of transverse colon. In case of malignant disease, greater omentum is also divided at the same line on the antimesenteric side to include the attached part of greater omentum in resection to give better clearance.

For all these procedures, vicryl is used. This dissection will produce a narrow rim of ileum and colon respectively, where no mesenteric or mesocolonic attachment will be present.

Excision of Segment

Usually, two crushing and two non-crushing clamps are required. Colon and/or ileum are divided in between crushing and non-crushing clamps at these rims. Non-crushing clamps are applied few inches inside on the healthy intestine. Crushing clamps are applied towards the devascularized side of intestine, which will be excised. This will help in anastomosis without the need to replace the clamps later reducing the chances of leakage of bowel content. To ensure vascularity further, line of resection can be made oblique so as to include more from the antimesenteric side of ileum or colon, with the excised segment. Any leakage of intestinal content needs attention and proper cleaning is necessary. Stapler can be used to resect the intestine as well.

This dissection will produce a narrow rim of ileum and/or colon on either side, where no mesenteric or mesocolonic attachment will be present.

Restoration of Continuity of Bowel

Before the anastomosis between transverse colon and ileum vascularity of the ends should be meticulously assessed, for this quick release of clamps for few seconds may be done with precaution to prevent leakage of intestinal content. Common method of restoration of the continuity of intestine is end-to-end anastomosis. However end-to-side or side-to-side anastomosis can also be done. During end-to-end anastomosis antimesenteric splitting of ileum may be necessary to match the lumen of colon (Figs 61.6 to 61.8). The terminal ileum is anastomosed to transverse colon in one or two layers using sutures or staples.

Anastomosis is done in two layers usually. Suturing is done in continuous fashion. Both layers can be done with 2-0 catgut. However, suturing of inner layer with continuous catgut and outer layers with interrupted vicryl is also an accepted method. Some advocate single layer interrupted vicryl suture. Silk is used for the anastomosis by some surgeons in the outer layer. Anastomosis can also be done with stapler.

Stapled Anastomosis

Divide the colon using a linear cutter stapling device and perform an end-to-side anastomosis or a functional end-to-end anastomosis using the same linear cutter stapling device.

Final Check

After the anastomosis, the vascularity is checked again. It is checked that there is no tension at the anastomosis. Hemostasis is checked as well. Closure of mesenteric rent is necessary to avoid internal herniation.

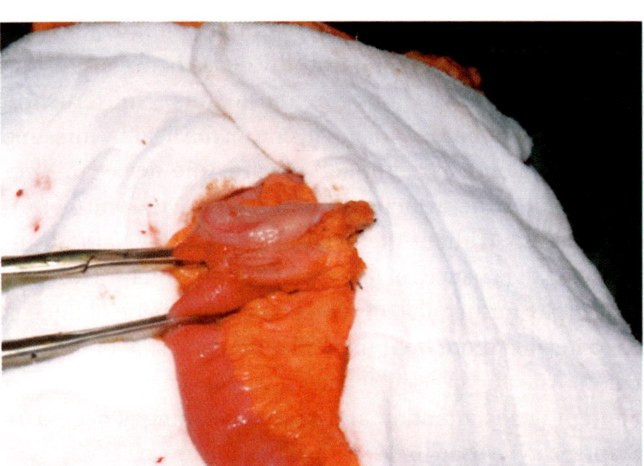

Fig. 61.6 Anastomosis end-to-end

Drain

It is better to drain the intraperitoneal area near the site of resection or any dependent area near to it with a drain of suction or passive type. The use of drain in right hemicolectomy is controversial. Some prefer and some do not. The author personally prefers to put a drain.

Closure

Nowadays midline incision is used very often. Mass closure with non-absorbable suture like nylon or prolene is the method of choice. Loop suture gives some extra advantage and security possibly. In case of paramedian or transverse incision, the wound is closed in layers using vicryl and non-absorbable monofilament suture materials. Wound drain is to be considered in case of gangrenous bowel resection or where contamination of wound could not be minimized.

Complications

- Anastomotic leak
- Ileus
- Abscess
- Wound infection
- Incisional hernia.

Extended Right Hemicolectomy

In this operation more is excised from the right side of transverse colon than what is included in right hemicolectomy.

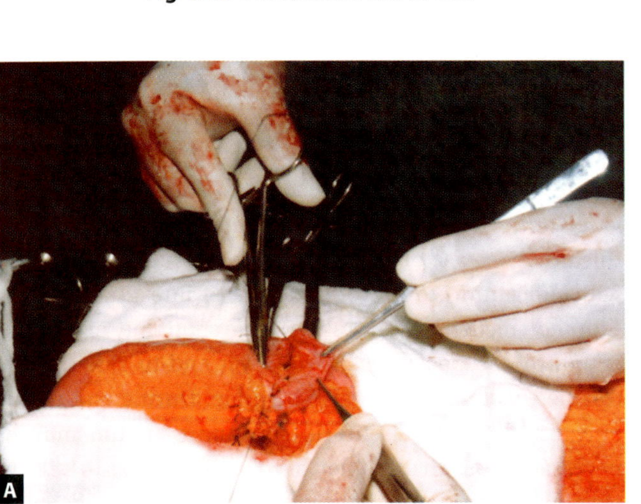

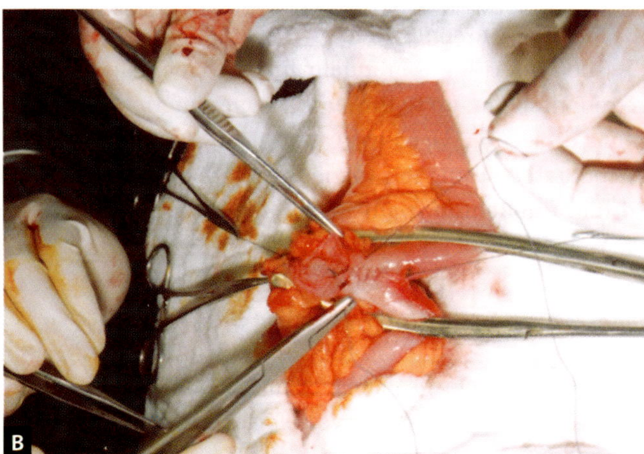

Figs 61.7A and B Anastomosis continued

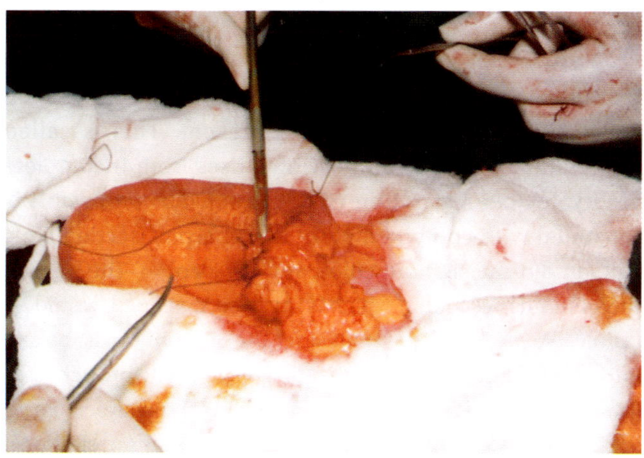

Fig. 61.8 Anastomosis completed

Almost the whole area supplied by the right branch of middle colic vessel is excised with the ileum and ascending colon. Greater part of greater omentum in the right side is excised.

Indications

Growth near hepatic flexure or right side of transverse colon.

Conservative Right Hemicolectomy

In this operation only the ascending colon with small part of terminal ileum is excised. The territory of right branch of middle colic artery is spared usually. The continuity is restored with ileo-ascending anastomosis. The descending colon is mobilized by division of peritoneal attachments at the white line of Toldt to level of splenic flexures.

Indications

Benign localized lesion near cecum like tuberculosis, gangrenous appendicitis with cecal involvement, Crohn's disease.

Left Hemicolectomy

In this procedure, the descending colon, upper part of sigmoid colon, small part of the left side of the transverse colon are excised in continuity. The actual length varies from patient to patient due to the location of pathology and other factors. In standard left hemicolectomy, the ascending left colic, descending left colic and some upper sigmoid arterial territory are excised.

Indications

Elective: Tumors of descending colon and proximal sigmoid colon. Diverticular disease, ischemic colitis, local trauma.

Emergency: Obstruction, perforation, hemorrhage or ischemia.

Mobilization of Left Colon

Peritoneum in the left paracolic gutter is incised. The lower end of this is curved medially around the upper lip of inverted V-shaped attachment of sigmoid mesocolon. Most of the time so-called congenital adhesion (Dyszygosis) is encountered between left side of sigmoid mesocolon and adjoining parietal wall. This needs to be separated. The upper side of the incision is curved medially around the splenic flexure to the left side of transverse mesocolon. Here the phrenocolic ligament is divided carefully. An attachment of left edge of omentum with spleen is also noted. Inadvertent pull on this might cause tear of spleen. Adequate mobilization near the splenic flexure is necessary to reduce tension on the anastomosis. The sigmoid colon, descending colon and splenic flexure are gradually lifted off medially and slightly downwards with blunt dissection. Apart from division of greater omentum no significant blood vessels are encountered during this maneuver. Great care must be taken to avoid injury to spleen, left ureter, gonadal vessels, pancreas and fourth part of duodenum.

Division of Blood Vessels and Ligation

Identify the inferior mesenteric artery and left colonic branches. These are isolated, ligated and divided.

Resection of bowel segment: The bowel is clamped and divided.

Restoration of continuity: Anastomosis is done in two layers usually. Suturing of inner layer with continuous 2-0 catgut and outer layers with interrupted 2-0 vicryl is an accepted method. Some advocate single layer interrupted vicryl suture. Silk is used for the anastomosis by some surgeons. Anastomosis can also be done with stapler.

Closure

Mass closure of the abdominal wall can be perforated after putting a drain. Skin closure is connected with sutures.

Radical Excision of Left Colon

In this operation, the whole territory of inferior mesenteric artery is excised. Descending colon, sigmoid colon with part of transverse colon and upper rectum are excised with the lesion.

Indications

Single most common indication for this operation is malignant tumor of the left colon.

Procedure

Peritoneum in the left paracolic gutter is incised. The lower end of this is curved medially around the upper lip of inverted V-shaped attachment of sigmoid mesocolon to the upper mesorectum. Inferior mesenteric vessel are divided close to midline. Left branch of middle colic vessels or its branches are divided at suitable area. Vicryl is used for this. Division line of mesentery of colon near rectosigmoid and left side of transverse colon should gradually proceed to the mesenteric side of colon to include the vascular arcades. In case of malignant disease, greater omentum is also divided at the same line on the antemesenteric side of left side of transverse colon up to the greater curvature of stomach to give better clearance. Mobilization is done up to midline.

This should devascularize descending colon with splenic flexure and sigmoid colon with upper rectum.

In case of colonic tumors, some surgeons favor the division of inferior mesenteric artery at origin before this mobilization begins, to minimize tumor embolization.

Sigmoid Colectomy

In this procedure sigmoid colon is excised. Adjoining part of descending colon or upper rectum may be included. The territory supplied by the sigmoid branches of inferior mesenteric artery with part supplied by lower branches of descending left colic artery is excised.

Indications

The indications to perform this operation are localized growth or polyp at or near the apex sigmoid loop, volvulus of the sigmoid colon, traumatic injury, colonoscopic injury.

Procedure

Usually, some adhesion between the left side of the sigmoid mesocolon and parietal wall is present. This is called congenital adhesion and possibly arises from incomplete embryological separation (dyszygosis). This adhesion is separated with combined blunt and sharp dissection. This will fan out the sigmoid colon and mesocolon. The base of the sigmoid mesocolon which is inverted V-shaped, would be visible. Near the base on both sider the peritoneum is incised and sigmoid colon is mobilized. The sigmoid branches of inferior mesenteric vessels will be seen. These are secured with 1-0 or 1 vicryl or other materials of surgeon's preference. The continuity of inferior mesenteric vessel is maintained after this division.

In elective cases, the colon should be prepared. It should be empty and clean. If it contains significant amount of stool primary anastomosis should be avoided. Defunctioning transverse colostomy or Hartmann's operation may be necessary as part of staged procedures.

Total Colectomy

In this procedure, whole of colon from ileocecal junction to rectosigmoid junction is excised. Continuation is restored with ileorectal anastomosis.

The indications for this operation are advanced ulcerative colitis, toxic megacolon, adenomatous polyposis, left-sided growth with perforated cecum.

POSTOPERATIVE CARE

Prophylactic antibiotics should be used almost routinely. A combination of later generation of cephalosporin and metronidazole is an accepted combination. For three to five days, patient is kept nil by mouth until the dependable function of intestine returns. Indwelling urinary catheter is used to monitor the urine output and hydration status. In many cases, Ryle's tube decompression is helpful.

COMPLICATIONS

Common and related complications encountered are excessive bleeding during operation, inadvertent damage to ureter and other structures, leakage from anastomosis, intraperitoneal and systemic infection, wound infection, burst abdomen, intestinal fistula, etc.

FURTHER CARE

In case of malignant disease, adjuvant therapy needs to be considered.

RECENT ADVANCES IN COLECTOMY AND COLON SURGERY

At present, to restore the continuity, more stress has been placed on single layered interrupted anastomosis, particularly in distal colonic operations. Synthetic mono-filament suture like PDS is being used increasingly.

Though somewhat expensive, stapled anastomosis has certain advantages in selected cases. It can reduce the duration of procedure. As an extra-lumina procedure, it can be used to do side-to-side anastomosis saving time. Anastomosis can also be done with specially designed circular staplers through anus, as an intraluminal procedure. In anterior resection, stapler anastomosis is less time consuming and much lower lesion of middle third of rectum can be dealt with successfully.

Compression anastomosis with proprietary 'Colon Ring' device has been reported with good results.

Recently an increase in tendency to employ laparoscopic or laparoscopy-assisted methods in colonic surgery has been noted. This is said to improve the postoperative recovery in terms of time and comfort. However, in many cases this increases the operation time significantly. This method needs endo-stapler, harmonic scalpel and some other sophisticated instruments, which are expensive.

Even if curative surgery is not possible, palliative surgery to reduce the symptomatic distress of the victim is necessary. Two of the most distressing symptoms are bleeding and obstruction.

Transanal excision of fulguration of endophytic growth can control bleeding. Arterial embolization procedure is considered in some.

To relieve obstruction, endoscopic colonic stents have been used successfully in place of traditional colostomy procedures.

CHAPTER

62

Total Colectomy with Mucosal Proctectomy and Ileal Pouch: Anal Anastomosis

Niraj Khetan, Peter J Billings, X Escofet

INTRODUCTION

Total colectomy with mucosal proctectomy and ileal pouch–Anal anastomosis or restorative procto-colectomy—is a well-established *elective procedure for ulcerative colitis (UC) and familial adenomatous polyposis (FAP).* Parks and Nicholls first described the technique in 1978. It avoids a permanent ileostomy and eliminates colonic mucosa, the source of inflammation and potential malignancy. The technique originally described involved a mucosectomy of the anal canal with a hand-sewn pouch and ileoanal anastomosis. A totally stapled approach has evolved more recently.

INDICATIONS

The main indications are:

- Ulcerative colitis
- Familial adenomatous polyposis.

Acutely unwell patients with colitis should have an initial colectomy followed by the elective restorative procedure if they so desire. Restorative proctocolectomy is the operation of choice in patients with chronic UC where medical therapy has failed. Follow-up surveillance shows high-grade dysplasia or malignant transformation or rarely in pediatric patients with features of retardation of growth. It is also the operation of choice for many patients with FAP requiring prophylactic or curative surgery.

The role of the ileoanal pouch in indeterminate and Crohn's colitis is controversial. The majority of surgeons would exclude Crohn's disease or patients with anal involvement. Pezim et al. showed good short-term results in indeterminate colitis. Long-term results in world literature are not so promising. Panis et al. have reported a low failure rate (7%) in a highly selected group of patients with Crohn's colitis. The majority of the published data have failure rates above 20%.

No age group is excluded from the procedure although caution should be exercised in older patients. The selection is based on medical suitability (fit to undergo major surgery, not acutely unwell, ability to achieve local clearance in patients with cancer and intact anal sphincters), technical feasibility (adequate small bowel mobilization for a tension-free anastomosis) and most importantly an informed choice by the patients. The alternative to restorative surgery is a panproctocolectomy and permanent end ileostomy.

PREOPERATIVE PREPARATION

The preoperative preparation of these patients can be broadly classified into:

- Assessment of operative suitability.
- Informed consent.
- Optimization of medical and nutritional status.

Restorative proctocolectomy is a major procedure with a high associated morbidity but a low mortality. Fitness for major surgery should be assessed. Patients with malignant disease need preoperative staging and assessment of resectability for cure especially in rectal cancers. Adequacy of anal sphincter needs clinical evaluation and manometry in selected patients. Ileoanal pouch construction in patients with anal sepsis or ulceration is contraindicated.

The decision to undergo restorative proctocolectomy is made after a full discussion with the patient. The potential benefits are the avoidance of a permanent ileostomy and associated perineal wound complications. The patients need to understand the possible short- and long-term morbidity associated with the operation. Pouch failure is reported in 4–19%. Poor functional results, especially incontinence (2%) and pouchitis (cumulative risk 18% at 1 year), have been reported. Patient support groups and specialist nurses provide invaluable information and support.

The majority of these patients are on multiple medications including steroids and immunosuppressants and may be in a poor nutritional status. A gastroenterologist's input to optimize the drug therapy and correction of a poor nutritional status by the dietician prior to surgery will have a positive influence on the outcome of surgery.

Standard preoperative measures include bowel preparation, deep vein thrombosis, antibiotic prophylaxis and sitting of an ileostomy by the stomatherapist.

OPERATIVE PROCEDURE

We have described the conventional open technique though a laparoscopic approach to restorative proctocolectomy has been described.

General Principles

Position of patient: The Lloyd Davies position is standard and the bladder is catheterized.

The abdomen and perineum are both cleaned and draped.

Incision

The abdomen is accessed by midline incision. The anterior abdominal wall is thus preserved for future stomas, if necessary. If an ileostomy is planned, the trephine for this is made up to the peritoneal cavity prior to the midline incision. This enables a direct tract without any distortion of the abdominal wall.

Total Colectomy and Proctectomy

Mobilization of the colon and rectum depends on presence or absence of malignant transformation. In presence of malignancy or dysplasia, the colonic resection is performed with radical clearance and high ligation of the lymphovascular pedicles. The mesorectal excision (TME) is performed for the rectum. In absence of malignant transformation ligation of vessels closer to the bowel may be performed.

The bowel is divided distally just above the puborectalis (down to pelvic floor) (Fig. 62.1).

The small bowel mesentery is dissected and the mobility assessed by performing a trial descent of the anastomosing part of the ileum to the anal canal. Further mobilization can be achieved after dividing the selected vessels in the mesentery. Potential ischemia can be checked and avoided by clamping the target vessels with vascular bulldog clamps prior to division.

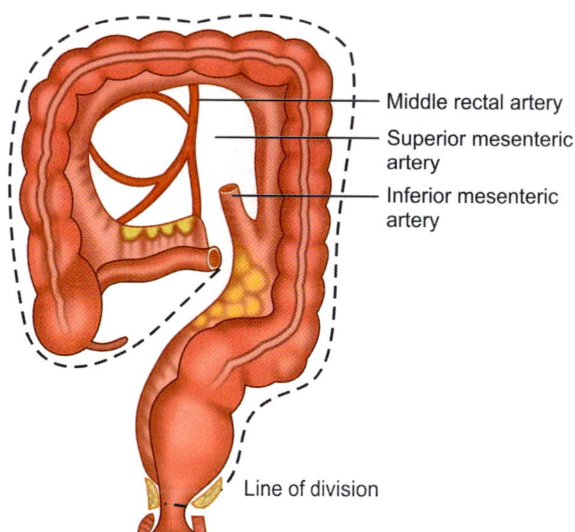

Fig. 62.1 Showing extent of total colectomy

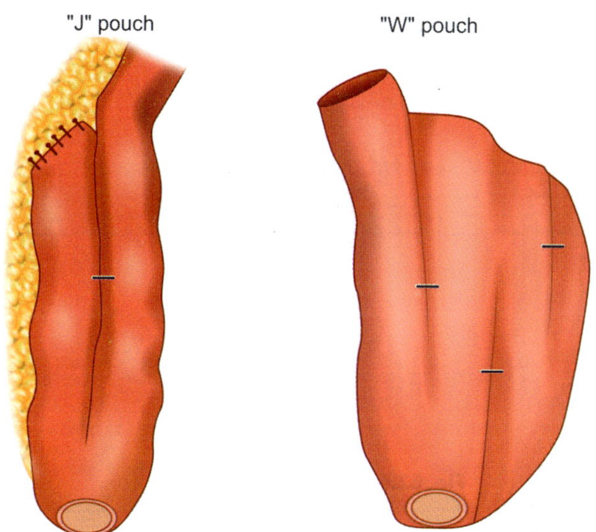

Fig. 62.2 Ileal reservoirs

Construction of the Ileal Pouch

Various pouches have been described based on the number of loops and nature of anastomosis. The "J" pouch (2 loops) is easy to construct. The terminal 30–40 cm of small bowel is folded into two limbs of 15–20 cm (Figs 62.2 and 62.3).

The two limbs of the terminal ileum are approximated using two or three stay sutures. An incision is made in the apex of the limb and a GIA instrument is inserted into the limbs of the J (Fig. 62.4).

The instrument is then fixed creating a common reservoir between the two limbs of the bowel.

A hand-sewn technique can also be used. The "W" pouch (4 loops) theoretically has a greater capacity. Selvaggi

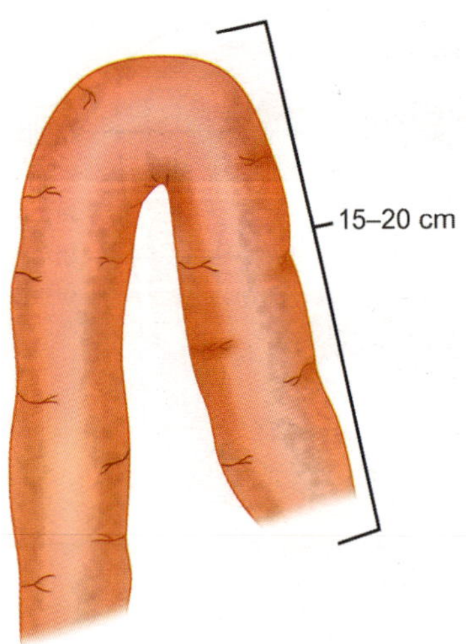

Fig. 62.3 Construction of ileal loop

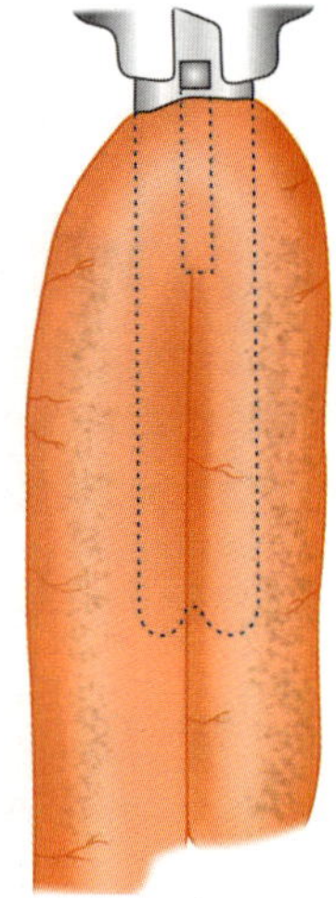

Fig. 62.4 Construction of ileal pouch

et al. reported better functional results with "W" pouch in comparison with "J" pouch though another study did not show any significant difference. The original "S" pouch is now rarely used due to evacuation difficulty. We routinely perform a staple "J" pouch.

Mucosectomy

Rectal mucosectomy removes the residual mucosa above the transitional zone of the anal canal. Anorectal mucosectomy removes all the mucosa above the dentate line. The transitional zone is lined by cuboidal epithelium and differs from the columnar rectal mucosa and squamous mucosa below the dentate line. It extends 1 cm (Fig. 62.5) above the dentate line. The procedure is performed "via the perineal route and a circular anal retractor facilitates the procedure". It carries a risk of injury to the anal sphincters either directly or indirectly during excessive retraction and the operating time is longer. Studies have shown lower resting anal canal pressure measurements but its impact on continence has not been significant. The above disadvantages have to be weighed against leaving residual anorectal mucosa and the potential for malignant transformation in the nonmucosectomy patients with the need for long-term surveillance.

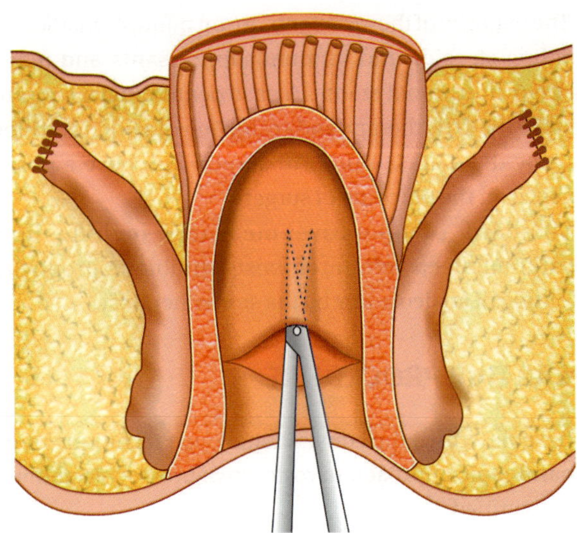

Fig. 62.5 Mucosectomy

Ileoanal Anastomosis

The apex of the J-loop is utilized for anastomosis at the dentate line. In order to construct a hand-sewn ileoanal anastomosis the self-retaining retractor is placed in the anus and the apex of the pouch is brought down to the anal canal. Interrupted full thickness 2-0 vicryl *(Ethicon)* or 3-0 PDS *(Ethicon)* sutures are used to fashion a side-to-end ileoanal anastomosis. However, a stapled technique without mucosectomy is easier and possibly has a lower morbidity in low volume centers. We routinely construct a stapled ileoanal pouch and anastomosis without mucosectomy (Fig. 62.6).

The majority of the surgeons divert the ileoanal pouch anastomosis with a proximal loop ileostomy. It has the potential advantage of limiting pelvic sepsis but its reversal is associated with significant morbidity. Major centers have reported an ileostomy anastomosis leak rate of up to 10%. It is fashioned in the right iliac fossa at the preoperatively marked site.

Closure

A closed suction drain is placed in the pelvis prior to closure of the abdominal wound.

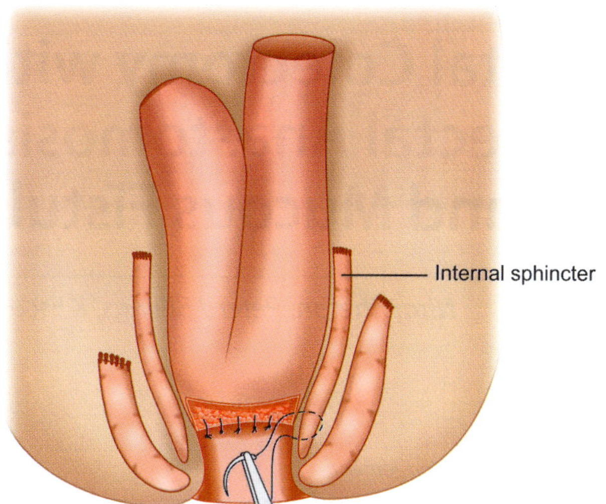

Fig. 62.6 Ileoanal anastomosis—hand-sewn

POSTOPERATIVE CARE

The immediate postoperative care is standard as for any other abdominal surgery. Special areas where closer attention is needed include fluid and electrolyte balance, nutrition, early detection and management of an anastomotic leak, stoma care, tapering of steroids and psychological support. After the patients have recovered from the primary operation further care depends on the clinical progress and assessment of functional outcome. Pouch failure, pouchitis and other complications as discussed later, are the major management issues in follow-up period.

COMPLICATIONS AND THEIR MANAGEMENT

Early Complications

Pelvic sepsis is a serious early complication following pouch surgery. The reported incidence varies between 5-14% and it presents clinically as fever, leukocytosis, and abdominal tenderness. A low threshold of suspicion is mandatory in postoperative patients and confirmation with a gastrograffin enema and computerized tomography is the key to early diagnosis. A diverting ileostomy may decrease the consequences of pelvic sepsis although the incidence remains unaltered. In selected cases, broad-spectrum antibiotics alone or in combination "with computed guided drainage, may be helpful, however, the majority require operative intervention if the patient does not have a proximal diverting loop ileostomy. Abdominal wound infection and transient urinary retention have been reported in 3 and 7% of patients respectively. Small bowel obstruction following pouch surgery is observed frequently and varies from 12 to 24%. It can present early or late. The cumulative probability of developing bowel obstruction increases significantly for up to 10 years. The majority will respond to conservative management.

Stool frequency and continence defines the functional outcome. A mean stool frequency of 4-6 per day and 1 per night with normal continence at discharge is generally accepted as a good outcome. Patients with increased frequency will benefit from anti-diarrheal medication or stool bulking agents. Some patients may need to wear protective pads.

Pouch function generally improves over the first year following surgery then remains stable during long-term follow-up. Poor functional outcome is the second commonest cause of pouch excision.

Late Complications

The specific late complications include sexual dysfuction, anastomosis stricture, pouchitis and pouch vaginal fistula. Impotence (1%) and retrograde ejaculation (2%) have been reported in men. Women record dyspareunia (3%) and fear of leakage of stool (3%), sexual activity improves substantially during long-term follow-up. An anastomotic stricture may require intermittent dilatation.

Pouchitis manifests itself as frequent watery, often bloody stools, urgency, incontinence, malaise, abdominal cramps and fever. A pouchitis activity index includes clinical, endoscopic and histological findings and may accurately predict the true incidence. The etiology of pouchitis is unknown although it occurs in ulcerative colitis but is very rare in patients with FAP. 14-18% patients were reported to suffer from pouchitis in the first year following surgery. The cumulative probability increases subsequently after the first episode during long-term follow-up. Most affected patients will respond to short courses of metronidazole, ciprofloxacin and augmentin.

Wexner et al. reported an incidence of 7.5% for pouch-vaginal fistula. Pouch salvage can be achieved in 40% of cases with diversion ileostomy and local repair.

Patients who require a permanent ileostomy or in whom the diversion ileostomy cannot be reversed are considered to have suffered pouch failure. It increases with prolonged follow-up and has been reported to range from 4-19%. The predominant causes of pouch failure are chronic pelvic sepsis, poor functional outcome and Crohn's disease. A failure to close a diverting ileostomy due to pelvic sepsis or because of patient choice has been reported in 1% of patients.

CHAPTER

63

Subtotal Colectomy with Ileorectal Anastomosis, Ileostomy and Mucous Fistula

Niraj Khetan, Peter J Billings, X Escofet

INTRODUCTION

The first proctocolectomy with permanent ileostomy was described approximately half a century ago. Since then surgical treatment for ulcerative colitis has been aimed at avoiding a permanent ileostomy. Colectomy with ileorectal anastomosis and restorative proctocolectomy are the two surgical options for those wishing to avoid a permanent stoma. Current dilemmas on the relative indications for these procedures, the indications for surgery against medical treatment and particular aspects of surgical technique are discussed in this chapter.

EMERGENCY SURGERY

Acute fulminant colitis, with or without toxic megacolon or perforation occurs in ulcerative colitis but also in Crohn's or indeterminate colitis. About 10% of patients with ulcerative colitis will eventually come to operation. Surgery should have a low operative mortality and enable the patient to return to as normal a life as possible health minimizing medication. The introduction of new drugs such as cyclosporin and infliximab may induce remissions resulting in fewer operations but a number of both acutely ill and chronically unwell patients cannot be brought into remission.

Colectomy with Ileostomy

The operation of choice is a total colectomy with ileostomy and preservation of the rectal stump. It has a low mortality and full recovery is achieved in most cases. Severe persisting disease in the rectum is rare, but when improvement does not occur, then subsequent rectal excision is indicated. Persistent rectal bleeding rarely occurs but if it does, it is an indication for proctocolectomy.

Preoperative management:

- Intravenous steroids: 100 mg of hydrocortisone 6-hourly.
- Broad spectrum antibiotic prophylaxis started with induction of anesthesia and continued for a maximum of three doses
- Venous thromboembolism prophylaxis
- Marking of ileostomy site
- Urinary catheter.

Operative Procedure

Position: Lithotomy Trendelenburg (Lloyd-Davies position) using Lloyd-Davies (Seward Medical, London, UK) or Allen (Allen Medical, Cleveland, OH) stirrups.

Anesthesia: General anesthesia with endotracheal intubation.

Incision: Long midline incision.

Exposure:

- *Assess peritoneal cavity:* The presence of free fluid or gas may indicate colonic perforation. Careful assessment of the colon is made, if a perforation has occurred, it should be closed if possible with a purse-string suture although this can be difficult as the colon may be edematous, hyperemic and friable. Adhesions between the colon and the omentum or abdominal wall are commonly present and may be the site of sealed perforations. Assessment of the small bowel is performed for presence of Crohn's disease and the mesentery for enlarged lymph nodes. The solid organs are examined.

Technique

- The colon is mobilized completely from the cecum down to the rectum. The omentum is preserved if possible, but

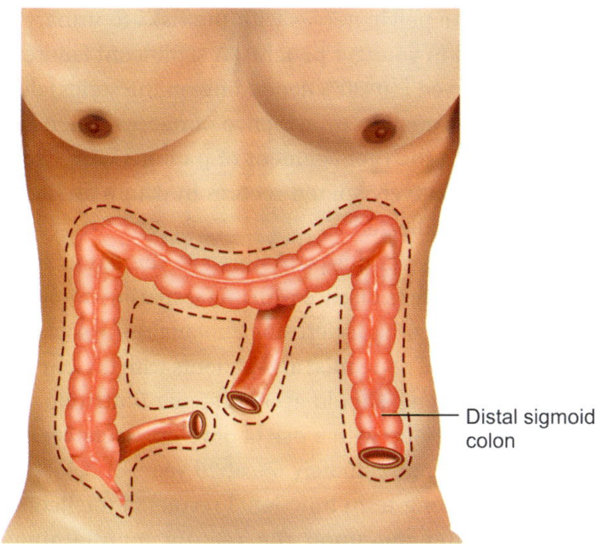

Fig. 63.1 Shows extent of dissection in subtotal colectomy

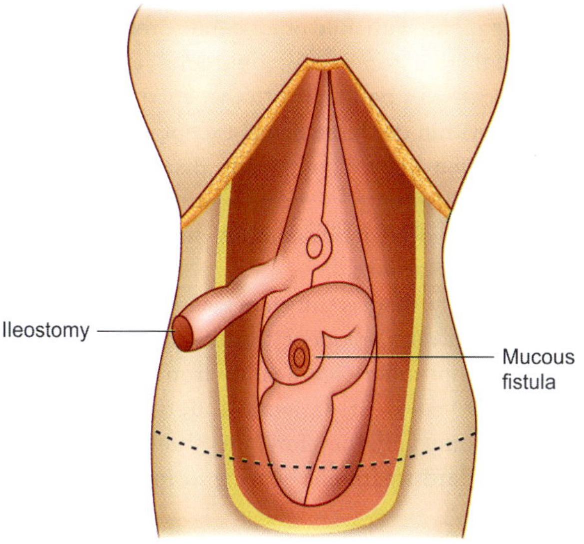

Fig. 63.2 Creation of mucous fistula and ileostomy

in grossly inflamed cases attempting to dissect it away from the colon may lead to perforation. The mesentery is transilluminated and the blood supply divided at a convenient point (Fig. 63.1).

- The terminal ileum is mobilized sufficiently to prevent any tension on the ileostomy. The small bowel is transected; a linear stapling gun may be used to prevent spillage (Fig. 63.1).
- If a mucous fistula is to be constructed, the distal sigmoid colon is divided at a convenient point between crushing bowel clamps (or a further firing of a linear stapler is used) to bring the open end of the rectosigmoid colon through the lower end of the laparotomy wound (Fig. 63.2).

  If closure of the rectal stump is the preferred option, a linear stapling gun is fired across the rectosigmoid junction, a continuous seromuscular non-absorbable suture is used to reinforce the stapled closure line.
- Hemostasis is secured and a warm saline washout of the peritoneal cavity performed.
- The terminal ileum is brought through a 2 cm in diameter circular trephine at the previously marked ileostomy site and the mesentery sutured to the lateral abdominal wall. The ileostomy is constructed with a 2 cm everted spout.

Mucus Fistula/Closure of Rectal Stump

Exteriorization of the rectosigmoid stump as a mucus fistula or closure inside the abdominal cavity remains controversial. Wojdemann et al. reported a retrospective review of 147 consecutive emergency colectomies for ulcerative colitis with 3% mortality and 2% pelvic sepsis due to leakage of the stump. No deaths were related to the rectal stump in this series and closure of rectal stump may be regarded as a safe procedure. There are no prospective trials comparing both options.

Mucus fistula formation is a safer option when the risk of leakage from the rectal stump is significant in acutely ill patients with poor nutrition and on high dose steroids. Mucus fistulas can be difficult for the patient to manage, often even more troublesome than the ileostomy itself. A balanced approach has been advocated in high-risk patients whereby the rectosigmoid stump is closed just under the anterior abdominal wall so that if leakage occurs, this should discharge through the laparotomy wound.

Length of Rectosigmoid Stump

A long rectal stump should be left which is either exteriorized through the abdominal wall (mucus fistula) or closed. The long stump is, in most cases, easy to locate at re-operation and avoids unnecessary pelvic dissection in an acutely ill patient. Transecting the rectum at the level of the pelvic peritoneum should be avoided. A short rectal stump will prevent a subsequent ileorectal anastomosis being constructed and can be difficult to locate. Only in cases of massive rectal bleeding it is justified to remove the rectum to stop the hemorrhage.

Elective Surgery

Indications

Indications for surgical intervention can be grouped in three categories:

1. Failure of medical treatment which includes recurrent acute exacerbations, evidence of chronic ill health, severe

symptoms, steroid dependence and extra-intestinal manifestations.
2. Evidence of dysplasia and/or malignancy.
3. Retardation of growth in children.

A large number of factors need to be taken into consideration when considering surgery in the elective setting. Social factors, family history, professional circumstances such as loss of time from work or type of job, number of hospital admissions all give the patient a prime role when deciding to proceed with surgery. Evidence of anemia, osteoporosis (bone densitometry) and malnutrition should be also documented.

Colonoscopic cancer surveillance in patients with ulcerative colitis still remains controversial. The difficulty in defining dysplasia and reaching uniform criteria to differentiate between low and high-grade dysplasia and when to perform a colectomy is still a matter of debate. There is evidence in the literature to confirm that the presence of low-grade dysplasia is not as likely as high-grade dysplasia to be associated with the presence of malignancy (54 vs 67%) when obtaining multiple colonic biopsies in patients with colitis. If colectomy is applied to low-grade dysplasia then a surveillance program can be cost-effective.

Which Operation?

Three main surgical procedures should be considered in the elective setting: proctocolectomy with permanent ileostomy, subtotal colectomy with ileorectal anastomosis, and restorative proctocolectomy with ileoanal anastomosis. A total colectomy is necessary, as partial colonic resections have resulted in high incidence of colitis in the remaining colon. The conventional proctocolectomy has increasingly been replaced by the restorative procedure over the past 25 years as shown in the St Mark's Hospital (London) series: a reduction from 60 to 21% in conventional proctocolectomy and increase from 7 to 52% in restorative proctocolectomy was observed in 422 patients undergoing surgery between 1976 and 1990. Also a fall from 28 to 11% was observed in patients undergoing colectomy with ileorectal anastomosis during that period. The indications and technical aspect of the restorative proctocolectomy are discussed elsewhere.

Subtotal Colectomy with Ileorectal Anastomosis

This procedure comprises leaving rectal mucosa with possible persisting inflammation or even malignant transformation in order to avoid a permanent stoma. This operation has a low morbidity and mortality, without the need of creating a defunctioning stoma in elective cases. It also avoids the risk of damaging the pelvic nerves with the risks to urinary and sexual function in younger patients. A significant failure rate has been observed (10–30% depending on the series) due to persisting inflammation or evidence of neoplastic changes. It has a place in the management of patients with Crohn's colitis with a relatively spared rectum in whom an ileoanal pouch is contraindicated.

The indications for this procedure are, therefore, limited. They include: Crohn's disease with rectal sparing, some cases of indeterminate colitis, sclerosing cholangitis (associated to a high incidence of pouchitis) and patients with disseminated malignancy. Patients should accept regular indefinite yearly endoscopic follow-up with a risk of developing cancer in the rectal stump of approximately 6% at 20 years and 15% at 30 years. Also the long-term functional results of the ileorectal anastomosis depend upon the rectum maintaining its capacitance, expansibility and the anal sphincter function being adequate. Anorectal studies with volume manometry to assess capacitance and contrast proctography will be helpful in patients with mild or moderate proctitis.

Subtotal colectomy with ileorectal anastomosis is contraindicated in patients with evidence of dysplasia or carcinoma within the large bowel except when the patient has established distant metastatic disease. If surgery is indicated in this group of patients, provided local cancer clearance is achieved, it becomes the best option because of the associated low morbidity.

In the elderly, there is sufficient evidence in the literature that continence rates, frequency of defecation and functional outcome do not differ significantly from the younger age groups (<50 years) in patients undergoing restorative proctocolectomy and, therefore, this should be considered as gold standard treatment bearing in mind the patient's comorbidity.

Technique

The mobilization of the colon is carried out in the same fashion as previously described in this chapter. The terminal ileum is transected as close to the ileocecal valve as possible, except in cases of Crohn's disease, where terminal ileum is involved. The caliber of the ileum can be gauged against the rectum. Occasionally, a cheatle antimesenteric incision in the ileum is necessary to accommodate the discrepancy in size between the ileum and the rectum. A non-crushing clamp is applied to the ileum avoiding clamping of the mesentery.

As a general rule, the rectum is transected at the level of the sacral promontory, avoiding the need for presacral space dissection (Waldeyer's fascia) with the potential risk of injury to the presacral nerve plexus. A linear stapling gun

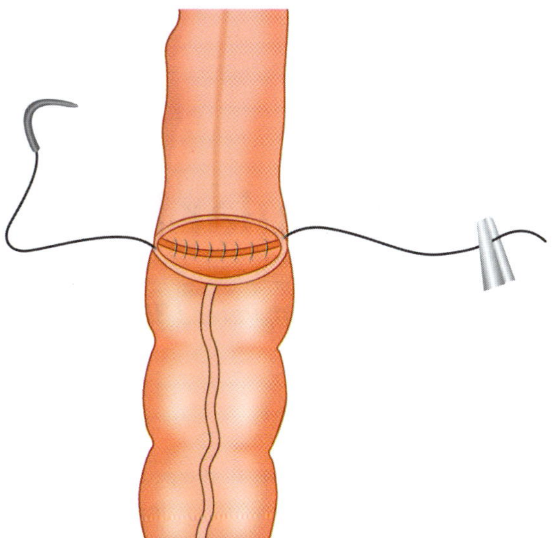

Fig. 63.3 Posterior continuous suture (Full-thickness) ileorectal anastomosis

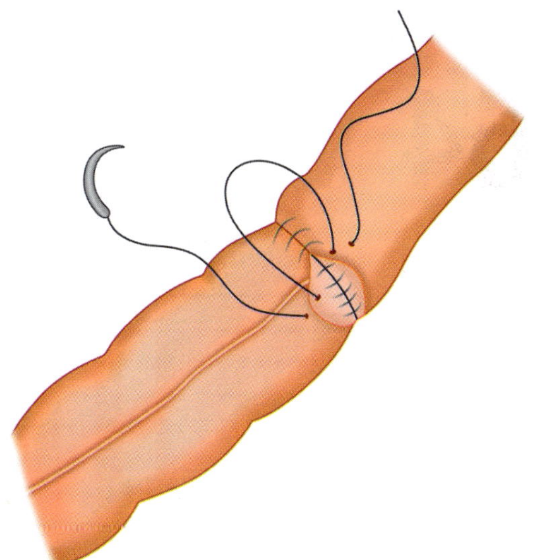

Fig. 63.5 Interrupted seromuscular suture

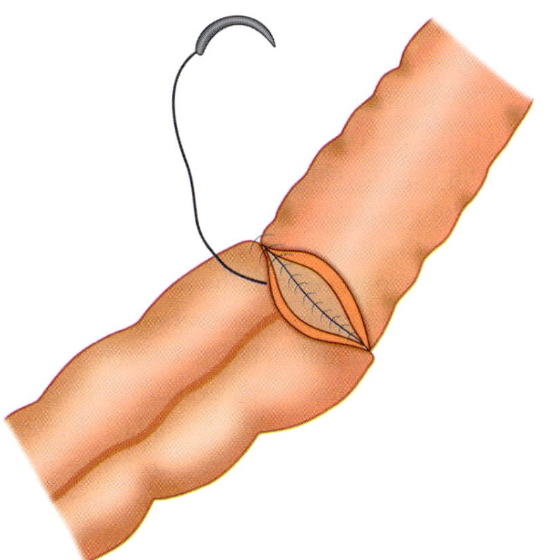

Fig. 63.4 Anterior continuous suture (full-thickness)

(TA, United States Corp., Norwalk, CT or TC, Ethicon Endosurgery Cincinnati, OH) is commonly used to transect the rectal stump.

Anastomosis (Figs 63.3 to 63.5)

A safe anastomosis, tension-free, circumferentially intact and well-vascularized can be achieved either by a two-layer hand sutured technique or, as preferred by the author, using an intraluminal circular stapler (CEEA, United States Surgical Corp, CT or LCA Ethicon Endosurgery Inc., Hamburg, Germany) to achieve an end-to-end anastomosis. All anastomosis to the rectum are leak tested by air (Jacuzzi test) intraoperatively. If a circular staple is used, both tissue 'doughnuts' are checked.

CHAPTER

64

Operations for Diverticular Disease

Niraj Khetan, Peter J Billings, X Escofet

SURGICAL MANAGEMENT OF DIVERTICULAR DISEASE

Diverticular disease is common in the western population with an incidence of 50% by the age of 60. Although diverticular disease may be widespread in the colon, the sigmoid colon is the site of most symptomatic disease. Clinical symptoms are usually accompanied by smooth muscle hypertrophy, thickening and shortening of the sigmoid colon.

Even in elective resections, the disease may be associated with marked pericolic inflammation and edema with pericolic abscess formation in the mesentery. Surgery is indicated in patients in good general health who have severe attacks of left-sided and suprapubic abdominal pain with marked diverticular on a barium enema X-ray, smooth muscle hypertrophy and narrowing of colonic lumen which is unresponsive to dietary change and antispasmodic drugs. The barium enema findings and symptoms do not always correlate and patients often have prolonged conservative management before being offered surgery. Indications for surgical treatment include:

- Male patients under the age of 50 years with symptomatic disease, over 80% will eventually come to surgery, many with complicated disease.
- Patients with urinary infection associated with their attacks indicating a colovesical fistula.
- Patients with two or more attacks of acute diverticulitis with a short period of time associated with a fever, mass and radiological signs of a pericolic abscess.
- Recurrent bleeding in patients fit for operation. A single episode does not make surgery mandatory.
- Complete colonic obstruction.
- Coexistent peritonitis.
- Spreading or generalized peritonitis.
- Massive continued colonic hemorrhage.

It is unnecessary to remove all the proximal diverticulae. The sigmoid colon is resected with the anastomosis between the middle or upper descending colon and the upper third of the rectum below the sacral promontory.

MANAGEMENT OF ACUTE DIVERTICULITIS

Acute sigmoid diverticulitis typically presents with fever, leukocytosis and pain in the left lower quadrant of the abdomen. The patient may or may not have a palpable mass in the lower abdomen or pelvis.

The best imaging technique for diagnosing a diverticular mass is a computerized tomographic scan. Initial therapy is conservative with intravenous antibiotics and nasogastric suction. After two to three days, the patient is usually much improved and the tenderness and fever will have diminished. If present, the abdominal/pelvic mass may no longer be palpable after a week. After three weeks, a barium enema may be performed. If it is the patient's first attack, surgery is not generally indicated unless the X-ray shows an extravasation of contrast media outside the lumen of the colon.

In most patients, acute diverticulitis is caused by intramural and pericolonic cellulitis, rather than an abscess. For this reason many patients will respond to conservative management. Conservative therapy often avoids the need for surgery and enables the surgeon to perform a one-stage resection as an elective operation instead of a two- or three-stage procedure.

In those patients in whom conservative therapy has failed, performing a proximal colostomy and local drainage will prove inadequate for control of spreading sepsis because of the column of stool in the left colon situated between the colostomy and the perforation. The progression of sepsis is likely if there is a continuing leak, and also the surgeon may fail to identify retroperitoneal or intermesenteric abscess.

In planning the surgical management of complicated diverticulitis, it is important to recognize and differentiate diverticulitis associated with abscess or phlegmon and diverticulitis with free perforation. The first condition falls into two categories:

1. Pericolic abscess
2. Distant abscess

The treatment of these patients as suggested by the Standard Task Force of the American Society of Colon and Rectal Surgeons is determined by the size and location of the abscess, as well as the clinical condition of the patient at the time of diagnosis.

Not all these patients require urgent or emergency surgical treatment. A small pericolic abscess may resolve with medical treatment. In some patients, a larger diverticular abscesses may resolve with CT-guided drainage allowing subsequent resection and primary anastomosis avoiding a temporary colostomy. Patients in which peritoneal drainage is not technically feasible (an absence of a radiological "window" or a multilocular collection with persistent sepsis in spite of drainage) should undergo surgery. In these cases, primary resection and anastomosis with or without a covering stoma may be performed if there is not substantial contamination. Resection of the affected bowel is undertaken with the proximal end brought out as an end colostomy and closure of the rectal stump (Hartmann's procedure) as the standard surgical procedure.

Free perforation is a surgical emergency that requires prompt operative treatment. Mortality appears directly related to several factors, such as the degree of fecal peritoneal contamination, severity of sepsis and the timeliness of surgical intervention. In this condition, the intervention of choice remains a Hartmann's procedure, whereas drainage alone or combined with colostomy should be abandoned. Hartmann's procedure is also advisable in the treatment of immunocompromised patients (patients with renal insufficiency, transplant patients and patients with acquired immune deficiency syndrome) in whom free perforation occurs more frequently than in non-immunocompromised patients with an accordingly high postoperative mortality rate (40%).

MANAGEMENT OF COLONIC OBSTRUCTION

A few patients who have diverticular disease, present with signs of complete colonic obstruction. In the absence of localized tenderness, fever and leukocytosis the diagnosis can be confirmed with a water-soluble contrast enema. Patients should be resuscitated and taken to theater for resection of the diseased segment with on-table colonic lavage and primary anastomosis. This has several advantages including resection of the diseased colon and cleansing of the proximal colon, which most surgeons believe to be an important factor in successful anastomotic healing. Intraoperative colonic lavage, resection and primary anastomosis has been described as a safe and expedient method of providing bowel preparation adequate for single-stage resection and anastomosis. It is a widely accepted, safe procedure for treatment of left-sided colonic obstruction. Performing a primary anastomosis ensures that further surgery is avoided. It should be born in mind that closure of a temporary stoma has its own set of potential surgical complications.

MANAGEMENT OF MASSIVE COLONIC HEMORRHAGE

Diverticular disease only accounts for a small proportion of cases of massive lower gastrointestinal bleeds. It occurs more frequently in elderly individuals with associated atherosclerotic and hypertensive cardiovascular disease. It is more common for these symptoms to be present in patients without diverticulitis and it is now generally agreed that patients who have massive lower gastrointestinal hemorrhage and diverticular disease are bleeding from vessels in the base of the diverticulae which are not themselves inflamed. Patients with hemorrhage from diverticulae characteristically present with sudden onset of profuse bleeding per rectum. The blood is usually bright red in color. Often the patient has a previous history supportive of diverticular disease. The bleeding usually stops spontaneously in at least 70% of patients and is rarely recurrent.

Bleeding from diverticular disease needs to be differentiated from other causes of lower gastrointestinal bleeding, principally angiodysplasia. Angiography is mandatory to identify the site of bleeding prior to surgery. Continuing life-threatening hemorrhage from diverticular disease requires an excision of the bleeding segment, which is usually in the sigmoid colon, a primary colonic anastomosis can be constructed.

MANAGEMENT OF COLOVESICAL FISTULA

Colovesical fistula presents infrequently in general surgical practice. Diverticular disease accounts for the underlying pathology in approximately two-thirds of the patients. Other causes include cancer, Crohn's disease, radiation and trauma. The management of colovesical fistula is associated with morbidity ranging from 4 to 45%. Recognized complications of surgical treatment include fistula recurrence, anastomotic leakage and abdominal sepsis.

Patients are treated according to a standard protocol whereby all diseased bowel, including the origin of the fistula and any colorectal stricture, is resected with construction of a primary colorectal anastomosis unless contraindicated by gross sepsis. The colon is prepared with a standard bowel cleansing regime with perioperative antibiotic prophylaxis. After division of healthy proximal and distal bowel, the resected specimen is sent for histological examination. A primary anastomosis is constructed in a standard fashion with interrupted seromuscular submucosal absorbable sutures. Only in cases where there is gross intraperitoneal sepsis or severe diverticulitis of the remaining bowel is an anastomosis not constructed and a colostomy performed. The bladder defect is closed with interrupted absorbable sutures and omentum mobilized to separate the colonic suture line from the bladder. A self-retaining urinary catheter is left to drain the bladder for 10 days following surgery.

PRIMARY RESECTION AND ANASTOMOSIS

Operative Strategy

The operative technique for the resection of the left colon and for the anastomosis is similar to that described for left colectomy for cancer, but with a number of important exceptions.

In the absence of cancer, there is no need to perform a high lymphovascular dissection and the mesentery may be divided closer to the bowel, unless the mesentery is so inflamed and edematous that it cannot hold sutures. It may be necessary to mobilize the rectum for the presacral space to construct the anastomosis at the level of the sacral promontory.

Ideally the majority of diverticulae should be removed, but it is not necessary to do an extensive colectomy as there will often be residual diverticulae in the ascending or transverse colon. At the site selected for anastomosis, however, there should be no diverticular disease or gross muscle hypertrophy.

Preoperative Preparation

In acutely ill septic patients, preoperative preparation involves rapid resuscitation using intravenous fluids, blood products and antibiotics. Patients being submitted to elective surgery should have the normal preoperative preparation with colonic cleansing. Diverticular disease only accounts for a small proportion of cases of massive lower gastrointestinal bleeds. It occurs more frequently in elderly individuals with associated atherosclerotic and hypertensive cardiovascular disease.

Operative Procedure

Incision

A long midline incision is made from the epigastrium to the pubis.

Dissection of the Sigmoid and Left Colon

The dissection is started in the region of the upper descending colon by incising the peritoneum in the paracolic gutter. The left hand is inserted behind the colon is in an area above the diverticulae to elevate the mesocolon. In order to safeguard the left ureter from damage, it is identified in the upper portion of the dissection where the absence of inflammation simplifies the maneuver. The ureter is then traced down into the pelvis and may have to be dissected off the side of the sigmoid colon. When the dissection has been completed, the sigmoid is free down to the promontory of the sacrum.

Division of Mesocolon

The mesentery generally may be divided at a point no more than 4 to 6 cm from the bowel wall. The proximal line of division is at a point on the left colon that is free of pathology, usually in the descending colon which may require mobilization of the splenic flexure and distal transverse colon. The dissection is continued to the rectosigmoid junction. The upper and middle thirds of the rectum may be mobilized to facilitate the anastomosis.

Anastomosis

The distal line of resection is at the rectosigmoid junction or beyond the affected area. If the anastomosis is at the rectosigmoid junction, an open hand-sewn anastomosis is constructed with an interrupted single layer extra-mucosal technique. An anastomosis constructed lower down the rectum is fashioned using a double-stapled technique.

Abdominal Closure

Mass abdominal closure is performed in a standard fashion with a monofilament synthetic non-absorbable or slowly absorbable suture.

Hartmann's Procedure

Hartmann's procedure is still a useful procedure to treat patients with advanced generalized peritonitis. In acute diverticulitis the rectosigmoid is not usually involved to a great extent in the inflammatory process. Mesenteric dissection should be terminated at this point. If the thickness of the rectosigmoid is not excessive, the rectum may be closed by the application of linear stapler. If edema and inflammation are present, it may not be possible to perform a stapled closure and the rectal stump should be closed by a continuous layer of absorbable sutures. The apex of the rectum is sutured to the pelvic fascia near or, if possible, higher than the promontory of the sacrum in order to prevent retraction into the pelvis, which would make re-anastomosis more difficult. The end colostomy is brought out through a trephine incision through the lateral portion of the left rectus muscle. The incision should admit two fingers. The cut end of the colon is brought out and immediately sutured with interrupted sutures to the subcuticular layer of the skin incision.

Laparoscopically-assisted Reversal of Hartmann's Procedure

Since Hartmann's procedure was first described in 1921, the need for a subsequent laparotomy to close the colostomy has been its greatest disadvantage. Median postoperative stay for a conventional reversal of Hartmann's procedure has been reported as 9 to 15 days.

Laparoscopic-assisted reversal of Hartmann's was described in 1993 and again in 1994, with the median postoperative stay of 8 days.

Patients who have their colostomy reversed laparoscopically appear to suffer less physiological upset and require little opiate analgesia, and return to their normal activities promptly. These points are better indications of improved recovery than the speed at which the patient leaves the hospital. As yet, no patient has been excluded from having attempted laparoscopic reversal of Hartmann's, nor has obesity proved a contraindication as it has in other forms of laparoscopic colorectal surgery. During the procedure, dissection of the ureter is unnecessary. It is a procedure well suited to bring the benefits of laparoscopic surgery to colorectal patients.

Preoperative rigid sigmoidoscopy or radiological contrast studies are used to assess the length of the rectal stump. The colon is prepared in a standard way by routine bowel preparation with laxatives together with a rectal washout.

All patients are given subcutaneous heparin, perioperative intravenous broad spectrum antibiotics with a urethral catheter *in situ*. Postoperative care is standard as for major abdominal surgery and the patient is allowed to home when fully recovered.

Surgical Technique

The patient is placed in the modified lithotomy position with the legs in stirrups. The stoma is mobilized through an elliptical incision approximately 6 cm in size and freed from its adhesions to the anterior abdominal wall and other intra-abdominal structures, allowing approximately 10–12 cm of colon to extend out of the abdominal cavity. The distal end of the descending colon is then excised and the lumen sized. The anvil of a circular stapling device is inserted and held in position by a purse string suture with 3-0 prolene and a curved needle. The descending colon is returned to the abdomen and a Trendelenburg tilt applied.

Adhesions between the greater omentum, small bowel and anterior abdominal wall are freed, particularly those below the umbilicus. Using a Rampley sponge holder with a swab, the small bowel is pulled out of the pelvis, and any adhesions are broken down. A sizer is then introduced into the rectal stump and moved from side to side while a finger is placed in the wound and the rectum palpated bimanually to assess for strictures adherent to the rectal stump. A 10–12 mm port is positioned just below the umbilicus under direct vision and a second 10–12 mm blunt port is placed in the colostomy wound, which is closed with 3-0 prolene, taking care to achieve an air-tight seal. The pneumoperitoneum is then established and a third 10–12 mm port inserted in the right iliac fossa. Any final adhesions in the pelvis are then freed laparoscopically. When the uterus is present, a straight prolene suture is placed through the anterior abdominal wall, the fundus of the uterus and once more out through the abdominal wall, to lift the uterus anteriorly. After ensuring sufficient length of descending colon to reach the rectum without tension, the circular stapler is introduced into the rectum attached to the anvil under direct vision, closed and fired. The integrity of the anastomosis is determined by inspection of the doughnuts, and by an insufflation test. Following removal of the ports, closure of the colostomy wound site is completed and the skin closed with clips over a drain.

CHAPTER

65

Management of Rectal Cancer

Marc D Bullock, Alexander H Mirnezami

INTRODUCTION

One third of colonic malignancies arise within the rectum. The rectum is clinically with the sigmoid colon and begins approximately at the level of the sacral promontory. Its distal margin is defined by the anorectal junction; the point at which puborectalis is traversed and the anal canal begins. The rectum is subdivided for descriptive purposes and as an aid in decision making into upper, middle and lower thirds. Although the precise definition of what constitutes the rectum varies in the literature from 12, 15 and even 16 cm from the anal verge, in the modern era of high-resolution pelvic imaging, consensus may be achieved using MRI measurements with the rectum defined as the portion of the large bowel below the sacral promontory that is associated with a definable mesorectum posteriorly.

Surgery remains the mainstay of treatment for rectal cancer (RC). Traditionally, newly diagnosed rectal tumors were clinically assessed and staged by digital examination and proctoscopy to determine treatment strategies. In more recent times, however, substantial advances in diagnostic imaging, neoadjuvant and adjuvant therapies, surgical treatment options, and pathological indicators of disease stage, have led to increasingly complex decision making in the management of patients with rectal cancer, and engendered an increasingly multidisciplinary management approach.

In the present chapter, we summarize the contemporary management of rectal cancer focusing on preoperative considerations, operative principles and techniques, and postoperative care.

PREOPERATIVE PLANNING

Multidisciplinary Team (MDT)

The management of patients suspected of having RC, should optimally be coordinated through an MDT meeting. Whenever possible, this could convene prior to surgery once preliminary investigations have been performed. Standard preoperative investigations include: colonoscopy in order to provide histological confirmation and rule out synchronous lesions; Computed tomography (CT) of the chest, abdomen, and pelvis to stage for distant disease, and high-resolution magnetic resonance imaging (MRI) of the pelvis for the purpose of loco-regional tumor staging and assessment of the tumor relationship to the putative circumferential resection margin (CRM).

Role of Radiologist

Accurate preoperative imaging is an indispensable tool, not only influencing the nature of the surgery but also guiding the use of neoadjuvant therapy.

Compared with colonic tumors, surgery for RC is associated with a higher rate of local recurrence. Key prognostic indicators are the extent of local tumor invasion (T-stage), lymph node status (N-stage), the distance of the tumor from the mesorectal fascia (the CRM), and the height of the tumor from the anal verge. The combination of these indices helps to stratify recurrence risk ahead of surgery and identify patients who might benefit from preoperative radiotherapy or combined chemotherapy.

MRI is the preferred technique for assessing these parameters, and has dramatically altered the management of rectal cancer. MRI imaging with a 1.5 Tesla unit device and a pelvic phased array wrap-around surface coil provides optimal images, and offers high overall T-staging accuracy between 65% and 86% depending on stage. MRI imaging is of particular importance as it provides important information about the relationship of the tumor to the mesorectal fascia (and therefore the all-important CRM); aids in differentiating between T3 and T4 tumors; and assessing tumors which may have invaded contiguous organs (reviewed by Beets-Tan RG et al., 2011; Valentini C et al., 2008).

Lymph node (LN) status, which includes the absolute number of LNs within the resection specimen as well as the number of LNs containing micro-metastases and the ratio of positive to negative LNs, has important prognostic value. However, none of the conventional radiological techniques at our disposal is able to accurately distinguish between benign and malignant LNs, and as emphasis moves towards provision of neoadjuvant therapy for RC, the categorization of LNs in advance of surgery has become increasingly important. Nodes greater than 10 mm with an irregular border and heterogeneous signal intensity on MRI are highly suspicious of malignant infiltration, but as many as 94% of those smaller than 5 mm may also be involved, which presents a considerable diagnostic challenge.

MRI is highly accurate for preoperative identification of tumor encroachment into the CRM. Tumor extending to within 1 mm of the radial margin of the resection specimen is associated with poor survival and an elevated risk of local recurrence. Preoperative prediction of a threatened or involved CRM enables the targeted use of neoadjuvant therapy which is intended to facilitate the complete excision of the specimen at the time of surgery and consequently, improve patient outcome (Figs 65.1 to 65.6).

Endorectal US (EUS) is another highly sensitive imaging technique, particularly, when discriminating between early stage (T1 / T2) lesions, but is limited in some contexts such as high or stenosing tumors where probe positioning becomes a challenge. Furthermore, sensitivity is operator-dependent

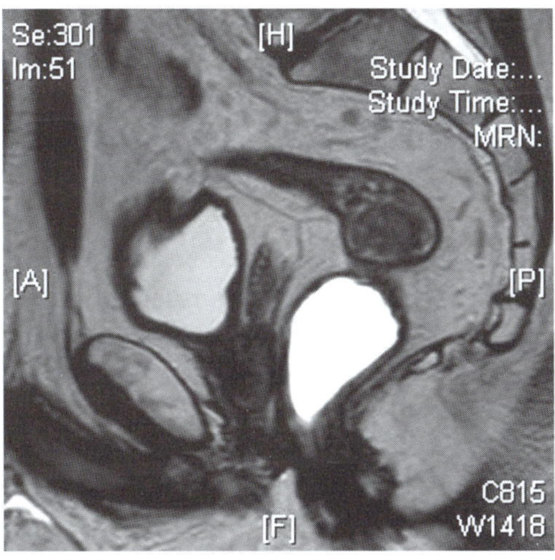

Fig. 65.1 Normal male pelvis on MRI

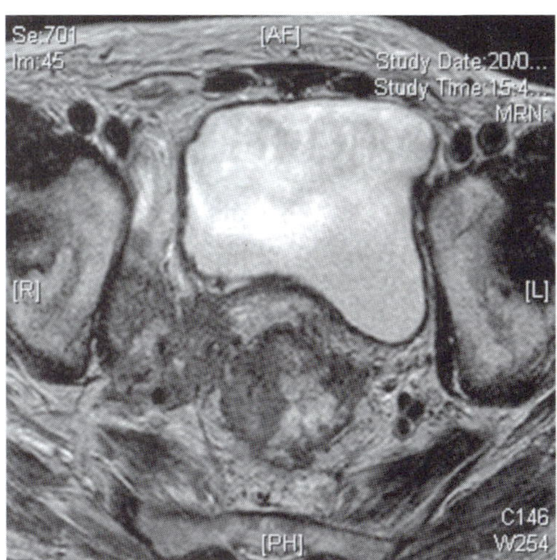

Fig. 65.2 Midrectal cancer with threatened lateral margins on pelvic MRI

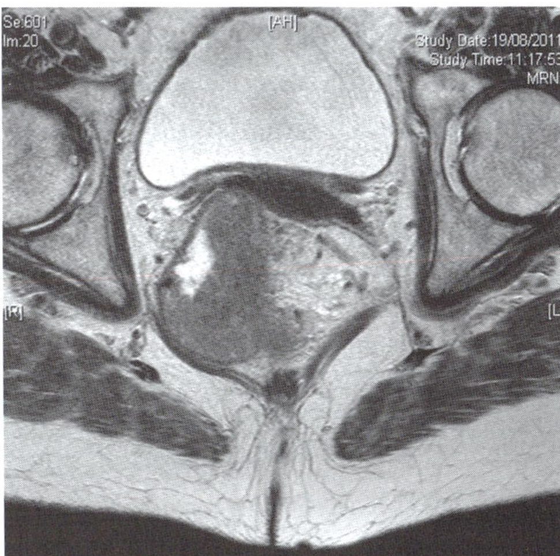

Fig. 65.3 Rectal cancer with threatened anterior and lateral margins on pelvic MRI

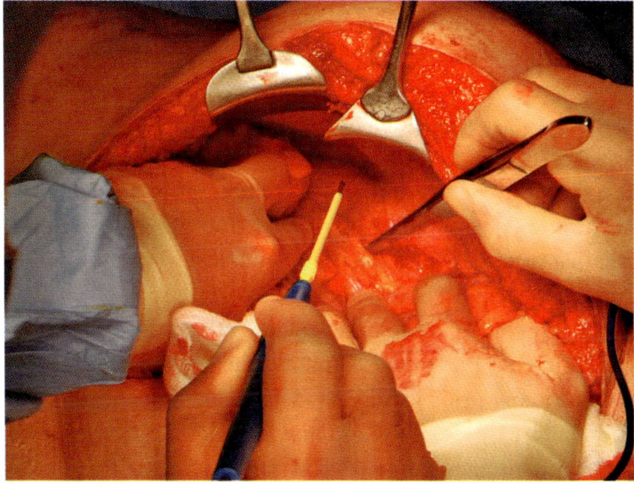

Fig. 65.4 Mobilization of colon. Left paracolic gutter

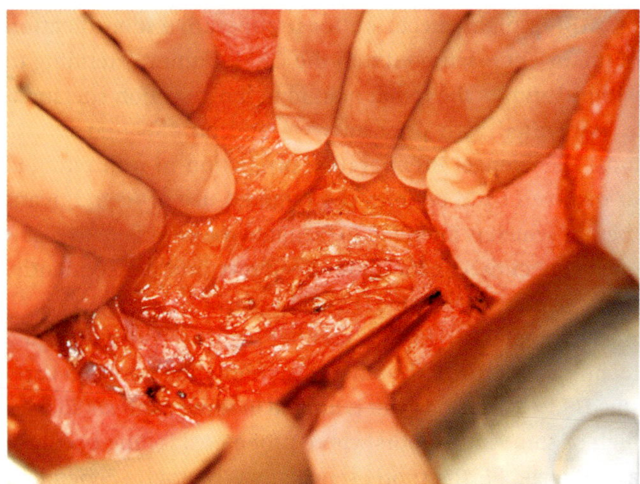

Fig. 65.5 Identification of left ureter and nerve plexus

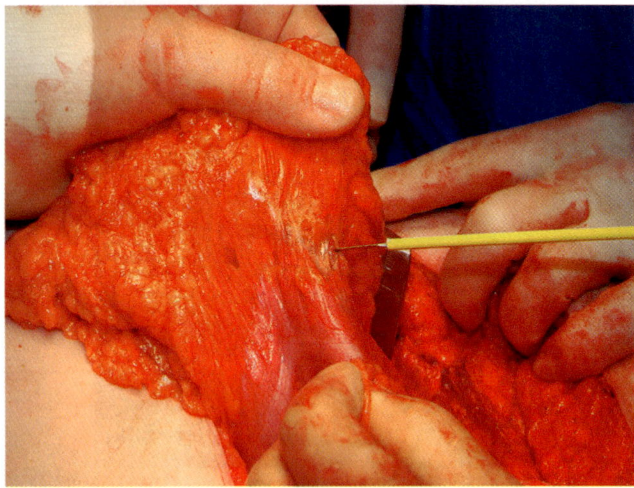

Fig. 65.6 Splenic flexure dissection: Entry to the lesser sac

and images less accessible to other members of the MDT for the purpose of therapeutic planning.

Role of Oncologist

Six neoadjuvant radiotherapy reduces the risk of local recurrence in resectable RC; however, the timing of irradiation relative to surgery and the use of concurrent chemotherapy remain the subject of debate.

A large scale systematic review of radiotherapy trials including 42 RCTs and 3 meta-analyses concluded that radiotherapy prior to surgery decreases the overall risk of local failure by 50 to 70% and may improve survival by about 10%. Advantages compared to postoperative irradiation include superior tumor radiosensitivity and a more favorable toxicity profile.

Neoadjuvant radiotherapy is also used to downstage disease, to facilitate complete resection of locally advanced tumors or to make sphincter preserving surgery more likely.

Short-course radiotherapy, administered in 5 fractions to minimize delay to surgery, is the method favored by some units for resectable RC, and is supported by trial evidence.

An alternative approach is long-course radiotherapy which is frequently administered with concurrent chemotherapy. It is particularly useful for downstaging tumors which threaten the CRM but inevitably leads to surgical delay.

Two randomized trials have examined the efficacy of concurrent chemotherapy, the largest of which, the EORTC trial, compared radiotherapy and surgery with radiotherapy, surgery and 3 concurrent pre and/or postoperative chemotherapy regimens, and demonstrated reduced rates of local recurrence in all three chemotherapy groups compared with radiotherapy and surgery alone. The lowest rate of local recurrence was achieved in the group receiving both preoperative and postoperative chemotherapy although overall survival at 5 years did not differ significantly between the groups.

Postoperative radiotherapy has become less frequently performed in recent years and is reserved for situations where tumour is found unexpectedly at one or more surgical resection margin, in a patient who had not previously received pre-operative radiotherapy.

Role of Surgeon

Surgery is the mainstay of treatment for RC. There are a number of important surgical considerations which impact upon clinical outcome and quality of life and should be at the forefront of the surgeon's mind as preparations are made for surgery:

Local Recurrence

In the 1980s, RJ Heald described the resection technique known as Total Mesorectal Excision (TME), which involves dissecting along the embryonic 'holy' hind-gut plane under direct vision to the level of the levator muscles and excising tumor en-bloc with the entire visceral mesentery of the rectum. TME highlighted the importance of meticulous surgical technique and has now become the gold standard approach to RC, radically reducing the rate of local recurrence.

Intramural RC spread is rarely found further than a few millimeters beyond the distal margin of palpable tumor however, metastatic deposits can be found in LNs up to 4 cm away. For this reason, 5 cm was traditionally considered the minimum resection margin in terms of acceptable oncological clearance, effectively meaning TME is required for all cancers arising in the middle or lower third of the rectum.

For upper rectal cancer, many surgeons choose to perform a 'subtotal TME', with transection of the mesorectum and at a suitable point below the tumor, thus avoiding a low anastomosis which is associated with elevated leak rates and typically requires a defunctioning stoma. While a proximal defunctioning stoma does not reduce the likelihood of an anastomotic leak, it does appear to mitigate the clinical impact.

Mesorectal LNs are removed en-bloc with TME, however, up to 11% of patients with RC will also present with metastases in the lateral pelvic LNs which run along the internal iliac vessels and which are not addressed by TME. For those patients, the Japanese in particular advocate supplementing TME with an extended pelvic lymphadenectomy (EPL), an approach which has not found favor in the west and remains controversial.

Although data suggests lateral pelvic LNs are pathologically relevant (reviewed by Georgiou et al., 2009) meta-analysis demonstrated the EPL accounts for significantly greater rates of sexual and urinary dysfunction without influencing survival or local recurrence. Importantly, the only randomized prospective trial included in the analysis, concluded that EPL was not necessary for patients with RC who undergo neo-adjuvant radiotherapy; which is the preferred approach in the UK. It is our practice to subject radiologically suspicious sidewall lymph nodes to PET scanning prior to any neoadjuvant treatment. If these prove to be FDG-avid and show little response to downstaging treatment, after careful discussion with patients, an EPL is considered.

Thirty to forty percent of patients with RC will have lymph node metastases within the inferior mesenteric LN chain which follow the course of the inferior mesenteric artery (IMA). The IMA can either be divided flush with the aorta (high ligation) or distal to the origin of the left colic artery (low ligation) and some controversy remains as to which method is superior. Many surgeons perform high vascular ligation, however, numerous studies have failed to demonstrate any survival benefit associated with this approach. High ligation does provide greater maneuverability and is sometimes obligatory to avoid anastomotic tension, while low ligation is associated with superior anastomotic perfusion as the descending colon continues to be supplied by the intact left colic artery via the marginal artery (reviewed by Lange MM et al, 2008).

In practice, the level at which ligation occurs is usually determined by technical rather than oncological considerations.

Sexual and Urinary Dysfunction

Genitourinary dysfunction, resulting from damage to the presacral autonomic nerve plexus (PANS) is a recognized complication following surgery for RC. The PANS receives sympathetic and parasympathetic contributions via the superior hypogastric (SHP) and inferior hypogastric (IHP) plexus. Parasympathetic innervation maintains erectile function and sympathetic innervation is important for ejaculation. Both are required for maintenance of urinary continence.

The left and right hypogastric nerves form a 'wishbone' like shape as they exit the SHP and descend into the pelvis along the mesorectal fascia. They can be identified at the pelvic brim at the beginning of the posterior rectal dissection. The HIP is located on the pelvic sidewall anterior-lateral to the rectum. Careful endeavor to identify and preserve these structures intraoperatively can reduce the risk of sexual and urinary dysfunction following surgery.

Sphincter Preservation for Low Rectal Cancer

It is almost a century since W Ernest Miles described the Abdominoperineal Resection (APE), a surgical approach which, at one stage, was the standard of care for all rectal tumors. Later, anterior resection (AR) becomes acceptable for high tumors and ubiquitous sphincter sacrifice was superseded by the concept of the safe margin of oncological clearance. Later still, the introduction of the circular stapling device meant that performing anastomoses deep in the pelvis and even onto the sphincter complex itself became technically feasible, raising the question: what is the minimum margin of oncological clearance for low rectal cancer?

Over a thirty-year period which has seen the universal adoption of TME and the introduction of adjuvant chemoradiotherapy, the margin of distal clearance considered safe has fallen. Excellent local control can be achieved by combining TME with radiotherapy and macroscopic margins below 1 cm have been shown not to increase the burden of local recurrence provided microscopic tumor encroachment at the level of the rectal transection and CRM and avoided.

As a result, sphincter preserving surgery has become increasingly popular, encouraged by the sense that a permanent colostomy may be detrimental to quality of life (QoL). The literature does not clearly support this association, however, recent studies and a Cochrane review have suggested that poor functional results after sphincter preserving surgery also compromise QoL, and QoL after AR can be similar or worse than after an APE. Indeed, if the condition of the anal sphincter complex is poor, and continence is already an issue in the preoperative stage, an APE (for a low tumor) or Hartmann's procedure (for a high tumor) may produce a better functional outcome than sphincter preservation 'at any cost'.

Factors such as co-morbid status, tumor size, and radiotherapy response, also sway the decision towards sphincter sacrifice or sphincter preservation, however, if tumor encroaches into the anal sphincter complex itself, APE is almost always indicated.

Locally Advanced Rectal Cancer

Tumors predicted to extend beyond the TME plane on MRI and involving adjacent viscera are deemed to be locally advanced, although this definition is not consistently applied in the literature. These cases are particularly challenging and multi-modal therapy incorporating radical exenteration surgery should be considered following careful discussion with the patient and MDT colleagues.

Laparoscopic Considerations

Laparoscopic TME is safe and effective for RC. Meta-analysis reveals that key oncological indicators such as the rate of local tumor recurrence, disease-free survival and cancer-related mortality are equivalent to open surgery and improved short-term outcomes such as time to oral diet ad length of hospital stay have meant that the laparoscopic approach has become increasingly popular for both AR and APE.

There are perhaps as many variations of technique as there are surgeons, however, laparoscopic TME is generally conducted with the patient in the lithotomy position with varying degrees of Trendelenburg tilt. Access to the peritoneal cavity is achieved via an infra-umbilical incision by sharp dissection under direct vision (Hasson technique). The camera is introduced through a 10 or 12 mm port enabling a further 3 to 5 ports to be inserted under direct vision. Typically, a 12 mm port is inserted in the RIF and 5 mm ports in the right flank and LIF.

Following a thorough inspection of the abdominal cavity and viscera to evaluate for occult metastatic spread, the respectability of the tumor, and the degree of colonic mobilization required, surgery may begin.

The authors find it useful to subdivided laparoscopic TME into the following 10 steps:

1. Mobilization of the sigmoid colon in a medial-to-lateral or lateral-to-medial approach, followed by preparation of the IMA and identification of PANS.
2. Identification and preservation of the left ureter and gonadal vessels.
3. Ligation of the IMA, carefully avoiding the left ureter.
4. Ligation of the inferior mesenteric vein (IMV).
5. Mobilization of the descending colon in the left paracolic gutter (lateral-to-medial).
6. Mobilization of the splenic flexure (medial, lateral and omental).
7. Mobilization of the rectum along the mesorectal 'holy' plane.
8. Division of the rectum using an endostapler.
9. Extracorporeal delivery of tumor through a minimal LIF muscle-splitting incision.
10. Formation of anastomosis with a transanal stapling device (for AR) including 'air-leak' or endoscopic test of integrity.

OPERATIVE PROCEDURES

Local Excision

TME is the fold standard surgical approach to RC, however, for small (<2 cm) well to moderately differentiated pT1 tumors, local excision only by transanal excision (TE) or transanal endoscopic microsurgery (TEMS) may be considered adequate in highly selected cases and with careful discussion of the risks and benefits with patients. Routine imaging with MRI is needed to help in planning and decision making, and if histopathology suggests poor differentiation or deeper tumor involvement, more radical surgery may be indicated.

Tumors located within 8 cm of the anal verge are usually amenable to excision using a 'standard' open TE technique which involves a full or partial thickness excision of the tumor with a 1 cm circumferential cuff of tissue. Partial thickness excision has the advantage of leaving tissue planes undisturbed if more radial surgery is subsequently required, but is less likely to result in complete tumor excision. The rectal defect can be repaired with interrupted mattress sutures or left open provided the peritoneal cavity has not been breached.

Tumors in the upper third of the rectum are less accessible and can be difficult to excise completely per anus. TEMS involves dilating the anal sphincter with a large diameter (4 cm) operating sigmoidoscope, and with the rectum insufflated, excising the tumor using endoscopic dissecting instruments. TEMS is safe, reliable and increasingly popular and may result in fewer recurrences than the conventional TE-technique.

Radical Procedures

The initial operative steps involved in APE, AR, and Hartmann's procedures are similar and are described together under the heading 'Colonic dissection'. Divergent elements of each operation are discussed in detail in subsequent sections.

Preoperative Considerations

The patient's fitness for surgery should be assessed and optimized preoperatively and informed consent obtained on the day of surgery. If an ileostomy or colostomy is anticipated, this should also be discussed during the consent process. Whenever possible, preoperative stoma marking should be conducted by a specialist nurse or trained clinician to take into account patient body habitus during different positions, relationship to clothes and belts, and to identify the optimal stoma position.

Preoperative work-up will vary according to local protocols. Important considerations include the use of mechanical bowel preparation, antibiotic prophylaxis and thromboprophylaxis: Using oral laxatives or retrograde enemas to purge the bowel prior to elective surgery has fallen out of favor as increasing evidence suggests it does not protect against infectious complications or anastomotic dehiscence and can lead to serious complications related to electrolyte disturbances and dehydration (Reviewed by Matsou et al., 2011). However, some surgeons may be reluctant to alter their practice as the outcome from early anastomotic dehiscence in bowel that has not been purged, can be catastrophic.

A Cochrane review concluded that optimal thromboprophylaxis for colorectal surgery is a combination of graduated compression stockings and low-dose unfractionated heparin.

Antibiotic prophylaxis is also recommended to reduce postoperative wound infection although the best choice of antibiotic and the timing and route of administration are not clearly defined.

Colonic Dissection

Patient preparation: The patient is placed in the modified Llyod-Davies position with arms optimally tucked at the patient's side. Legs are adjusted to allow for slight flexion and minor hip flexion particularly if a laparoscopic approach is planned. A urinary catheter is inserted and taped to the right thigh to permit clear access to the anus. Anti-embolism compression stockings and pneumatic calf compression devices are used.

For conventional APE, it may also be appropriate to elevate the pelvis using a sandbag.

The abdomen, upper thighs and perineum are prepared and draped routinely.

The abdominal incision: For open surgery, a midline incision is made from the symphysis pubis to a point approximately 5 cm above the umbilicus. Superior extension may be needed to mobilize a high splenic flexure.

Assess: Once the abdomen is open, a systematic examination of the peritoneal cavity and visceral organs is performed and tumor resectability assessed.

The wound edges are retracted with a self-retaining device, providing a clear view of the pelvis and the opportunity to exclude the small intestine from the field of surgery using warm, and wet packs (Fig. 65.7).

Mobilization of colon and pedicle ligation: The sigmoid colon is retracted medially to produce tension in the congenital peritoneal folds between the lateral aspect of the mesocolon and the lateral wall of the abdomen. These fibrous band are released with electrocautery along the entire length of the sigmoid in a continuous motion which simultaneously allows the left ureter and gonadal vessels to be swept laterally and inferiorly, and the sigmoid mesentery containing the vascular pedicle to be drawn medially.

In order to ensure the safe execution of the following steps, the left ureter should always be identified prior to ligation of the vascular pedicle (Fig. 65.8).

The sigmoid colon is then drawn back into the left paracolic gutter and the medial peritoneum of the mesosigmoid incised at the level of the pelvic brim, creating a window in the colonic mesentery. This window is extended cranially to the origin of the vascular pedicle, thereby permitting access to the IMA and IMV from both sides.

This vascular pedicle is isolated by creating a second mesenteric window above it. The IMA and IMV are then double legated and divided in turn (Fig. 65.9).

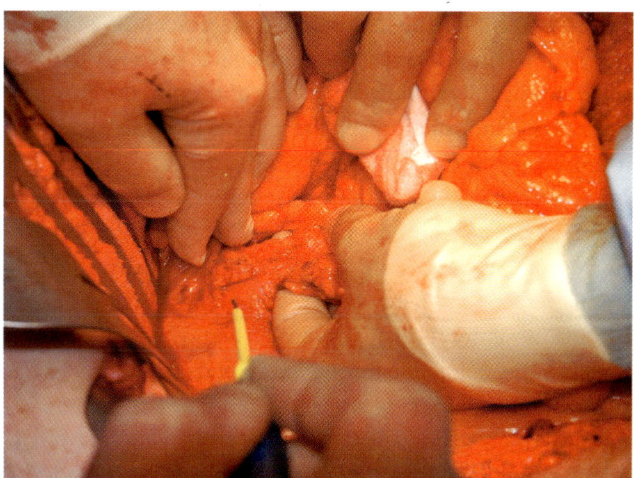

Fig. 65.7 Dissecting the vascular pedicle

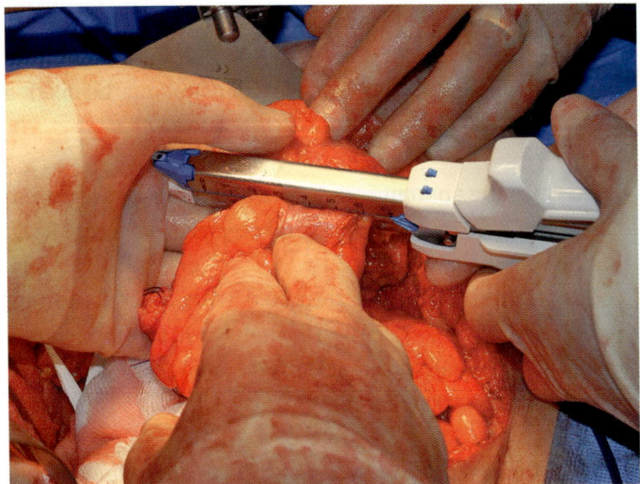

Fig. 65.8 Transection of colon: Division of convenience

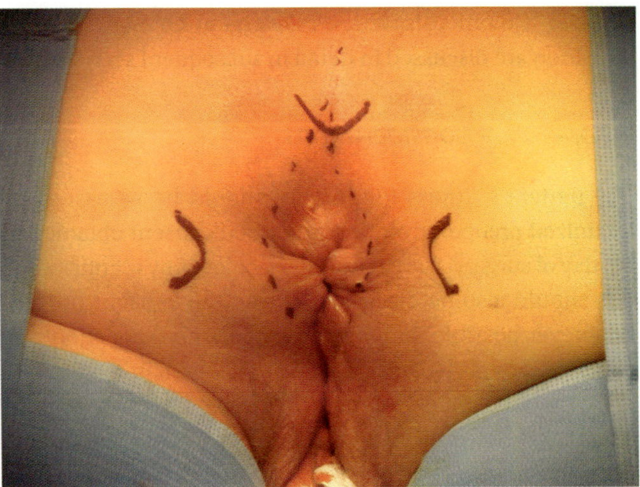

Fig. 65.10 Preoperative markings for teardrop perineal incision with patient in the prone position

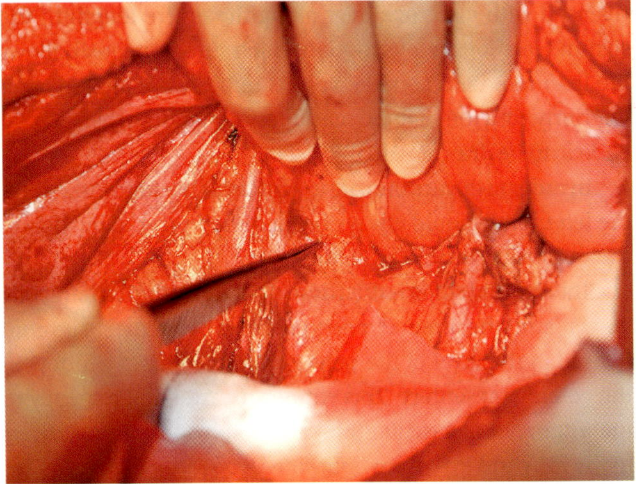

Fig. 65.9 Mobilization of the rectum: Entering the TME plane

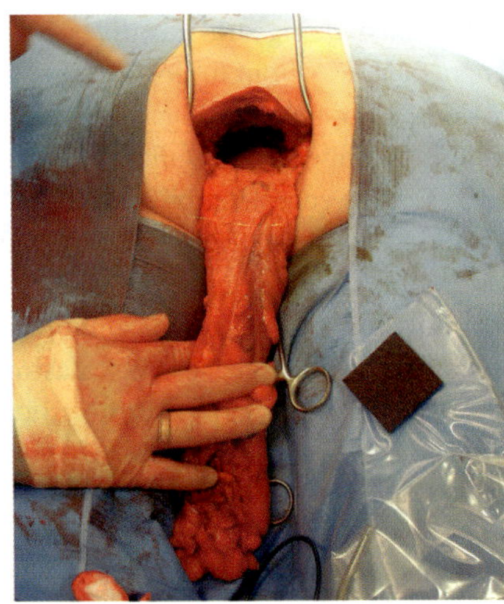

Fig. 65.11 Specimen is delivered via perineal defect facilitating dissection of anterior attachments

Division of colon: The length of usable descending colon is determined once the vascular pedicle has been divided and the colon is fully mobile. As a rule of thumb, the proximal limb must comfortably reach the pubic symphysis to produce a tension-free anastomosis or end colostomy depending on what is required. If there is insufficient length, it may be necessary to mobilize the colon further by dividing the peritoneal attachments of the splenic flexure. This is frequently the case if low AR is required (Fig. 65.10).

The mesentery is divided between hemostatic clips at right angles to the colon in a line which extends from the vascular pedicle to the colonic serosa at the point of transection. The colon is then divided with a linear cutter stapling device which simultaneously partitions and isolates the lumens and provides effective hemostasis (Fig. 65.11).

The distal colonic limb is now untethered which facilitates pelvic dissection. The proximal limb is temporarily packed away in the upper abdomen until it is required for construction of the coloanal/colorectal anastomosis or end colostomy.

Pelvic dissection and TME: The rectosigmoid is lifted forward to 'tension' the mesorectum. An incision at the level of the sacral promontory allows access to the pre-sacral space, defined posteriorly by the presacral fascia and anteriorly by the intact mesorectum. This place is developed with electrocautery to the level of the coccyx under direct vision.

Once the rectum has been freed posteriorly, the lateral peritoneal folds on either side are incised parallel to the rectum. The 'lateral ligaments' containing the middle rectal

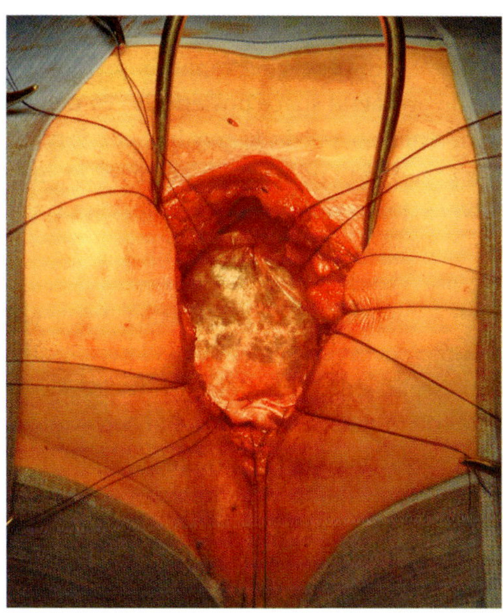

Fig. 65.12 Pelvic floor reconstruction with biological mesh

arteries encountered during lateral dissection should be legated or cauterized appropriately (Fig. 65.12).

Traditional teaching suggests that the transverse incision freeing the peritoneum from the from of the rectum should be made 1 cm beyond the deepest point of rectovesical recess in men or rectouterine pouch in women. The proximity to the bladder should remind the surgeon to pay special attention to the course of the ureters during pelvic dissection.

A lipped St Mark's retractor is useful at this stage as it can be used to draw the rectum to the left or right, facilitating lateral dissection and to draw the seminal vesicles forward (or posterior vaginal wall in women) enabling dissecting along Denonvillier's fascia.

The development of cutter-stapling devices for low rectal division in ARs has meant that dissection can extend onto the pelvic floor if required. In APEs, the pelvic floor is the limit of the abdominal component of the operation.

Anterior Resection

The initial operative steps are described under 'Colonic dissection'.

The degree of pelvic dissection required at the right of the colorectal anastomosis will depend largely on the position of the tumor. As discussed previously, in order to reduce the risk of anastomotic dehiscence, the approach for high RCs is usually to form an anastomosis in the mid to lower rectum once 5 cm of distal clearance has been achieved rather than perform a full TME on each occasion.

In low RCs located in close proximity to the anal sphincteric complex, the dilemma remains whether an ultra-low anastomosis or even an intersphincteric dissection with partial or complete excision of the internal anal sphincter is superior in terms of oncological and functional outcome to APE. If a safe margin of oncological clearance can be achieved, rectal transection at the level of the pelvic floor is appropriate and by definition requires the formation of a coloanal anastomosis at or below the level of the anorectal ring.

Prior to transection with a linear cutter stapling device, a right angle occlusion clamp is applied beyond the lower margin of the tumor and an assistant washes the rectum with a saline/betadine mix, administered via an irrigation set using a proctoscope. Rectal washout using a cytocidal agent has the combined benefit of removing faucal residue and destroying viable tumor cells present in the rectum prior to anastomosis.

Several options are available to reconstitute colonic integrity. A Cochrane review did not demonstrate significant differences in performance between hand-sewn and stapled techniques, however, modern practice has seen the near ubiquitous adoption of the circular stapling device.

For the majority of mid-to-high rectal cancers, an end-to-end anastomosis is appropriate: The proximal colonic limb is prepared to receive the anvil of the stapler using a purse-string suture. The circular stapler is inserted through the anus and into the rectal stump and is opened, which has the effect of driving a trocar through the wall of the rectum. The anvil, protruding from the lumen of proximal colon is maneuvers into position and married with the stapler. Before the stapler is closed and fired, the orientation of the proximal colon is verified to ensure it is not twisted.

Once formed, the integrity of the anastomosis is assessed either endoscopically or by insufflating air into the rectum whilst the anastomosis is submerged in water; the so-called 'air-leak test'. The 'donuts' formed by the cutting action of the device should also be checked for completeness and sent for histological analysis if this is required by local protocol.

Once the anastomosis is formed, it is important to consider whether it should be protected with a defunctioning stoma. The sequelae of anastomosis dehiscence can be devastating both in terms of morbidity and functional outcome. There is an association between proximity to the anal verge and leak rate and meta-analysis clearly demonstrates that a defunctioning stoma is effective in mitigating the clinical impact of a leak and reducing the need for reoperation. Various reviews conclude that defunctioning should be considered for all anastomoses within 5 cm or even 7 cm of the anus, but other relevant factors should also be considered, including comorbid status; particularly steroid use, immunosuppression, and the presence of diabetes, as well as whether the pelvis has been previously irradiated.

Abdominoperineal Resection

In recent years, the nature of surgery for RCs has evolved. Increasing use of adjuvant therapy has permitted ever lower ARs as the margin of oncological clearance considered 'safe' has narrowed. As a consequence, the comparative clinical outcome measures for patients undergoing low ARs and APEs have come under increasing scrutiny.

Importantly, a conventional APE has been shown to be associated with higher rates of CRM involvement and intraoperative perforation (IOP) which may impact significantly on oncological outcome. To some extent, this difference may be attributable to the normal anatomical tapering of the distal mesorectum, with smaller tissue volumes surrounding lower tumors, resulting in 'surgical wasting'; thereby increasing the risk of a positive CRM and/or IOP. A further factor may be the modest operative view that one may obtain during the conventional perineal phase of an APE in the supine position.

One solution to offset these tissues is to perform an 'Extra-levator' (or cylindrical) APE (ELAPE), which requires a wider resection including a cuff of levator muscle around the anorectal junction, without separating the levators from the rectum from above. This technique is rapidly gaining popularity as multicentre experience suggests it is associated with a reduced CRM involvement and IOP compared with standard surgery, with little impact a QoL or short-term outcomes.

Both conventional APE and ELAPE consist of 2 stages (abdominal and perineal). Conventional APE is performed with the patient in the lithotomy position permitting 2 surgeons to operate in tandem. The abdominal phase, described under the heading 'Colonic dissection', concludes with the formation of an end-colostomy in the LIF and closure of the abdomen. The perineal phase involves 'en-bloc' resection of the perianal soft tissue, anal sphincter complex, rectum, and intact mesorectum. In ELAPE, the abdominal phase is typically combined with a subsequent extended prone component to remove the rectum en bloc with the levator ani.

'Standard' APE

At the beginning of the perineal phase, the anus is closed with a purse string suture. An elliptical or shield-shaped incision is made extending from the perineal body anteriorly, to the tip of the coccyx posteriorly, and the ischial spines laterally. The cut skin edges are grasped with Allis tissue forceps or a Lone Star Retractor System™, to facilitate retraction as the incision is depended into the ischiorectal fossa bilaterally, staying outside of the external anal sphincter. Once the coccyx is exposed, the anococcygeal raphe is divided to permit access to the presacral space posteriorly. To deliver a large tumor from a narrow pelvis, it may be necessary to remove the coccyx in full or in part. This is achieved by incising the sacrococcygeal joint, which is held in flexion using forceps, whilst simultaneously lifting the rectum to protect it from injury (Fig. 65.13).

A finger is inserted into the presacral space to guide division of the coccygeal attachments laterally. The lateral dissection is deepened on to the levator muscles: Iliococcygeus is divided close to the lateral wall of the pelvis on both sides exposing the rectal fascia of Waldeyer, behind which lies the mesorectum. Once divided, the fascia of Waldeyer and the mesorectum are retracted forward, separating them from the presacral fascia and allowing the posterior abdominal and perineal resection planes to be joined.

The rectum is retracted posteriorly and the incision extended superiorly until the superficial and deep transverse fibers of transverses perinea are encountered. Importantly, the vagina penetrates the pelvic floor at this level and in men the urethra is close by. The anterior place of dissection must therefore, lie posterior to these muscles unless excision of the vaginal wall is planned for oncological reasons.

Once the aperture created by the posterolateral dissection is large enough, the proximal end of the divided rectum is delivered via the perineal defect, everting the specimen and facilitating anterior dissection. During the anterior dissection, the bladder, seminal vesicles, and prostate or uterus and vagina, are retraced upwards to avoid injury. The anterior

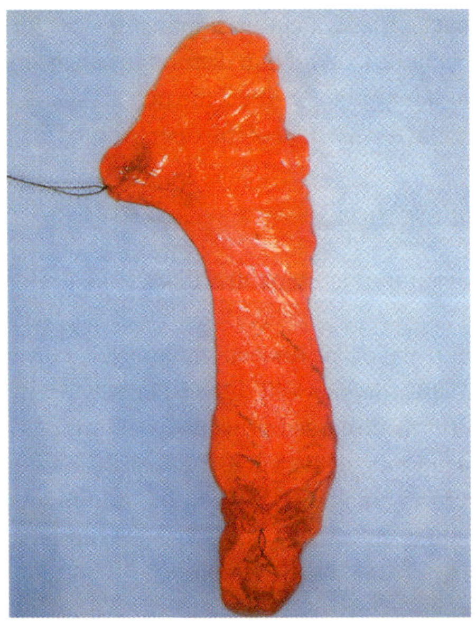

Fig. 65.13 Extra-levator APE resection specimen

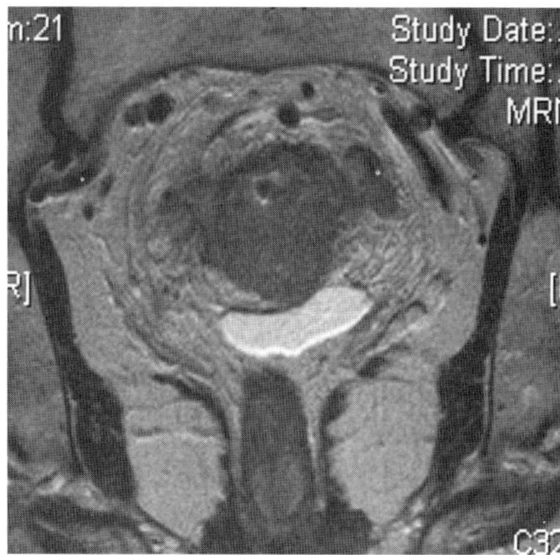

Fig. 65.14 Anterior dissection of rectum

dissection proceeds along the external sphincter and anterior rectal wall posterior to transverses perinea. The two limbs of pubococcygeus are encountered anterolaterally either side of the rectum as they loop behind to form a sling. The muscle and underlying fascia are divided as far laterally as possible leaving only tough fibromuscular attachments tethering the rectum in the anterior midline. Once these have been divided, the specimen can be delivered (Fig. 65.14).

Perineal closure is achieved in layers but in most cases the levator muscles will not approximate: Subcutaneous fat is brought along the length of the wound and the skin closed using vertical mattress sutures. Biological meshes may be used to reconstruct the perineal defect, however, there is little high quality data to support this approach. A suction drain may be brought out lateral to the wound, if required.

ELAPE

There are a number of key differences between ELAPE and the 'standard' surgical approach.

Firstly, during the abdominal phase of the operation, the TME is not extended to the pelvic floor. To prevent coning, the dissection terminates at the upper border of the coccyx posteriorly, the level of the seminal vesicles or cervix anteriroly, and just below the inferior hypogastric plexus anteriolaterally. Secondly, due to the larger perineal defect after ELAPE surgery and the risk of perineal herniation, the abdominal phase is typically combined with an omentoplasty where possible. After completion of the abdominal phase, the patient is usually turned to a prone jack-knifed position to facilitate visualization of anatomical structures during the perineal phase. During the perineal phase, a longitudinal tear-drop shaped incision is made around the anus. Unless the tumor is predicted to breach the levator complex or involve external anal sphincter (EAS) or ischiorectal fat, a skin and fat-sparing approach is adopted. The levator muscle is identified by following the plane lateral to the EAS, and dissection continued along its superficial border onto its origin on the pelvic side wall. The coccyx is disconnected from the sacrum and Waldeyers fascia divided to allow entry into the posterior pelvic cavity. The levator muscles are divided at their lateral attachments in a posterior to anterior direction. The specimen is delivered into the wound at an opportune moment, facilitating the remainder of the anterior dissection. Pelvic floor reconstruction is performed using a combination of biologic mesh and omentoplasty, and supplemented by retroverting the uterus in women. Alternative options reported for closing the larger perineal wound in ELAPE surgery include myocutaneous flap closure (gracilis, rectus abdominus and gluteal), and are particularly advantageous for cases where a perineal skin or ischiorectal fat-sparing approach cannot be approved. Nevertheless they add to the duration of the procedure, and carry the risk of longer bed rest, flap-related complications, and do not site morbidity.

Construction of Colostomy

The end colostomy is created before the perineal dissection begins unless the operation is being performed synchronously by 2 surgeons. A 2 cm circular cuff of skin is excised in a premarked position in the LIF. A cruciate incision is made in the anterior fascial sheath of rectus abdominus and the muscle fibers split to expose the posterior rectus sheath. A second incision through the posterior sheath and peritoneum allows access to the abdominal cavity. A Babcock forceps is introduced though the incision and draws the divided end of proximal colon through the abdominal wall, with care to avoid rotation or tension.

To mature the stoma, the colonic lumen is reopened by cutting immediately proximal to the linear staple line with diathermy or scissors. The mucosa should look pink and well perfused. The whole thickness of colon is sutured to the surrounding skin using 2.0 absorbable interrupted sutures.

Hartmann's Procedure

Hartmann's procedure, where the proximal colon is brought out as an end colostomy and the distal colonic remnant is closed over or brought out as a mucous fistula, is usually reserved for scenarios when reconstituting colonic integrity is unlikely to succeed due to sepsis, peritoneal contamination, or patient comorbidity. It may also be adopted in patients with high and mid-rectal tumors where for reasons of continence and function, it is undesirable to reconstitute intestinal continuity.

In the presence of obstruction, Hartmann's can often be avoided by decompressing the colon ahead of surgery with expanding metal stents, inserted under endoscopic and radiological guidance. This "bridging" technique can reduce the need for emergency intervention and improve conditions for primary anastomosis formation at a later date after appropriate staging and or bowel preparation. Surgical technique mirrors that described under the heading 'colonic dissection' however, in the acute setting, tissue planes are often profoundly corrupted by intra-abdominal contamination and particular care should be taken to avoid injury to other structures.

A midline laparotomy is performed with the patient in the supine position. The colon and rectum are mobilized and the IMA legated and divided as previously described. The colon is transected at a safe point beyond the distal margin of the tumor or otherwise corrupted colon using a linear cutter stapling device which simultaneously divides the rectum and closes the rectal stump. The rectal stump is left in-situ and the proximal colon brought out as an end colostomy. In the presence of gross intraperitoneal contamination liberal irrigation is essential and several large caliber drains should be left in-situ.

Closure of the Abdomen

Laparotomy wounds are closed using a mass closure technique incorporating all of the layers of the abdominal wall (except skin) as a single structure, in a simple running suture, using #1 or #2 absorbable monofilament sutures with a suture length to wound length ratio of 4 to 1. Skin is closed with a continuous absorbable #3 monofilament or clips.

During APE or Hartmann's procedure, the stoma is matured only once the abdomen is closed.

THE POSTOPERATIVE PERIOD

Enhanced Recovery

Enhanced recovery after surgery (ERAS) programs are designed to promote recovery and facilitate discharge following elective colorectal surgery by optimizing physiological function in the postoperative period. This is achieved by standardizing various aspects of perioperative care including preoperative patient education and preparation, analgesia and fluid balance, nutrition, bowel preparation, early mobility, and reduced use of drains, in a single integrated ERAS protocol.

ERAS programs benefit patients by reducing primary and overall hospital stay and may improve overall morbidity, however, they have not been shown to impact upon mortality or hospital readmission rates.

Postoperative Follow-up

It is standard practice to follow up patients after surgery for colorectal cancer with curative intent. Aims of follow up include the early detection of recurrent local and/or distant relapse which may be amenable to further surgery, or identification of metachronous disease. In addition, follow up also provides psychological support and facilitates clinical audit and quality assurance analysis. Nevertheless, the nature and optimal duration of follow up are not clearly defined.

To address this issue, a number of large scale randomized trials have been established. The UK FACS (Follow-up after colorectal surgery) trial, which is closed to recruitment but has not been reported, randomized patients with Duke's A, B and C tumors treated with curative intent into 4 groups:

Group 1 received a CT scan between 12 and 18 months following surgery and a colonoscopy after 5 years. Group 2 had a CEA blood test every 3 months for 2 years and then every 6 months for a further 3 years, a CT between 12 and 18 months following surgery and a colonoscopy after 5 years. Group 3 received a CT scan every 6 months for 2 years and then every year for a further 3 years and a colonoscopy at 2 and 5 years ad Group 4 had both scans (as for group 3) and blood tests (as for group 2).

The primary objective of the study is to compare the rate of treatable recurrences detected in each group. Secondary objectives are to assess whether the method of follow-up impacts on survival, quality of life, or cost per life-year saved.

Results are awaited and are likely to have a significant impact on further clinical practice.

CHAPTER

66

Operations for Rectal Prolapse

Dhiraj Choudhury

Prolapse of the rectum may be partial or mucosal prolapse or complete (Procedentia). Partial prolapse, particularly in children, may be successfully treated by conservative methods. Complete prolapse requires operative treatments. *The aim of operation for complete rectal prolapse should be to correct the prolapse avoiding fecal incontinence and constipation.* A number of operations have been introduced—some carried out through abdominal route while others through perineal route. This suggests that doubt still exists regarding the ideal choice. The anatomical defects observed with rectal prolapse include diastasis of the levator ani muscles, loss of adhesion to sacrum, coccyx and pelvic wall, an abnormally acute anorectal angle, patulous anal sphincters and redundant sigmoid colon with deep cul-de-sac. No single procedure had achieved reconstruction effectively of all the defects.

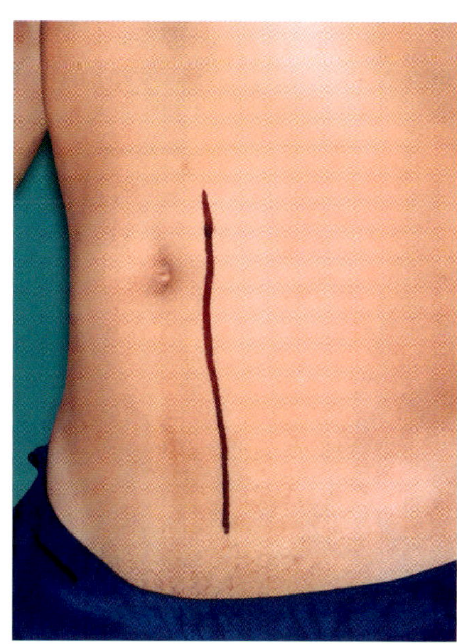

Fig. 66.1 Skin incision

ABDOMINAL PROCEDURES

Indication

Whenever the patient is fit, an abdominal rectopexy is the procedure of choice for complete rectal prolapse. The principle of the operation is to fix the rectum firmly to the sacrum by inserting polyvinyl alcohol sponge or prolene mesh between them.

Preoperative Preparation

- Full bowel preparation.
- Prophylactic antibiotic.

Operative Procedure: Wells Procedure: Rectal Fixation

This procedure is well-tolerated, even by elderly patients.

- *Position:* The patient lies supine with some Trendelenburg tilt.
- *Anesthesia:* General anesthesia with endotracheal tube. A Foley's catheter is introduced into bladder.
- *Incision:* Left paramedian or midline incision is preferred (Fig. 66.1).
- *Exposure:* Full laparotomy is performed. The small bowels are pushed into upper abdomen.

Mobilization of Sigmoid Colon and Rectum

The sigmoid colon is freed of any attachment. Then the left leaf of the peritoneum (congenital white line) is incised and gonadal vessels and left ureter are pushed laterally (Fig. 66.2).

The right leaf of the pelvic mesocolon is now incised from a point just below the superior hemorrhoidal artery, keeping close to the sigmoid colon and rectum.

The two peritoneal incisions on two sides are extended downwards and joined together in front of the rectum at the

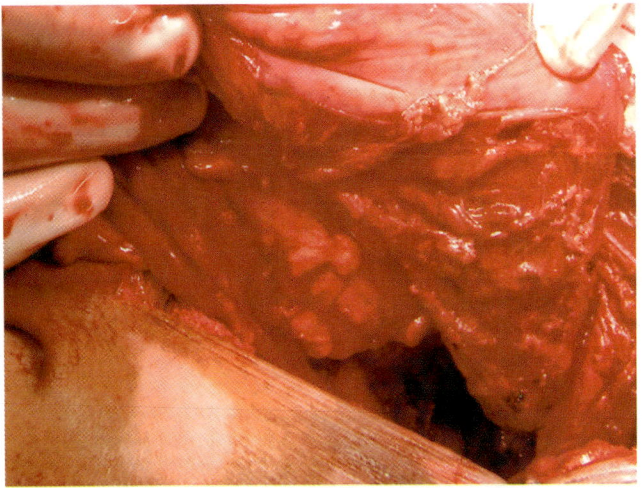
Fig. 66.2 Mobilization of sigmoid colon and rectum

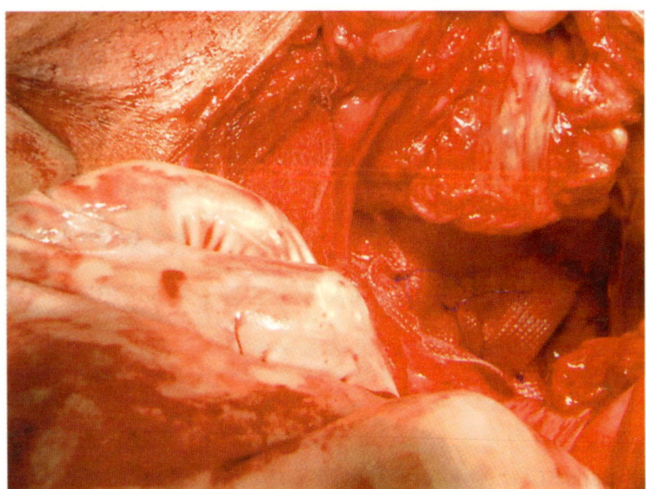
Fig. 66.3B Fixation of mesh to presacral fascia

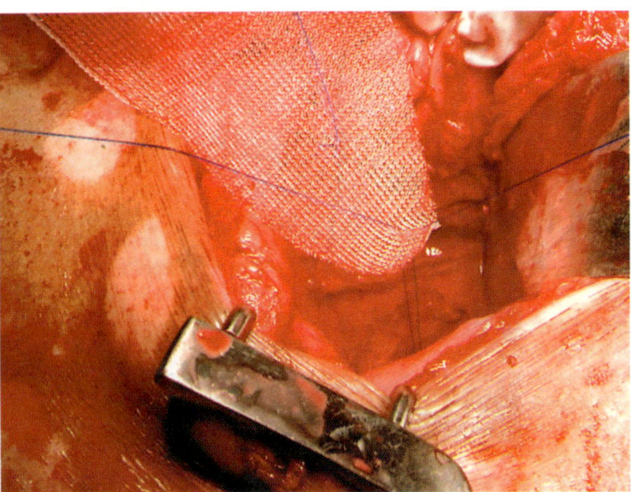
Fig. 66.3A Placement of mesh

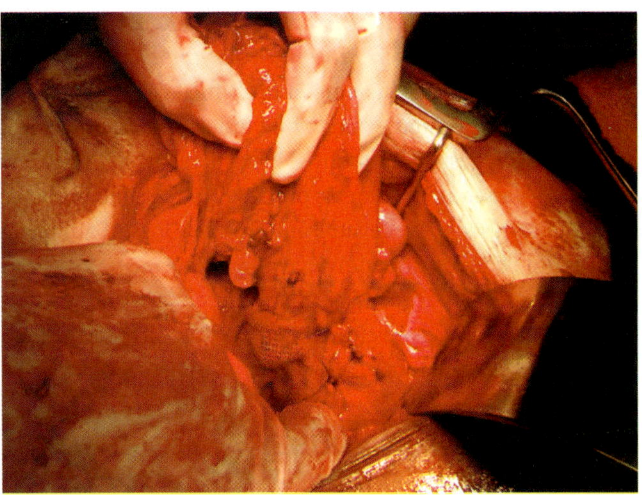
Fig. 66.4 Fixation of mesh to rectal wall

bottom of the rectovesical or rectouterine pouch. The presacral space is opened.

The rectum is mobilized posteriorly by blunt finger dissection as low as sacrococcygeal joint and lifted up. Mobilization of the rectum in the mesorectal plane is carried down to pelvic floor. The lateral ligaments are not divided. Anteriorly, the plane between posterior vaginal wall and the rectum is opened in females.

Rectopexy

Once the sigmoid colon and the rectum have been mobilized, a sheet of prolene mesh (about 5 cm wide and 12 to 15 cm length) is placed in front of the sacrum and is fixed by series of 2/0 proline sutures to the presacral fascia (Figs 66.3A and B), avoiding injury to middle sacral vessels.

The mesh is then wrapped around the lateral sides of the mobilized rectum, leaving 1/3rd of the anterior circumference of the rectal wall uncovered. The free margins of the mesh are now sutured to the margin of the anterior wall by 2/0 proline sutures (Fig. 66.4). The pelvic peritoneum is then sutured.

Ripstein Procedure

The rectum is first thoroughly mobilized by dividing the lateral peritoneal reflexions and lifted up. Holding the rectum taught upwards a sling of Teflon mesh (5 cm wide) is passed round it and its ends are sutured to the fascia and periosteum on the front of the sacrum 5 cm below sacral promontory. This operation is simple; safe and effective, and is one of the commonly used rectal fixation operations in USA (Fig. 66.5).

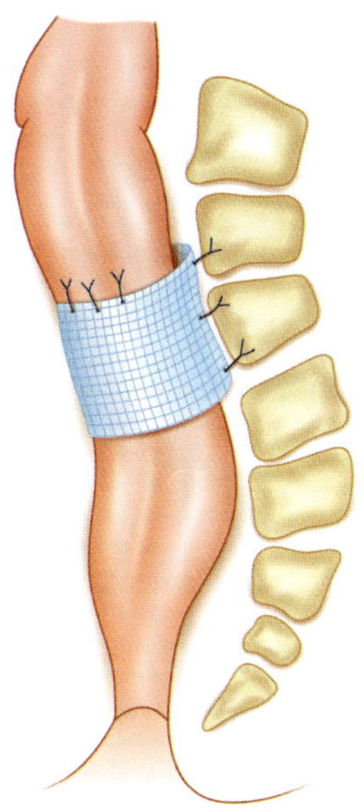

Fig. 66.5 Ripstein procedure

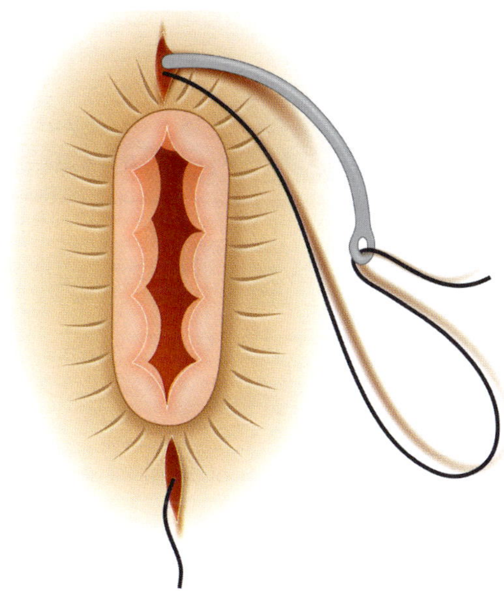

Fig. 66.6 Application of suture

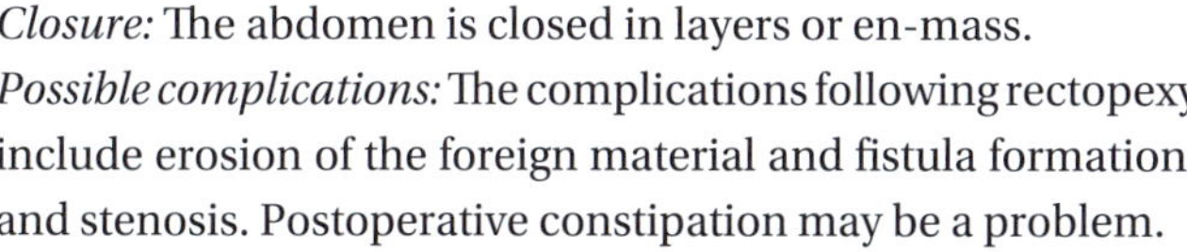

Closure: The abdomen is closed in layers or en-mass.

Possible complications: The complications following rectopexy include erosion of the foreign material and fistula formation, and stenosis. Postoperative constipation may be a problem.

Anterior resection has also been applied in the treatment of rectal prolapse. The principle in this procedure is the creation of fibrosis between the anastomosis and the sacrum. A major disadvantage of this procedure includes a possible decrease in continence secondary to decrease in rectal reservoir. There is also the problem associated with anastomosis.

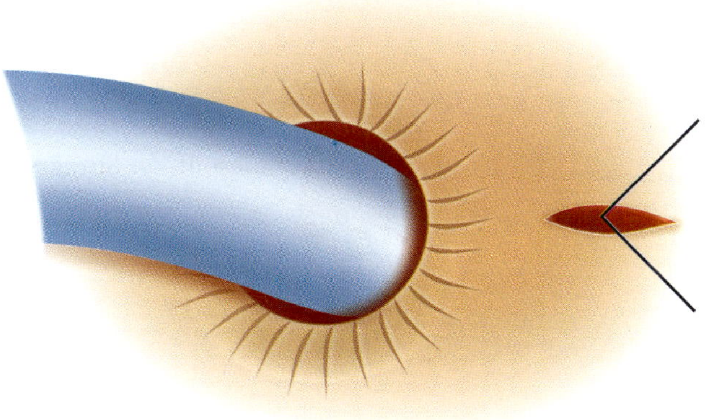

Fig. 66.7 Tightening of suture

PERINEAL PROCEDURES

Thiersch Operation

It was used for elderly frail patients as it involves a minimal degree of surgical trauma and can be done under local anesthesia. But, it does not cure the prolapse and hence not ideal for fit patient.

Procedure

- *Anesthesia:* It can be done under local anesthesia.
- *Position:* Lithotomy.

Technique

Thiersh originally used wire to tighten the anal orifice but the wire eventually breaks. Subsequently nylon and proline are used as suture material. A small incision is made 1 inch behind the anus and a long curved needle fitted with 1 proline is passed round 1/2 of the anus emerging through skin in front of anus through a small incision there also. The needle is withdrawn and reinserted through the same wound and passed round the opposite side of the anus to emerge through the same opening in front of the anus (Fig. 66.6).

The index finger of the surgeon is introduced through the anus and the assistant is asked to tighten the knot (Fig. 66.7).

Delorme's Procedure

This is the best perineal procedure, which has been successfully used in elderly patients.

- *Anesthesia:* General or spinal.
- *Position:* Lithotomy.

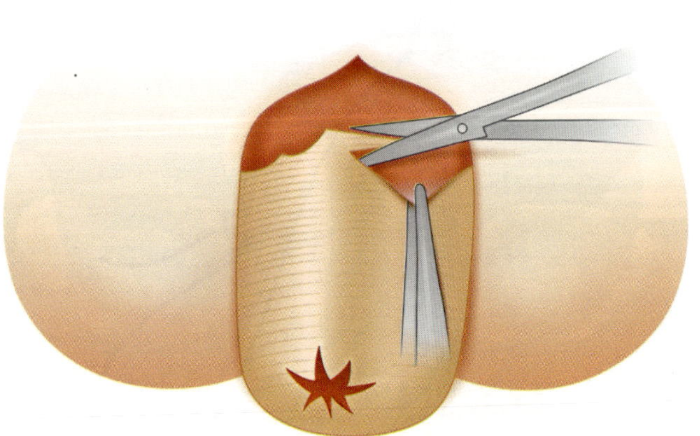
Fig. 66.8A Application of circular incision

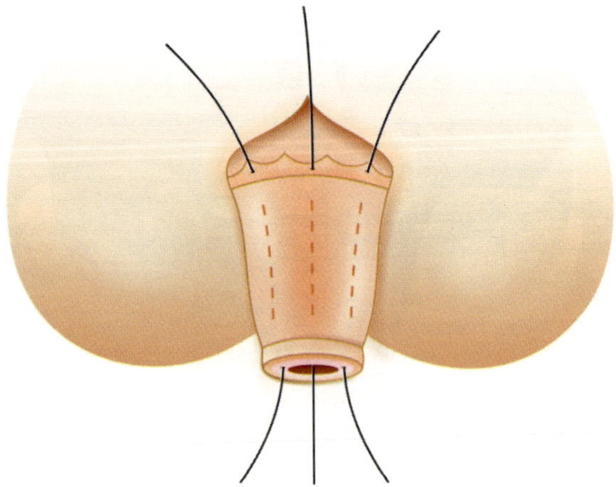
Fig. 66.8C Plication of muscles

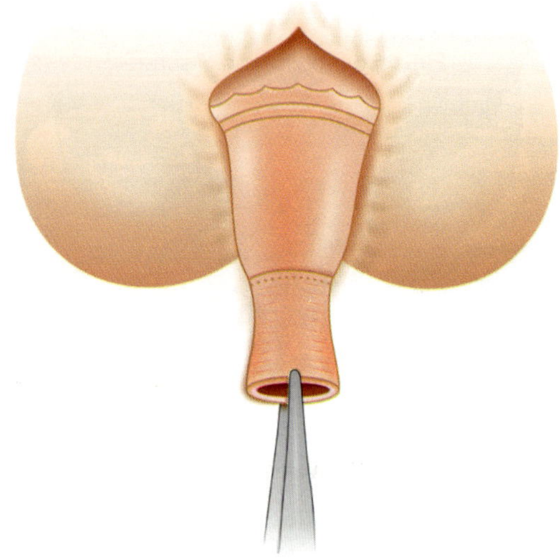
Fig. 66.8B Stripping of mucosa

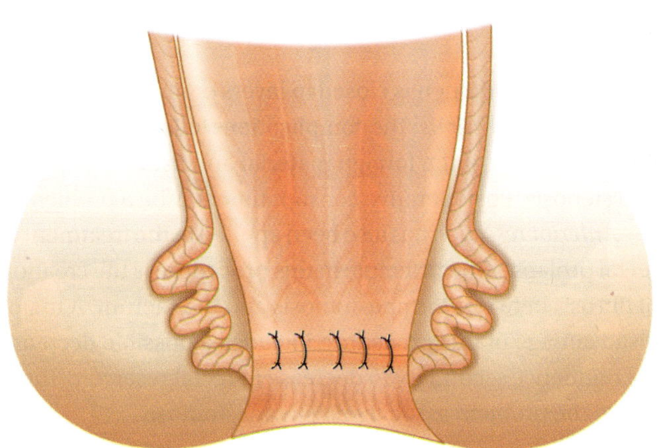
Fig. 66.8D Coloanal anastomosis

Technique

With the bowel fully prolapsed, a circular incision is made through the mucosa 1-2 cm from dentate line (Fig. 66.8A). The mucosa is then stripped circumferentially from the muscle coat as a sleeve (Fig. 66.8B). A length of 10-12 cm of the mucosa can be removed. The underlying muscle is plicated with 2/0 vicryl sutures (Fig. 66.8C). Then a coloanal anastomosis is carried out (Fig. 66.8D), by absorbable sutures.

POSTOPERATIVE CARE

- Intravenous fluids are given till flatus is passed.
- Systemic antibiotic.
- Laxative is given orally.

POSTOPERATIVE COMPLICATIONS

- Sepsis
- Fecal impaction
- Recurrence of prolapse.

Recent advances: The use of laparoscopic technique in the surgical treatment of rectal prolapse has several attractive features. Mobilization of rectum laparoscopically has been shown to be safe and feasible. Long-term results need to be assessed before widespread use.

SECTION

14

Anal and Perianal

CHAPTER

67

Treatments of Hemorrhoids

Dhiraj Choudhury

SURGERY FOR HEMORRHOIDS

Hemorrhoids are enlarged, displaced anal cushions. They may be primary (genetically determined) or secondary (may be due to gravid uterus, pelvic tumor).

Primary hemorrhoids are usually located at 3, 7 and 11 o'clock positions in lithotomy position. They are traditionally classified into four degrees, First degree hemorrhoids cause painless bleeding during defecation. Second degree hemorrhoids prolapse through anal canal at the time of defecation but are reduced spontaneously. Third degree hemorrhoids protrude during defecation and require manual reduction. Fourth degree hemorrhoids remain permanently prolapsed.

Treatment

First and second degree hemorrhoids can be treated by conservative measures such as change of defecating habit, use of stool softener. Active methods include injection, banding, infrared coagulation or combination of methods.

Injection of phenol in almond oil acts by causing submucosal fibrosis which shrinks and anchors anal cushion to normal position.

Barons banding is effective for more bulky second degree piles. The Barons bander is used to apply tight elastic bands onto the base of the pedicle of each hemorrhoid. The band causes ischemic necrosis of piles by 7 days.

Cryotherapy (Lloyd Williams) freeze tissue causing thrombosis of submucosal veins by application of liquid nitrogen or nitrous oxide.

Photocoagulation delivers energy in the form of light applied through a quartz obturator.

Third and *fourth* degree hemorrhoids require hemorrhoidectomy.

HEMORRHOIDECTOMY—OPEN METHOD/ MILLIGAN MORGAN METHOD

Indications

- Surgery offers the best chance of permanent cure of hemorrhoid particularly third degree and fourth degree.
- Failure of nonoperative treatment of second degree hemorrhoid is also an indication for hemorrhoidectomy.
- Fibrosed hemorrhoid
- Interno-external hemorrhoids.

Preoperative Preparations

- Bowel preparation with laxative is sufficient. Enema or bowel wash is not necessary.
- Metronidazole 400 mg orally thrice daily may be given.
- Shaving is not necessary.

Contraindications

- In presence of inflammatory bowel disease
- Intestinal tuberculosis.

Operative Procedure

- *Position:* Lithotomy, with buttocks lifted over the edge of table.
- *Anesthesia:* General endotracheal or spinal. But hemorrhoidectomy can also be done with sedation and local anesthesia. Locally, on 1% xylocaine with 1 in 20,000 adrenaline is injected subcutaneously into the piles.
- *Procedure:* Confirm the positions of the piles by proctoscopic examination. Mild anal stretching is done.

- *Triangle of exposure*: Apply a curved artery forceps to the perianal skin just outside the mucocutaneous junction at 3, 7, and 11 o'clock positions, opposite the primary pile groups and gently pull outwards. As a result, the mucosa covered part of the piles protrude out. Now apply a second artery forceps individually to the hemorrhoidal tissue of the three main piles which are drawn downwards to produce triangle of exposure of Milligan (Fig. 67.1).
- *Ligation and excision:* The left lateral pile or largest pile is dealt first. With a blunt pointed scissors, a V-shaped cut is made around the pile on mucocutaneous junction (Fig. 67.2).

  The hemorrhoidal mass is dissected with scissors from the transverse fibers of the internal sphincter. The dissection is continued just beyond the dentate line. The pedicle is transfixed doubly at the apex with silk and catgut which are cut long and held by hemostat.

  The pile tissue is excised distal to the ligature with scalpel (Fig. 67.3).

  The procedure is repeated for the remaining major piles. Any bleeding from the perianal skin or submucosal veins secured by diathermy.

  The three major hemorrhoidal group are excised, mucosal and skin bridges must be preserved. When the operation has been completed, the wound will present a '*tri-foil*' *appearance* (Fig. 67.4).
- *Dealing with additional hemorrhoids:* Additional hemorrhoids can be removed by filtering it out by undermining the skin bridge or by dividing the skin bridges, removing the underlying veins and stitching the trimmed flap back into position by suturing with 3/0 catgut.
- *Dressing:* A large pad of roller gauze smeared with betadine lotion and xylocaine jelly is applied to the anus and secured with a T-bandage (Fig. 67.5).
- *Recurrent hemorrhoids* are usually treated by injection.

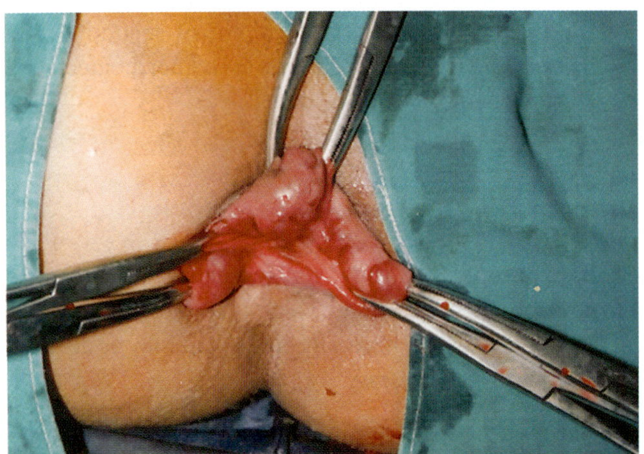

Fig. 67.1 Exposure of hemorrhoids and application of artery forceps

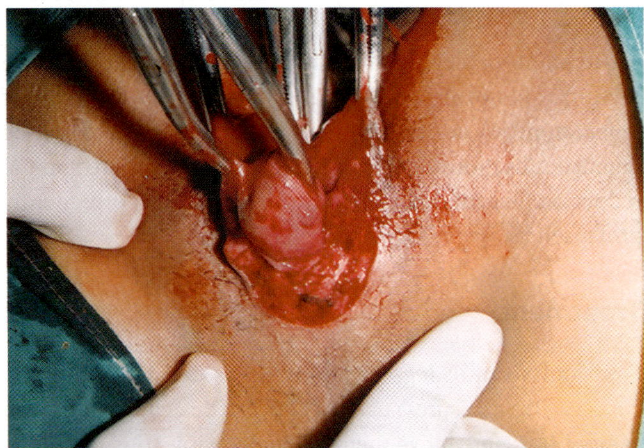

Fig. 67.2 Ligation and excision of piles

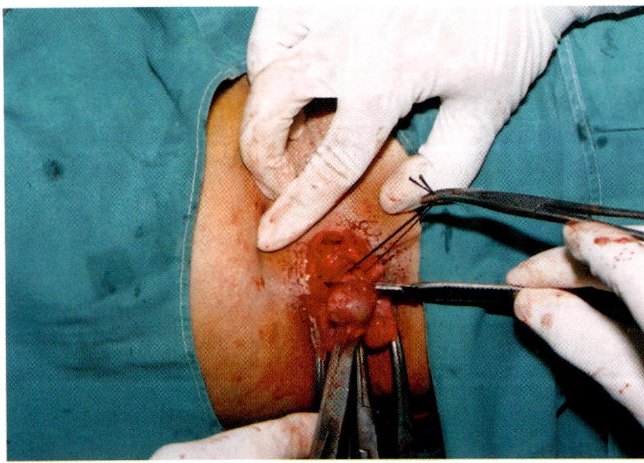

Fig. 67.3 Ligation and excision of piles

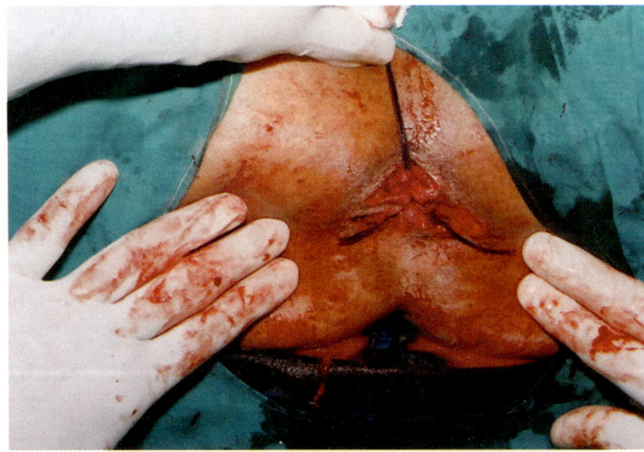

Fig. 67.4 Posthemorrhoidectomy. Tri-foil appearance

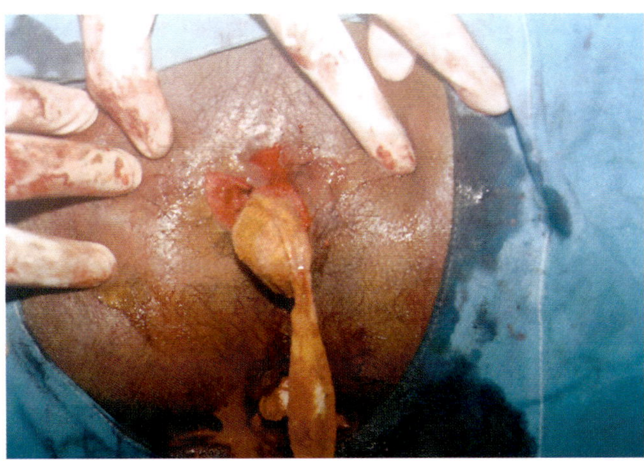

Fig. 67.5 Application of roller gauze

Postoperative Care

- The dressing is changed after 24 hours and the patient is put into sitz bath twice daily. Some topical preparation is applied each time after sitz bath and T-bandage is re-applied.
- Analgesic and stool softener are advised in postoperative period.
- The patient can be discharged after 4–5 days.

Postoperative Complications

- Reactionary hemorrhage should be avoided by transfixing pedicle twice. In case of serious bleeding, re-exploration and further transfixation may be necessary.
- Secondary hemorrhage should be treated by blood transfusion and antibiotic. In most cases the bleeding stops.
- *Retention of urine:* The condition usually responds to simple measure like adequate privacy, analgesic and removal of pack. Catheterization may be necessary in elderly patients.
- *Anal stenosis:* This can be treated by anal dilator. Sometimes anal stretching under anesthesia may be necessary.

MINIMALLY INVASIVE PROCEDURE FOR HEMORRHOIDS

Minimally invasive procedure for hemorrhoids (MIPH) is a short procedure that offers:

- Reduced pain
- Shorter hospital stay
- Reduced blood loss
- Faster return to normal activity.

Surgical kit required for the procedure consists of:

- Purse-string suture anoscope
- Circular anal dilator
- Purse-string suture threader
- Hemorrhoidal circular stapler.

Procedure

Anesthesia: Spinal or general
Position: Lithotomy.

Steps

- The purse-string suture is applied several centimeters above the dentate line.
- The anvil of the fully opened stapling gun is inserted endoanally so that it is above the purse-string suture.
- The purse-string suture is now tied around the shaft of the gun.
- The gun is closed and fired.
- After firing, a 3–4 cm strip of mucosa and submucosa containing the hemorrhoid is excised and the mucosal edges are simultaneously stapled together.

CHAPTER

68

Surgical Procedures for Anal Fissure

Dhiraj Choudhury

An anal fissure is a longitudinal split in the anoderm of the distal anal canal, close to midline. In man, 95% are close to posterior midline, while in women, 80% are close to posterior midline. Most anal fissure heal spontaneously and only require some stool softener and sitz bath locally. Surgical intervention is indicated if there is failure of conservative treatment in acute anal fissure deep chronic fissure associated with sentinel tag also requires operative treatment.

ANAL STRETCHING

- *Position:* Lithotomy
- *Anesthesia:* General endotracheal or spinal. Muscle relaxation is desirable.

Procedure

'Four-finger' anal stretch of the internal sphincter is carried out slowly and gently. Well-lubricated index fingers are initially inserted in the anus one by one and internal sphincter is dilated laterally (Fig. 68.1A). Subsequently, four-finger dilation is carried out (Fig. 68.1B). The stretching is maintained for 2–3 minutes.

Postoperative Care

- Prescribe stool softener.
- Application of anesthetic ointment after sitz bath.

Result: Achieves healing in up to 90% of patients, though it may be associated with minor incontinence in up to 50% of patients. The risk of incontinence has made it unpopular.

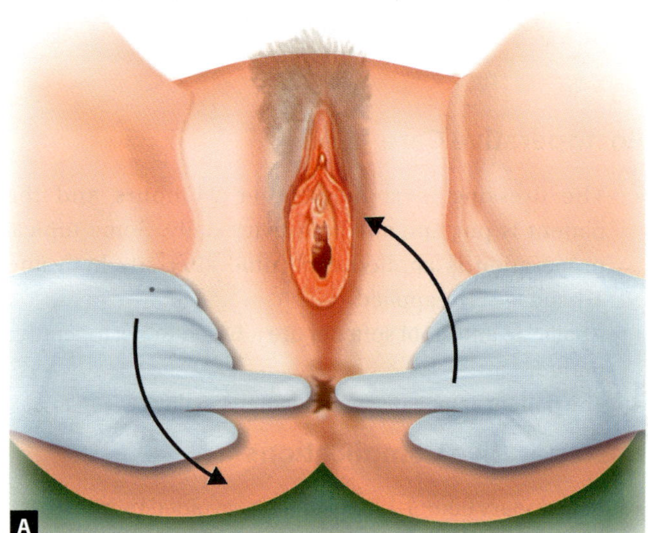

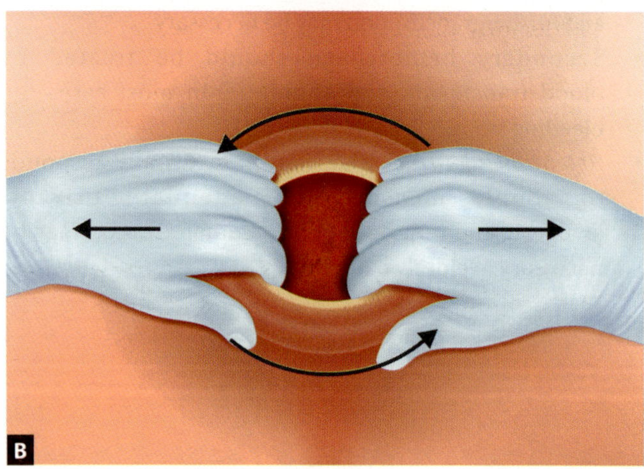

Figs 68.1A and B Anal stretching

LATERAL INTERNAL SPHINCTEROTOMY

It divides the lower two-thirds of the internal sphincter. About 98% of the fissures heal following sphincterotomy. In this procedure, the internal sphincter is divided away from the fissure either in the right or left lateral positions.

Operative Procedure: Open Method

- *Position:* Lithotomy.
- *Anesthesia:* General endotracheal or spinal.

Technique

The perineum is prepared and draped. Examine anorectal region under anesthesia. A bivalve anal speculum is introduced into anal cavity and gently opened.

Palpate the internal sphincter.

A transverse incision is made into the perianal skin 5 mm lateral to the groove on one side. Hold the upper end of the incision with tissue forceps and separate the anoderm with hamostat from the internal sphincter by blunt dissection (Figs 68.2 and 68.3).

The exposed internal sphincter (recognized by white fibers) is then picked up with tissue forceps and divided by narrow scalpel blade (Figs 68.4 and 68.5).

Closure

The wound may be closed with interrupted absorbable sutures. A lubricated roller gauze pack is left in anal canal and secure it with T-bandage.

Result: Low recurrence rate about 30% incontinence particularly in women who have weaker, shorter sphincter complex.

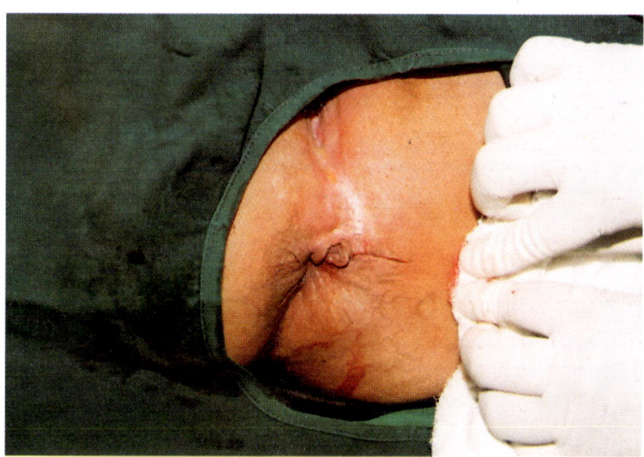

Fig. 68.2 Transverse incision

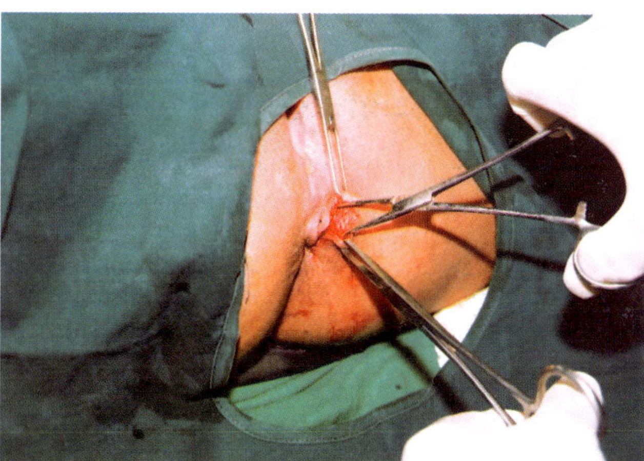

Fig. 68.3 Exposure of sphincter

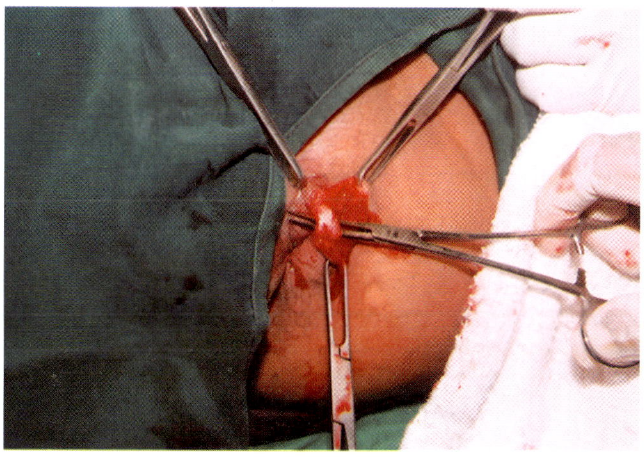

Fig. 68.4 Identification of sphincter

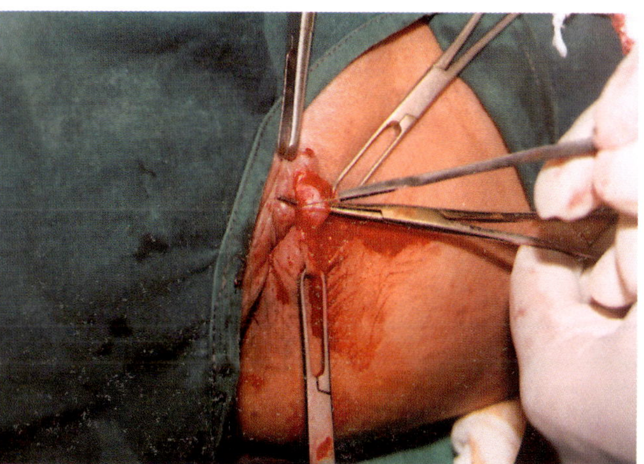

Fig. 68.5 Division of sphincter

CLOSED LATERAL INTERNAL SPHINCTEROTOMY

A subcutaneous closed sphincterotomy may be done using a narrow-bladed knife inserted through a skin puncture into the inter-sphincteric groove. A finger is placed in the anal canal to feel the fibers as they are cut. A bivalve speculum is introduced in such a way that the blades are positioned anteriorly and posteriorly. The von Graefe's cataract knife is introduced through the perineal skin vertically upwards up to pectinate line. A knife is then rotated and the internal sphincter is cut with gentle stroke.

Fissurectomy with Dorsal Sphincterotomy

Resistant and recurrent cases can be treated by dorsal sphincterotomy with fissurectomy. A traingular skin is excised around the anus. This exposes the lower third of the internal sphincter which is then divided under direct vision. This can produce a key hole deformity and hence not applied nowadays.

Postoperative Care

- Sitz bath and application of ointment.
- Prescribe analgesic and stool softener.

CHAPTER

69

Incision and Drainage of Anorectal Abscess

Dhiraj Choudhury

More than 95% of all anorectal abscess result from infection in anal glands that communicate with anal crypts. Anorectal abscess may be perianal, ischiorectal and submucous of which perianal abscess is most common. Ischiorectal is next common one.

OPERATIVE PROCEDURE: INCISION AND DRAINAGE

Perianal and Ischiorectal Abscess

- *Position:* Lithotomy.
- *Anesthesia:* General endotracheal or spinal, but perianal abscess and some ischiorectal (anal) abscess can be drained under local anesthesia.

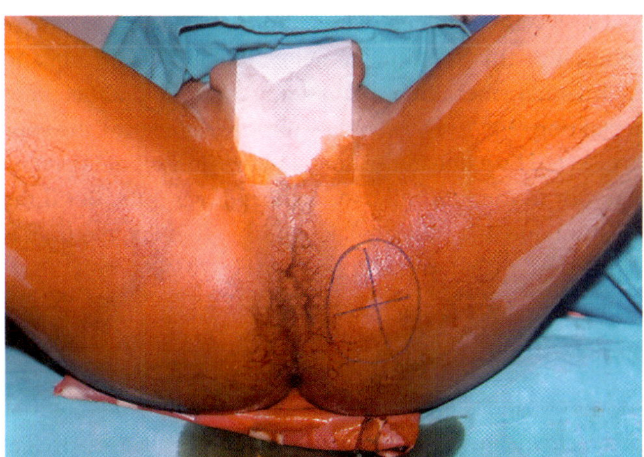

Fig. 69.1 Slowing cruciate incision

Technique

An assessment of the abscess by careful examination is carried out. Now, open the abscess at the most fluctuant part by a cruciate incision or single incision (Fig. 69.1).

Pus is allowed to escape and a sample is sent for culture and sensitivity test. Explore the abscess cavity with finger and break the loculi. The incision may require extension depending on the direction of the abscess. To ensure continued drainage, some overlying skin may require removal. The supralevator abscess can be difficult to diagnose and treat; fortunately, it is rare.

In horse-shoe abscess, pus tracks circumferentially around the anus. Drainage of pus from both ischiorectal (anal) fossae by separate incisions is required.

- *Packing:* The wound is packed loosely with roller gauze soaked in povidone iodine. A firm pressure dressing is applied and maintained by T-bandage.
- *Submucous abscess*: It can be diagnosed by examination under bivalve speculum and drained by incision.
- *Pelvirectal abscess:* These are usually pelvic abscess and treated accordingly.
- *Primary fistulotomy:* There are several arguments against fistulotomy at the time of abscess drainage. Between one-third and two-thirds of patients was present for the first time with anorectal abscess will not develop a fistula. Hence, fistulotomy in these patients will be unnecessary Moreover, in more than one-half of the patients, internal opening cannot be found at the time of abscess drainage.

POSTOPERATIVE CARE

- Systemic antibiotic should be given.
- Analgesic.
- The dressing is changed and re-dressed, after sitz bath.
- Bowel movement is allowed from 3rd day. Some stool softener is given.

POSTOPERATIVE COMPLICATIONS

- Persistent fistula will require fistulectomy. The wound should be examined after infection has subsided for fistulous opening and treated accordingly.

CHAPTER

70

Operation for Fistula in Ano

Dhiraj Choudhury

Fistula in ano has been classified into low fistula, where internal opening is situated below the anorectal ring; and high fistula where internal opening is situated above ano-rectal ring (Fig. 70.1). According to Goodsall's law, if the anus is bisected by a line in the frontal plane, an external opening anterior to the line will have a short direct tract. But if the external opening is located posterior to the line, the tract is curved and may be horse-shoe type (Fig. 70.2).

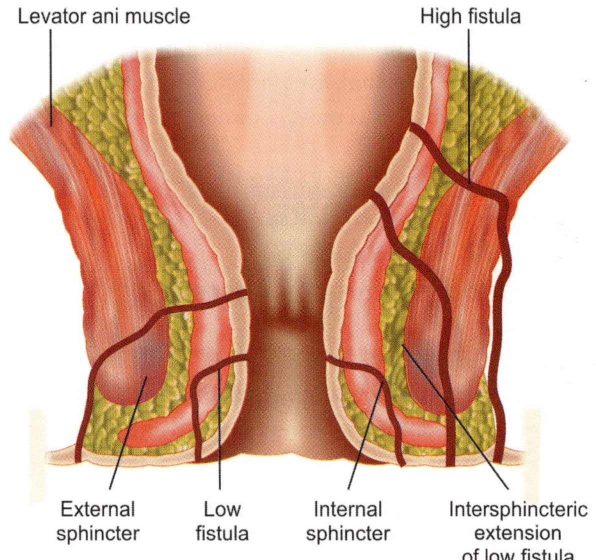

Fig. 70.1 Types of fistula in ano

LOW FISTULA

Most low fistulae may be adequately treated by *fistulotomy* or *fistulectomy*. Fustulectomy has two disadvantages. Surgical wounds are larger and time for wound healing is significantly prolonged. But recurrence rate is similar in both types of operations.

Preoperative Preparations

- A fistulogram or MR scanning may be helpful to define the fistulous tract. It may be helpful in evaluation of recurrent fistula.
- A proper bowel-wash is desirable to empty anorectal region.

Operative Procedure and Technique

- *Position:* Lithotomy.
- *Anesthesia:* General endotracheal or spinal.

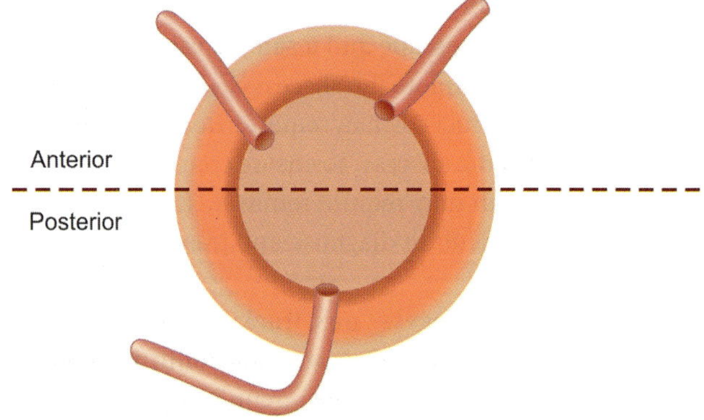

Fig. 70.2 Goodsall's rule

Procedure

Identify the internal opening as a localized area of induration commonly in midline posteriorly through a proctoscope. Now insert a probe pointed director through the external opening along the tract until it emerges through the internal opening. The director should never be passed forcefully through the tissues (Fig. 70.3).

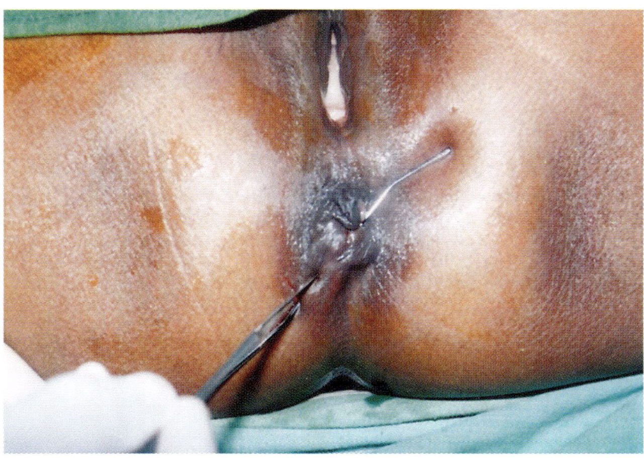

Fig. 70.3 Introduction of probe

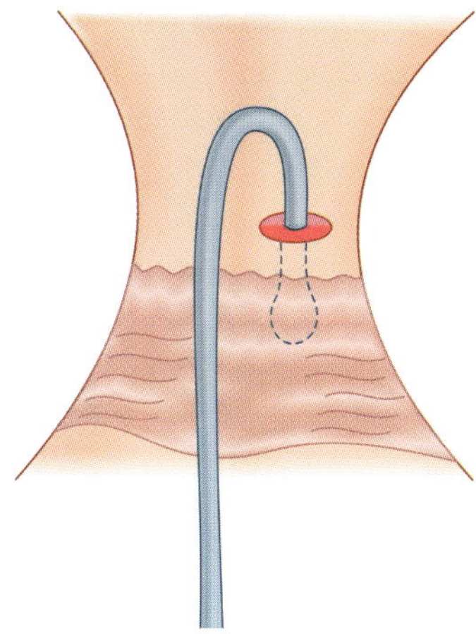

Fig. 70.4 Retrograde probing

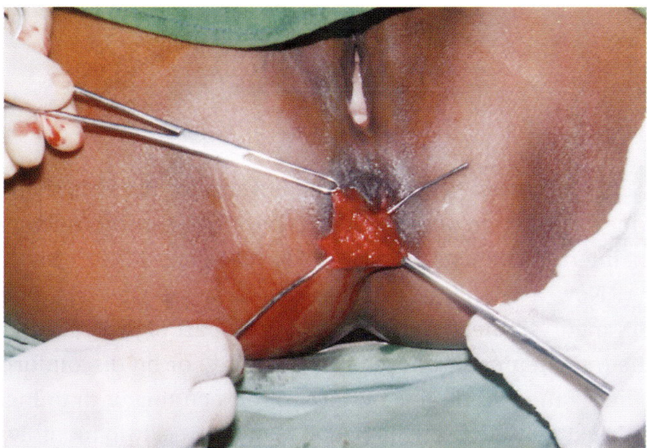

Fig. 70.5 Fistulotomy

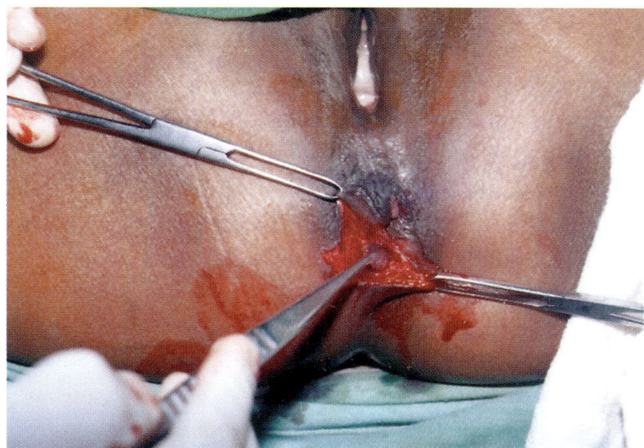

Fig. 70.6 Curettage

Technique

If the internal opening cannot be seen, retrograde probing through a crypt can be attempted (Fig. 70.4).

Fistulotomy: The track is laid open by cutting all the tissues between the director and skin surface. Divide all those structures lying between external and internal openings (Fig. 70.5). Curette the granulation tissue lining the track and send the materials for histopathology. The margins of the tract are trimmed. A search should be made for any other tract passing from the (secondary tract) main wall. If present, it is also laid open (Fig. 70.6). Primary fistula may be adequately treated by fistulotomy.

It provides better anatomical definition of fistular anatomy, but has longer healing time than fistulotomy.

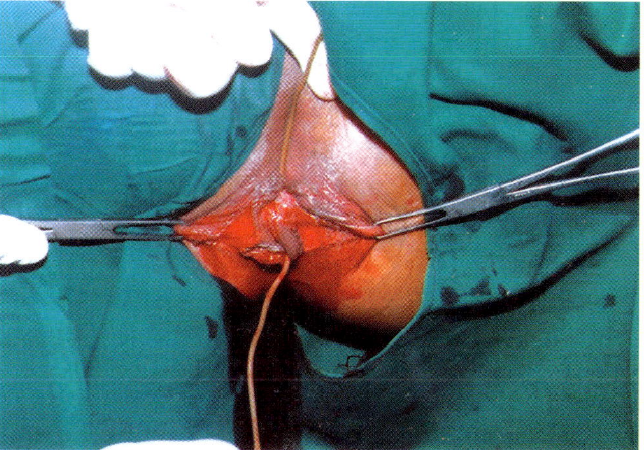

Fig. 70.7 Introduction of probe

Fistulectomy: Introduce a malleable probe gently through the external opening of the fistula and allow the probe to emerge through internal opening into anal canal, as in case of fistulotomy (Fig. 70.7).

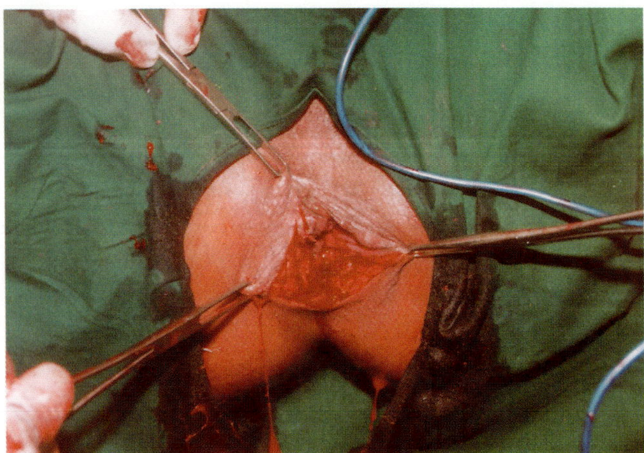

Fig. 70.8 Fistulectomy

Thus the entire tract may be defined. Now excise the subcutaneous tract with some internal sphincter. The wound is usually pyriform or traingular in shape with its broader part externally (Fig. 70.8). Fistulectomy wounds are larger and time for wound healing is significantly prolonged. Moreover, incontinence to flatus is more. Fistulectomy provides histologic material.

Trim the margins with scissors to leave a shallow conical area with its apex entering the anal canal.

Closure

The wound is packed with roller gauze soaked in povidone iodine to allow healing by secondary intention under supervision. This is the widely accepted method.

Alternative methods

- Primary suture has been advocated after fistulectomy but has not been widely accepted.
- Primary split skin graft has also been practiced by some surgeons.

Operative Procedure for Horse-Shoe Fistula

The short posterior portion of the tract is unroofed and involved crypt is excised. The anterior portions are curetted and drained through secondary incisions along the tracts.

HIGH FISTULA

These are fistulae in which the internal opening is situated above the ano-rectal ring. Operative interventions in these varieties may cause damage to the sphincter resulting in incontinence.

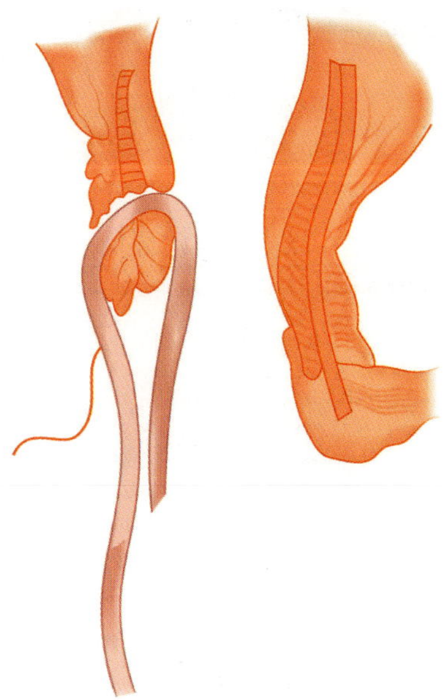

Fig. 70.9 Application of stout silk

Seton placement technique: The lower part of the fistulous tract is laid open or excised with division of superficial fibers of internal sphincter as in case of low fistula.

Now, a seton (ligature of stout silk) is passed on a probe or aneurysm needle through the deep part of the tract and tied, tightening of the seton causes little or no discomfort. The seton takes on one of the two roles cutting or draining. The cutting seton is tightened at regular (weekly to monthly) intervals to slowly cut through the sphincter allowing the track to become more and more superficial while scar tissue prevents significant separation of sphincter muscle. The drainage seton is left loosely in place to prevent the track or cavity from closing (Fig. 70.9).

Endorectal Advancement Flap Repair

Anterior midline anal fistula are better treated by endorectal advancement flap repair because fistulotomy may be associated with increased risk of anal incontinence particularly in the women. It aims to preserve both anatomy and function.

A mucomuscular flap with its base pointing proximally is raised. The apex of this flap should extend approximately 1 cm below the internal opening. The base of the flap should be approximately twice as wide as the width of the flap. The internal opening in the muscle should be closed with absorbable sutures after debridement of the fistula. The tip of the flap containing the internal fistulous opening is excised, and the flap is sewn down over the internal opening with absorbable sutures, so muscular repair and mucosal repair do not overlap.

Postoperative Care

- Sitz bath and dressing daily.
- Stool softener at night.
- Systemic antibiotic.
- Careful wound dressing.

Postoperative Complications

- Sepsis.
- Recurrence.

- *By additional methods:* Application of the glues, attempts are being made to plug and seal the tract (once lining granulation tissue has been removed) and allow ingrowth of healthy tissue by application of fibrin glue. Long-term result is still not encouraging.
- *Video-assisted anal fistula treatment (VAFT):* This is a new, radical approach to treatment of fistula in ano. The fistula tract is entered with a small 3 mm endoscope. The fistula is cleansed and the lining of the tract is cauterized. The internal opening is closed per rectum with a stapler.

SECTION

15

Hernias

- **Operation for Epigastric Hernia**
  Dhiraj Choudhury
- **Operation for Umbilical Hernia in Infants and Children**
  Dhiraj Choudhury
- **Operation for Adult Umbilical Hernia or Paraumbilical Hernia**
  Dhiraj Choudhury
- **Operation for Incisional Hernia: Open Method**
  Dhiraj Choudhury
- **Operation for Inguinal (Groin) Hernias: Open Method**
  Dhiraj Choudhury
- **Operations for Femoral Hernia**
  Dhiraj Choudhury
- **Inguinal Hernia: Laparoscopic Repair**
  C Palanivelu

CHAPTER

71

Operation for Epigastric Hernia

Dhiraj Choudhury

Epigastric hernia is a midline hernia through a defect in the linea above the umbilicus.

INDICATION

Large ones and symptomatic ones should be operated.

OPERATIVE PROCEDURE

- *Position:* The patient is placed on supine position.
- *Anesthesia:* General anesthesia with endotracheal intubation is preferred but the operation can be done under local anesthesia.
- *Incision:* A small transverse incision over the bulge gives the best cosmetic result (Fig. 71.1).
- *Exposure:* Deepen the incision to expose the herniated fat (Fatty hernia) or sac (Fig. 71.2).
- *Dealing with sac:* An empty sac can be returned to the abdomen, but if the sac has content, it should be opened. If the content is omentum it can be excised with sac. The sac is ligated at the neck and excised (Fig. 71.3).
- *Repair:* The defect in the linea alba can be closed with few interrupted sutures using 1/0 proline, taking (Fig. 71.4) generous bites of edges (anatomical repair). Mayo's repair by overlapping is also being done, if the defect is large.
- *Closure:* The skin is closed by interrupted 2/0 ethilon stitches.

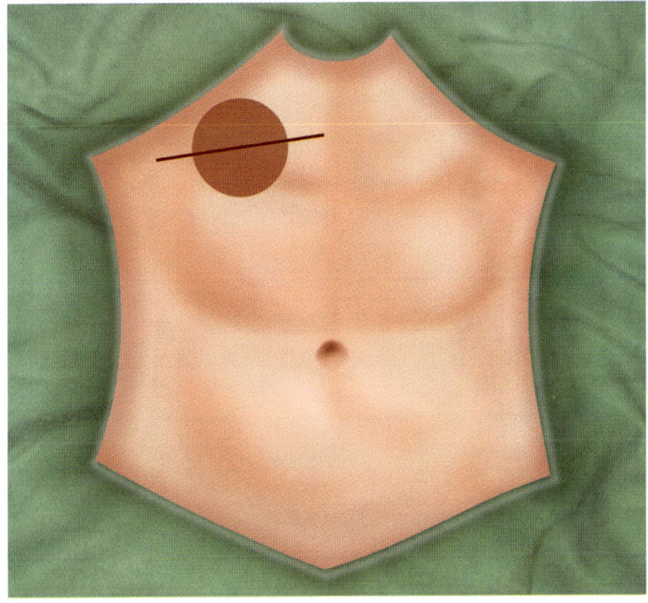

Fig. 71.1 Skin incision

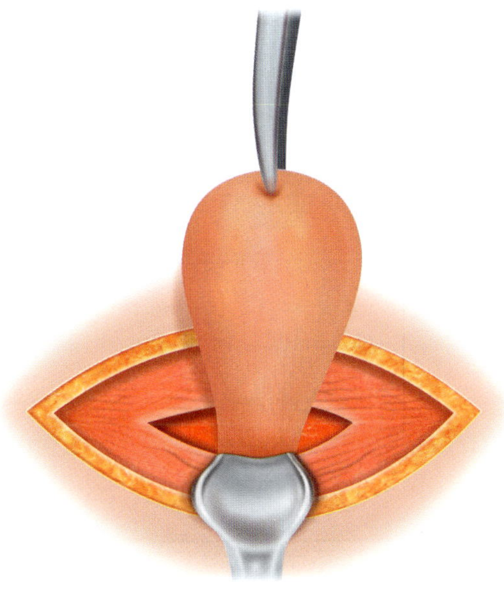

Fig. 71.2 Dissection of sac

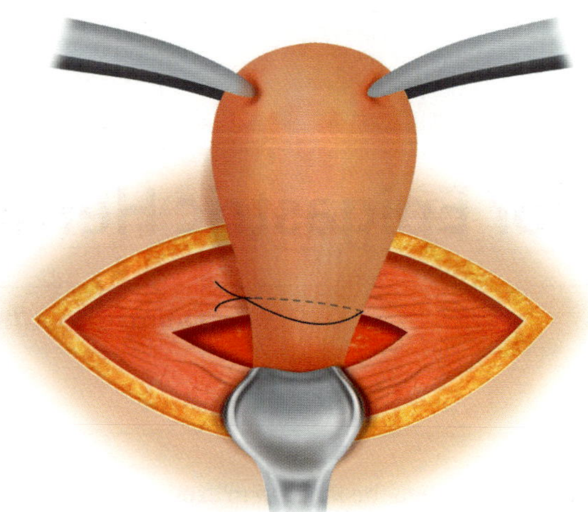

Fig. 71.3 Dealing with sac

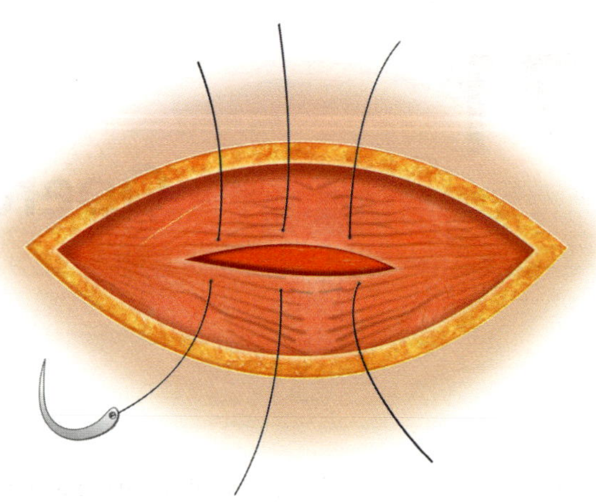

Fig. 71.4 Anatomical repair

POSTOPERATIVE CARE

- Oral feeds can be started when the patient is fully alert
- Oral analgesic is given for control of pain.

POSTOPERATIVE COMPLICATIONS

- Hematoma
- Sepsis.

CHAPTER

72

Operation for Umbilical Hernia in Infants and Children

Dhiraj Choudhury

Infantile umbilical hernia is a true umbilical hernia occurring through weak umbilical scar. Majority of these umbilical hernia closes spontaneously by 3–4 years. Hence, operation is recommended for those persisting beyond the age of 4 years.

INDICATION

Persisting and enlarging umbilical hernias after the age of 4 years should be surgically repaired.

OPERATIVE PROCEDURE

- *Position:* The patient is placed in supine position.
- *Anesthesia:* General anesthesia with endotracheal intubation.
- *Incision:* A curved incision is made below the umbilicus, after adequate skin preparation and application of sterile drapes (Fig. 72.1).
- *Exposure:* The incision is deepened through subcutaneous tissues. The umbilical scar is pulled upwards with Alli's tissue forceps and the dissection is carried upwards to expose the hernial sac up to the neck (Fig. 72.2).
- *Technique: Exposure of the sac*—The sac is freed on either side by blunt dissection. A fine artery forceps is now passed around the superior aspect of the sac and used as a retractor to clear the rest of the sac. The distal end of the sac is freed from the skin by sharp dissection (Fig. 72.3).
- *Dealing with the sac:* An empty sac can be inverted into the abdomen. In presence of content, open the sac, reduce

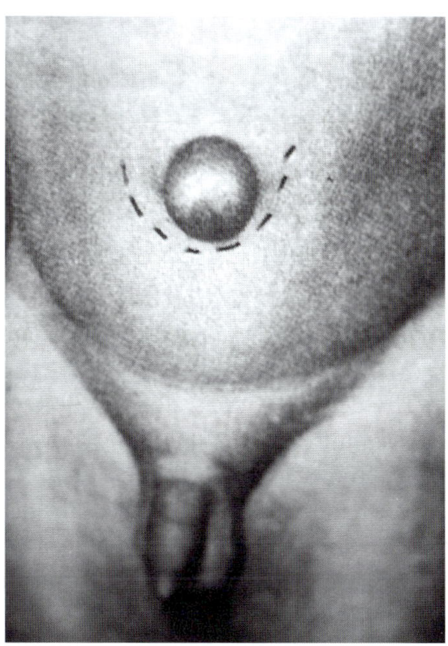

Fig. 72.1 Skin incision. Curved infraumbilical skin incision

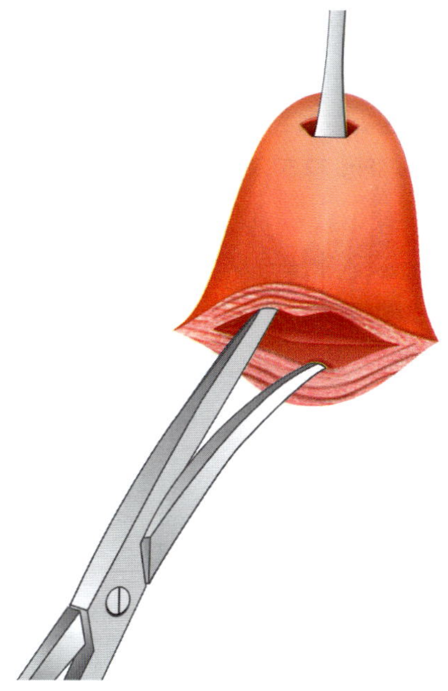

Fig. 72.2 Exposure

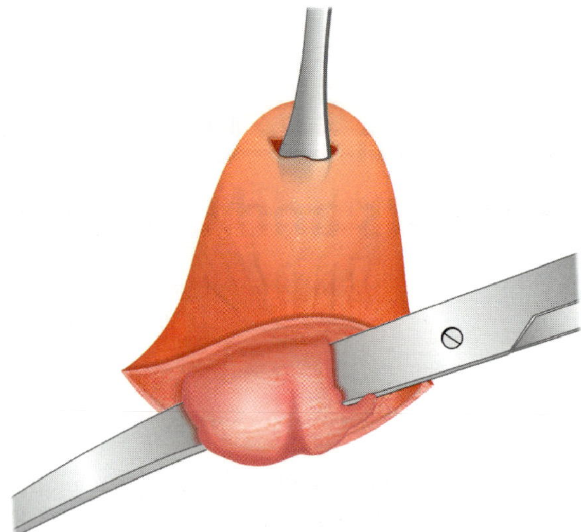

Fig. 72.3 Exposure of sac

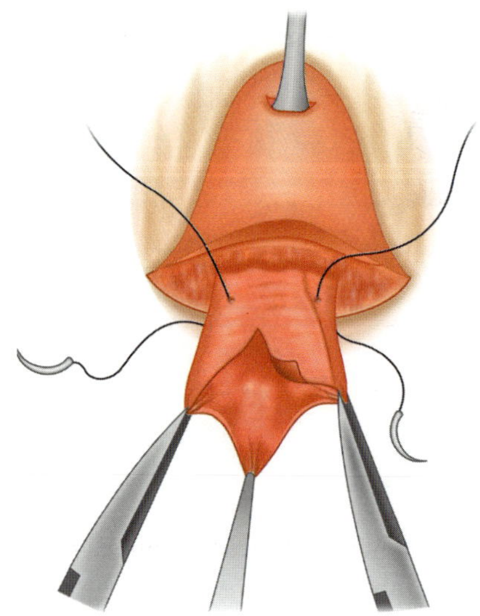

Fig. 72.4 Dealing with sac

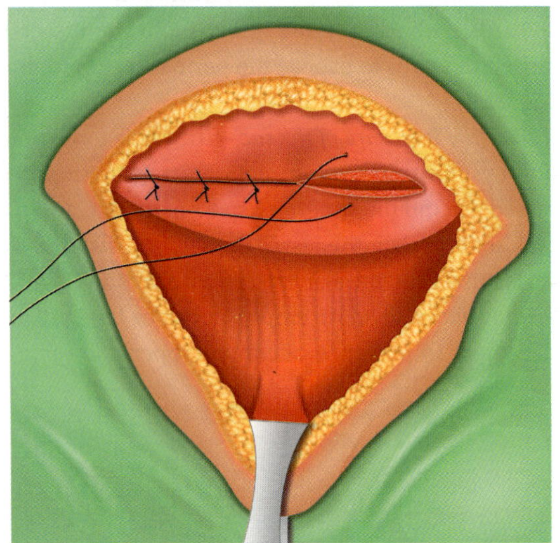

Fig. 72.5 Repair of linea alba

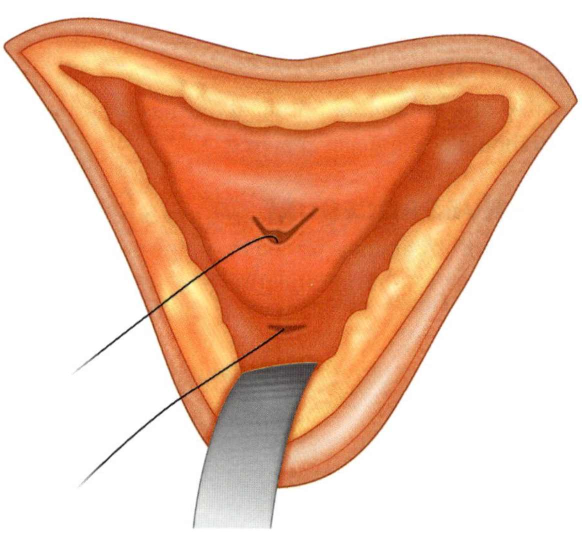

Fig. 72.6 Umbilicoplasty

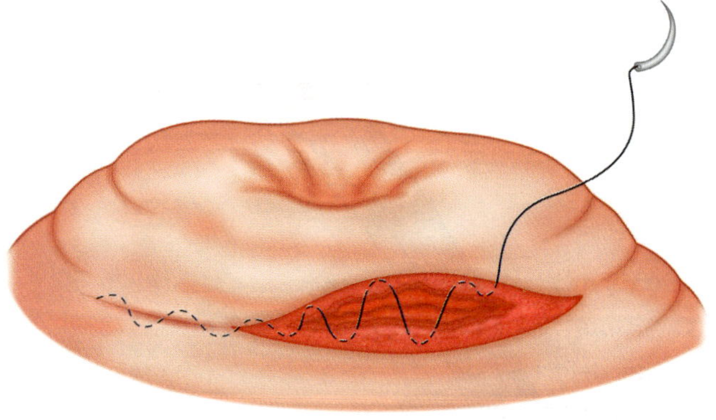

Fig. 72.7 Closure of skin

the content and ligate the neck of the sac and excise it (Fig. 72.4).

- *Repair:* The defects in linea alba can be repaired with interrupted sutures with 2/0 proline/vicryl (anatomical repair). Recurrence is rare (Fig. 72.5).
- *Closure:* Stitch the apex of the umbilicus to linea alba with absorbable sutures to invert the umbilicus for cosmetic reason (Umbilicoplasty) (Fig. 72.6). Subcuticular closure of skin is preferred but it can be closed with interrupted 3/0 ethilon sutures (Fig. 72.7).

CHAPTER

73

Operation for Adult Umbilical Hernia or Paraumbilical Hernia

Dhiraj Choudhury

Most umbilical hernias in adults are paraumbilical, protruding above or below the umbilicus through linea alba.

INDICATION

All paraumbilical hernias should be operated as they are liable to undergo complication. Irreducibility is frequent due to adhesion between the content and the sac. Strangulation occurs in 20% cases because of narrow neck.

PREOPERATIVE STEPS

- Reduction of obesity—if any
- Anti-DVT prophylaxis.
- Antibiotic prophylaxis.
- Cardiovascular and respiratory care.

OPERATIVE PROCEDURE

- *Position:* The patient is placed in the supine position.
- *Anesthesia:* General anesthesia with endotracheal intubation.
- *Incision:* An elliptical incision is made to remove overstretched skin including the umbilicus (Figs 73.1A and B).
- *Exposure:* Deepen the incision until the aponeurosis is exposed. Identify the sac and continue dissection until the neck of the sac is evident. The anterior rectus sheath is cleared of subcutaneous fat around the neck of sac (Figs 73.2A and B).
- *Dealing with sac:* The sac is opened near its neck were adhesion are least likely to occur. The contents are (Figs 73.3A and B) freed and returned to abdomen. Omentum can be excised with ligation of omental vessels. The whole circumference of the neck is gradually incised. The fundus of the sac with redundant skin is now removed.

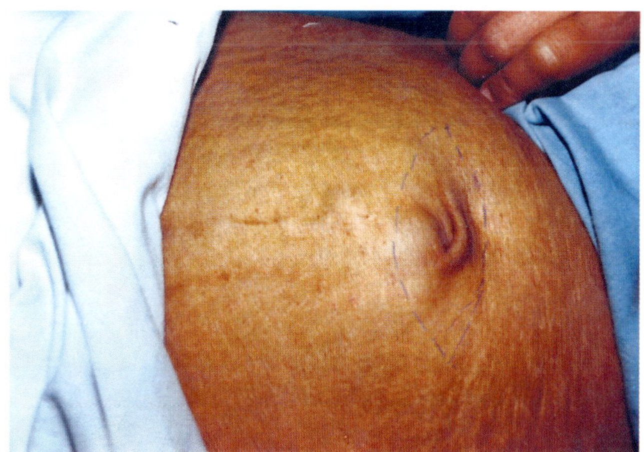

Fig. 73.1A Paraumbilical hernia large infraumbilical swelling

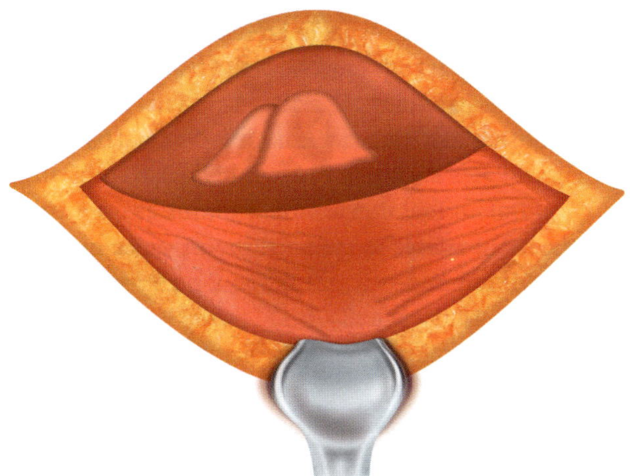

Fig. 73.1B Skin incision schematic diagram

- *Repair:* A standard Mayo-type of repair is suitable if the defect is not large. The gap containing peritoneum, posterior rectus sheath and aponeurosis is held in large

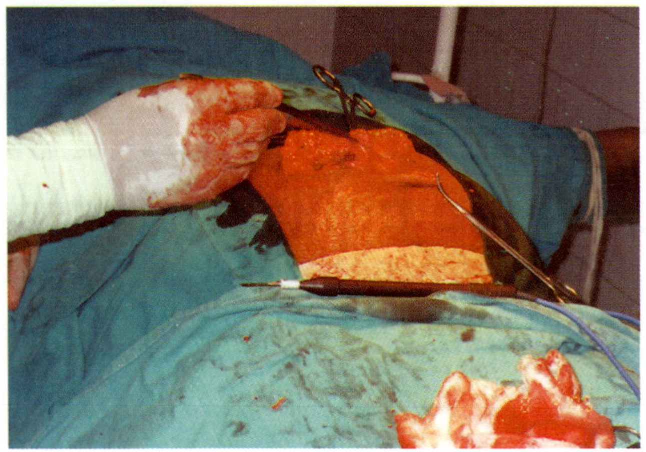

Fig. 73.2A Paraumbilical hernia: excision of umbilical scar

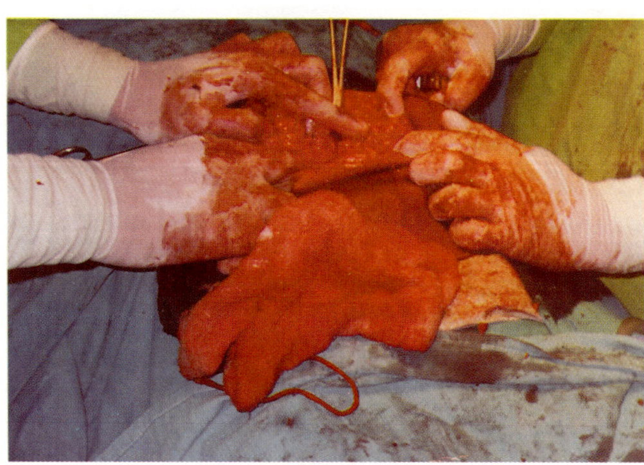

Fig. 73.3B Paraumbilical hernia: contents pushed in

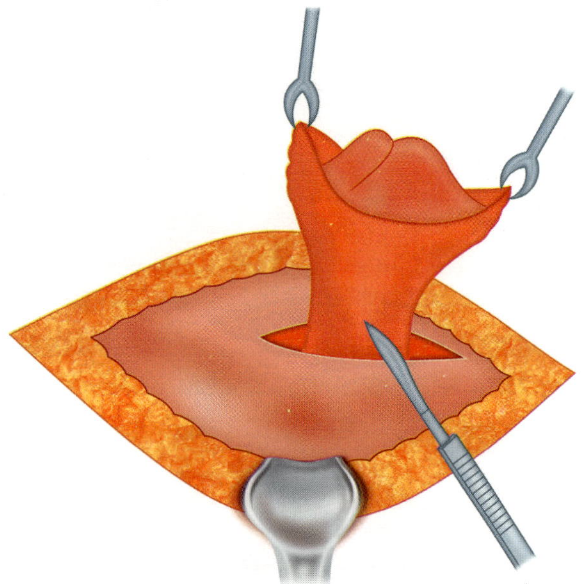

Fig. 73.2B Exposure of sac

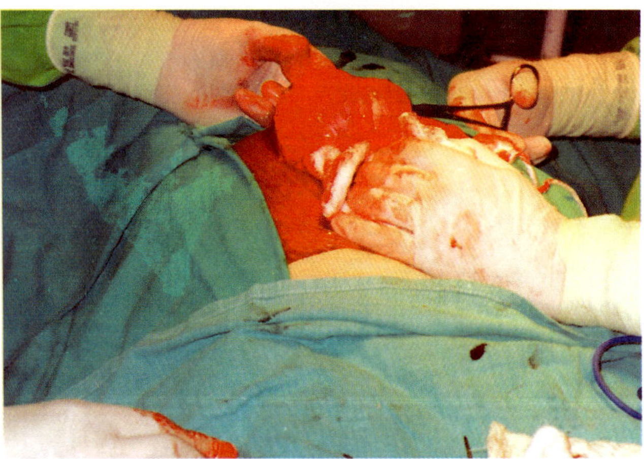

Fig. 73.3A Paraumbilical hernia: infraumbilical sac with omentum and small gut

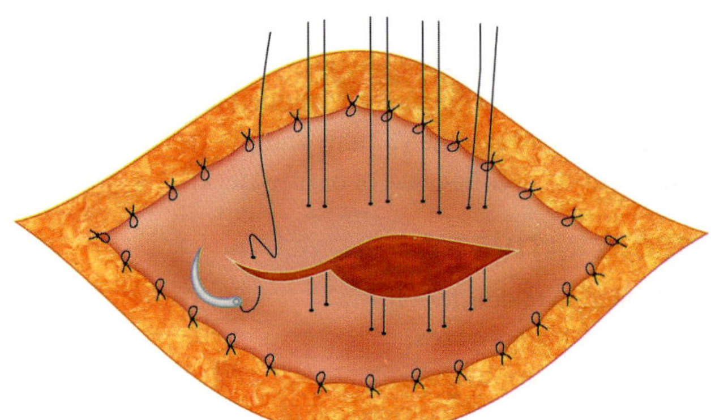

Fig. 73.4A Mayo's repair, schematic diagram

hemostats by the assistant. The first layer of the suture with 0 proline is passed through the upper flap 2–3 cm from its margin. The needle is then re-introduced through the lower flap from outside and finally brought through the deep surface of the upper flap. The sutures are initially held in hemostats to be tied when all are applied. A fine suction drain is inserted between two flaps of the aponeurosis. The margin of the upper flap is now sutured continuously to the anterior surface of the lower flap with 0 proline (Figs 73.4A and B).

- *Proline mesh repair:* Fascia defects >4 cm would require reinforcement with placement of an onlay mesh. The mesh is sutured on the anterior rectus sheath and laterally to external oblique aponeurosis. The mesh must overlap the fascial closure by at least 3 cm in all directions (Fig. 73.5).
- *Closure:* The skin can be closed with subcuticular absorbable sutures or interrupted ethilon sutures.

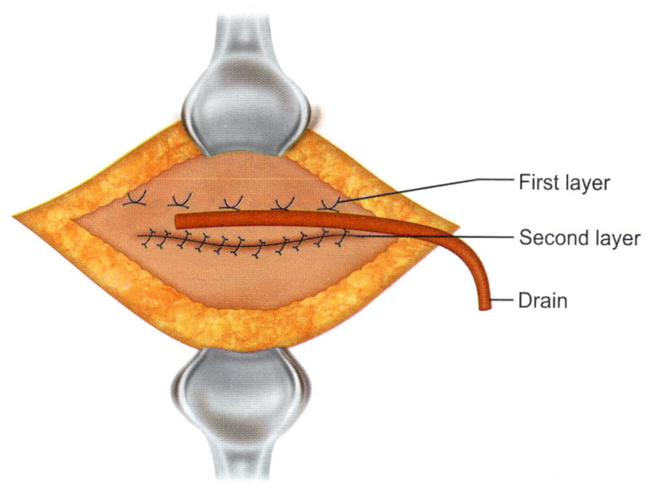

Fig. 73.4B Mayo's repair completed

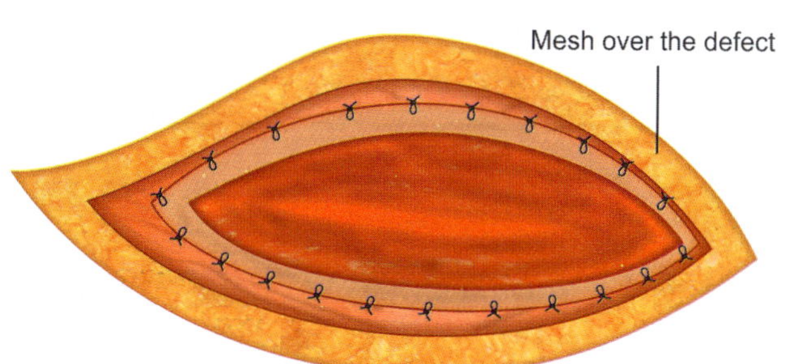

Fig. 73.5 Application of proline mesh

POSTOPERATIVE CARE

- Oral feed is started early
- Systemic antibiotic is particularly required if there is a chest problem
- Drain is removed after 48 hours
- Stitches are removed on 7–8 days.

POSTOPERATIVE COMPLICATIONS

- Respiratory complication
- Wound sepsis
- Recurrence.

CHAPTER

74

Operation for Incisional Hernia: Open Method

Dhiraj Choudhury

Incisional hernia is iatrogenic occurring through operative scar. They appear to occur after 3–5% of all abdominal operations. An incisional hernia may develop through any abdominal incision, but commonly through midline or paramedian incision. They can present as early hernias or late hernias (Fig. 74.1).

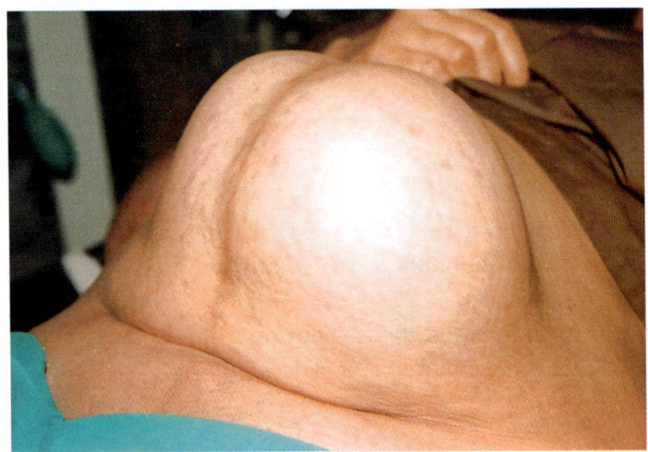

Fig. 74.1 Incisional hernia following midline incision

INDICATION

Operation is necessary if the defect is narrow (liable to strangulation), if there is evidence of obstruction or if there is discomfort (symptomatic). Wide neck hernias rarely strangulate and hence abdominal corset may be sufficient in these cases particularly in elderly people.

PREOPERATIVE PREPARATIONS

- Reduction of obesity, if any
- Control of blood sugar, if any
- Respiratory care
- Correction of anemia.

OPERATIVE PROCEDURE

- *Position:* Supine.
- *Anesthesia:* General endotracheal.
- *Incision:* An elliptical skin incision is made enclosing old scan and redundant skin which are removed (Fig. 74.2).
- *Exposure:* The outer edges containing skin and subcutaneous tissue are undercut with great care and reflected beyond the hernial protuberance (Fig. 74.3).

  The incision is deepened until the aponeurosis is reached, and then dissection is continued towards the margins of the hernia defects or the neck of the sac. Hemostasis must be perfect (Fig. 74.4).
- *Dealing with the sac:* The peritoneal sac is carefully dissected free and neck of the sac is cleared of fibro-fatty tissue. An empty sac can be invaginated by buried mattress sutures. An adherent sac is better opened, if the content is omentum, it is better ligated and removed with sac. Adherent bowels should be separated gently and returned to the abdomen. The sac is transfixed at the neck and

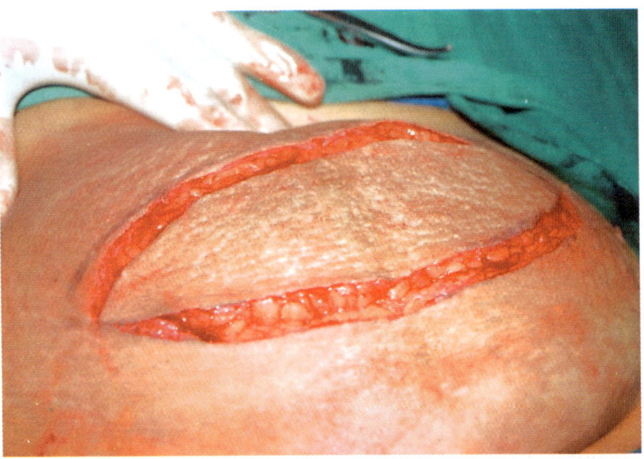

Fig. 74.2 Skin incision

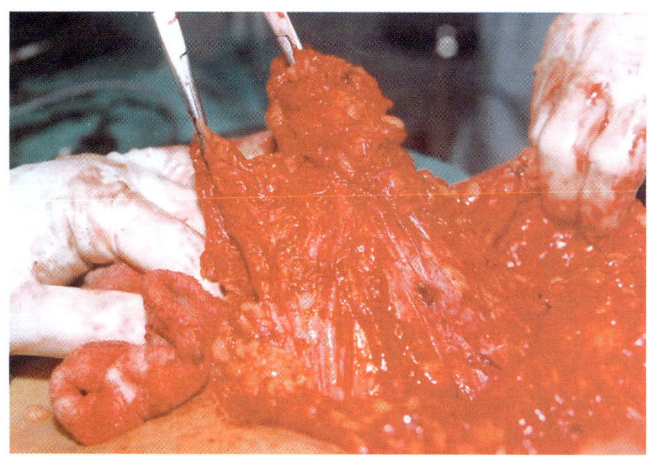

Fig. 74.3 Raising skin flaps

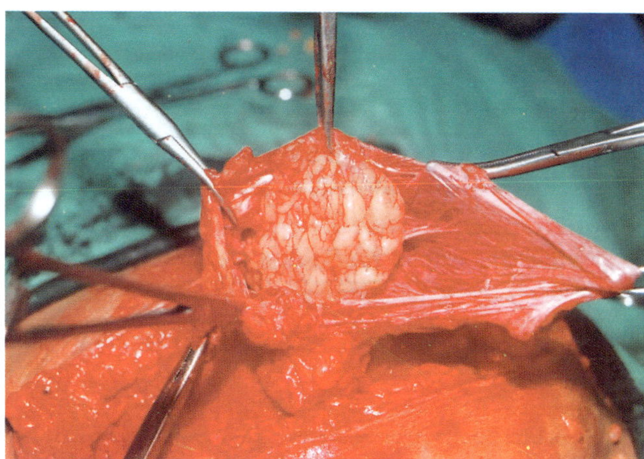

Fig. 74.5 Dealing with sac and content

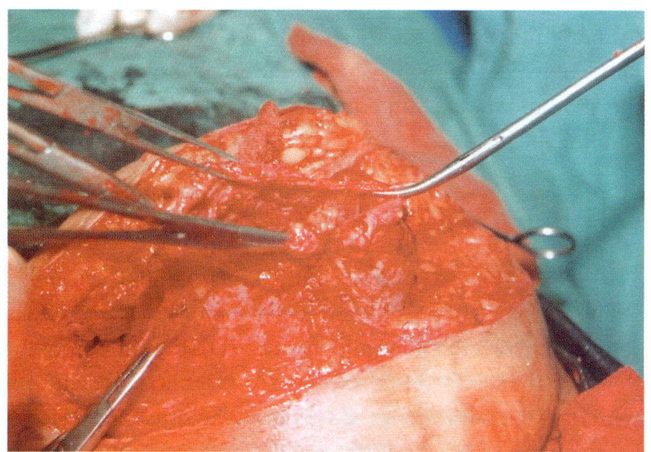

Fig. 74.4 Exposure

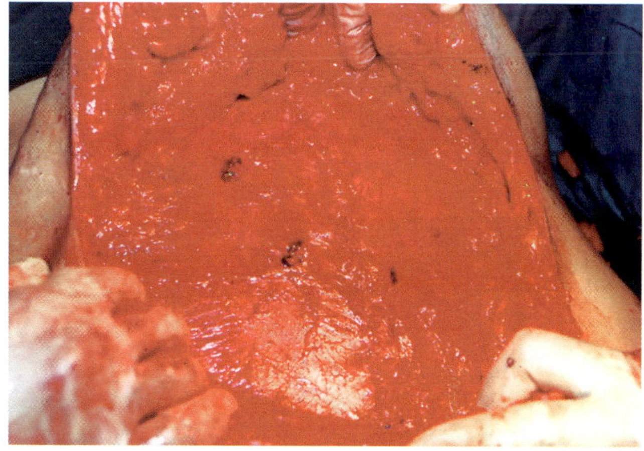

Fig. 74.6 Application of proline mesh

excised. Multiple defects in abdominal wall (Button hole tears) can be corrected by uniting them and repairing the resulting larger defect with 2/0 proline sutures (Fig. 74.5).

Repair

Simple Anatomical Repair

This can be used for repair or small incisional hernia with minimal scarring and small defect. The peritoneum and aponeurosis are sutured separately without tension using nonabsorbable (0-proline) suture.

Complex Anatomical Repair

These have been rendered obsolete nowadays since introduction of proline mesh.

Repair by Proline Mesh

This is considered the *best option* for repair of incisional hernia with larger defect or poor tissue to avoid recurrence. Following excision of the sac the peritoneum and the sheath can be closed with continues sutures taking large bites using number 1 proline (Fig. 74.6).

A proline mesh of adequate size (slightly oversize than the defect) is placed (Figs 74.7A to C) shows three alternative levels of application of mesh: (A) onlay, (B) extraperitoneal, (C) intraperitoneal.

Onlay Patch Repair

This is the simplest method. The proline mesh is placed anterior to the aponeurosis. It should extend 4 cm beyond

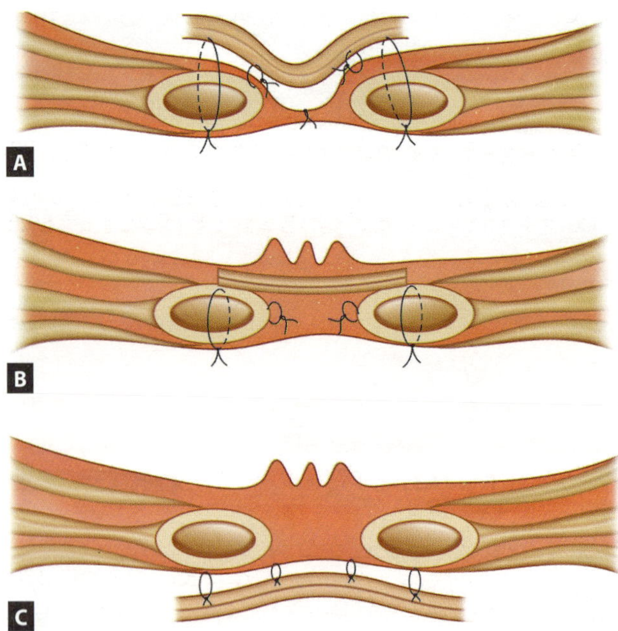

Figs 74.7A to C Onlay (A), extraperitoneal (B), intraperitoneal (C), Mesh placement (diagrammatic)

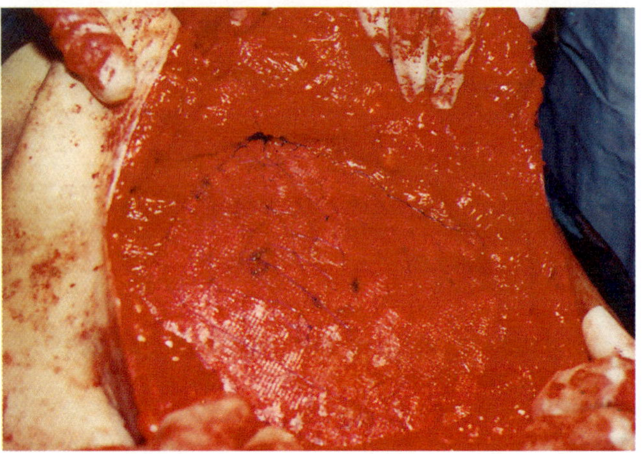

Fig. 74.8 Fixation of onlay mesh

the margin of the defect. The mesh is secured with (Fig. 74.8) interrupted 2/0 proline sutures at 2 cm intervals. This may be further strengthened with a over and over stitches. The mesh may be fixed to the margin of the defect by continuous sutures.

Extraperitoneal Mesh Repair: Rives Stoppa Techniques

In this method mesh is placed behind the rectus muscle and laid on to the anterior aspect of closed posterior rectus sheath and peritoneum. The mesh is fixed by few nonabsorbable

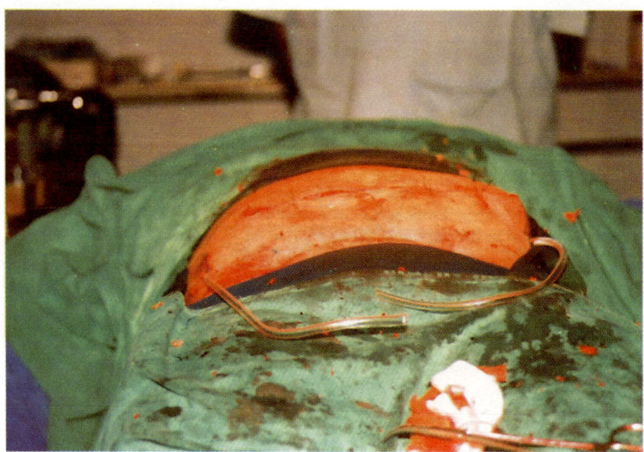

Fig. 74.9 Skin closure after application of suction drain

monofilament synthetic sutures. The sutures are passed through the edge of the mesh and then along the line of the lateral edge of the rectus sheath, through whole thickness of the abdominal wall. Surgeons have also developed method of stapling the mesh.

Intraperitoneal Mesh Repair

The sac is opened and any adhesions present are freed. Prepare a piece of mesh 2 cm larger than the defect in each direction. Draw the margin of the mesh under the rim of the defect with a series of U-sutures of 2/0 proline. The sutures penetrate the peritoneum 2–3 cm from the rim. The mesh can be reinforced with a continues over and over suture taking care to avoid the bowel.

Closure

- Hemostasis is checked
- A subcutaneous suction drain is inserted
- Skin wound may be closed with interrupted 2-0 ethilon suture or subcuticular sutures (Fig. 74.9).

POSTOPERATIVE CARE

- The drain is left until daily loss is less than 30 mL
- Systemic antibiotic is administered
- Early ambulation is encouraged
- Stitches are removed after 7 days.

POSTOPERATIVE COMPLICATIONS

- Hematoma formation
- Sepsis
- Recurrence.

CHAPTER

75 Operation for Inguinal (Groin) Hernias: Open Method

Dhiraj Choudhury

GENERAL PRINCIPLES

Hernia is as old as mankind. An inguinal hernia should be treated, because it will not go away on its own. And left untreated, hernias can develop severe-even life-threatening complications. The only way to cure hernia is with surgery. The only contraindication for operation is terminal illness or no consent for operation.

An indirect inguinal hernia is not simply congenital defect represented by a persistent patent processus vaginalis because except in infant and children simple removal of the hernial sac (herniotomy) results in unacceptably high recurrent rate. This indicates failure of fascia transversalis as an additional factor. Incase of direct hernia there is no peritoneal sac and the incidence is more related to failure of the posterior inguinal wall. Hence, except in infant and children herniotomy should be accompanied by some form of repair of the posterior wall.

TYPES OF REPAIR

There are two main categories of surgical hernia repair:

1. Tension repair/pure tissue repair/sutured techniques
2. Tension free repair.

Till first half of the 20th century, pure tissue repairs (Bassini, Marey, Mevay, Shouldice) were considered gold standard for treatment of groin hernias. By second half of this century, surgeons were rapidly changing towards tension free repairs, following routine use of prosthetic materials.

Tension Repair/Pure Tissue Repair/Sutured Techniques

For this type of hernia repair the surgeon makes an incision over the hernia site, deals with sac or contents and than stitches the hernia closed. The shouldice operation is the most effective technique of all sutures repairs. Meticulous anatomical four-layered repair of fascia transversalis with nonabsorbable sutures is the mainstay of this operation.

A tension repair is recommended for young patient if the hernia is small but this technique has several disadvantages. First, the level of discomfort following a tension repair is greater and recovery period is longer (about 4–6 weeks).

In addition, there is approximately 10–15% chance that the hernia will recur again.

Tension Free Repair/Mesh Repair

Tension free hernioplasty with mesh was introduced in 1984 and reported by Irving Lichtenstein and colleagues in 1989. The operation is simple, rapid, almost pain-free and allows early rehabilitation. Results from this type of repair are good, with only 1–3% recurrence rate. Recovery is quick and there is less discomfort following surgery. Furthermore this procedure can be done under local anesthesia. It is relatively costly procedure.

In 2007, the best practice in groin hernia repair is proline mesh hernioplasty. The debate is whether by open method or by laparoscopy.

INGUINAL HERNIOTOMY IN INFANTS AND CHILDREN

Infantile inguinal hernia is mostly due to failure of obliteration of processus vaginalis. Inguinal hernia in infants and children are indirect type and should be operated as early as possible because of the risk of complication like obstruction or strangulation. Emergency surgery is required in 10% if it is not reducible. This is not a minor procedure in a neonat. The incidence of irreducibility is highest in first 3 months. Prompt elective surgery prevents morbidity secondary to strangulation.

Operative Procedure

- *Position:* The patient is placed in supine position.
- *Anesthesia:* General anesthesia is employed.
- *Incision:* A transverse crease incision is made just above the symphysis pubis (Fig. 75.1).

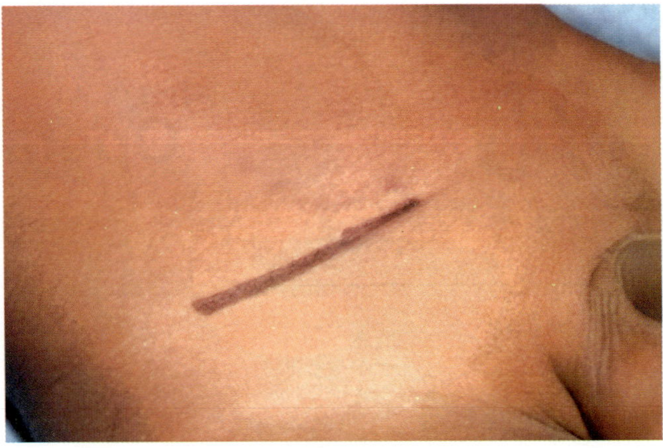

Fig. 75.1 Skin incision

Exposure

Deepen the incision through subcutaneous fat and superficial fascia to expose the superficial ring and the cord. Since the superficial and deep rings are almost superimposed at this age, splitting of external oblique aponeurosis is not necessary.

Divide and ligate the superficial epigastric vessels at this stage.

Dissection of the Cord

Identify, lift-up, and isolate the cord just distal to superficial ring (Fig. 75.2).

Separate the coverings of the spermatic cord (external spermatic fascia, cremasteric fascia and internal spermatic fascia) by blunt dissection with mosquito forceps. The contents of the cord are gently separated from the sac by gauze dissection. Care is taken not to damage fragile testicular vessels.

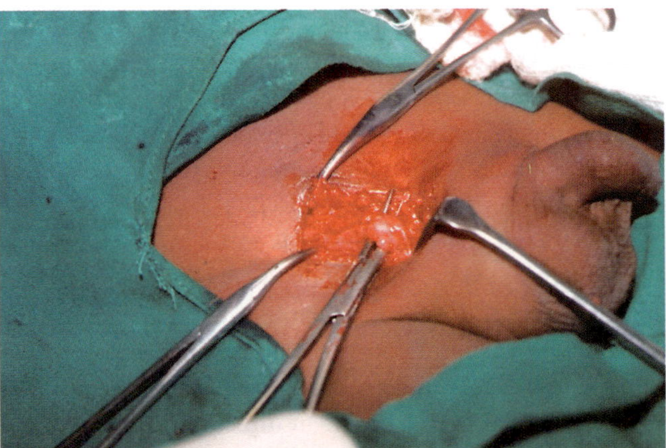

Fig. 75.2 Dissection of cord

Isolation of the Sac

The thin fragile sac can be identified as a glistening structure lying on the anterosuperior aspect of the cord having a white curved distal edge. Hold the fundus of the incomplete sac with hemostatic forceps. Carefully dissect the sac proximally up to the neck which is evident from the presence of extraperitoneal fats. Free the sac distally with similar care. A sac extending into the scrotum should not be dissected distally but transected leaving the distal end open (Fig. 75.3).

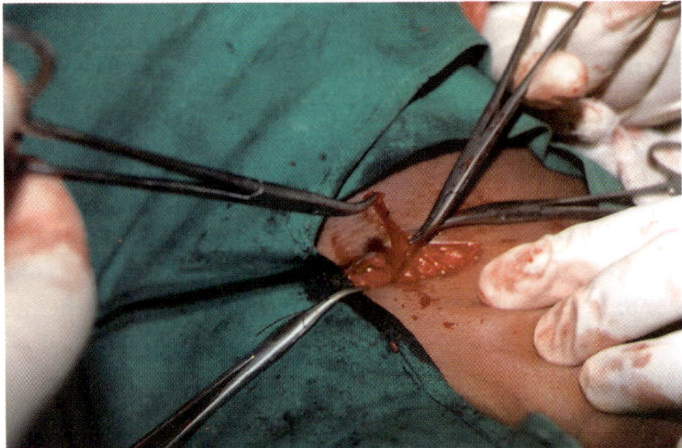

Fig. 75.3 Isolation of sac

Herniotomy

The sac is opened and contents are examined and pushed back into abdomen. Transfix, ligate and divide the neck of the sac at the level of superficial ring (Fig. 75.4).

Repair

Repair is not necessary in infants, but if the superficial ring has been stretched by large sac it can be narrowed by one or two catgut stitches. The coverings of the cord can be repaired by few interrupted fine stitches.

Closure

Close the subcutaneous tissues with 3/0 chromic catgut stitches. The skin is closed with subcuticular stitches with absorbable sutures.

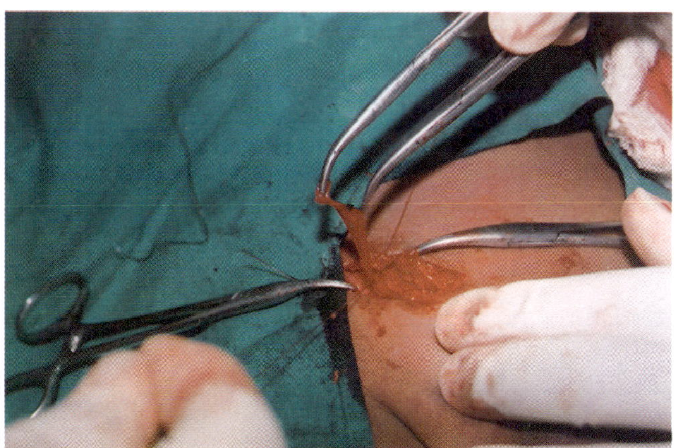

Fig. 75.4 Herniotomy

Bilateral herniotomy can be done in infants and children as this is simple and quick, but routine exploration of contralateral side is controversial.

HERNIA REPAIR: PROCEDURES IN ADULTS

Preoperative Preparations

- Treat medical conditions particularly chronic bronchitis, bronchial asthma, diabetes adequately if present.
- Deep vein thrombosis (DVT) prophylaxis in high-risk cases.
- Care of the bowel and bladder.
- Dealing with giant hernia. In case of giant hernia sudden returning of contents (loops of bowel) into abdomen during operation may cause respiratory embarrassment due to diaphragmatic compromise. This should be avoided by following preventive measures, (i) Preoperative gradual reduction of content by raising foot end of the bed for some days, (ii) Repeated abdominal pneumoperitoneum will increase the capacity of the intra-abdominal cavity, (iii) Respiratory support with ventilator in immediate postoperative period.

Operative Procedure

- *Position:* The patient is placed in supine position.
- *Anesthesia:* The operation can be performed under general anesthesia, spinal anesthesia or even local anesthesia. Most cases can be operated on day case basis.

Local anesthesia: With a fine needle inject initially about 10 mL of 1% xylocaine along the line of incision raising a continues bleb and then inject deeply along the same line with a larger needle. Iliohypogastric and ilioinguinal nerves are blocked by injecting 5 mL of 1% xylocaine deep to external oblique at a point 3 cm above and medial to anterior superior iliac spine. Drape the patient exposing only operative site.

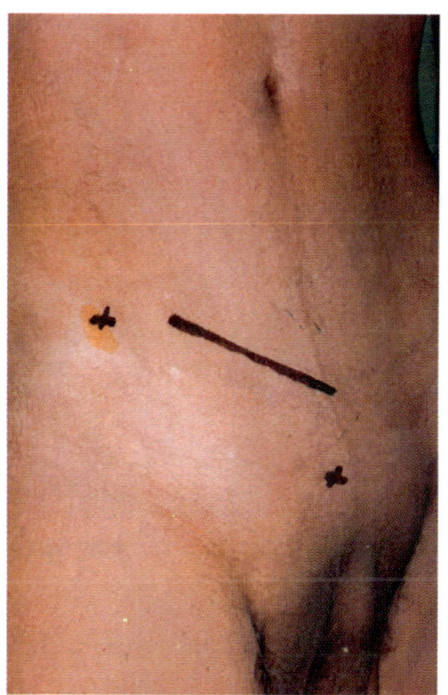

Fig. 75.5 Skin incision

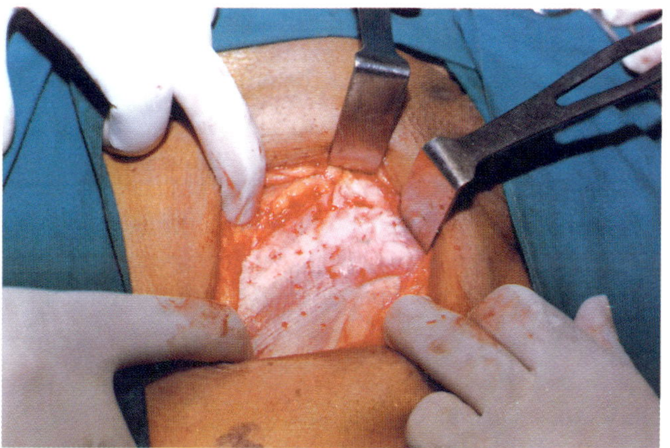

Fig. 75.6 Exposure

Incision

A crease incision (2–3 cm) is made 1 cm above the medial part of inguinal ligament. The pubic tubercle and anterior superior iliac spine are important landmark (Fig. 75.5).

Exposure

The incision is deepened through sub-cutaneous tissue and Scarpa's fascia, until the external oblique aponeurosis with its glistening fibers is exposed (Fig. 75.6).

The superficial epigastric and superficial external pudendal veins are divided and ligated at same time.

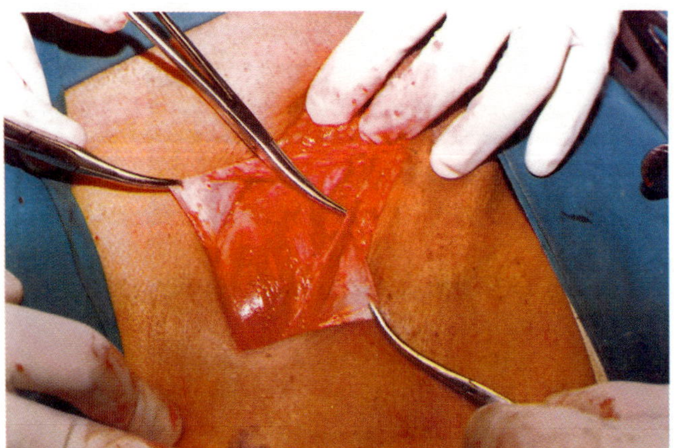

Fig. 75.7 Isolation of ilioinguinal nerve

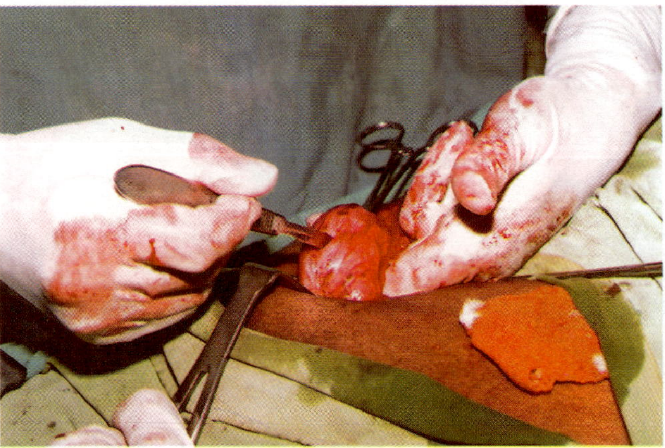

Fig. 75.8 Dissection of cord

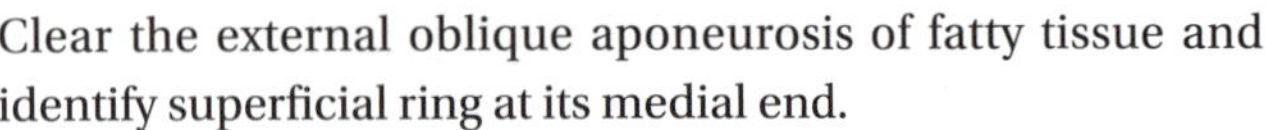

Clear the external oblique aponeurosis of fatty tissue and identify superficial ring at its medial end.

Incise the external oblique aponeurosis in the line of its fibers at the level of apex of the external ring. Initially a small cut is made in the external oblique aponeurosis—which is then extended medially through superficial ring and laterally for 5 cm. At the medial end the superficial ring will be opened now.

Retract the cut edges of external oblique aponeurosis with hemostats to expose conjoined muscle arching over the cord, and glistening upper surface of inguinal ligament. Identify the ilioinguinal nerve lying on the anterior aspects of the cord and preserve it to avoid postoperative pain and numbness (Fig. 75.7).

Dissection of the Cord (Fig. 75.8)

Life the structures of the spermatic cord and hernial sac with left index finger and spread it over the fingers. Incise the coverings (cremasteric muscle) of the spermatic cord longitudinally. Separate the coverings by blunt dissection with nontoothed dissection forceps taking care of spermatic veins. Any lipoma present is excised. Encircle the spermatic cord with a sling or cord holding forceps. An indirect sac will now be exposed.

Dissection of the Sac

An *indirect sac* is easily identified as a pearly white pyriform structure on the anterosuperior aspect of the cord. In case of small sac a white curved edge may be seen, if it is an incomplete hernia. Hold the fundus of the sac with a pair of hemostat and gently separate it from vas and testicular vessels up to the neck (Fig. 75.9). If the hernia is complete the sac should be purposefully divided at the level of superficial ring and proximal portion dissected up to the neck. The distal part is left open.

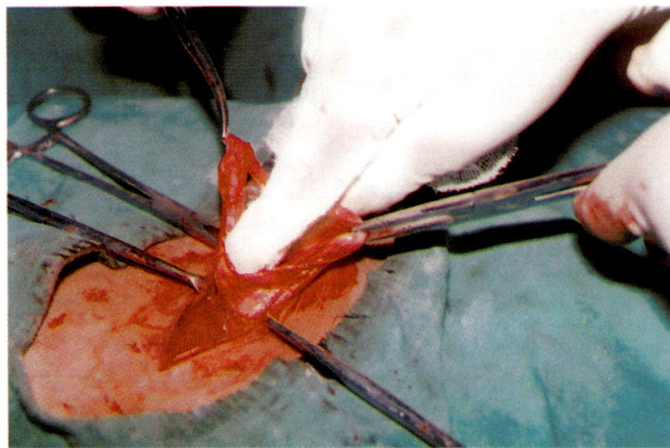

Fig. 75.9 Dissection of sac

The neck of the sack is identified by the following features (Fig. 75.10):

- Narrowest part of the sac
- Presence of collar of extraperitoneal fat
- Pulsatile inferior epigastric artery medially.

Direct sac: A direct sac is usually a broad based bulge of the peritoneum on the posterior wall which can be seen once the cord is retracted laterally and downwards. Incase of direct hernia always look for indirect sac first by dissection of the cord (Fig. 75.11).

Dealing with the Sac

Indirect sac: Herniotomy: Open the fundus of the sac, examine the contents and reduce it. The sac is then twisted at the neck to occlude the lumen (Fig. 75.12). Apply transfixation suture

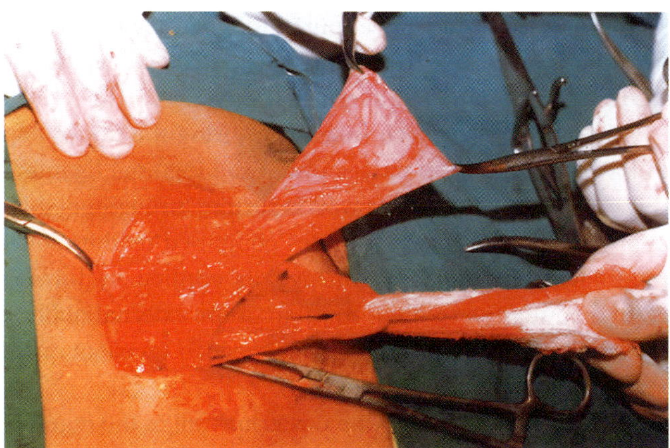

Fig. 75.10 Dissection of sac and identification of neck of sac

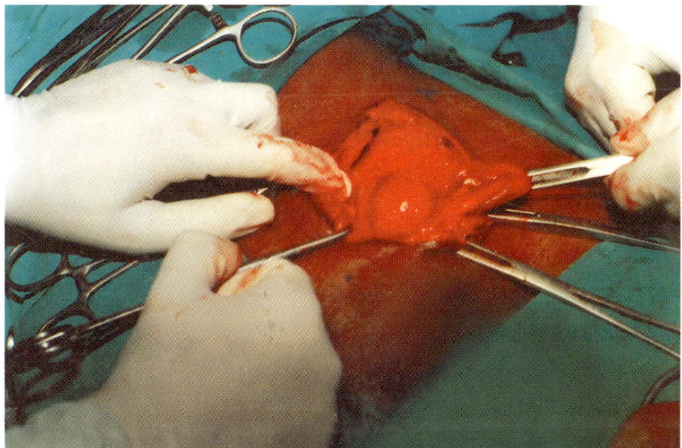

Fig. 75.11 Direct sac

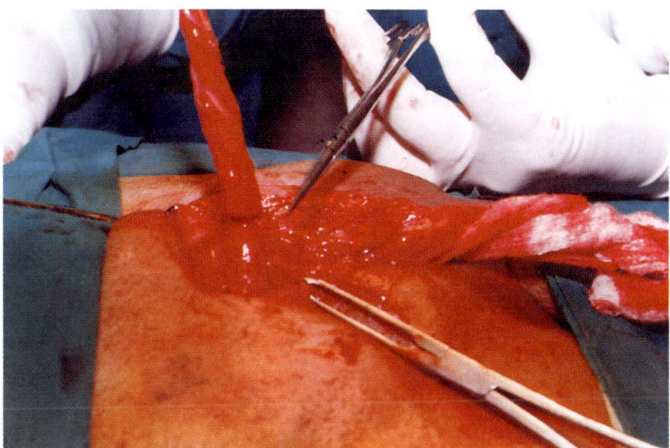

Fig. 75.12 Dealing with indirect sac. Herniotomy after ligation of neck

with 0 chromic catgut as high as possible and excise the sac distal to ligature. Do not cut the ends of the ligature before the redundant sac has been excised. The stump of the sac usually

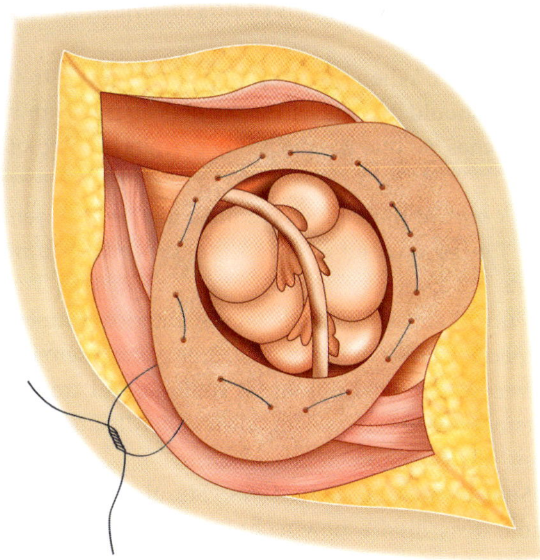

Fig. 75.13 Dealing with sliding hernia sac

retracts through the deep ring. In case of giant hernia (scrotal abdomen) methods of dealing with the sac has already been described under preoperative care. For a large inguino-scrotal hernia, dissect the hernia sac to deep ring. The distal sac in scrotum is not disturbed. Open the sac deal with contents. Ligate the sac at its neck leaving the open distal sac in the scrotum.

Direct sac: It does not require a formal herniotomy. The sac is simply pushed back.

Sliding hernia sac (Fig. 75.13): Incase of sliding hernia clear the peritoneal sac as far as possible without dissecting the gut and then close it by applying an inside-out purse string suture.

Repair

Pure Tissue Repairs

The Bassini method: Edoardo Bassini (1884), an Italian surgeon, was first to realize that the key to normal inguinal canal was the integrity of the posterior wall, and in particular, the fascia transversalis. He opened the fascia transversalis from pubic tubercle to beyond deep ring, and sutured the conjoined tendon and upper half of transversalis fascia in one layer, to lower half of transversalis fascia and inguinal ligament. In our younger days, the Bassini operation, we used to practice consisted of suturing conjoined tendon to inguinal ligament behind the cord. The incidence of recurrence varied from 2.9% to 9.6%.

Additions and Alterations of Bassini Method

Lyttle's stitches: When the deep ring is weak and stretched, the repair should include narrowing of deep ring with two or three stitches, so that the deep ring permits only tip of little finger.

Tanner's muscle slide: Since Bassini's method is a tension-repair, Tanner advised muscle slide' procedure to reduce tension.

A curved incision is made on the anterior rectus sheath near medial border of the muscle. This will cause relaxation of lower border of the internal oblique and transversus abdominis, which can lie alongside inguinal ligament without tension.

The Shouldice repair: In 1953, Shouldice of Ontario, Canada, described a new technique which is basically a multilayered Bassini operation. Bassini's essential concept was rediscovered just after World War II by Shouldice who advocated a multilayered technique of repair of the posterior wall of the inguinal canal.

The fascia transversalis forming the posterior wall of the canal is incised from deep ring to pubic crest. Divide the medial margin of the deep ring and proceed medially splitting the transversalis fascia as far as pubic tubercle midway between the conjoined tendon and inguinal ligament (Fig. 75.14).

Raise the upper flap from extraperitoneal tissue to expose its shinny white deep surface at the level of conjoined tendon. Similarly separate the lower flap down to inguinal ligament (Fig. 75.15).

The 'first layer' of suture unites the cut edge of the lower flap to the under surface of the upper flap with '0' proline suture. Start a suturing at the level pubic tubercle taking bites at irregular levels. Once the lateral is reached the deep ring is reconstructed around the spermatic cord (Fig. 75.16).

The 'second layer' consists of suturing the upper flap to lower flap where it passes under the inguinal ligament (Fig. 75.17). The posterior wall is further strengthened by applying third layer which unites conjoined tendon down inguinal ligament. A fourth layer is applied by joining conjoined tendon to the lower flap of the external oblique aponeurosis. The Shouldice repair provided excellent result in the hands of dedicated surgeons.

Cooper's ligament repair: The posterior wall of the inguinal canal is split widely open. The hernial sac is dealt with and the Cooper's ligament is cleared. A series of sutures with proline

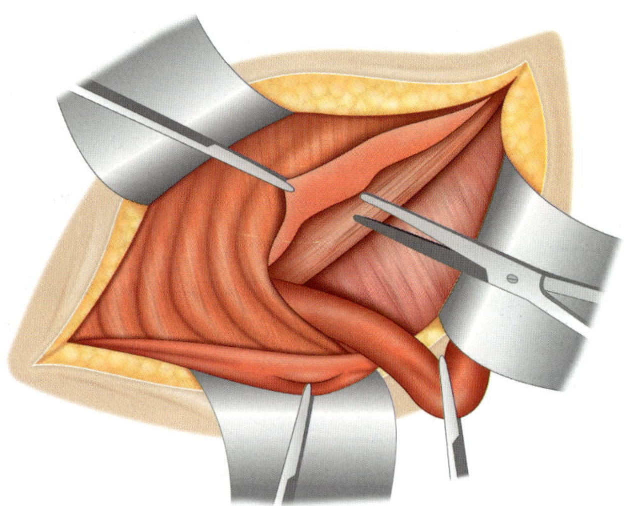

Fig. 75.15 Raising flaps of fascia transversalis

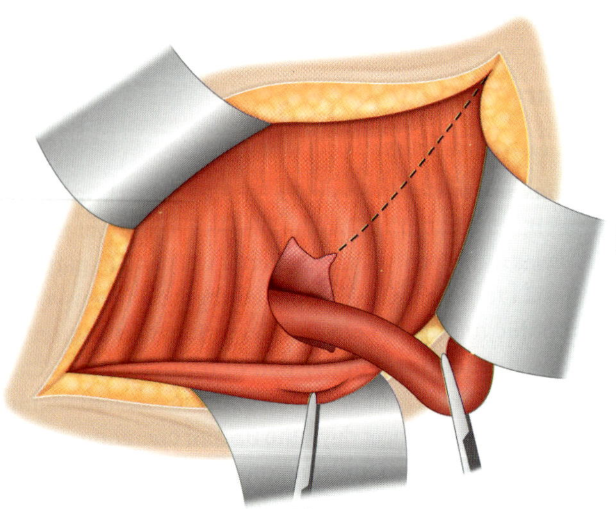

Fig. 75.14 Splitting transversalis fascia

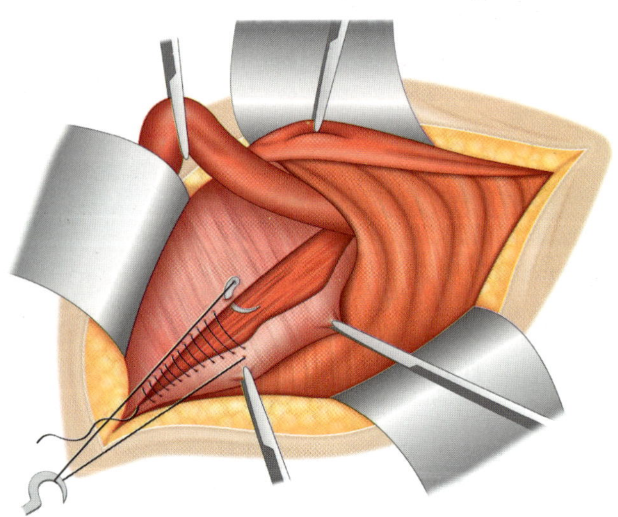

Fig. 75.16 First layer

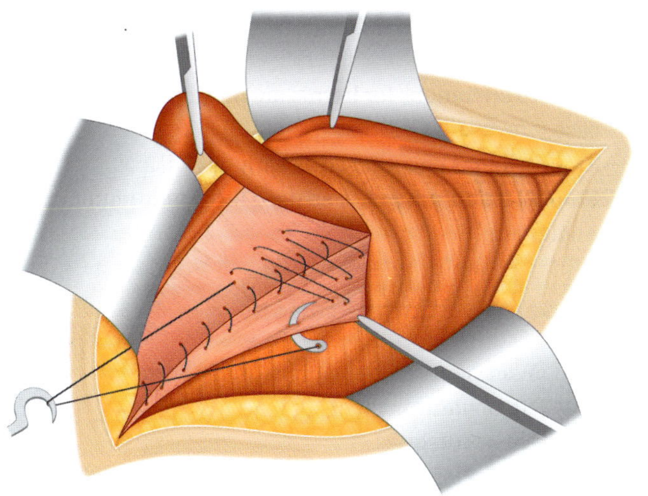

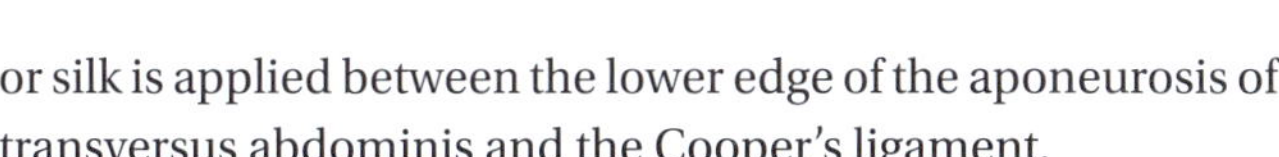

Fig. 75.17 Second layer

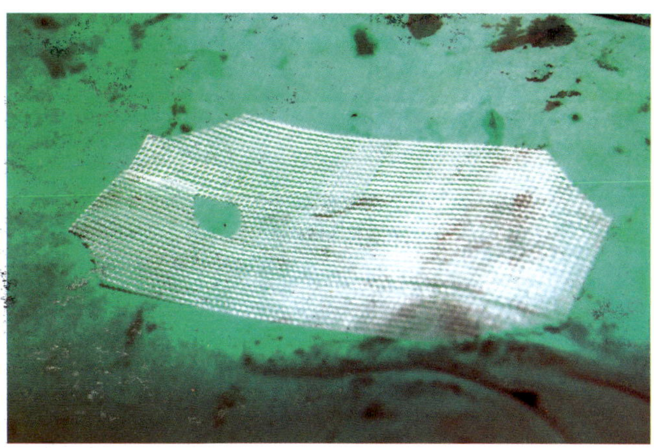

Fig. 75.18 Mesh

or silk is applied between the lower edge of the aponeurosis of transversus abdominis and the Cooper's ligament.

Closure: Close the inguinal canal by suturing external oblique aponeurosis with absorbable suture starting laterally and ending medially by reconstructing the superficial ring. Close the skin with absorbable subcuticular suture or 2/0 ethilon stitches.

Tension-free Repair

Lichtenstein proline mesh repair: At present this remains the gold standard for primary inguinal hernia repair in adults. This is particularly indicated for inguinal hernia in elderly and in recurrent hernia. Recurrence rate following Lichtenstein repair is less than 1%. The sac of the hernia has already been dealt with.

Technique: Now, take a proline mesh of appropriate size (Fig. 75.18) and fashion it to the shape of the floor of the inguinal canal. An opening is made on the lateral aspect of the mesh to allow it to pass around the spermatic cord at the level of the deep ring.

Place the mesh over the floor of the inguinal canal (fascia transversalis) behind the cord (Fig. 75.19) and secure it to pubic tubercle. The lower edge is sutured to inguinal ligament by continuous proline suture. Fix the upper end to conjoint tendon and anterior rectus sheath.

The excess mesh on the lateral side is trimmed leaving 3-4 cm beyond the deep ring which is inserted underneath external oblique aponeurosis. For the procedure to be successful the mesh must be large enough and must be correctly secured without tension on tissues particularly medially.

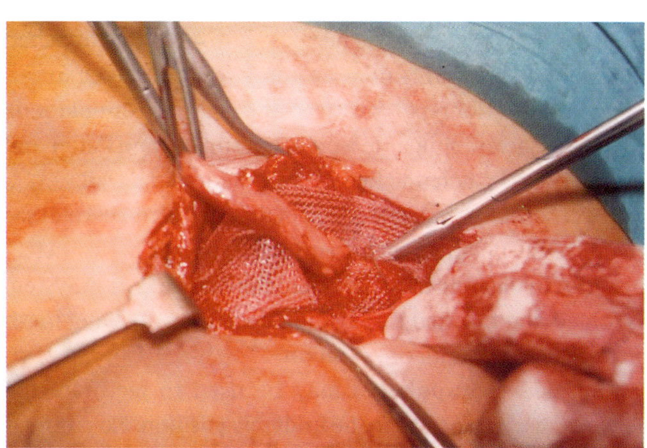

Fig. 75.19 Placement of mesh

Plug and Patch Repair

A premanufactured mesh plug is tailored to the hernia defect and inserted partially into preperitoneal space through the defect. The prosthesis is secured circumferentially to the defect using few interrupted sutures.

A flat mesh prosthesis is then placed on the top of the plug and overlaps the entire inguinal floor in a manner similar to Lichtenstein.

Three-dimensional Mesh Repair

Proline hernia system for repair: A device (Proline Hernia System—manufactured by Ethicon, a Johnson and Johnson Company) has been designed to overcome many of disadvantages of tension free repair techniques while incorporating the advantages of each (Fig. 75.20).

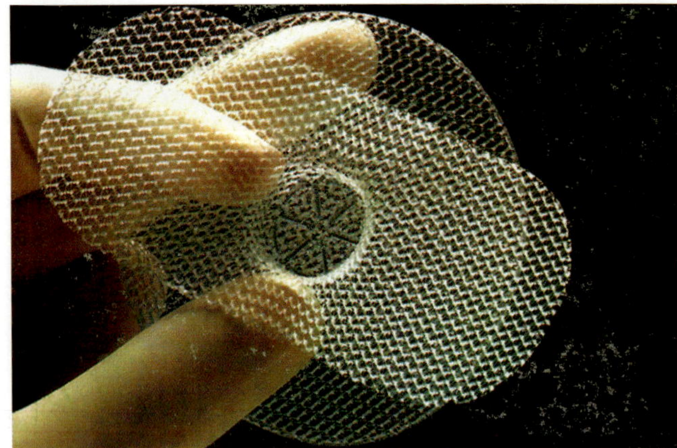

Fig. 75.20 Proline hernia system (Ethicon)

The device, which is currently used primarily to repair direct and indirect inguinal hernias consist of three attached components: (1) an "underlay patch" that provides for an effective posterior repair on the inside of the abdominal wall; (2) a "connector" similar to a plug, but smaller and flatter and (3) an "onlay" patch that files over the abdominal wall.

Indirect hernia: A high dissection of the neck of the hernial sac to utilize the potential of the peritoneal space is performed.

The circular underlay portion of the Proline Hernia System is folded and inserted through the deep ring, allowing mesh to expand to the underlay position.

Surgical manipulation may be used to facilitate the expansion of the device to the underlay position. No suture is necessary in the underlay patch.

The onlay patch, which is designed to cover the posterior wall (floor of the canal) is then modified as needed to accommodate the cord structures. If one end of the oval onlay patch is longer than the other, the Proline Hernia System is positioned so that the longer end covers the posterior wall (floor of the canal) and overlaps the pubic tubercle. Sutures or clips may be used to secure the onlay patch in place. The cord structure then lie on top of the medial portion of the onlay patch.

For *direct hernia* the defect is circumscribed at its base, the contents fully reduced, prior to insertion of the Proline Hernia System.

The circular underlay portion of the Proline Hernia System is folded and inserted through the defects, or internal ring, allowing mesh to expand to underlay position. The underlay portion should expand under the defect in the floor of the canal.

Surgical manipulation may be used to facilitate the expansion of the device to the underlay position. Sutures or clips may be used to secure the onlay patch in place.

Postoperative Care

- Elective operations for hernia are mostly done as day care case
- Ambulation is encouraged as early as possible
- Prophylactic antibiotic is advised for elderly patients
- Analgesic.

Postoperative Complications

General: Pulmonary complications are important, particularly in elderly.

Local: Hemorrhage
Testicular complications (Swelling orchitis), atrophy
Vas deferens injury
Neuralgia (iliohypogastric, ilioinguinal)
Wound infection.
Recurrence.

STRANGULATED HERNIA

Preoperative Preparations

- Nasogastric suction
- Intravenous fluid and electrolytes
- Systemic antibiotic.

Salient Steps

- The inguinal canal is exposed by steps similar to those described under elective operation. Dissect and isolate the sac, and open it near the fundus, before relieving obstruction to suck toxic fluids present in the sac.
- Relieve construction:
  At the neck of the sac most common: Feel the construction and divide it under guidance of a grooved director, upwards and outwards to avoid inferior epigastric artery, which lies medially.
  At superficial ring: It is divided in early part of the operation.
- Dealing with contents:
  Intestine:
  - Viable intestines are returned back into abdomen.
  - Nonviable intestines (color changes, loss of peristalsis and loss of mesenteric arterial pulsation) are treated by resection and anastomosis.
  - Doubtful gut is better excised if there is no color change after application of hot mops.
    Omentum: Devitalized omentum is excised.

Dealing with Sac

Standard herniotomy is done.

Repair

Repair of hernia is not mandatory, if condition of the patient and experience of surgeon permits, repair (herniorraphy or hernioplasty) can be done at the same time.

Prosthetic implant is better avoided, if resection of the bowel is done, because chance of wound infection is high.

Closure

The wound is closed in layers.

Postoperative Care

- Early ambulation is encouraged
- Prophylactic antibiotic in elderly
- Early discharge from hospital
- A two weeks postoperative leave for a sedentary worker and three weeks for a manual worker.

Postoperative Complications

General: Pulmonary complications are important.
Local: Hemorrhage.
Testicular complications (Swelling, orchitis) Vas deferens injury.
Neuralgia (Iliohypogastric, ilioinguinal) wound infection.

Concluding Remarks about Surgery of Groin Hernia

- "No disease of the human body belonging to province of surgeons require in its treatment of greater combination of accurate anatomical knowledge with surgical skill than hernia is all its varities." Sir Astley Cooper 1804.
- The outcome of hernia surgery is to or large extent surgeon dependent.
- For most surgeons open mesh repair remains the gold standard for primary inguinal hernia repair is adults.
- There is no clear answer from literature about at what age should mesh repair replace childhood herniotomy, a recent consensus reckoned 18 years was the watershed.
- *Laparoscopic approach has following advantages*: Less postoperative pain, an earlier return to normal activities and lower incidence of chronic pain. However, laparoscopic hernia repair requires experience and is relatively expensive.
- The open mesh technique remains the clear procedure of choice for massive, obstructed and irreducible hernia.
- Laparoscopic approach has clear advantages for patients with recurrent or bilateral hernias. Total extraperitoneal approach is favored.

CHAPTER

76

Operations for Femoral Hernia

Dhiraj Choudhury

Femoral hernias constitute only 5% of all abdominal wall hernias. They are more common in females (F : M 4: 1).

SURGICAL ANATOMY

The femoral sheath, a prolongation of fascia transversalis (anteriorly) and fascia iliaca (posteriorly) into thigh has three compartments: in lateral compartment contains femoral artery and intermediate one femoral vein. The most medial compartment is femoral canal whose internal opening is called femoral ring. The femoral ring is bounded anteriorly by inguinal ligament posteriorly by pectineal ligament laterally by femoral vein and medially by lacunar ligament. The femoral hernia enters through the femoral ring passes through femoral canal and then turns forward through saphenous opening (Fig. 76.1). The neck of the hernial sac is below the inguinal ligament, and lateral to the pubic tubercle, which helps to distinguish this type of hernia from an inguinal hernia.

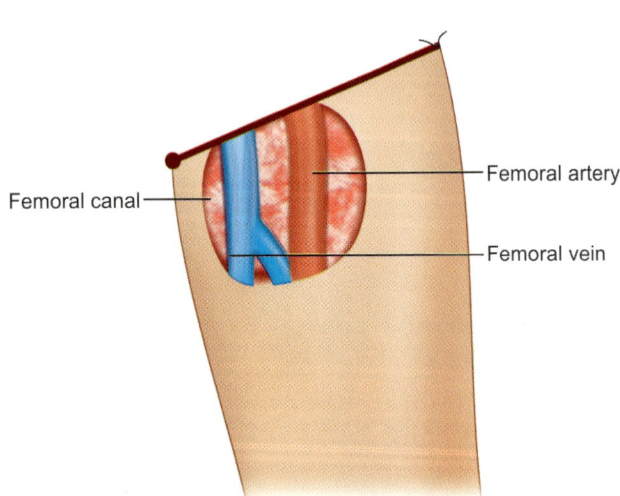

Fig. 76.1 Anatomy of femoral canal (L)

The femoral hernia sac is covered by extra-peritoneal fat, fascia transversalis, cribriform fascia, superficial fascia and skin.

INDICATION FOR OPERATION

All femoral hernias should be operated, as these are liable to undergo obstruction or strangulation. Even elderly frail patients can be operated under local anesthesia. Femoral hernias are often irreducible because of the rigid margins of the femoral ring, contributing to the risk of strangulation.

OPERATIVE PROCEDURE

- *Position:* The patient is placed in supine position.
- *Anesthesia:* General anesthesia is preferred, but can be done under spinal or even local anesthesia.

Approaches

Low or crural approach—Lockwood: This is the usual approach for elective repair of femoral hernia. It allows direct assess to the hernia sac.

High or preperitoneal approach—McEvedy: This is preferred for strangulated hernia.

High or inguinal approach—Lotheissen's approach is rarely used because it weakens the inguinal canal.

Low Approach

Lockwood approach.

Incision: An oblique incision is made directly over the hernia, parallel to medial half of inguinal ligament (Fig. 76.2).

Exposure: The incision is carried through subcutaneous tissues till hernial sac is exposed. Secure hemostasis by ligating small tributaries of long saphenous vein (Fig. 76.3).

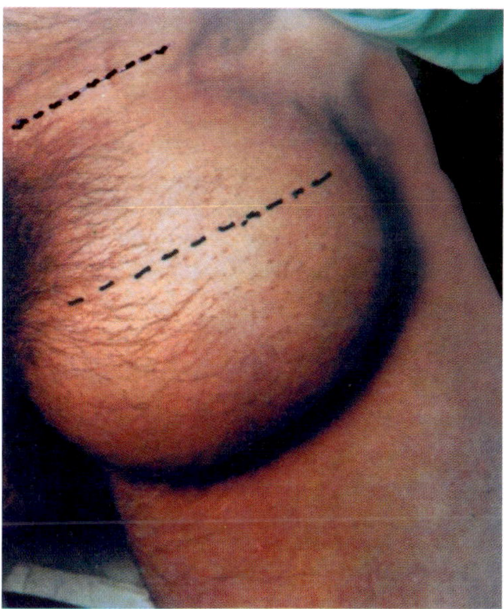

Fig. 76.2 Skin incision. Parallel to inguinal ligament

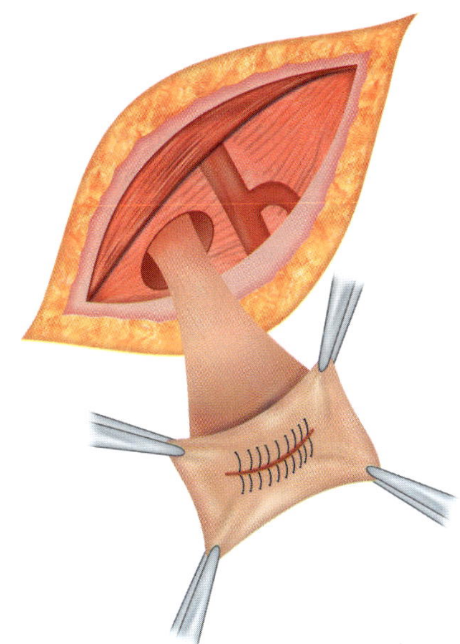

Fig. 76.4 Dealing with the sac

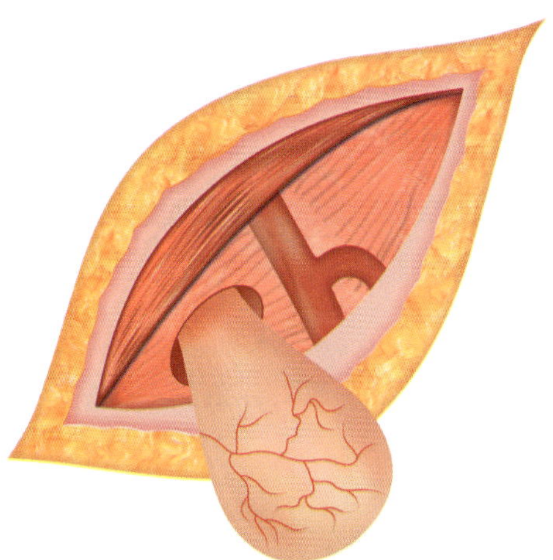

Fig. 76.3 Exposure of sac

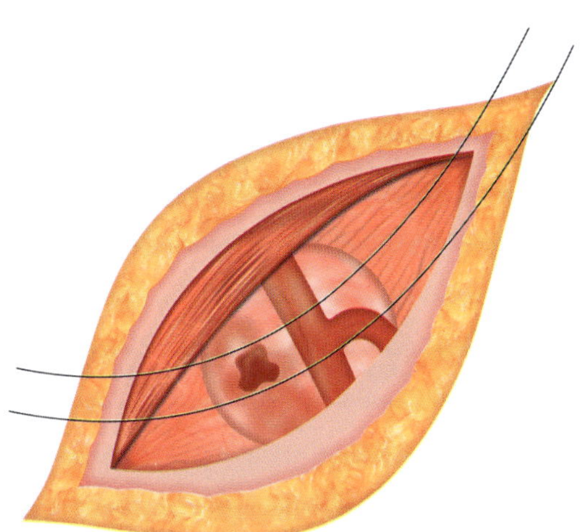

Fig. 76.5 Repair

Operative technique

- *Dealing with the sac:* The sac covered by extraperitoneal fat is cleaned by blunt dissection. Hold the sac with artery forceps and dissect it up to neck below the inguinal ligament. The sac is opened cautiously taking care that the bladder may form the medial wall of the sac. Examine the contents and reduce it if it is viable (Fig. 76.4).

  Transfix the neck of sac and excise the redundant parts, taking care not to injure bowel or bladder. The femoral veins lies laterally and should be retracted during this step.
- *Repair:* Ideally the repair is done by suturing the inguinal ligament (Cooper's ligament) to pectineal with 1/0 proline suture. But technically this is difficult from below. The simplest alternative is obliteration of the space previously occupied by hernia by 2 or 3 stitches passing through fascia forming the floor and lateral margin of the saphenous opening. A purse string repair taking bite through inguinal ligament then alternately through lacunar ligament, the pectineal fascia, the fascia over medial aspect of femoral vein and then through inguinal ligament is also been recommended. Alternatively, the femoral canal can be closed with a 'plug' of rolled mesh, secured with sutures using 2/0 proline, to surrounding fibrous tissue (Fig. 76.5).
- *Closure:* Close the skin with 2/0 ethilon.

Preperitoneal Approach: McEvedy

This approach is preferred in case of strangulated femoral hernia. It does not weaken the inguinal canal.

Incision: The femoral hernia can be approached through a suprainguinal, Pfannenstiel, midline or pararectal (McEvedy) incision.

Exposure: Deepen the incision to reach the anterior rectus sheath. The anterior rectus sheath is incised and the rectus muscle retracted medially.

Open the preperitoneal space by blunt dissection continue the process downwards towards the inguinal ligament and identify sac.

Operative technique

- *Dealing with sac*: If the sac is empty, reduce it back into abdomen by pushing from below and gently pulling from above.

  If there is difficulty in reducing hernia, medial edge of femoral ring can be sharply divided, taking care of aberrant obturator artery.

  The sac is opened and contents examined. Nonviable gut should be treated by resection and anastomosis. The sac is excised.
- *Repair:* The femoral ring is now obliterated by stitching inguinal ligament to pectineal ligament by 2/0 proline stitches. The plug repair is an alternative in which a strip of mesh is anchored to femoral canal by 4/5 stitches.
- *Closure:* The anterior rectus sheath is closed with 0 proline. The skin is stitched with ethilon.

High Approach—Lothisen

This approach is now seldom used as it damages the inguinal canal. The inguinal canal is opened and the transversalis fascia is divided to reach the femoral hernia sac.

POSTOPERATIVE CARE

- Early oral feed should be started
- Early ambulation
- Systemic antibiotic.

POSTOPERATIVE COMPLICATIONS

- Sepsis
- Injury to femoral vein
- Injury to bladder
- Recurrence.

Laparoscopic preperitoneal femoral hernia repair is possible but not widely used.

CHAPTER

77

Inguinal Hernia: Laparoscopic Repair

C Palanivelu

INTRODUCTION

The revolutionary success of laparoscopic cholecystectomy, has resulted in an intense effort to apply this concept of minimally invasive surgery to other operative procedures like inguinal hernia. Unfortunately the initial enthusiasm in laparoscopic herniorrhaphy, was met with a disappointing early recurrence rates, which was as high as 25% in some series. But, now with the decade of experience in laparoscopic hernia surgery, the dust seems settling down more towards accepting the superiority of the laparoscopic repairs over conventional surgeries. This is mainly due to the proper understanding of endoscopic inguinal anatomy, effacement of initial procedures like plug and patch technique, refinement of the techniques, introduction of the preperitoneal placement of mesh, etc.

The laparoscopic hernioplasty represents an amalgamation of principles of conventional preperitoneal hernia repair and minimally invasive surgery. The mesh is placed in the preperitoneal layer covering the entire myopectineal orifice. The preperitoneal mesh uses the forces available from within the preperitoneal space to keep the mesh in position between the abdominal layers. It is very difficult to dislodge a mesh in the preperitoneal space, as the intra-abdominal pressure equally exerts on the entire prosthesis helping to fix the prosthesis within the abdominal layer overlying the defect.

Laparoscopic hernioplasty has several advantages over its "open" counter part. First, and often the most important from the patients point of view, the reduced postoperative pain and very short recovery period. Second, the entire myopectineal orifice can be inspected bilaterally, allowing for repair of any unexpected hernias thereby reducing the chance for recurrence. Third, laparoscopic hernioplasty avoids the previous operative scar site in patients with recurrent hernias.

ANATOMY

Till recently most of the descriptions of the surgical anatomy of the inguinal region began with the anterior layer proceeding to deeper layers. Now, the same anatomy from the laparoscopic surgeon's perspective begins with the inner most aspect and proceeds to superficial layers. Certain structures such as iliopubic tract, Coopers ligament are more obvious from inside while certain structures like inguinal ligament, pubic tubercle are more evident in the conventional dissection from anterior layer. For the purpose of brevity, we will keep the description of conventional inguinal anatomy to minimum and concentrate on the anatomy from laparoscopic perspective.

CONVENTIONAL ANATOMY

The inguinal canal is an oblique space measuring 4 cm in length, and extending 2–4 cm above the inguinal ligament between the superficial and deep inguinal rings. It appears triangular in cross-section and it courses from lateral to medial, deep to superficial and cephalad to caudal. The deep inguinal ring is an opening in the transversalis fascia at the level of the mid-point of the inguinal ligament. The external ring is a small slit like opening in the aponeurosis of the external abdominal oblique located just above and lateral to the pubic tubercle. The inguinal canal envelopes the spermatic cord in males and the round ligament in females. The inguinal ligament is the folded inferior portion of external oblique aponeurosis that extends from anterosuperior iliac spine to pubic tubercle. The inguinal ligament forms a bridge across the iliopsoas muscle underneath which the femoral vessels and nerves pass from the pelvic cavity to the thigh compartment. The fan shaped medial expansion of the inguinal ligament is called as the *lacunar ligament*. This forms the most medial part of the inguinal canal.

Laparoscopic Anatomy

Having familiarized ourselves with the conventional anatomy, we will discuss the laparoscopic anatomy of the inguinal canal. A person may be perplexed by a totally new view of anatomy, when he sees a laparoscopic hernia repair being performed for the first time. This view of posterior wall of the groin is in total contrast with what the general surgeon is familiar. We will restrict ourselves to the most relevant anatomical landmarks, which are of practical importance. As soon as the laparoscope is inserted into the peritoneal cavity and turned to inguinal region, the surgeon faces the peritoneal landmarks, which need to be identified. Once these landmarks are identified, the orientation becomes much clearer.

Median umbilical ligament is the peritoneal fold, which is present in the midline from the fundus of the urinary bladder to the umbilicus. This represents the obliterated urachus. As we move the scope from the midline to lateral aspects, the first fold to be visualized on either side is the *medial umbilical ligament.* This represents the obliterated umbilical artery through with the fetal circulation was maintained. This fold varies size from person to person and from side to side in the same patient. Further lateral to the medial umbilical ligament is the inferior epigastric artery which courses from the external iliac vessel towards the lateral border of the rectus muscle to form the *lateral umbilical ligament.* This fold is usually seen well, but is not clearly seen in obese patients as this area is covered with fat.

The area between the median and medial umbilical ligament is known as *supra vesical fossa* which is usually protected by the rectus muscle. The area between medial and lateral fold is the *medial fossa* through which direct hernia passes and the area lateral to the lateral fold is termed as *lateral fossa* through which indirect hernia passes through.

Triangle of Doom

Once the folds and the fossa are identified the scope is directed towards the caudal aspect of the inferior epigastric artery. This is the area of the internal inguinal ring where the vas deferens from the seminal vesicle and the testicular vessels from the aorta converge to form the cord structures. The triangle formed by these structures is known as *Triangle of doom.*

Triangle of Pain

The area bounded superiorly by the iliopubic tract and medially by the testicular vessels is a dangerous area where all the branches of lumbar plexus (genital and femoral branches of genitofemoral nerve, femoral nerve and lateral femoral cutaneous nerve) are present. Any staple or suture placed in this area is likely to produce a transient neuropraxia, permanent neuralgias or weakness of the muscles supplied by these nerves.

Inferior epigastric artery forms an important landmark. The *Hasselbachs triangle* is formed by inferior epigastric artery as lateral border, rectus sheath as the medial border and inguinal ligament as the inferior border.

Cooper's ligament is the shiny fibrous structure covering the superior pubic ramus is a blend of fibrous periosteum, recurved fibers of iliopubic tract and inguinal ligament. It is one of the most useful landmarks to the surgeon as a strong anchoring structure for both open and laparoscopic herniorrhaphy.

The anatomy of the inguinofemoral canal is much more detailed once the peritoneum is incised and preperitoneal space is reached. The deep inguinal ring, iliopubic tract, Cooper's ligament and femoral canal all are exposed after the peritoneal reflection. Once deep inguinal ring is identified the structures such as iliopubic tract, Cooper's ligament and the inferior epigastric vessels can be identified easily. Iliopubic tract is seen coursing from lateral to medial aspect in the same direction of inguinal ligament. The space above iliopubic tract and medial to the inferior epigastric vessels is the area of direct hernia. The space above the iliopubic tract and lateral to the inferior epigastric vessel is the area of indirect hernia. The femoral hernia passes through the defect between the iliopubic tract anteriorly and superior ramus of pubis posteriorly. The femoral canal is bounded the medially the recurved fibers of the iliopubic tract and laterally by the femoral vein.

LAPAROSCOPIC HERNIOPLASTY

Laparoscopic hernia repair can be performed in two ways, the TAPP (transabdominal preperitoneal) and TEP (Totally extraperitoneal) approach. A surgeon must be experienced in conventional anterior approaches as well as both laparoscopic approaches (TAPP and TEP) in order to make a rational decision on which hernioplasty best fits an individual patient. For most patients we prefer the TEP approach because it avoids entering the peritoneal cavity, requires less operative time, and has less potential complications than the TAPP approach. I choose TAPP for selective indications where TEP cannot be done such as incarcerated hernia, very large scrotal hernia, etc. The laparoscopic approach is ideally suited for recurrent hernias, whether TAPP or TEP approach should be dependent upon the expertise of the surgeon. The dissection of the recurrent hernial sac can be difficult using the TEP approach and requires more skill than that of a primary repair.

Transabdominal Preperitoneal Hernioplasty

The transabodinal preperitoneal (TAPP) approach can be performed in almost all types of inguinofemoral hernia depending on the level of expertise of the surgeon. Patients unsuitable for general anesthesia, presence of active infection or inflammatory process like peritonitis, incarcerated hernia and large irreducible long standing scrotal hernia (scrotal abdomen) are absolute contraindications for this type.

Operative Technique

The patient is placed in supine position with arms by the side. The patient is given 10° head down position at this time to allow the bowel loops to fall away from the groin region. The position of the surgeon and the camera assistant is always on the same position regardless of the side of the hernia as shown in Figure 77.1.

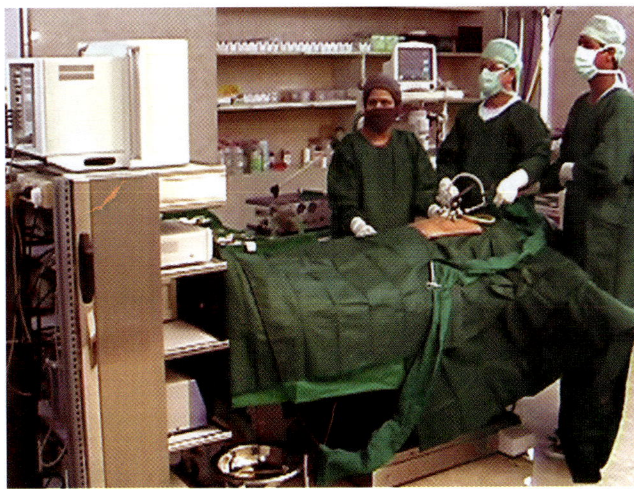

Fig. 77.1 Position of patient, surgeon and assistant

Pneumoperitoneum is created either by Veress needle technique or open laparoscopy technique. In the absence of operative scar, periumbilical site (thinnest site) is the most preferred site for Veress needle insertion. Depending on the shape of umbilicus either transverse or vertical stab is made, the Veress needle is inserted perpendicular to the abdomen with a slight degree of tilt so that tip of the needle feces the pelvis. Aspiration test is used to confirm the position of the needle in the abdominal cavity. Five milliliter of saline is injected through the Veress and aspirated. If aspiration does not yield the injected solution, then the position of the needle in the peritoneal cavity is confirmed. If the saline is aspirated back into the syringe then it indicates that the needle is within the layers of the abdominal wall or the presence of adhesions. In patients who had undergone surgeries before, we prefer insertion of the Veress needle in either right or left hypochondrium (Palmar's point) for creation of pneumoperitoneum. We routinely use 3 mm scope initially through the first port and under vision we create the umbilical port, subsequently changing the scope to 10 mm. The epigastric and the right iliac fossa are the other sites for needle insertion. After creating the pneumoperitoneum with Veress needle, 1 cm transverse or vertical incision according to the shape of the umbilicus is made and the camera trocar is inserted. Some surgeons use Hasson's technique with specialized cannula to decrease the incidence of visceral injuries. We place the camera port in the umbilicus in majority of the patients and the two working trocars just lateral to rectus sheath on either side of umbilicus, few cms below the camera port (Fig. 77.2).

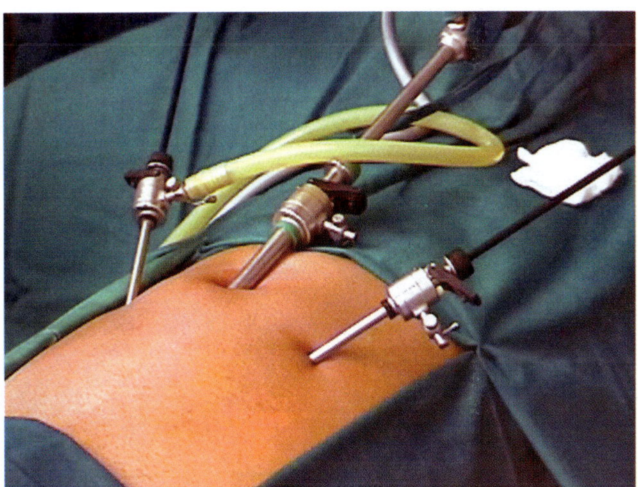

Fig. 77.2 Trocar position

The basic technique consists of reduction of contents, peritoneal incision and dissection of the entire myopectineal orifice, placement and fixation of mesh (Fig. 77.3).

After creation of ports the contents of the sac are gently pulled into the abdominal cavity with the help of instruments from the two working ports. A horizontal peritoneal incision is made above the defect to extending from the medial umbilical ligament to the level of anterior superior iliac spine (Fig. 77.4). The peritoneal flaps are dissected above and below to expose the entire area.

Dissection: Dissection in the area of direct hernias is relatively an easy task. The thinned out transversalis fascia termed as pseudosac, can be readily identified by its glistening appearance. The peritoneum and the preperitoneal fat can

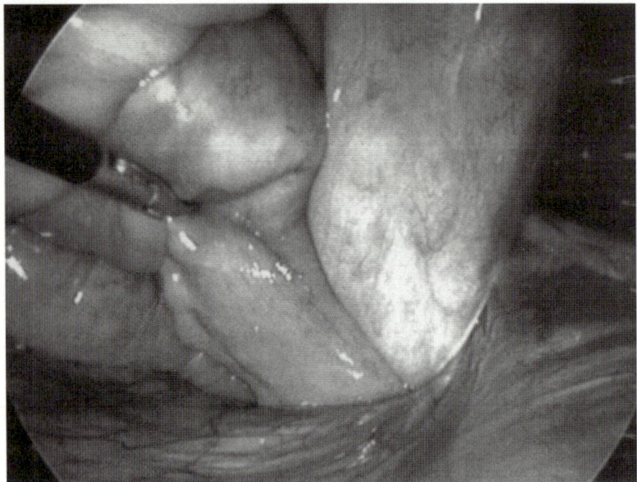

Fig. 77.3 Reduction of contents

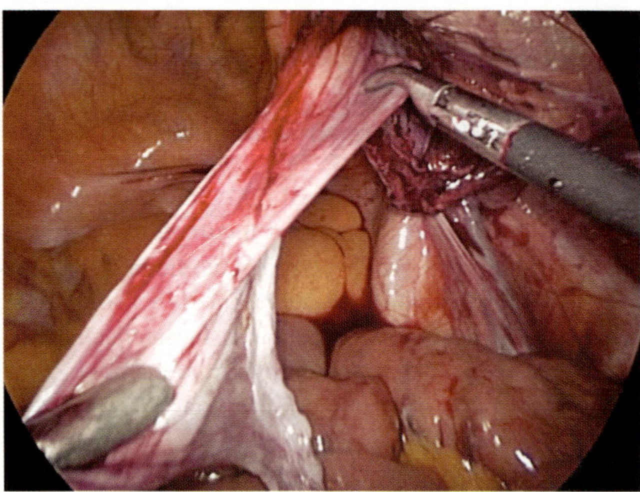

Fig. 77.5 Dissection of sac from cord structures

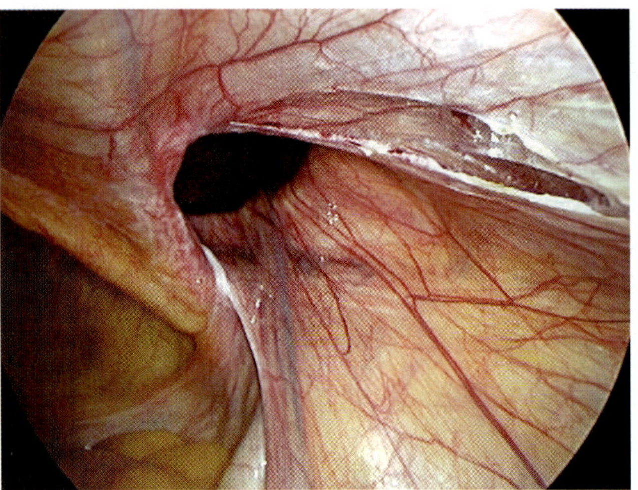

Fig. 77.4 Peritoneal incision above the defect

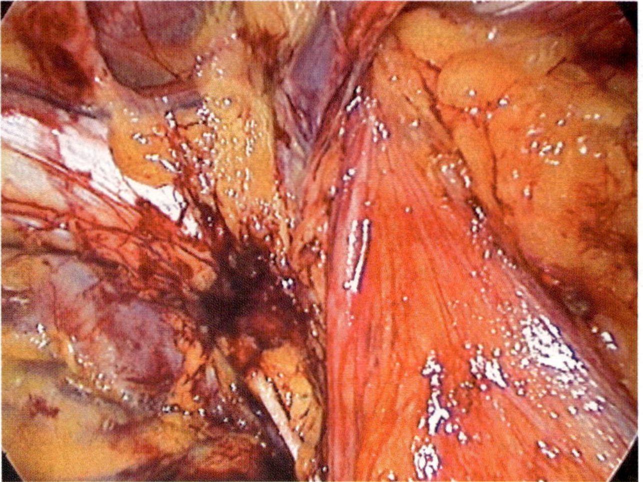

Fig. 77.6 Completion of medial dissection

be easily separated from this pseudosac by gentle traction. The medial aspect of the myopectineal orifice is dissected by gentle atraumatic dissection. Early identification of certain anatomical structures at this stage is considered vital for safe completion of the surgery. Epigastric vessels, symphysis pubis, pubic ramus and Cooper's ligament are the important structures that require prompt recognition. Care is taken during dissection beneath the iliopubic tract to avoid injury to nerves (Triangle of Pain) and vessels (Triangle of Doom).

The dissection in the lateral compartment is more challenging as the sac is densely adherent to the cord structures in long standing hernias. The relationship of the hernial sac and cord structures is usually constant. The hernial sac is usually present above and lateral to the spermatic cord. At the level of the deep ring the vas deferens curves medially over the iliac vessels after emerging out of the pelvis. The testicular vessels are located on the lateral aspect. The sac is carefully separated from the cord structures and divided at the highest possible level (Fig. 77.5). For larger sacs extending deep into the scrotum, particularly congenital type, complete mobilization of the sac is more traumatic and chances of injury to cord structures are increased. In these situations, hernial sac is divided beyond the internal ring within the canal, leaving the distal end of the sac *in situ* (Fig. 77.6).

Once the hernial sac is reduced or divided, the peritoneum is separated from the vas and gonadal vessels towards the cranial aspect. This procedure is known as parietalization (Fig. 77.7). Extensive parietalization is important to position the currently recommended larger sized (15 × 12 cm) unslit mesh. Inadequate mobilization leads to displacement and folding of the mesh and eventually to recurrence. The dissection should be at least 1–2 cm beyond the edges of the mesh on all sides.

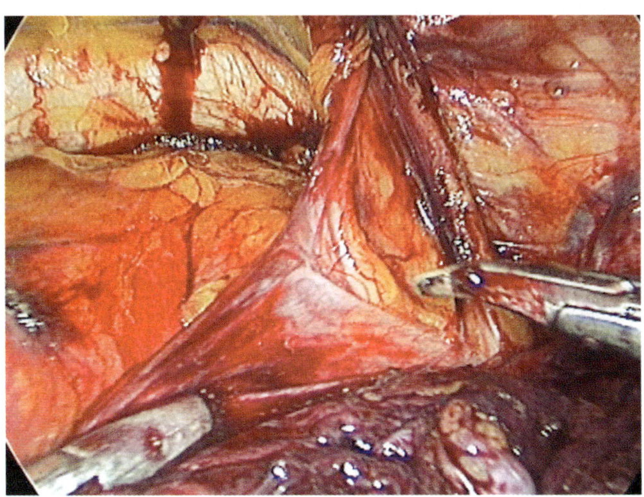

Fig. 77.7 Parietalization

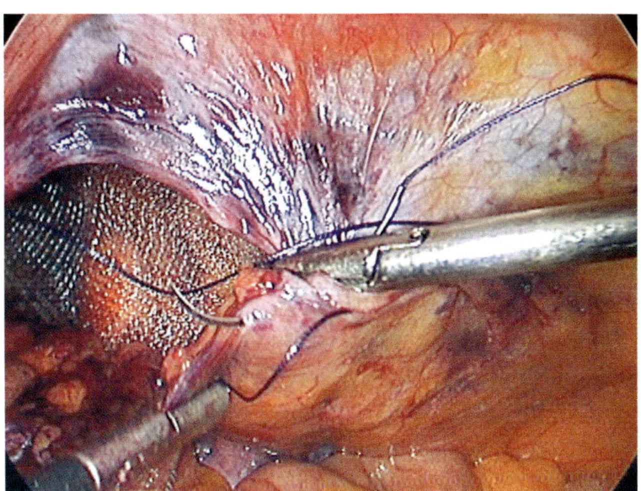

Fig. 77.9 Suturing of peritoneum over the mesh

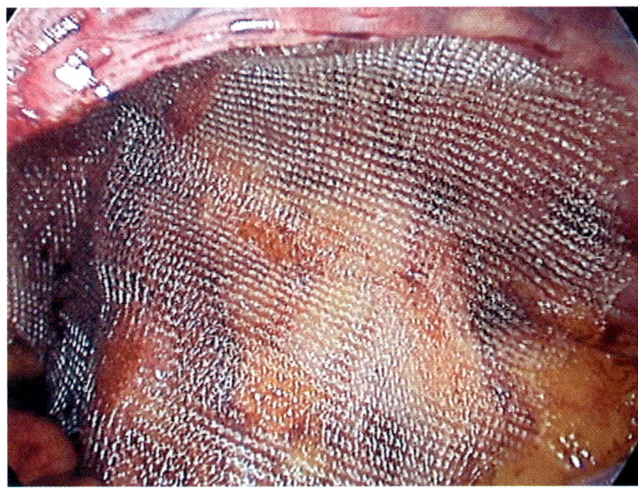

Fig. 77.8 Placement of mesh

Before placement of the mesh flap should be lifted and the extent of dissection verified. The dissected space should extend beyond the midline on the medial aspect, beyond the anterosuperior iliac spine exposing the psoas muscle on the lateral aspect, inferiorly up to the symphysis pubis and the level of obturator foramen and superiorly up to the level of working trocars. The peritoneum should be free from the vas deferens and testicular vessels. This wide dissection is needed to ensure problem free placement a 15 × 12 cm mesh.

Placement and fixation of mesh: The corners of a 15 × 12 cm polypropylene mesh are trimmed and taken into the abdominal cavity by reverse loading technique as shown in Figure 77.8 through the 10 mm camera port. Once inside the dissected space, the mesh most often unfolds by itself and spreading of the mesh becomes much easier. The mesh is positioned to cover the entire myopectineal orifice of Fruchaud (direct, indirect and femoral defects).

The conventional needle of 1-0 polypropylene suture material is slightly straightened, and taken into the peritoneal cavity in a similar fashion as mesh. The mesh is fixed to the Cooper's ligament inferiorly and to the rectus muscle on the superomedial aspect of the mesh, by intracorporeal suturing method. Apart from these areas, we do not fix the mesh on the lateral aspect. As the area of triangle of Doom and triangle of pain are totally avoided, the incidence of vascular injuries and neuralgias are negligible following this approach. Alternatively the mesh can be fixed with the mechanical fixation devices such as hernia stapler, tacker and anchors if the surgeon is not well versed in intracorporeal. We prefer suturing as it is more effective and reduces the cost of surgery (Fig. 77.9).

After the placement of the mesh the peritoneum is sutured over the mesh to prevent adhesions of bowel or omentum. The peritoneal flap can be closed either by suturing with absorbable sutures or with the help of hernia staplers or tackers. A long acting local anesthetic can be injected into the peritoneal space at this stage to reduce postoperative discomfort.

The 5 mm trocar sites are closed with subcuticular sutures while the camera port requires closure of the rectus sheath separately before closing the skin to prevent trocar site herniation.

The TAPP is more widely used because of its relative ease to learn this technique. Invasion into the peritoneal space for treatment of defect in the abdominal wall is one of the major drawbacks of this technique. Insufficient closure of this incision will lead to formation of internal hernias with its antecedent complications. Because of these concerns, laparoscopic surgeons are now switching towards TEP repair. Still TAPP will remain as an ideal approach for management of difficult inguinal hernias such as incarcerated hernias, sliding hernias and other complex hernias.

Extraperitoneal Approach

The extraperitoneal approach is made possible by the fact that the peritoneum in the suprapubic region can be easily separated from the anterior abdominal wall. This space can be enlarged to help in dissection of the hernial sac and insertion of mesh. Several techniques have been used to create this space, e.g. Phillips, McKernan and Dulucq's technique. Our approach is the posterior rectus sheath approach, where the trocar enters the plane between the rectus muscle and posterior rectus sheath just above the preperitoneal space. A 2 cm infraumbilical incision is created and the rectus sheath is exposed. The rectus sheath is lifted and incised vertically exposing the rectus muscles. Retractors are placed beneath the rectus muscle and a tunnel is developed between the rectus muscle and the underlying posterior rectus sheath.

Operative Technique

Incision: With the patient in the supine position, we begin the procedure with a 12 mm subumbilical incision extending up to linea alba. The skin and subcutaneous tissue are retracted to the side of the hernia or to the dominant side (usually the right). The subcutaneous tissue is dissected to expose the anterior rectus sheath. The specially designed retractor helps to retract the subcutaneous tissue and fat. The anterior rectus sheath is incised transversely and it is separated with a curved hemostat to expose the rectus muscle. The entire rectus muscle is retracted to anterolateral side to enter the space between the muscle and posterior rectus sheath. The curved hemostat is inserted and the space is widened for introduction of the trocar. The outer cannula of a 10 mm reusable trocar with its oblique end is carefully guided into the space between muscle and the rectus sheath. The wound is approximated with a thick suture material. Wet gauze is plugged between the suture and the wound to prevent leakage of gas. The same suture material is kept long and tied to the insufflation channel to prevent slippage of the trocar out of the incision. A 10 mm Hassons cannula is inserted into this tunnel and further space is created by blunt introduction of the 0° scope and the additional ports are created.

Extraperitoneal dissection: A 10 mm telescope (0°) is introduced into the trocar. The scope is then moved downward on the sheath, allowing it to fall between the rectus muscle and the posterior rectus sheath. The telescope is moved forward and backward through the cobweb areolar tissue towards the pubic symphysis. These movements divide the transversalis fascia and the extraperitoneal space is entered. The dissected space is maintained by continuous CO_2 insufflation at 12–14 mm Hg. Moving the telescope at various directions widens the space created. We feel that use of balloon is not necessary and it also increases the cost of the surgery (Fig. 77.10).

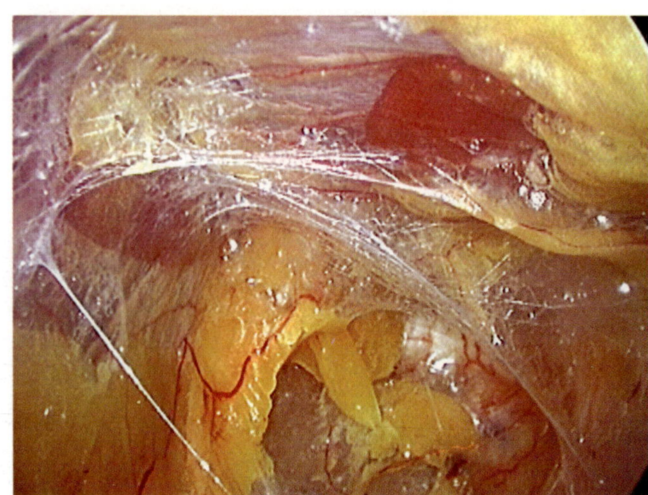

Fig. 77.10 Creation of pre-peritoneal space

Creation of working ports: In case of right inguinal hernia the left hand working port is made just lateral to the midline about 5 cm below the level of the camera port. The extraperitoneal space is widened on the right lateral aspect and the right hand working port is placed on the right pararectus as shown in Figure 77.10. In case of wide rectus muscle the lateral working port 5 mm is introduced in between the umbilicus and anterior superior iliac spine as laterally as possible (preferably just medial to the lateral rectus sheath fusion). The surgeon moves to the head end of the patient for the rest of the procedure.

Two hand technique: The position of the trocars in this technique is deserves special mention. Most of the techniques that have been described till now, have all the trocars in the midline. This arrangement of the trocars in the midline is associated with a relatively acute, unfavorable working angle resulting in crowding of the instruments. In our approach triangulation of instruments (70° angle between the working trocars) is maintained as in any other laparoscopic surgery. This arrangement follows the basic ergonomic principles of laparoscopy. Dissection of preperitoneal space and placement of mesh is easier in this two hand technique. Even difficult hernias can be dealt with ease by this approach.

Medial dissection: Further dissection is performed as in the TAPP approach and the entire myopectineal orifice

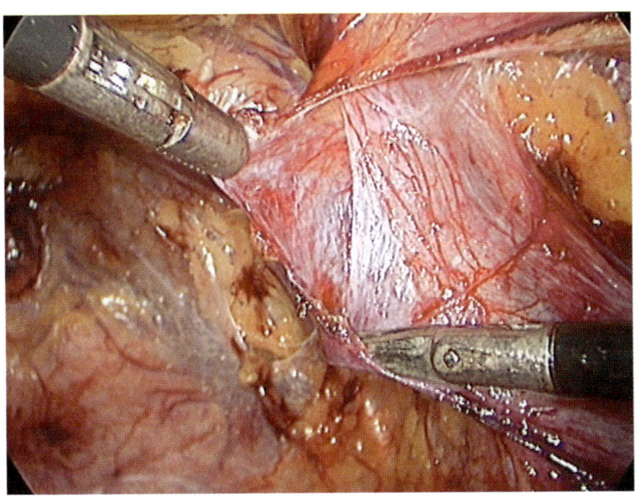

Fig. 77.11 Separation of sac from transversalis fascia sling

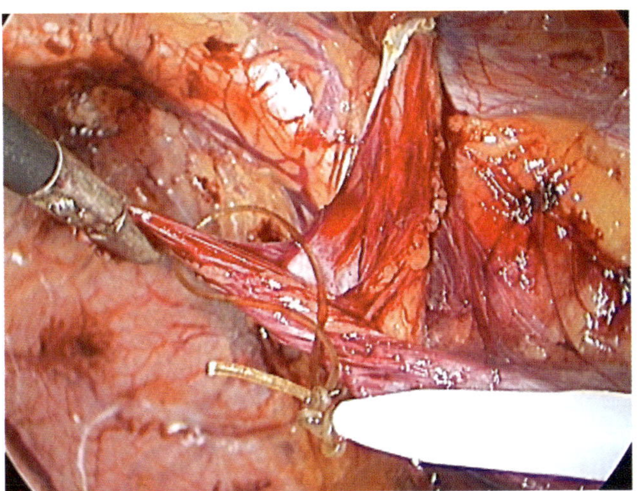

Fig. 77.12 Endoloop applied to the proximal sac after division

is dissected out. A similar sized mesh is taken inside and ancored to the Cooper's ligament and the anterior rectus sheath.

Lateral dissection: The dissection into lateral inguinal fossa begins by dividing the transversalis fascial extension. The left hand grasper gives traction on the sling and curved dissector is used to dissect between the sling and the sac (Fig. 77.11). In case of direct hernia, the peritoneal edge will easily separated from the internal ring. In indirect hernia, the sac should be separated from the cord structures which is usually seen on the posterior aspect.

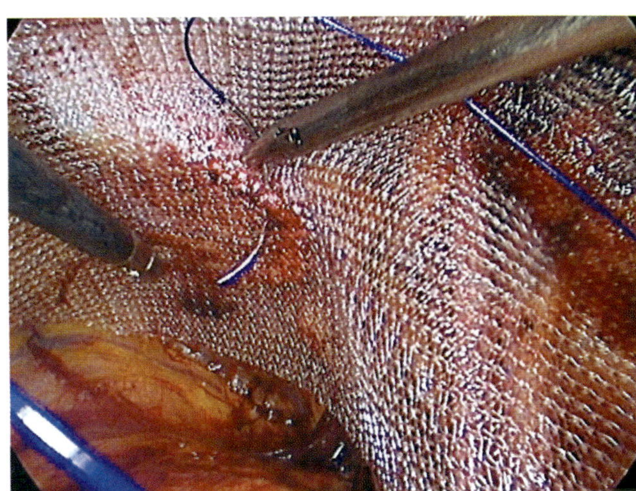

Fig. 77.13 Fixation of mesh

After the proximal sac is completely separated from the distal aspect and the cord structures, it is divided and ligated with as endoloop (Fig. 77.12).

Parietalization: The entire posterior floor should be dissected in all eases of TEP.

Placement of mesh and fixation: The mesh is trimmed and then introduced into the dissected space and fixed by suturing (Fig. 77.13).

POSTOPERATIVE MANAGEMENT

We allow the patient to take liquids after the recovery from general anesthesia and encourage moving in the room by evening. The patients usually use the toilet by evening. Adequate analgesia is given through rectal (diclofenac) suppositories. We tend to keep the patients for a day in the hospital and discharge them on the 1st postoperative day. Patients are allowed to take normal diet on the 1 postoperative day and advised to carry on with their normal routine work as per their level of comfort.

CONCLUSION

Out technique of extraperitoneal repair (TEP) is more comfortable and highly effective in the laparoscopic management of inguinal hernias. Our port placement and 2 hand technique maintains the triangular orientation which is considered vital as per the ergonomics of laparoscopy. Nearly 98–99% of inguinal hernias can be treated by TEP approach.

SECTION

16

Genitourinary Surgery

CHAPTER

78

Surgical Approaches to Kidney

Dhiraj Choudhury

ANATOMY

The kidneys measuring 10 cm long, 5 cm wide and 2.5 cm thick, are retroperitoneal organs situated in the upper parts of the paravertebral gutters on the sides of the D, L, L and L, vertebrae. The upper pole of the right kidney lies at a lower level than the left.

The kidney is enclosed by (inside outwards) (a) fibrous capsule, (b) perirenal fat, (c) renal fascia (fascia of Zukar Kandal which also encloses suprarenal) and (d) pararenal fat.

The hilum is a vertical slit on the medial (concave) border of the kidney situated in the transpyloric plain 1-½" from midline. It transmits—ureter, renal artery and renal vein placed posteroanteriorly. Each renal artery arises from aorta, and each renal vein drains into inferior vena cava.

Posteriorly, the upper part of the kidney lies on the diaphragm and is related to pleura and 12th rib. The lower part lies on psoas, quadratus and transversus from medial to lateral side. Between kidney and quadratus are subcostal vessels, and subcostal, iliohypogastric and ilioinguinal nerves.

Anteriorly, right kidney is directly related to 2nd part of the duodenum and right colic flexure; the left kidney to pancreas and splenic vessels. Laterally, the right kidney is related to the ascending colon; the left kidney to left colic flexure and descending colon.

SURGICAL APPROACHES TO KIDNEY

Posterolateral Approach

The patient is placed in a lateral position on the healthy side with the lower limb flexed and upper limb extended. An axillary roll is placed under the lower dependent arm. The position is maintained by applying adhesive tape or strap. Kidney rest is elevated (Fig. 78.1)

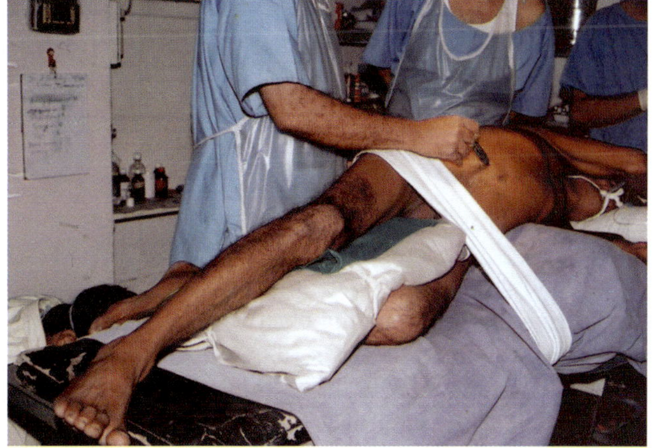

Fig. 78.1 Position of patient for posterolateral approach

Nagamatsu's Thoracolumbar Approach

Here the lumbar incision is extended vertically upwards towards the chest wall. This is an extrapleural extension of the lumbar incision or incision excising 12th rib.

Anterior Transperitoneal Approach

This is indicated for malignant tumors of the kidney for carrying out radical nephrectomy. By this approach the blood vessels can be dealt with before mobilization of the kidney. A transverse muscle cutting incision is preferred. A paramedian incision can be used to open peritoneal cavity.

CHAPTER

79

Nephrostomy

Dhiraj Choudhury

INDICATIONS

Acute pyonephrosis (obstructed infected kidney) requires urgent drainage which can be carried out in the following ways:

Percutaneous Nephrostomy

Ultrasound-guided percutaneous nephrostomy is usually the best method to drain the obstructed infected kidney, under local anesthesia and under ultrasonographic guidance a fine bore hollow needle is introduced through flank. Through parenchyma into expended collecting system of the obstructed kidney. A wire is inserted through the lumen of the needle to act as guide for insertion of number of dilators to enlarge the track. A suitably sized nephrostomy tube is now inserted.

INSERTION OF J-STENT

This allows drainage of ureter into bladder. Under fluoroscopic control a guidewire is introduced through cystoscope and guided into renal pelvis. The J-shaped stent is rail roaded over the guidewire until its distal and lies within the renal pelvis above the site of obstruction. When the guidewire is removed the end of the stent curl to form J-shape. The stent can be left in position for several months.

OPEN NEPHROSTOMY

It is indicated when percutaneous method could not be established or pus is too thick to be drained by small caliber tube.

Preoperative Preparations

Adequate rehydration and administration of broad spectrum antibiotic. The site to be operated should be marked.

Steps

The operation is done under general anesthesia.

Position: The patient is placed in lateral position with side to be operated upper most. Lower limb flexed and upper limb extended. Kidney rest is elevated.

Incision: A standard posterolateral (loin) incision is made.

Expose the kidney which appears swollen, make a small transverse pyelotomy and insert the tube.

CHAPTER

80

Treatment of Renal Stones

Dhiraj Choudhury

Renal stones can be treated by the following methods:

- Extracorporeal shock wave lithotripsy (ESWL)
- Percutaneous nephrolithotomy (PCNL)
- Open surgery.

Extracorporeal shock wave lithotripsy (ESWL): Calcium stones and magnesium ammonium phosphate stones can be successfully treated by ESWL. Because of the physical properties of the crystal lattice ESWL is not effective in fragmenting cystine stones. The shock wave produced by the electrode are focused and directed at the stone by two dimensional radiographic systems. The average patient receives 100–1500 shock wave pulses. After 200 pulses the stone begins to fragment. The small fragments are passed in urine. Less than 10% of patients treated with ESWL require endourological or surgical treatment.

PERCUTANEOUS NEPHROLITHOTOMY

In selected patients percutaneous stone removal may be successful. A percutaneous tract enters the renal collecting system through an appropriate calyx (percutaneous nephrostomy). The tract is then dilated and endoscopic extraction of stone is carried out. Pulverization by means of ultrasonic, electrohydraulic or laser probe passed through nephrostomy tract may be useful. The advantages include local anesthesia, no incision and rapid recovery. The disadvantage is that there may be need for multiple treatment.

Open Surgical Removal

Endourologic intervention and ESWL have markedly decreased the indications for open surgery. Now-a-days open surgery is rarely required when PCNL and ESWL are not available.

Procedure

- *Position:* The patient is placed on operating table in lateral position
- *Anesthesia:* General endotracheal

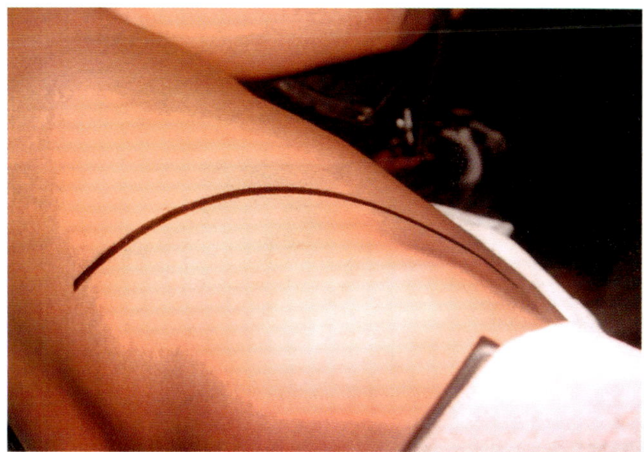

Fig. 80.1 Loin incision

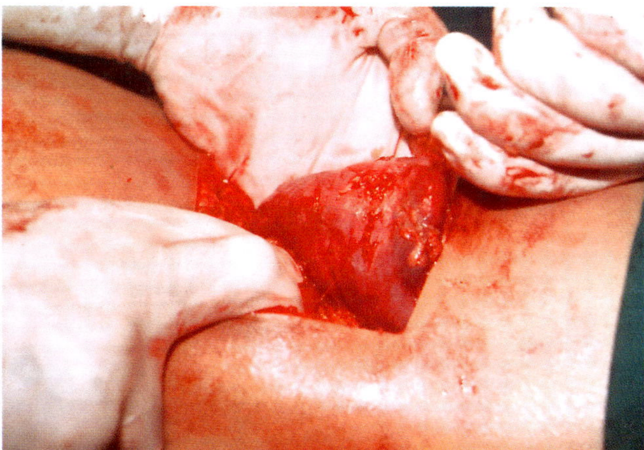

Fig. 80.2 Exposure of posterior surface of pelvis of the kidney

- *Incision:* The kidney is exposed by standard loin incision described in (Fig. 80.1)
- *Exposure:* The kidney is exposed and delivered to the wound by steps similar to those described under nephrectomy. The posterior surface of the pelvis of the kidney is dissected free of the surrounding fat (Fig. 80.2).

Technique

Pyelolithotomy

This is indicated for stone in the renal pelvis. Palpate the stone in the pelvis and steady it between fingers. Two stay sutures with 3/0 catgut may be applied. A small posterior longitudinal incision is made directly over the stone. The stone is then extracted with Desjardin's forceps or any stone holding forceps. In case of intra-renal pelvis retraction of kidney substance will allow incision on the renal pelvis (Figs 80.3A to C).

Closure

- A ureteric stent is passed downwards through the ureter (Fig. 80.4)
- Close the rent in the renal pelvis with interrupted 3/0 catgut sutures
- A corrugated or tube drain is inserted.

Extended Pyelolithotomy

For removal of stag horn calculus Gil-Vernet technique may be used. Fully mobilize the kidney and gently remove the peripelvic fat from the posterior aspect of the renal pelvis. Apply small retractors under the parenchyma which is gradually pushed back off the renal pelvis with a peanut swab. The renal pelvis is opened longitudinally. The length and direction of the incision varies according to the shape of the contained stone. Remove the stone with the help of stone holding forceps (Fig. 80.5).

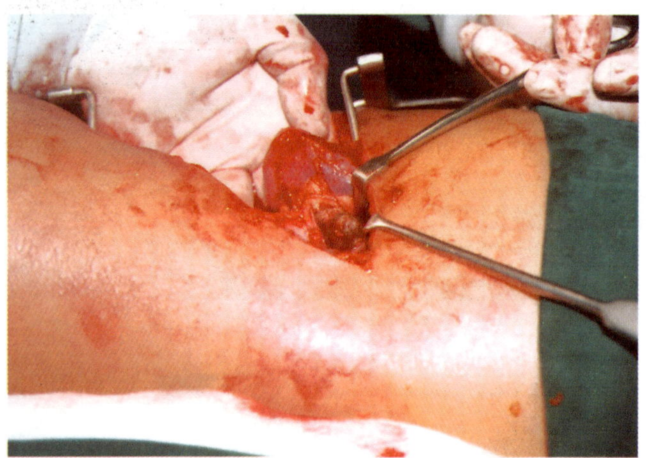

Fig. 80.3A Palpation of stone

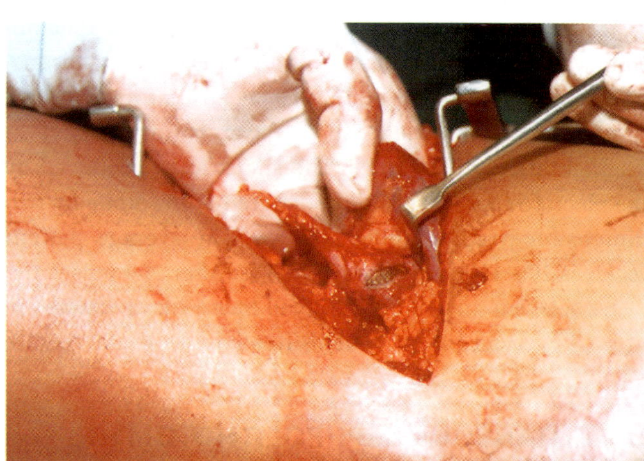

Fig. 80.3B Longitudinal incision on pelvis over the stone

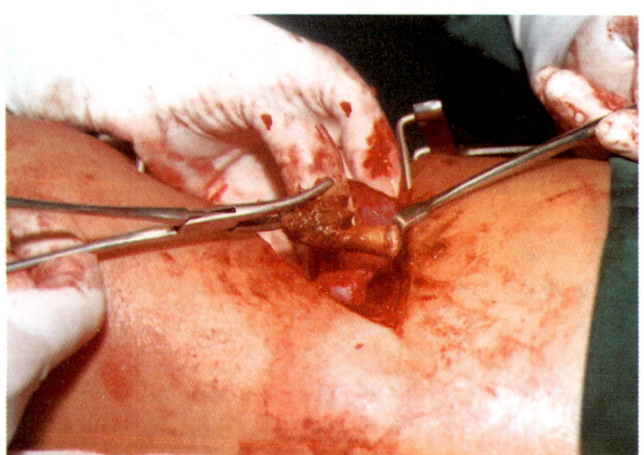

Fig. 80.3C Removal of stone from pelvis

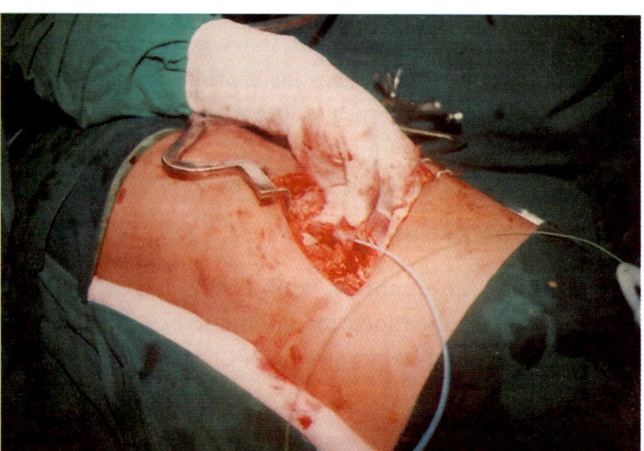

Fig. 80.4 Introduction of ureteric stent

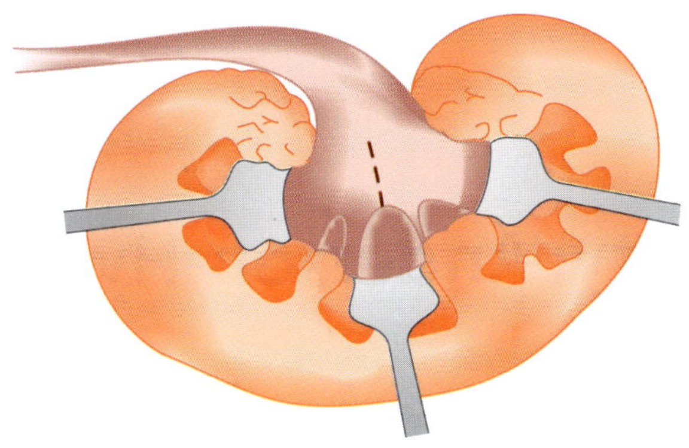

Fig. 80.5 Schematic diagram of extended pyelolithotomy

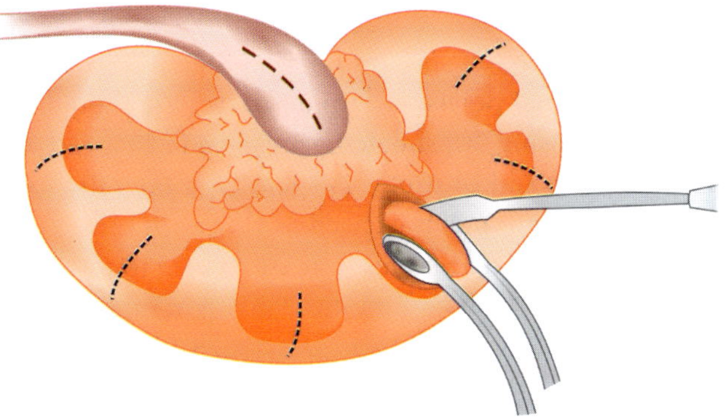

Fig. 80.6 Schematic diagram of pyelolithotomy and direct nephrolithotomy

Nephrolithotomy

This is indicated for removal of stones from the renal calyces.
Exposure: The kidney is exposed by standard lumbar incision.
Technique: A solitary stone in the calyx may be (Fig. 80.6) removed by direct radial nephrotomy.

The incision is then closed by interrupted catgut stitches. For removal of stag horn calculus or multiple stones, the kidney is cooled with sterile ice specks and the pedicle is temporarily clamped.

Make a nephrotomy through the Brodel's line (5 mm behind and parallel to convex border of the kidney). After removal of stones the open ends of the calyces are closed with 3/0 catgut stitches. The incision in the renal parenchyma is closed with interrupted 2/0 catgut sutures.

Pyelonephrolithotomy

A combination of pyelotomy and nephrotomy may be required for the removal of large stag horn calculus.

Nephrectomy

This is indicated when renal function has been grossly damaged by the stone and the opposite kidney is normally functioning. Steps of simple nephrectomy will be found in Chapter 82.
Closure: The loin incision is closed in layers with a corrugated or tube drain near the pelvis of the kidney.

POSTOPERATIVE CARE

- Start oral fluid as soon as the patient is stable
- Systemic antibiotic should be administered
- The drain is removed as soon as it stops draining.

POSTOPERATIVE COMPLICATIONS

- Pulmonary complications particularly atelectasis
- Hemorrhage
- Sepsis
- DVT.

CHAPTER

81

Pyeloplasty: Anderson-Hynes

Abhijit Chatterjee

INDICATION

Idiopathic pelvi-ureteric junction (PUJ) obstruction with hydronephrosis and at least 15% function on DTPA scan. Aim is to excise the PUJ and fashion a wide-dependent anastomosis.

OPERATIVE PROCEDURE

Anesthesia: General anesthesia with endotracheal intubation.

Approach

- Standard loin incision in kidney position detailed elsewhere or
- Upper transverse incision in supine position with sandbag, under loin—approaching kidney extraperitoneally or
- Laparoscopic transperitoneal approach.

Technique

The kidney, renal pelvis and upper ureter are mobilized. Any vessel crossing PUJ should be preserved PUJ is excised. The cut upper end of ureter is spatulated laterally for 3 cm and redundant pelvis excised as shown in (Figs 81.1A and B). The spatulated ureter is anastomosed to the lower half of the pelvis with continuous 3-0 catgut or 4-0 vicryl. A double-J ureteric stent (5 Fr) is placed from pelvis to bladder. Upper half of pelvis is closed with a continuous suture. Anastomosis should be anterior to any crossing vessel (Fig. 81.1C).

Closure

- 18 Fr suction drain is inserted
- Mass closure of all muscle layers with loop nylon
- 2-0 subcuticular proline to skin.

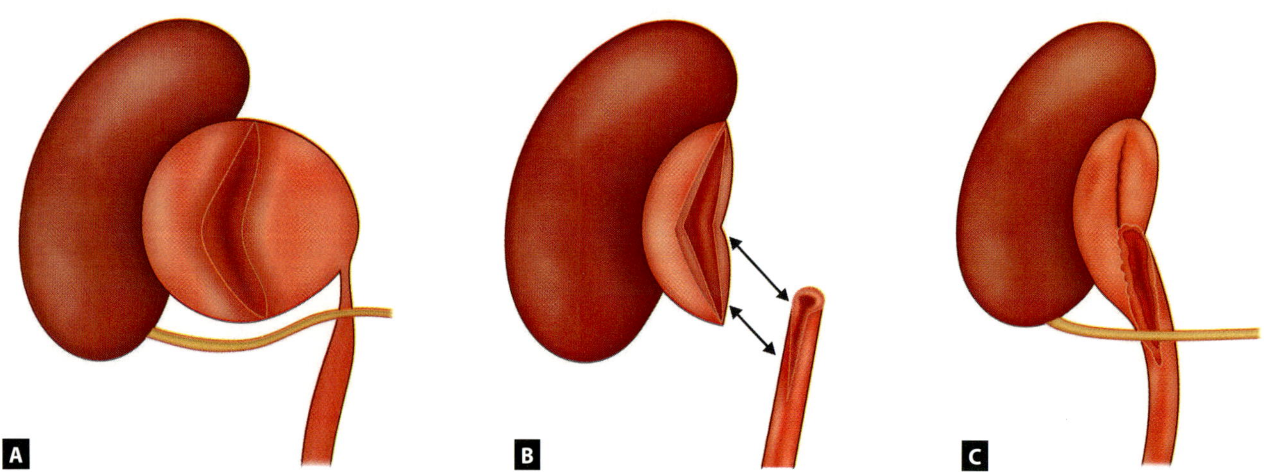

Figs 81.1A to C Anderson-Hynes pyeloplasty. (A) Excision of PUJ; (B) Spatulation of upper end of ureter and excision of redundant pelvis; (C) Anastomosis

POSTOPERATIVE CARE

- Allow sips of water 2 hr after surgery and IV fluids continued till flatus passed
- Systemic antibiotics and analgesia
- Remove drain when drainage less than 100 mL/24 hr
- Remove DJ stent cystoscopically under local anesthesia after 4 weeks.

POSTOPERATIVE COMPLICATIONS

- Hemorrhage
- Sepsis
- Leaking anastomosis
- Recurrent pelvi-ureteric junction (PUJ) obstruction.

CHAPTER

82

Nephrectomy

Dhiraj Choudhury

INDICATIONS

- Nonfunctioning kidney due to hydronephrosis, pyonephrosis, renal-tuberculosis and stag-horn calculus
- Malignant tumors of kidney
- Trauma causing severe laceration or vascular injury
- Donor's kidney for transplantation.
  The other kidney should be adequately functioning.

OPERATIVE PROCEDURE: SIMPLE NEPHRECTOMY

Anesthesia

General anesthesia with endotracheal intubation.

Position

The patient is placed in a lateral position. An axillary roll is placed under the lower-dependent arm. The lateral position is maintained by applying adhesive tape or strap. Kidney is elevated.

Incision for Posterolateral Approach

A standard lumbar (loin) incision is made. It starts below the posterior renal angle (angle between 12th rib and lateral border of sacrospinalis) and extends anteriorly up to lateral border of the rectus abdominis, 4–5 cm above the anterior superior iliac spine (Fig. 82.1). Many surgeons prefer *12th rib approach* by making incision over 12th rib and resecting anterior part of the 12th rib. This offers better access.

Exposure

The incision is deepened through skin and subcutaneous tissues. Divide *posteriorly* the latissimus dorsi and serratus posterior inferior muscles in the line of incision to expose lateral border of quadratus and lumbar fascia. Anteriorly the external oblique and internal oblique (Fig. 82.2) muscles are divided initially with diathermy. The subcostal vessels are divided between ligatures. Resection of anterior part of the 12th rib is favored by many as it offers better access (Fig. 82.3).

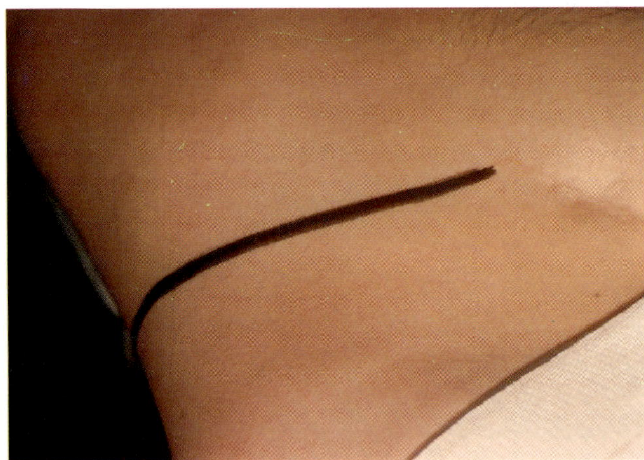

Fig. 82.1 Loin incision

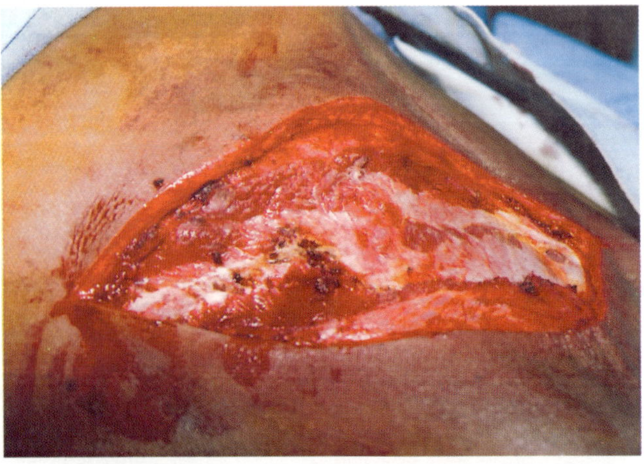

Fig. 82.2 Exposure: Posteriorly and anteriorly

The lumbar fascia is opened posteriorly and two fingers are introduced behind the transversus abdominis muscle to develop extraperitoneal plane of dissection. As the peritoneum is deflected, the transversus abdominis muscle is divided safely (Fig. 82.4). The renal fascia is identified and incised by a combination of blunt and sharp dissection. The kidney is freed from perirenal fat. At the upper pole division of fibrous band may be necessary. The kidney can be delivered to the wound. This can be assisted by passing a sling around the kidney and applying traction on hilum (Fig. 82.5).

Dealing with Renal Pedicle (Fig. 82.6)

The upper ureter is identified, divided between clamps and ligated. It is always desirable to secure the renal vessels individually away from the hilum and the artery should be ligated first. Gently clean the renal hilum by gauze dissection both posteriorly and anteriorly. The renal artery can be approached by mobilizing the kidney and retracting it up to the wound. The artery will be found in the angle between the upper medial border of the kidney and posterior abdominal wall. The artery should be clamped and ligated doubly with 1/0 silk. The renal vein is similarly dealt with subsequently. If the renal pedicle is short it may have to be clamped in one mass. When the pedicle is ligatured in one mass apply two clamps on the pedicle and divide the pedicle distal to both the clamps. A transfixing ligature is applied just proximal to the deeper clamp which is gradually released and then taken-off. A second ligature is then applied just proximal to superficial clamp which is gradually released and taken off. If the vessels are approached from the front, the renal vein is gently retracted to expose the renal artery, which is ligated first.

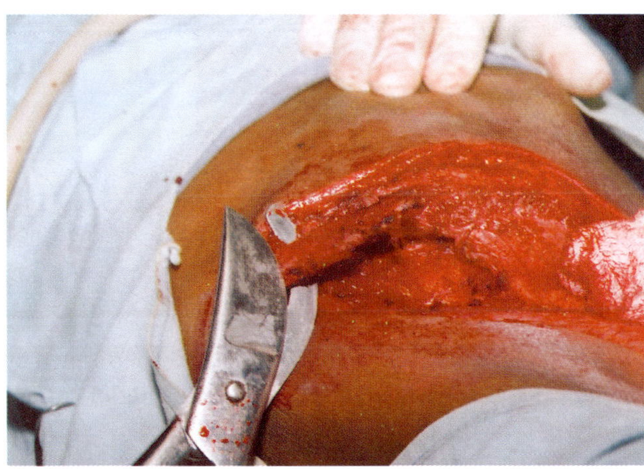

Fig. 82.3 Resection of 12th rib

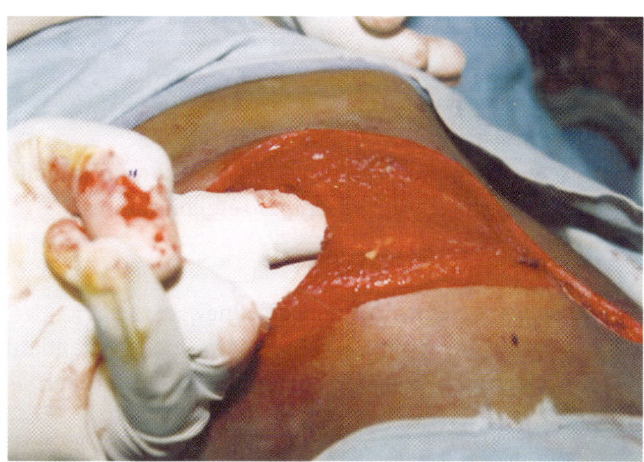

Fig. 82.4 Division of transversus abdominis muscle

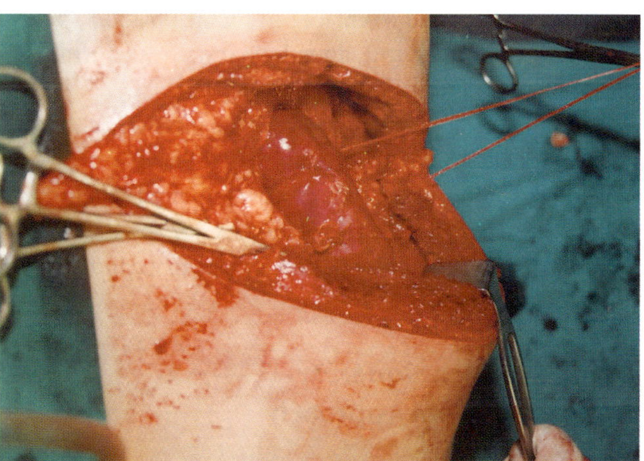

Fig. 82.5 Application of sling around kidney

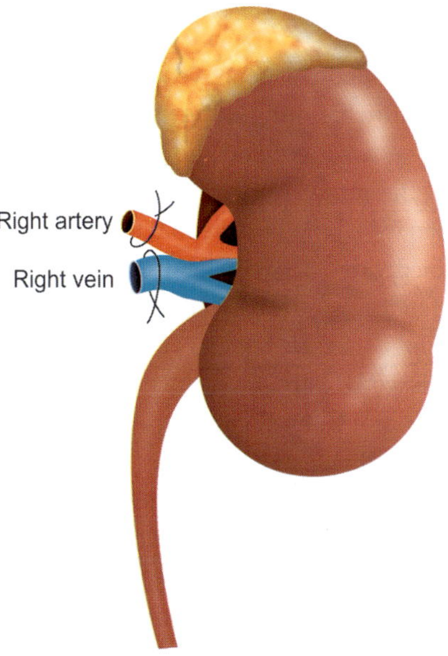

Fig. 82.6 Vascular pedicle from lumbar approach vessels ligated individually

Closure

- Ensure hemostasis
- Put corrugated rubber or tube drain
- Muscles are sutured interruptedly with 0 chromic catgut
- The skin is closed with interrupted ethilon sutures.

RADICAL NEPHRECTOMY

- *Indication:* Malignant tumors of kidney
- *Approach:* The operation can be performed by standard loin approach but a transabdominal approach is considered better.
- *Advantage:* The renal pedicle and inferior vena cava can be widely exposed and better dealt by transabdominal approach.
- *Position:* The patient is placed in supine position
- *Anesthesia:* General anesthesia with endotracheal intubation.
- *Incision:* A transverse muscle cutting incision on the side of nephrectomy is preferred.
- *Exposure:* The peritoneal cavity is opened by cutting a rectus sheath and muscles of the anterior abdominal wall. A thorough exploration is carried out to exclude distant (liver) metastasis.

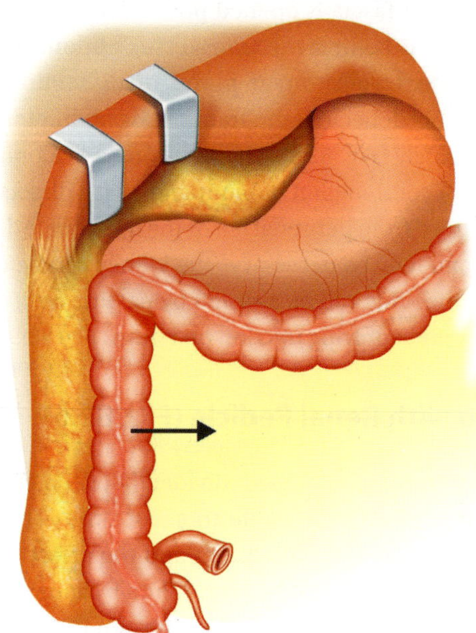

Fig. 82.7 Approach to right kidney by displacement of ascending colon medially

Operative Technique: Transabdominal Approach

Right-sided Nephrectomy

Incise the peritoneum along the lateral border of the ascending colon and hepatic flexure which are retracted medially (Fig. 82.7).

The vascular pedicle (renal vein, renal artery) should be ligated first before handling kidney.

The renal vein is identified and gently dissected to expose renal artery. The renal artery should be ligated in continuity. The renal vein is palpated for metastatic deposits. If it's lumen free, it can be divided between ligatures (Silk) (Fig. 82.8).

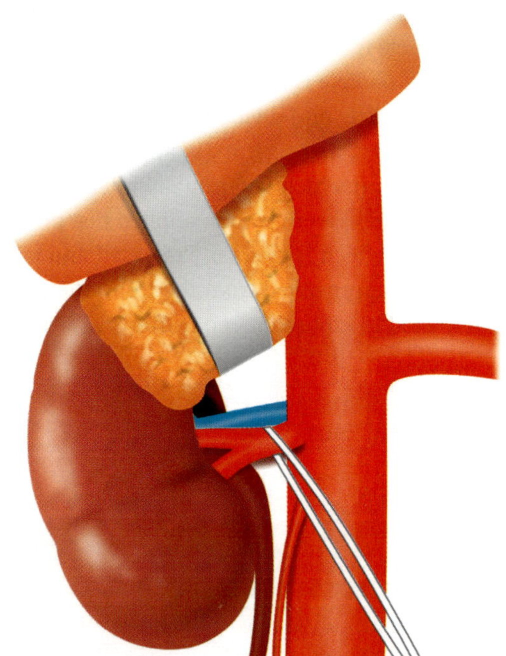

Fig. 82.8 Dealing with vascular pedicle

The dissection is now carried upward and downward in front of inferior vena cava and fibrofatty tissues and lymphatic tissues are dissected laterally.

The ureter and right gonadal vessels are now mobilized and individually divided and ligated.

Now divide the peritoneal reflection over the lateral aspect of the kidney from the level of aortic bifurcation to adrenal gland. The fascia of Gerota is dissected from renal bed.

Once the lower pole has been mobilized, the kidney can be displaced upwards and divided above the adrenal gland.

Additional lymphadenectomy can now be performed by carefully dissecting lymphatic tissues along anterior surface of aorta or vena cava.

Dealing with Venacaval Involvement

The involvement of the inferior venacava by malignant thrombus may be infrahepatic or suprahepatic. Vena caval tumor thrombectomy may be done through renal vein or by direct cavatomy. When the tumor thrombectomy is complete the cavatomy wound is repaired with a continues 5/0 silk or proline suture.

Left-sided Nephrectomy

Divide peritoneum on lateral aspect of descending colon and splenic flexure. The splenorenal ligament is divided to mobilize spleen upwards and to the right.

The colon is displaced medially until aorta and antero-medial aspect of inferior vena cava are exposed.

The structures at the hilum of the kidney are exposed and are ligated and divided individually.

Closure

- Put corrugated drain.
- Close the abdomen in layers.

POSTOPERATIVE CARE

- Intravenous fluid is administered until the condition of the patient is stable
- Systemic antibiotic is administered.

POSTOPERATIVE COMPLICATIONS

- Pulmonary complications particularly atelectasis
- Secondary or reactionary hemorrhage
- Sepsis
- Paralytic ileus.

CHAPTER

83

Treatment of Ureteric Stones

Dhiraj Choudhury

ANATOMY

The ureter is a thick muscular tube 28–30 cm long and less than 1 cm in diameter.

The *abdominal* part of the ureter lies on psoas muscle accompanied by genitofemoral nerve. It then crosses the bifurcation of the common iliac and is frequently lifted forward with peritoneum during iliac approach. At the upper end the right ureter is related to third part of the duodenum and is crossed by right colic, ileo-colic and the genital vessels at lower part. The left ureter is crossed by genital and left colic vessels.

The *pelvic part* of the ureter passes below the internal iliac artery along the side wall of the pelvis until ischial spine is reached. It then turns forward and medially in the fat above the levator ani to enter the bladder at the posterosuperior corner of its base. In male it is crossed by vas deferens near bladder. In female it lies above the lateral fornix of the vagina.

The *intramural* part (1 cm long) passes obliquely through the mascular wall of the bladder. The two ureteric orifices lie at the upper angles of the trigone 2–3 cm apart.

TREATMENT OF URETERIC STONES

Endoscopic stone removal–

- *Dormia basket*: This can be used for stones within 5-6 cm of ureteric orifice. A wire basket is introduced under image intensifier control and the stone is removed within the basket.

Ureteroscopic removal–

- *Push back*: The stone is pushed back into renal pelvis and then extracorporeal shock wave lithotripsy (ESWL) is used.

OPEN URETEROLITHOTOMY

Ureteric stones of 5 mm or less in size will pass spontaneously. Intervention is indicated for persistent colicy pain, deterioration of renal function and proximal infection.

Indication

Operative ureterolithotomy is indicated when endoscopic methods (Dormia basket, ureteroscopy) or lithotripsy is either not available or successful. Open ureterolithotomy is also indicated as first-line of treatment if there is ureteric stricture below the stone. For a large impacted stone in mid-ureter open surgery is probably better option.

Preoperative Preparation

- A plain X-ray of KUB region should be taken immediately before operation
- Urine culture and sensitivity
- Systemic antibiotic particularly in presence of infection.

Operative Procedure

Stone in the Upper Third of Ureter

- *Position:* Patient is placed in lateral position.
- *Incision:* Kidney is exposed by standard loin incision.
- *Exposure:* The upper ureter is gently exposed by blunt and sharp dissection taking care not to dislodge the stone.
- *Technique:* Once the stone is located apply two stay sutures with 3/0 chromic catgut. A longitudinal ureterotomy is made directly over the stone which is extracted with stone

holding forceps. After removal of the calculus ureteral patency is tested by passing ureteric catheter.

- *Closure:* The ureterotomy may be left open and drained but usually closed with few interrupted 3/0 chromic catgut sutures placed through the adventitia. Insert a tube drain and close the wound in layers.

Stone in the Middle Third of Ureter

- *Position:* Patient is placed in semirecumbent position with a sand bag behind the buttock.
- *Anesthesia:* General anesthesia with endotracheal intubation.
- *Incision:* An oblique muscle-cutting incision is made one inch above and parallel to iliac crest (Fig. 83.1).
- *Exposure:* The ureter is exposed by cutting the muscles and pushing the peritoneum medially by gauze dissection (Figs 83.2A and B).
- *Identification of ureter:* The ureter is identified crossing the bifurcation of common iliac vessels. Remember, the ureter is often found lifted with peritoneum during dissection. The ureter presents vermicular movements on touching (Fig. 83.3).
- *Technique:* The ureter is gently mobilized by gauze dissection and brought towards the surface and held by a sling of tape. A longitudinal incision is made directly over the stone which is then extracted with stone holding forceps (Figs 83.4A and B).
- *Closure:* The ureterotomy is usually closed with few interrupted 3/0 chromic catagut sutures.

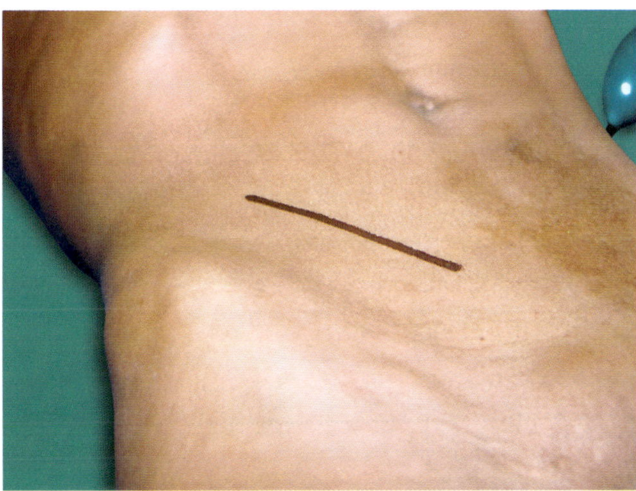

Fig. 83.1 Oblique muscle—cutting incision

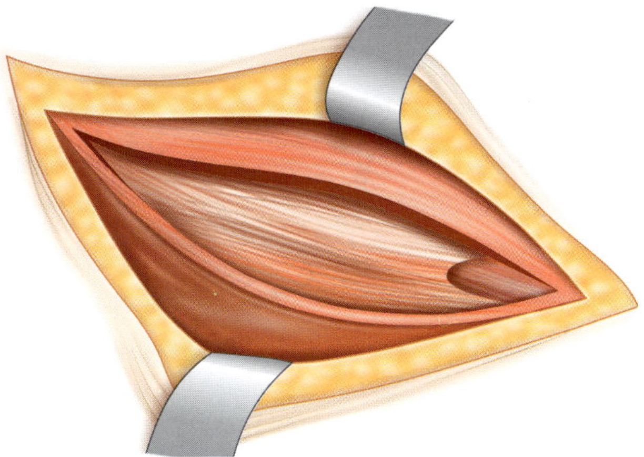

Fig. 83.2A Division of muscles along the line of incision

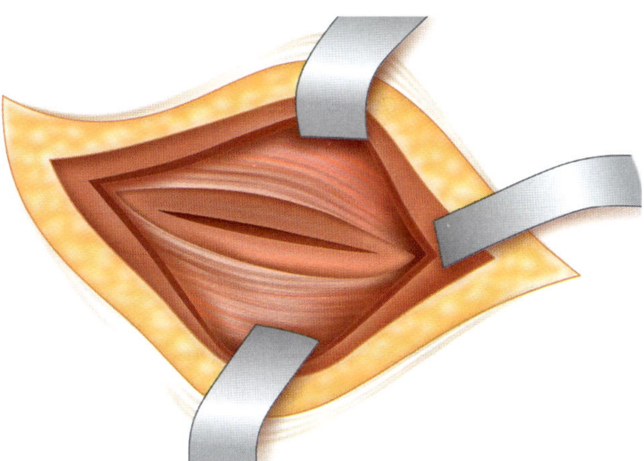

Fig. 83.2B Exposure of extraperitoneal space

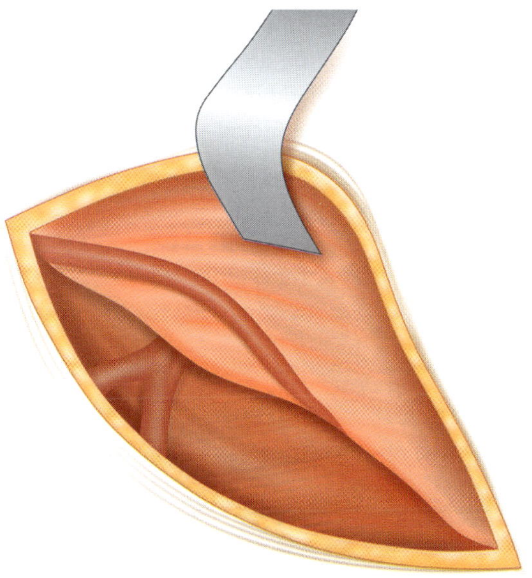

Fig. 83.3 Retraction of peritoneum to expose ureter

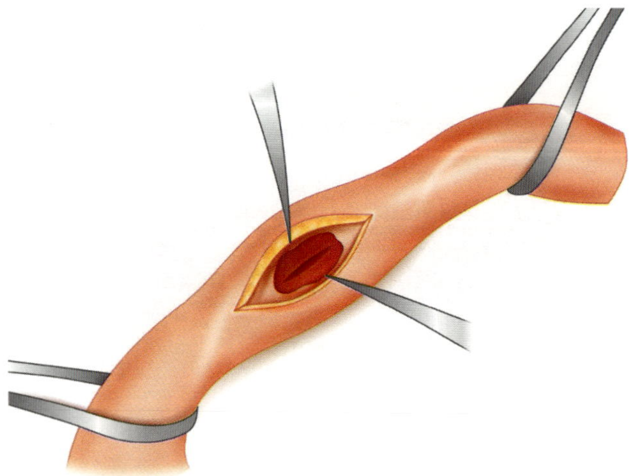

Fig. 83.4A Ureterotomy over stone

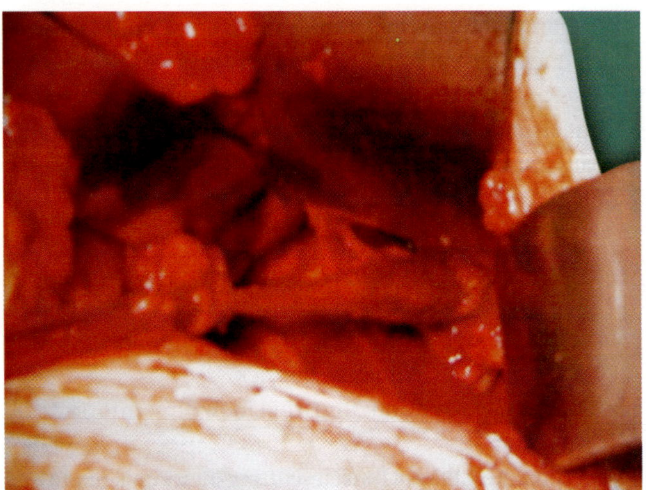

Fig. 83.4B Extraction of stones

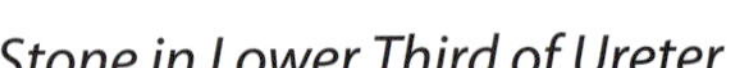

Stone in Lower Third of Ureter

- *Anesthesia:* General.
- *Position:* Patient is placed in recumbent position.
- *Incision:* Lower third of ureter can be approached by Pffannenstien or lower midline incision.
- *Exposure:* Following any of the above incisions the rectus sheath is divided along the line of incision. The rectus muscle in now retracted laterally. The peritoneum is gently raised from the bladder and side wall of the pelvis until bifurcation of common iliac vessel is seen. Identify the ureter and trace in downwards and palpate the stone. Subsequent steps of ureterolithotomy is identical to those described for middle third. In case of a stone impacted in intramural part of the ureter a transvesical approach may be used. The bladder is opened in the midline, a meatotomy on the effected side done and stone is extracted with forceps.
- *Closure:* The abdomen is closed in layers with a drain in the field of operation.

POSTOPERATIVE CARE

- Oral fluid is started as soon as the patient recovers from anesthesia.
- Systemic antibiotic.
- Drain is removed when it stops draining.

POSTOPERATIVE COMPLICATIONS

Early

- Temporary leakage of urine which usually stops by 7 days
- Sepsis
- Hemorrhage.

Late

- Ureteric stricture.

CHAPTER

84

Total Radical Cystectomy

Dhiraj Choudhury

INDICATION

Radical cystectomy with pelvic lymphadenectomy is the standard treatment for T2–T3 disease without evidence of secondary spread or of carcinoma *in situ* (CIS) that has not responded to bacillus calmette-Guérin (BCG).

AIMS

Radical cystectomy implies the en block removal of the anterior pelvic organs–the prostate, seminal vesicles, bladder and urethra in males and urethra, bladder, cervix, vaginal cuff, uterus, ovaries and anterior pelvic peritoneum in females. A pelvic lymphadenectomy and urinary diversion are parts of the operation.

PREOPERATIVE CARE

- Counseling for urinary diversion, usually ileal conduit.
- Bowel preparation, to offer a sterile internal tract.
- Prophylactic antibiotic to ensure a sterile urinary tract.
- DVT prophylaxis.

OPERATIVE PROCEDURE

- *Position:* The patient is placed in supine position.
- *Anesthesia:* General anesthesia with endotracheal tube is preferred.
- *Preparation:* A Foley's catheter is introduced after the draping. Site of ileostomy is marked on the skin on the right side of the abdomen.
- *Incision:* A long midline incision extending from mid-epigastric region to symphysis pubis is made.
- *Exposure:* On opening abdomen, perform full laparotomy to assess operability of bladder lesion and exclude liver metastasis. The peritoneal cavity is usually opened above the umbilicus and extended downwards taking care of urachal remnant. Insert self-retaining retractor and pack small bowel into upper part of abdomen.

Procedure

Ligation of Internal Iliac Artery

Mobilize sigmoid colon. Identify distal end of each ureter and divide overlying peritoneum. Mobilize ureter upwards. Ligate internal iliac artery in continuity with silk.

Transection of Ureters

Divide ureters close to bladder. Ligate distal end of each ureter. The proximal ends are used for urinary diversion (Fig. 84.1).

Mobilization of Bladder

This involves opening both retropubic and retrovesical (male) or retrouterine (female) spaces by incising peritoneum.

Lateral dissection lift the bladder forward and to opposite side by traction on urachal remnant, to define the superior and inferior vesicle vessels. Divide the vessels between clamps and tie them. Divide the lateral pedicle.

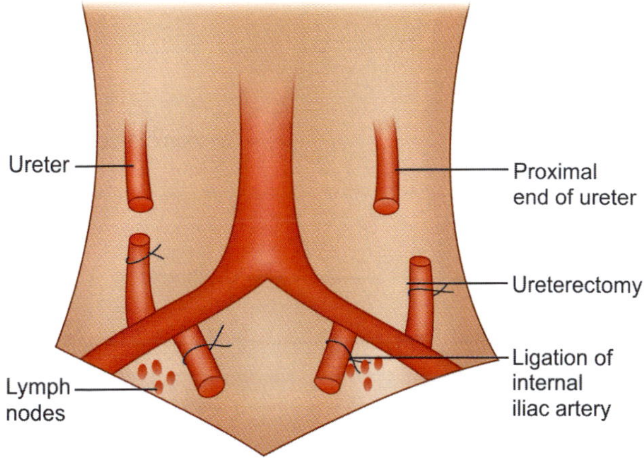

Fig. 84.1 Ureterectomy and ligation of internal iliac artery

Posterior dissection: The peritoneum lateral to rectum incised for visualization of pouch of Douglas. This allows entry into Denonvillier's space. In this plane, rectum is swept from bladder, seminal vesicles and prostate in men and posterior vaginal wall in women.

Anterior dissection: When posterior and lateral dissection have been completed, anterior dissection is started. The bladder is now held by puboprostatic ligaments and urethra. The dissection is continued into retropubic space. The puboprostatic ligaments are identified in men and divided. Next a right angled clamp is passed anterior to membranous urethra under dorsal venous complex. The venous complex is now ligated and divided.

Bladder is now attached by urethra inferiorly.

Dealing with Membranous Urethra

Clamp the urethra distal to prostate in males and bladder neck in females and divide the urethra (Fig. 84.2).

Urinary Diversion (Figs 84.3A to D)

Perform ileal conduit. Isolate and mobilize a loop of ileum 20 cm in length and approximately 50 cm from ileocecal valve on its vascular pedicle. Divide the bowels between clamps. Restore continuity of bowel with end to end anastomosis. Spatulate the ends of the ureters, suture them together along one edge to create a common orifice which is anastomosed to proximal end of the ileal loop with a single layer of continuous vicryl sutures. Ureteric catheters are inserted into each ureter before anastomosis is complete and other ends passed through ileal conduit. Secure the ileal loop by passing several interrupted sutures through the serosa of the bowel and peritoneum of posterior abdominal wall.

Bring the distal end of the ileal loop through the abdominal wall at the preselected site and fashion a spout as for an ileostomy.

Pelvic Lymphadenectomy

Bilateral pelvic lymphadenectomy is done now. A limited dissection extending from common iliac bifurcation is carried along medial aspect of external iliac artery to the beginning of femoral canal. All lymphatics and fatty tissues within the boundary are removed.

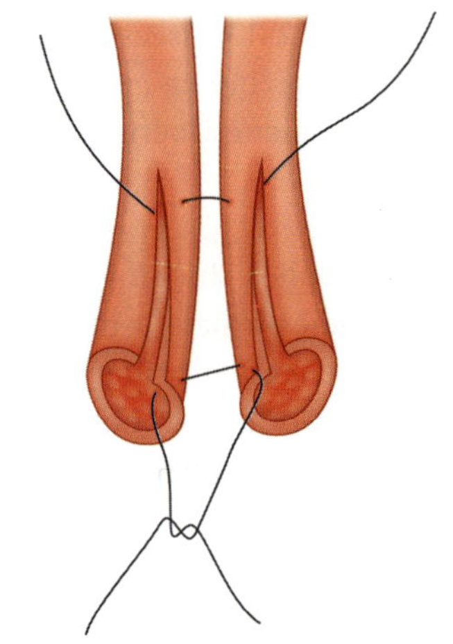

Fig. 84.3A Spatulation of ureteric ends

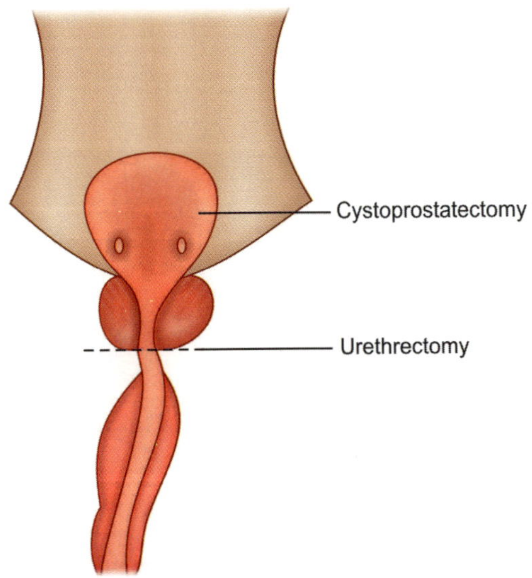

Fig. 84.2 Urethrectomy

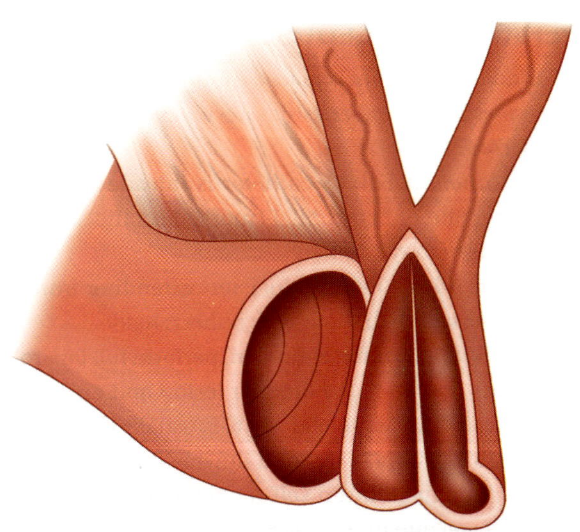

Fig. 84.3B Uretero-ileal anastomosis

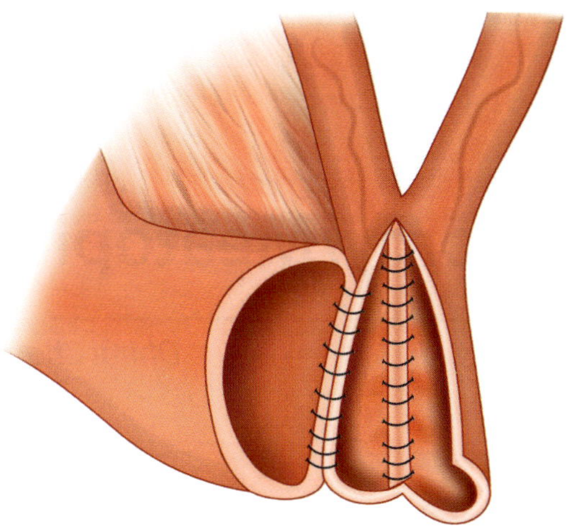

Fig. 84.3C Uretero-ileal anastomosis

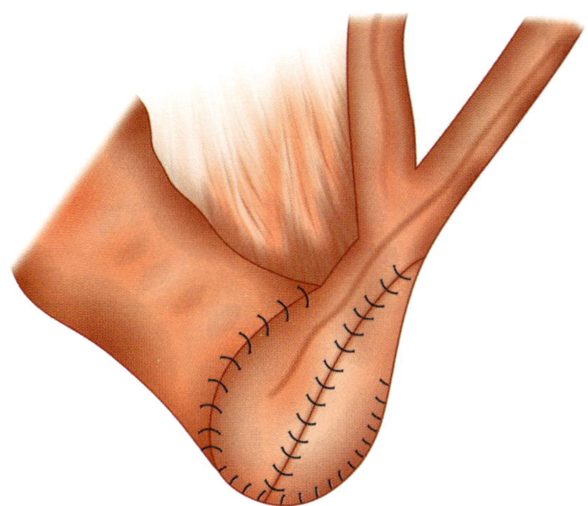

Fig. 84.3D Construction of ileal conduit

Closure

- Insert a suction drain
- Close the abdomen en-mass.

POSTOPERATIVE CARE

- IV fluid to continue, till flames is passed
- Nasogastric suction for 48–72 hours
- Systemic antibiotic
- Drain is removed when it stops draining.

POSTOPERATIVE COMPLICATIONS

Immediate

- Hemorrhage
- Sepsis
- Wound infection
- Pulmonary complications
- DVT.

Late

- Intestinal obstruction.

CHAPTER

85

Meatotomy/Meatoplasty

Dhiraj Choudhury

INDICATION

Pinhole meatus: This is a congenital condition—where the opening of the glans is excessively small. It may cause obstruction of the out-flow of urine.

OPERATIVE PROCEDURE

- *Position:* The patient is placed in supine position
- *Anesthesia:* General or spinal anesthesia.

Technique

Meatotomy

The tightened meatus is widened by cutting down external meatus with fine scissors (Fig. 85.1).

The cut-edge of urothelium and skin are stitched together (interrupted) with absorbable suture (Fig. 85.2).

Meatoplasty

This is considered better procedure. A curved C-shape flap of the skin is raised on the ventral surface of the penis (Fig. 85.3).

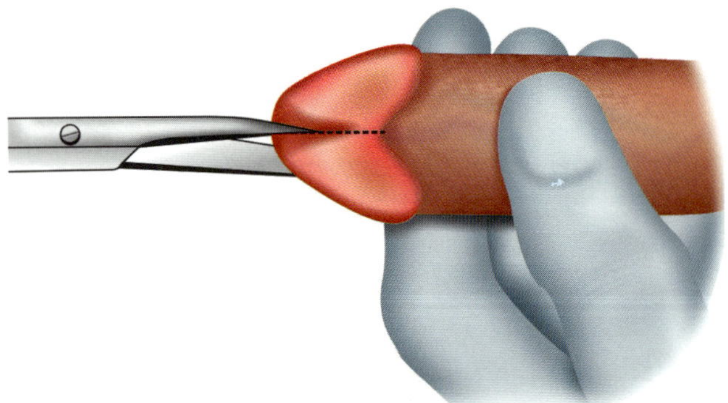

Fig. 85.1 Widening of meatus

A wide meatotomy is done (Fig. 85.4). The flap is now stitched to the defect with 4/0 chromic catgut (Fig. 85.5).

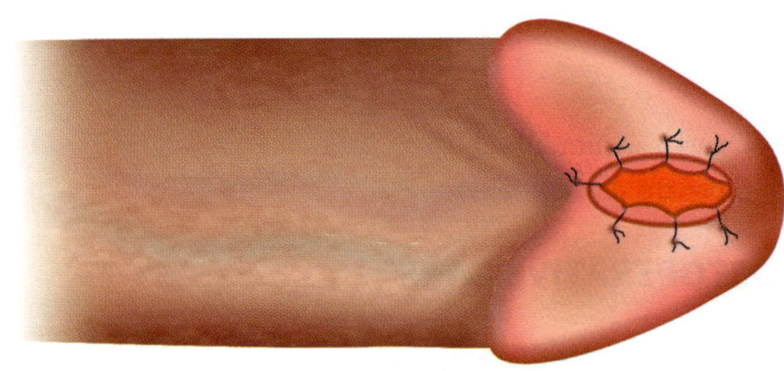

Fig. 85.2 Suturing of urothelium and skin

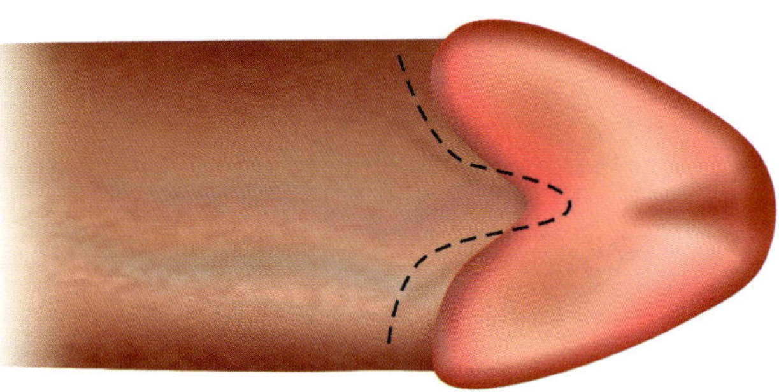

Fig. 85.3 Raising skin flap

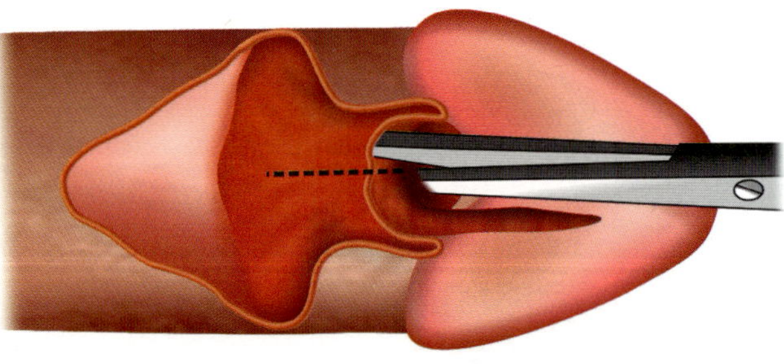

Fig. 85.4 Meatotomy

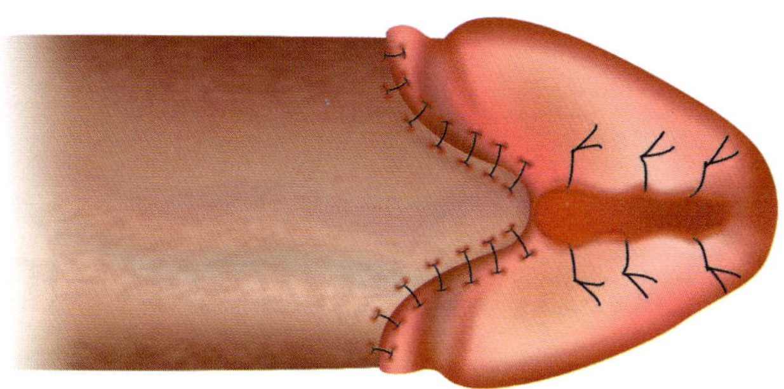

Fig. 85.5 Meatoplasty

POSTOPERATIVE CARE

- Administer systemic antibiotic
- Dilatation by suitable bougie may be required in case of meatotomy.

POSTOPERATIVE COMPLICATIONS

- Hemorrhage
- Sepsis
- Spraying of urine
- Re-stenosis. This is common after meatotomy.

CHAPTER

86

Circumcision

Dhiraj Choudhury

Circumcision means partial excision of penile foreskin.

INDICATIONS

Inability to retract the foreskin. A normal, nonretractic foreskin seen at birth usually separates spontaneously by the age of 5 years. So, circumcision is not indicated before the age of 5 years, for such physiological adhesion.

- Religious circumcision is performed in neonates or infants by Jews and Muslim.
- The vast majority of circumcisions performed on children and adults are for:
  - Persistent phimosis at the age of 5 years
  - Recurrent paraphimosis, recurrent balanoposthitis, carcinoma of penis confined to prepucial skin.

Contraindications: Hypospadias

OPERATIVE PROCEDURE IN CHILDREN

Guillotine Method/Forceps-guided

Position: The patient is placed in supine position
Anesthesia: General anesthesia
Procedure: The opening in the foreskin is gently opened with a probe or mosquito forceps (Fig. 86.1). The tip of the foreskin is held with hemostats, as the prepuce is now fully retracted to expose coronal sulcus and remove retained smegma. Return the prepuce to normal position and mark the skin at the level of corona.

Apply forward traction at the tip of prepuce with the hemostats (Fig. 86.2).

Apply a narrow clamp obliquely across the prepuce distal to the glans and parallel to corona (Fig. 86.3).

Divide the prepuce distal to the clamp (Fig. 86.4) with scalpel.

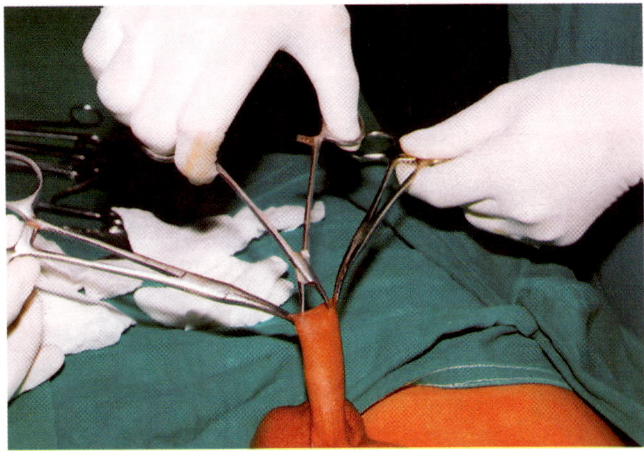

Fig. 86.1 Widening opening in foreskin

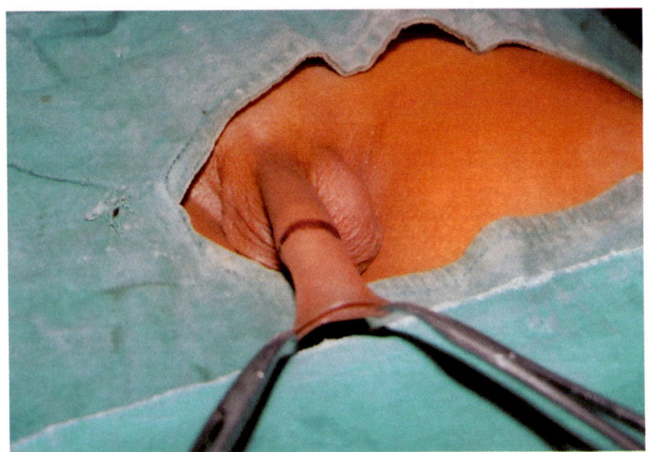

Fig. 86.2 Application of forward traction

The inner layer requires further trimming which can be done by making a dorsal incision from the free margin of the inner layer.

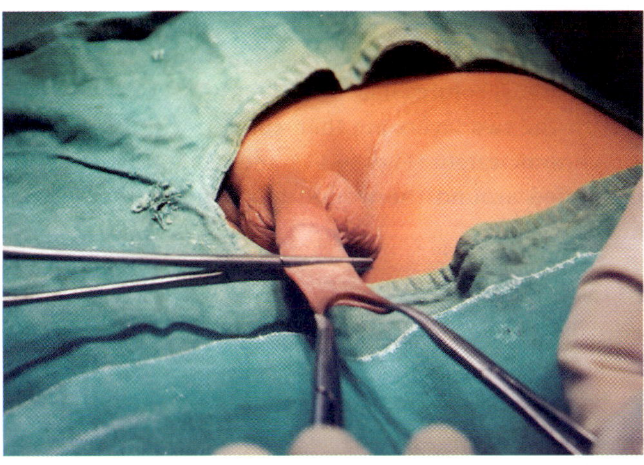

Fig. 86.3 Application of clamp

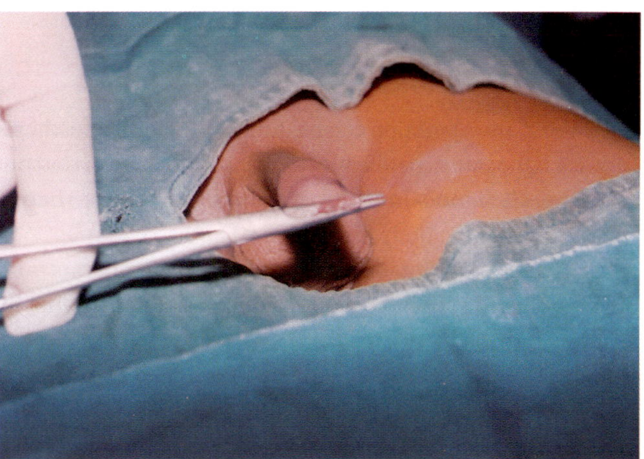

Fig. 86.4 Division of prepuce

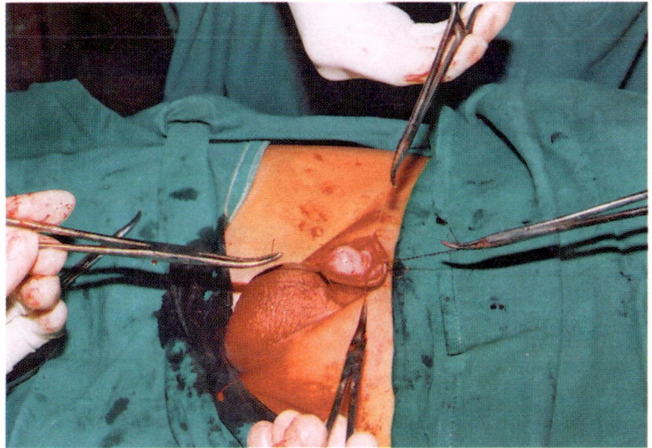

Fig. 86.5A Application of sutures

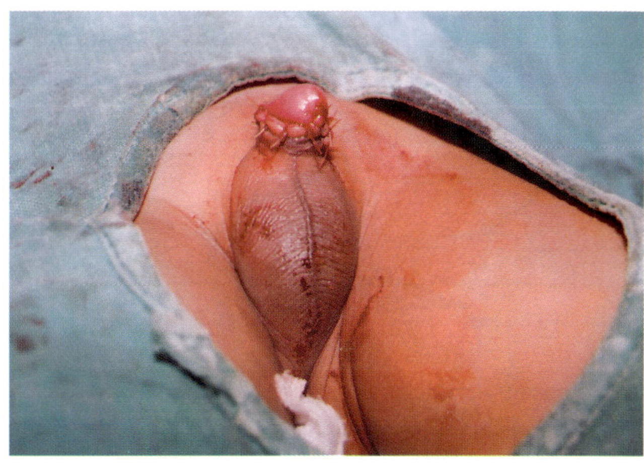

Fig. 86.5B Completion of suturing

Hemostasis is secured by ligating bleeding points with 3/0 chromic catgut. The frenal vessel may require ligation with 3/0 chromic catgut applying figure of eight stitch or three-in-one stitch. The two layers are the sutured by interrupted 3/0 chromic catgut (Figs 86.5A and B). This technique has been opposed in view of risk of injury of glans.

Dressing: Apply anesthetic jelly on to a strip of gauze or sofratulle and wrap it around the wound (Fig. 86.6).

Plastibel (Hollister) device is a safe method for circumcision in infants. The foreskin is freed and retracted. After the plastibel device has been slipped into place over the glans penis, the foreskin is ligated over the groove of the bell and redundant foreskin is cutway.

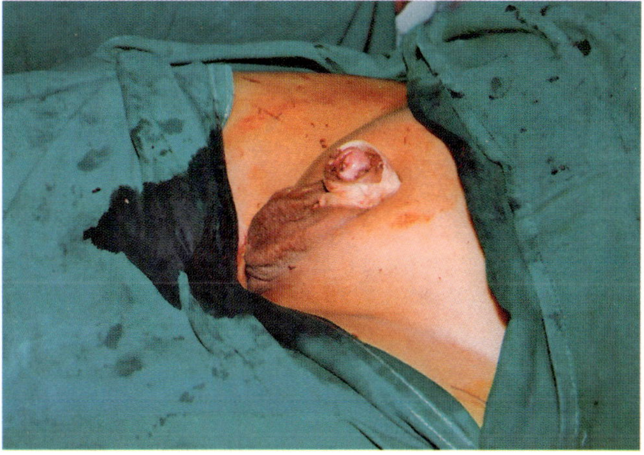

Fig. 86.6 Application of dressing

OPERATIVE PROCEDURE IN ADULT

Dorsal Slit Technique/Dissection Method

Anesthesia: The operation can be done under local anesthesia with 1% lignocaine (penile block). Penile block is carried out injecting 1% lignocaine subcutaneously in a ring-shaped fashion around the body of the penis (Fig. 86.7).

Procedure: Hold the prepuce with two hemostats and break any adhesions between prepuce and glans penis by introducing mosquito forceps.

Dorsal slit: A dorsal slit is made at 12 o'clock position with scissors up to corona (Fig. 86.8). The foreskin which is now in two halves is excised with scissor at the level of coronal sulcus (Fig. 86.9). Hemostasis is achieved by ligating frenal vessels and any bleeding points with 3/0 chromic catgut. Frenal sutures may be given as finger of eight (Fig. 86.10). The two layers are then sutured with interrupted 3/0 chromic catgut (Figs 86.11A and B). A gauze dressing is applied around the wound to prevent adherence to undergarment.

POSTOPERATIVE CARE

- Patient is discharged after completion of operation
- Systemic antibiotic is advised
- Analgesic is advised
- Removal of dressing after 48 hours.

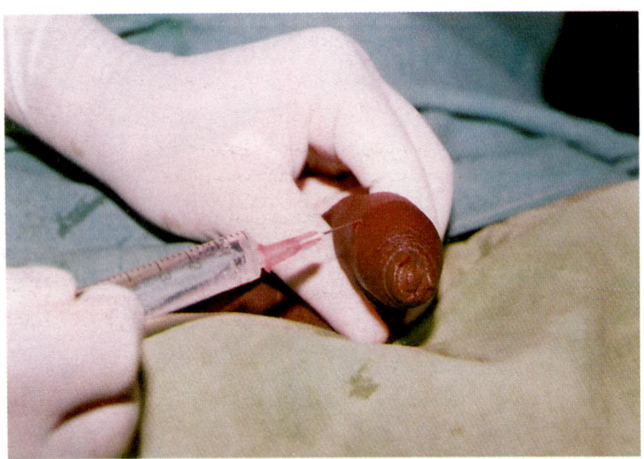

Fig. 86.7 Penile block

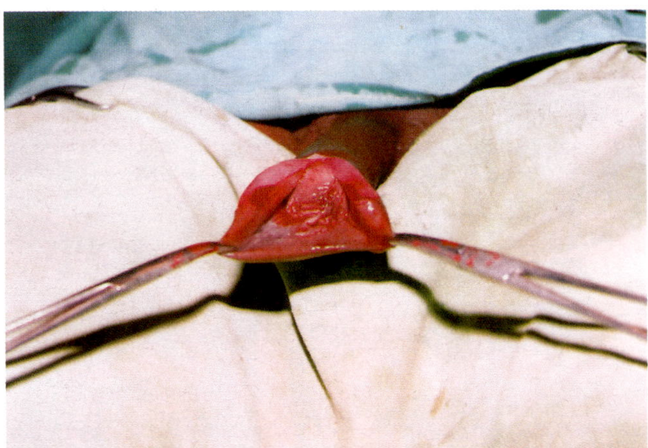

Fig. 86.8 Dorsal slit

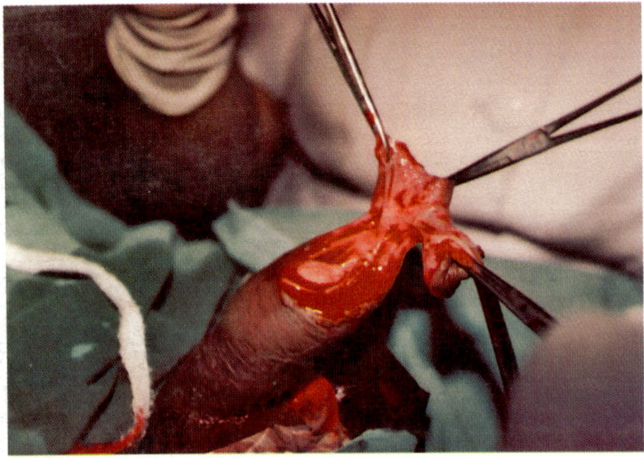

Fig. 86.9 Excision of foreskin

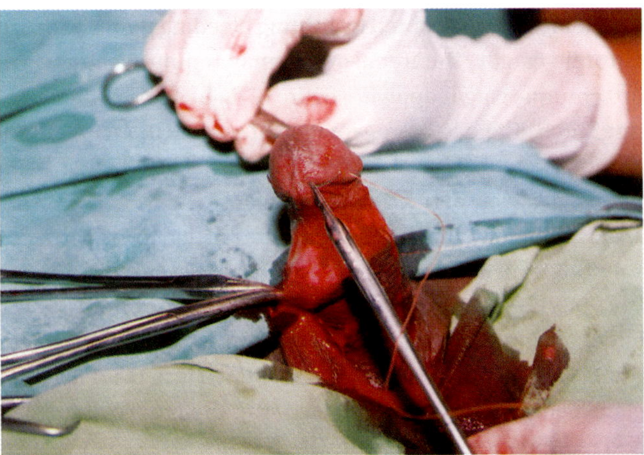

Fig. 86.10 Application of frenal suture

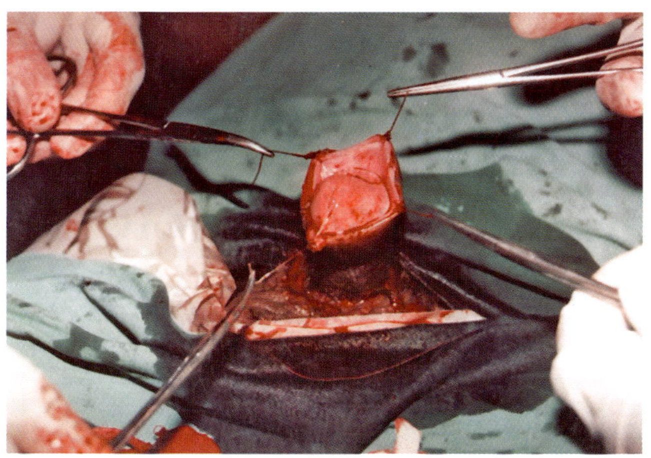

Fig. 86.11A Application of sutures uniting two layers

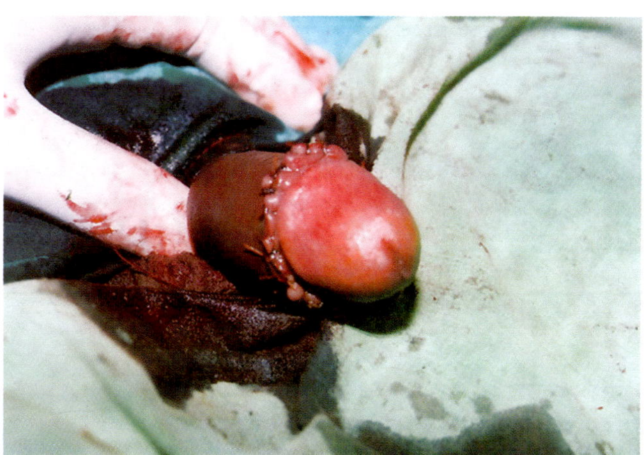

Fig. 86.11B Completion of sutures

POSTOPERATIVE COMPLICATIONS

Early

- Hemorrhage—this can be avoided by meticulous hemostasis particularly of frenal vessels (1–2%)
- Sepsis
- Urinary retention.

Late

- Meatal stenosis
- Stitch sinus.

CHAPTER 87

Amputation of Penis/Penectomy

Dhiraj Choudhury

The penis is divided into three parts—glans, body and root.

The glans is conically expanded anterior end of corpus spongiosum into which two corpora cavernosa are embedded. The glans contains external urinary meatus.

The body of penis is the remaining mobile part containing two corpora cavernosa and single corpus spongiosum.

The root consists of two diverging crura and the bulb of the penis.

The penis is covered by superficial (Scarpa) and deep (Buck's) fascia.

It is supplied by three sets of arteries on each side—dorsal artery, deep dorsal artery and artery of the bulb.

Lymphatics from the skin drains into superficial and deep inguinal nodes. Rest drain into deep inguinal and external iliac group of lymph nodes.

INDICATIONS

Carcinoma of the penis can be successfully treated by surgery or radiotherapy. Surgery is especially indicated for the followings:

- Large anaplastic growth
- Involvement of shaft of the penis
- Lesion developing over the leukoplakia
- Radio recurrent lesion.

OPERATIVE PROCEDURE

Partial Amputation of Penis/Penectomy

This is indicated for distal growths—involving glans or prepuce. A least 2 cm proximal clearance should be feasible. (Stage I and II)

- *Position:* Supine
- *Anesthesia:* Spinal or general endotracheal
- *Preparation:*
  - The field or operation is painted with betadine lotion
  - A tourniquet or fine catheter is applied around the base of the penis
  - Mark the site of amputation about 3 cm proximal to the growth
- *Incision:* Incisions are planned to produce a long U-shaped ventral flap and a short dorsal flap. The combined length of the two flaps should little more than the diameter of the penis (Fig. 87.1).

Exposure and Technique

The incision is deepened through subcutaneous tissue up to fascial sheath covering corpora cavernosa and corpus spongiosum. The superficial vessels particularly the dorsal veins are ligated with 3/0 catgut and divided. The two corpora cavernosa are now divided at the level of the base of the flaps starting dorsaly and extending downwards. The deep vessels in corpora cavernosa are now identified and ligated. The corpus spongiosum-containing urethra is dissected free and divided half inch distal to the line of section of corpora

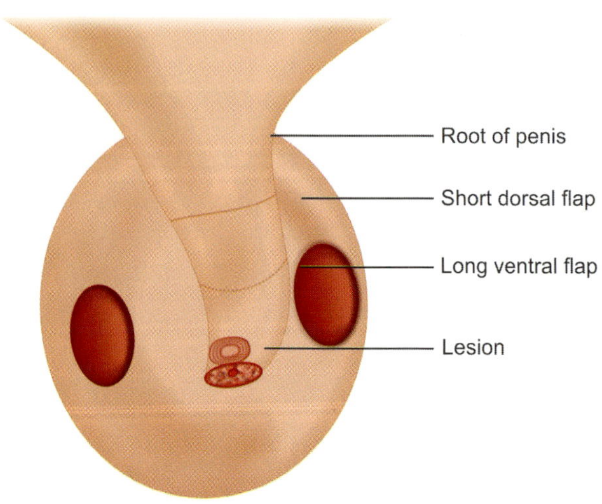

Fig. 87.1 Skin incisions making long ventral flap and short dorsal flap

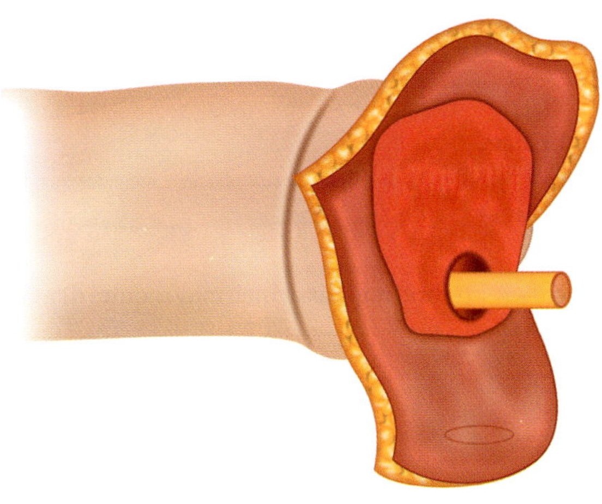

Fig. 87.2 Partial amputations of penis

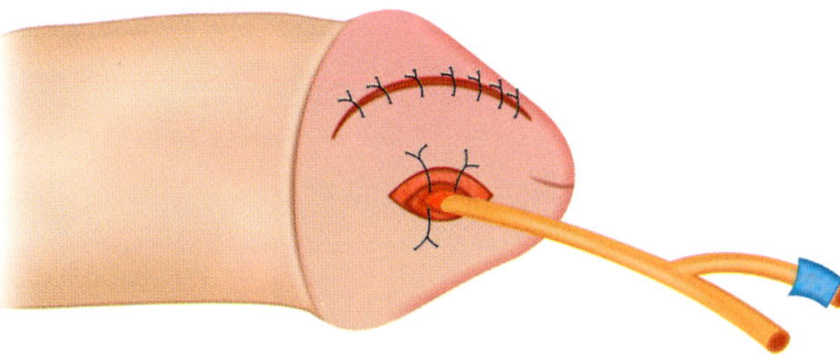

Fig. 87.3 Closure

cavernosa. The tourniquet is now removed and bleeding points are secured by suture ligation (Fig. 87.2).

Fashioning of Urethral Opening

A small opening is made in the ventral flap and the corpus spongiosum is brought out through the opening. The two flaps are now sutures together at the dorsum of the penis.

The end of the emerging urethra is split for a distance of 1 cm. Eversion of each flaps is followed by fixation of the flap margins to the skin with interrupted absorbable sutures 2 mm beyond the button hole edge to prevent stricture.

A fine Foley's catheter is left indwelling until wounds have healed up. The urethral stump is covered by a dressing (Fig. 87.3).

Total Amputation of Penis/Penectomy

This is a mutilating operation associated with psychological depression. This is indicated for lesion involving body of the penis. This is indicated for advanced cases.

- *Position:* The patient is placed in Lithotomy-Trendelenburg position.
- *Anesthesia:* Spinal or general endotracheal.
- *Preparation:* After application of betadine lotion and drapping, a metal bougie is passed per urethra.
- *Incision:* A racket-shaped incision is made encircling base of the penis and is extended vertically downwards in the midline of the scrotum to the perineum up to a point 1" in front of the anus.

Exposure

The scrotum is split into two halves by dissecting in the midline. The penis is now mobilized anteriorly by dividing the suspensory ligament. The dorsal vessels are secured by ligature. The perineal part of the incision is now deepened and its margins are retracted to expose the bulb of the penis and the two crura.

The bulb is now separated from the anterior part of the perineal membrane and the crura are detached from the ischiopubic rami with raspatory.

The bougie is now withdrawn and the bulb of the urethra is now divided about 2" distal to the perineal membrane, after dissecting it from muscular tissues at the bulb.

Closure

The wound is now closed by suturing the two flaps in the midline. The posterior part of the incision is closed round the stump of the urethra. A small drain is left in its anterior part.

Fashioning Urethrostomy

The urethral stump is split into two halves which are sutured apart to overlap the surrounding skin edges. A self-retaining catheter (Foley) is introduced and left for several days.

Dealing with Inguinal Lymph Nodes

There is controversy regarding management of inguinal lymph nodes in carcinoma of the penis. The following rational approach has been identified. In early cases without lymph node involvement, a wait and watch policy may be adapted. In presence of enlarged mobile lymph nodes bilateral block dissection can be done few weeks after the treatment of primary. Others believe that it is probably best to remove the growth together with intervening lymphatics en-block.

Metastatic fixed lymph nodes are treated by palliative deep X-ray therapy.

POSTOPERATIVE CARE

- Systemic antibiotic should be administered
- Indwelling catheter is removed after 5 days
- Stitches are removed on 7th day.

POSTOPERATIVE COMPLICATIONS

Early

- Hemorrhage
- Sepsis

Late

Stenosis of new urethral meatus, which may require dilatation.

CHAPTER

88

Orchidopexy/Orchiopexy

Dhiraj Choudhury

INDICATIONS

Undescended or ectopic testis, should be operated to avoid complications like loss of function (sterility in bilateral cases), malignant change (about 10%), trauma and infection. Though some pediatric surgeons are doing the operation at the age of 2 years, for most general surgeons, the ideal age of the patient for operation should be 3–4 years. Testis should be brought down to scrotum before the boy starts going to school. Orchidopexy consist of mobilization of testis and spermatic cord and retaining the testis in the scrotum, in a subdartos pouch. This can be undertaken as a day-care case.

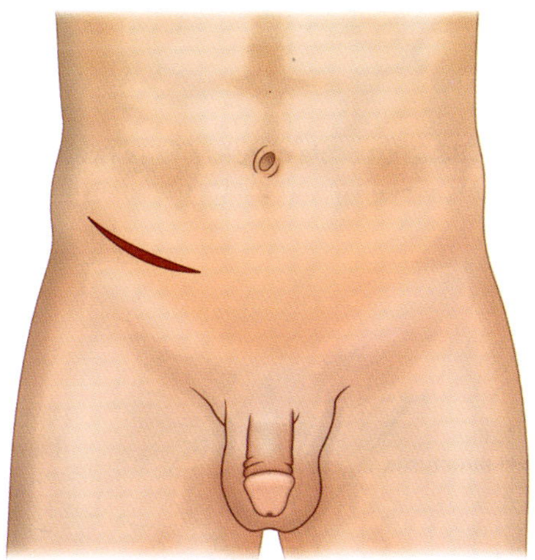

Fig. 88.1 Skin-incision over inguinal canal

PREOPERATIVE PREPARATIONS

- Ultrasonography or MRI can be done to localized the testis.
- A course of hormone (Pregnyl) can be given particularly in bilateral cases.

OPERATIVE PROCEDURE

- *Position:* The patient is placed in supine position.
- *Anesthesia:* General endotracheal anesthesia. The lower abdomen, genitali and upper thighs are prepared and drapped.
- *Incision:* A short transverse skin-crease incision is made over the deep inguinal canal ring (Fig. 88.1).
- *Exposure:* The incision is deepened through subcutaneous tissue and scarpa's fascia up to external oblique aponeurosis.
- *Identification of testis:* If the testis is ectopic, lying in superficial inguinal pouch, it can now be easily felt and seen. But if the testis in inguinal canal, it is exposed after opening the canal. Identify the superficial inguinal ring and incise the external oblique aponeurosis taking particular care to identify ilioinguinal nerve which should be preserved. The testis should now be obvious, if not already exposed (Fig. 88.2).

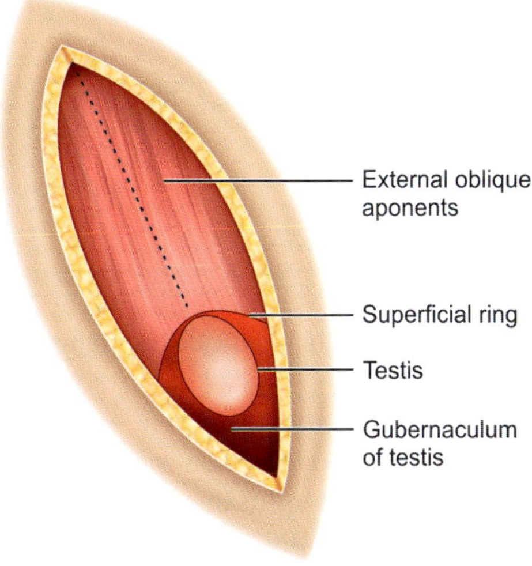

Fig. 88.2 Exposure of ectopic testis prior to opening of inguinal canal

- *Mobilization of testis and cord:* At the distal end of the testis, the gubernacular remnant is clamped, divided and

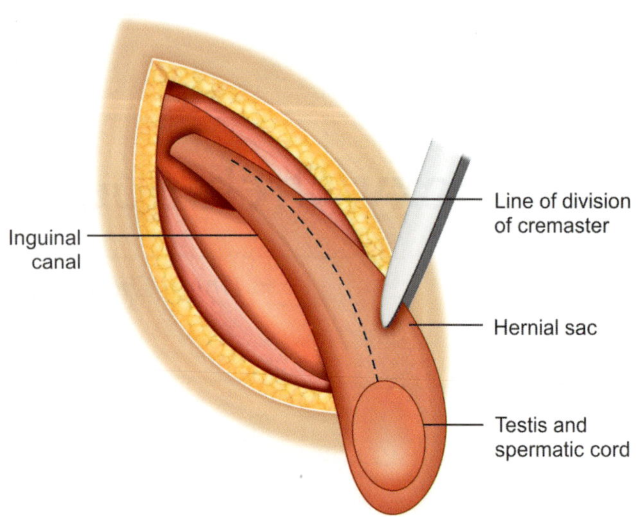

Fig. 88.3 Exposure of testis and its investing layer on opening inguinal canal

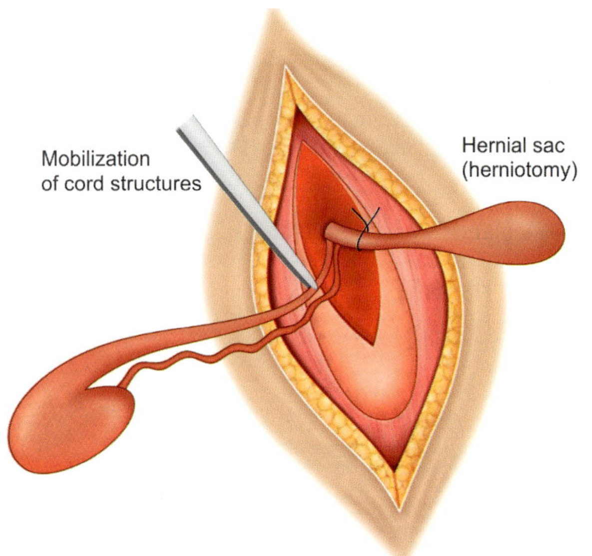

Fig. 88.4 Excision of sac and dissection of cord structures

ligated. Hold the testis and divide the cremasteric muscle (Fig. 88.3).

- *Identification of sac and herniotomy:* At the anterolateral aspect of the cord, identify thin walled hernial sac. It is freed from the cord up to the deep ring, twisted and transfixed at the neck with 3/0 chronic catgut. The excess sac is excised.
- *Mobilization of vessels and vas deferens:* Division of thin, relatively avascular fibrous bands, will straighten the path taken by testicular vessels, lengthen the spermatic cord and allow testis to reach scrotums (Fig. 88.4).

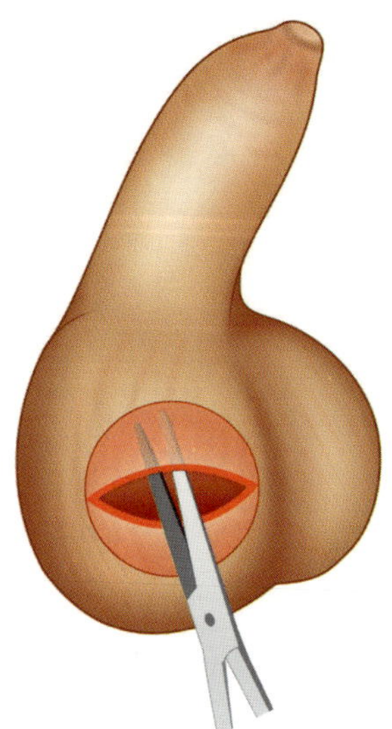

Fig. 88.5 Creation of subdartos pouch

If further mobilization is required, the deep ring can be opened on its medial border up to the level of inferior epigastric vessels.

- *Creation of subdartos pouch:* A transverse scrotal incision is made to enter the subdartos space which is developed by using forceps or scissors (Fig. 88.5).
- *Placement of testis in subdartos pouch:* An index finger is introduced from the inguinal canal to guide a mosquito forceps introduced from below through an opening made in loose fascia.

  Grasp the distal tunical covering of testis with the forceps and draw the testis gently through the 'button-hole' in subdartos pouch (Fig. 88.6).
- *Fixation of testis:* The testis can be anchored to midline tissue of scrotum by 3/0 catgut suture through tunica albugenia (Fig. 88.7).

Ombrédannés operation consists of taking the testis through the scrotal septum.

Problem

Failure to bring the testis into scrotum. When the testis cannot be brought down due to inadequate length of the cord, a two stage procedure is advised. The testis is mobilized as far as possible and fixed with a suture. After 6 months orchidopexy is completed.

Orchidectomy is indicated, if the other testis is normal, and the undescended testis is atrophied and the patient is past puberty.

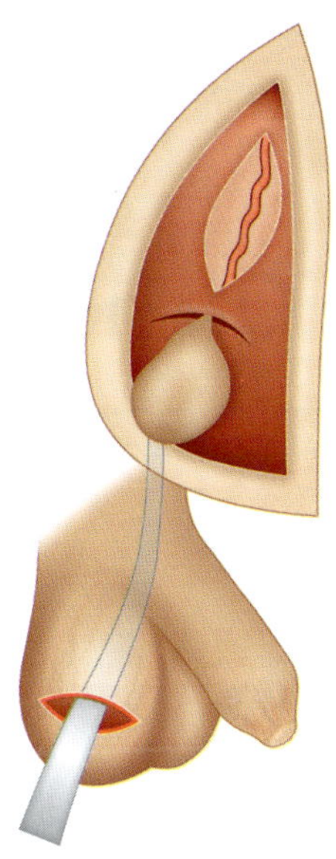

Fig. 88.6 Testis being drawn into scrotum

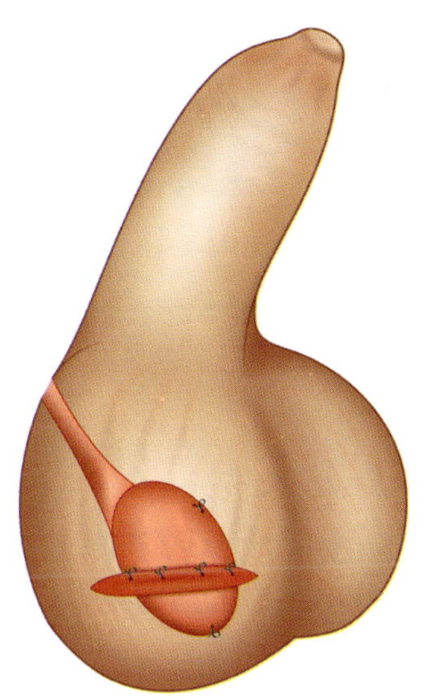

Fig. 88.7 Fixation of testis into subdartos

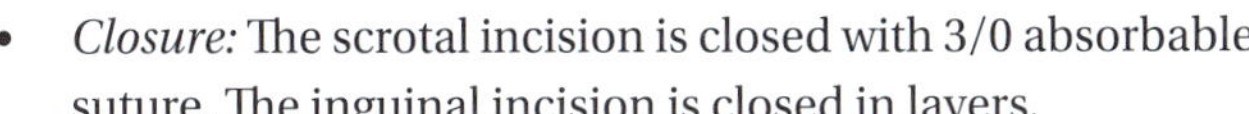

- *Closure:* The scrotal incision is closed with 3/0 absorbable suture. The inguinal incision is closed in layers.

POSTOPERATIVE CARE

- Early administration of oral fluid
- Systemic antibiotic
- Oral analgesic
- Physical activity after two weeks.

POSTOPERATIVE COMPLICATIONS

- Sepsis
- Testicular atrophy due to cord damage.

CHAPTER

89

Orchidectomy

Dhiraj Choudhury

SIMPLE ORCHIDECTOMY/ SCROTAL ORCHIDECTOMY

Indications

- Testicular torsion with nonviable testis
- Pyocele with degenerated testis.

Operative Procedure

- *Position:* The patient is placed in supine position
- *Anesthesia:* General endotracheal or spinal
- *Incision:* A vertical scrotal incision is made on the scrotal skin on the affected side
- *Exposure:* The subcutaneous tissue and dartos is divided with diathermy. The testis is delivered into the wound after incising tunica vaginalis
- *Technique:* The structure of the spermatic cord are exposed by dissection. The vas deferens and blood vessels are clamped, divided and ligated as high as possible, separately.

  In case of mass ligature transfixation suture should be applied. The testis is now removed.
- *Closure:* The dartos is closed with interrupted 2/0 catgut sutures. The skin is approximated with interrupted sutures.
- *Complications:* Hematoma.

RADICAL ORCHIDECTOMY/ INGUINAL ORCHIDECTOMY

Indication

Malignant tumors of the testis. Operation is performed on the basis of clinical diagnosis and ultrasonographic evidence.

Operative Procedure

- *Position:* The patient is placed in supine position
- *Anesthesia:* General or spinal
- *Incision:* An inguinal incision is made over medial two-thirds of inguinal ligament (Fig. 89.1)
- *Exposure:* The incision is deepened through subcutaneous tissue and superficial fascia until external oblique aponeurosis is exposed. The inguinal canal is exposed after division of external oblique aponeurosis (Fig. 89.2)
- *Technique:* The spermatic cord is identified, and freed by blunt dissection at the level of the deep ring (Fig. 89.3). A Sogi clamp applied across the cord stops dissemination of malignant cells as the testis is mobilized into the wound. The testis is pulled up from the scrotum and examined. If the tumor is confirmed by gross appearance, the spermatic cord is doubly clamped at the level of the deep ring and divided (Fig. 89.4)

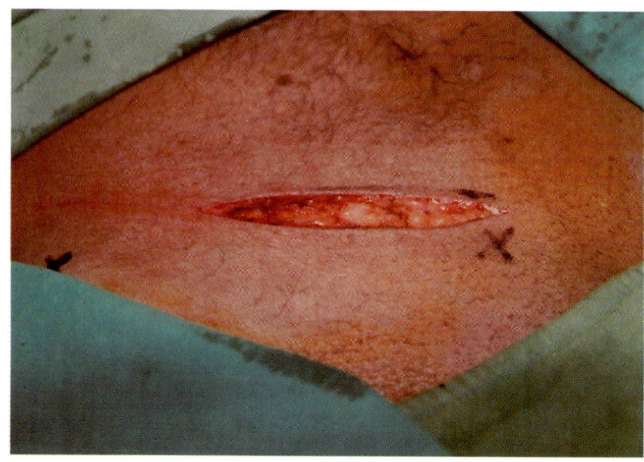

Fig. 89.1 Skin incision for radical orchidectomy (inguinal)

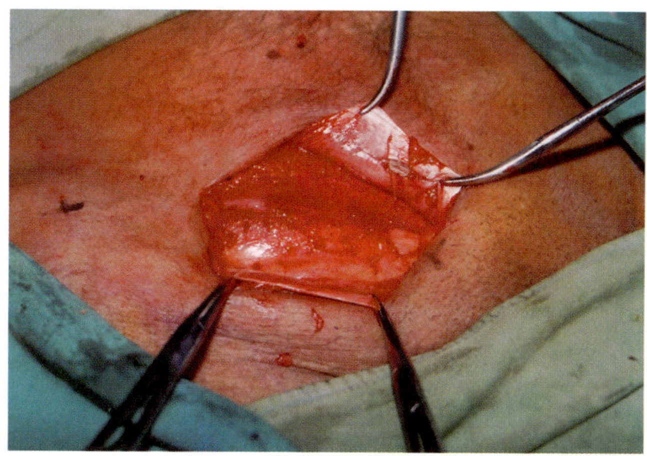

Fig. 89.2 Exposure of inguinal canal

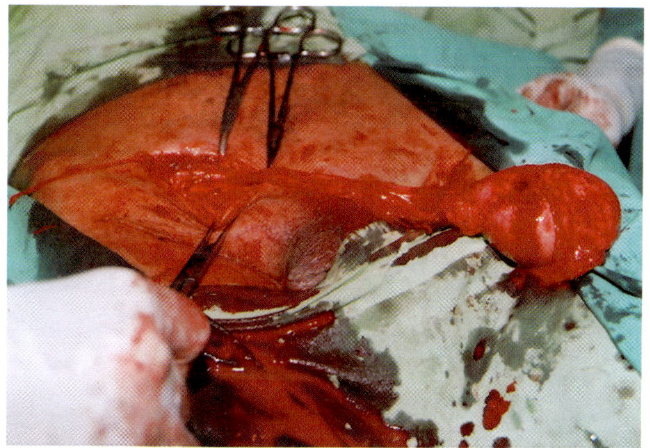

Fig. 89.3 Delivery of testis

The proximal end of the cord is ligated with 0 silk. An additional transfixation suture should be applied. The testis and cord is removed.

- *Closure:* The external oblique aponeurosis is closed with 2/0 chromic catgut. The skin is closed with interrupted nonabsorbable suture.

Complications:

- Bleeding from transected cord
- Scrotal hematoma
- Tumor seedling
- Damage to ilioinguinal nerve causing anesthesia over pubic bone.

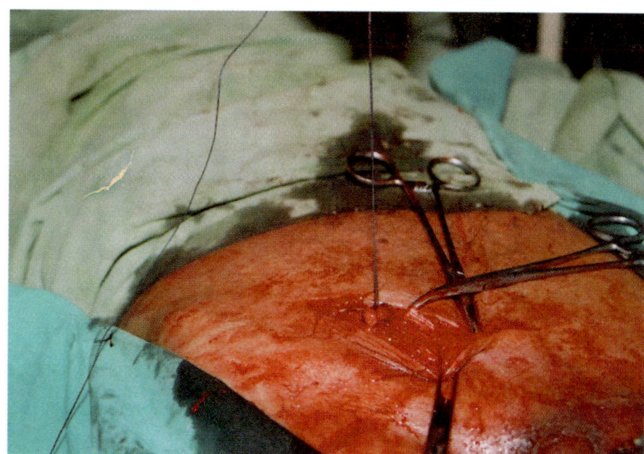

Fig. 89.4 Ligation of cord and division

SUBCAPSULAR ORCHIDECTOMY

Indication

Carcinoma of prostate as part of hormone manipulation.

Procedure

- *Position:* Supine
- *Anesthesia:* General or spinal
- *Incision:* A small vertical incision is made through lower part of scrotum
- *Exposure:* The incision is deepened to expose each testis in turn
- *Technique:* The testis is delivered through an incision in tunica albugenia. The glandular substance is scoped from each testis
- *Closure:* The scrotal incision is closed by interrupted sutures.

POSTOPERATIVE CARE

- Systemic antibiotic is advised
- Oral analgesic
- Removal of stitches after 7 days.

POSTOPERATIVE COMPLICATIONS

- Hemorrhage
- Sepsis.

CHAPTER

90

Operation for Hydrocele

Dhiraj Choudhury

Vaginal hydrocele is an abnormal collection of fluids in the tunica vaginalis.

INDICATIONS FOR OPERATION

- *Acquired hydrocele*
- Congenital hydroceles are treated by herniotomy not resolve spontaneously
- Symptomatic hydrocele should be operated. Sometimes operation is also indicated for medical fitness. Surgical treatment of hydrocele is curative.

PREOPERATIVE PREPARATIONS

- Scrotal ultrasound should be performed.

OPERATIVE PROCEDURE

- *Position:* Supine.
- *Anesthesia:* General endotracheal, spinal or local anesthesia may be used.
- *Incision:* A vertical incision is made on the scrotal skin avoiding superficial blood vessels, while the assistant holds the hydrocele to steady it and stretch the skin (Fig. 90.1). This compresses the small vessels in the scrotal skin and subsequent incision is usually bloodless.

  For large hydrocele a transverse elliptical incision with removal of part of redundant skin may be applied. This may be used also for bilateral operations.
- *Exposure:* Deepen the incision through subcutaneous tissue and dartos until tunica vaginalis is reached. At this point, the dartos muscle is gently pushed off the tunica to expose it for 5 cm length (Fig. 90.2).

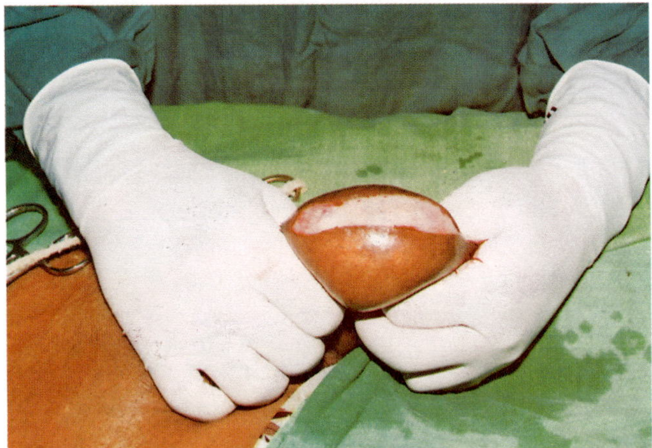

Fig. 90.1 Vertical scrotal skin incision

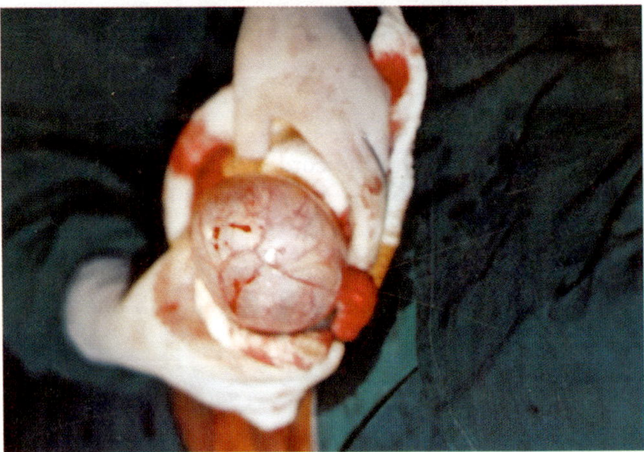

Fig. 90.2 Exposure of tunica vaginalis

Technique

The hydrocele sac is opened anteriorly by a small incision away from the testis in an avascular area (Fig. 90.3). Samples of hydrocele fluid may be collected for culture and cytology. A sucker may be inserted to aspirate the fluid to keep the operation site dry. The incision in the tunica is then enlarged and the testis is squeezed from below so that it exteriorizes through the defect in tunica vaginalis. The testis is examined for signs of pathology.

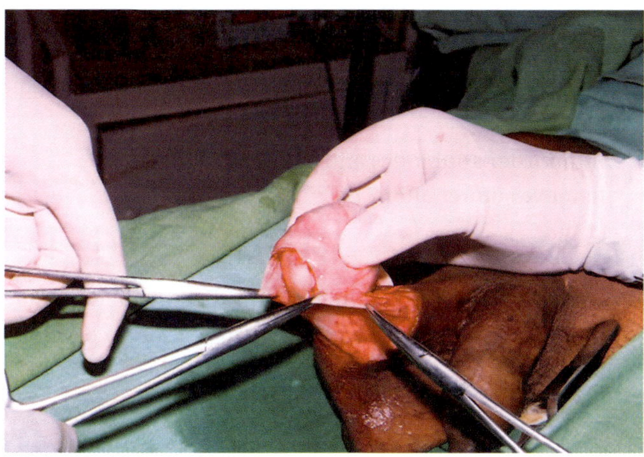

Fig. 90.3 Opening hydrocele sac

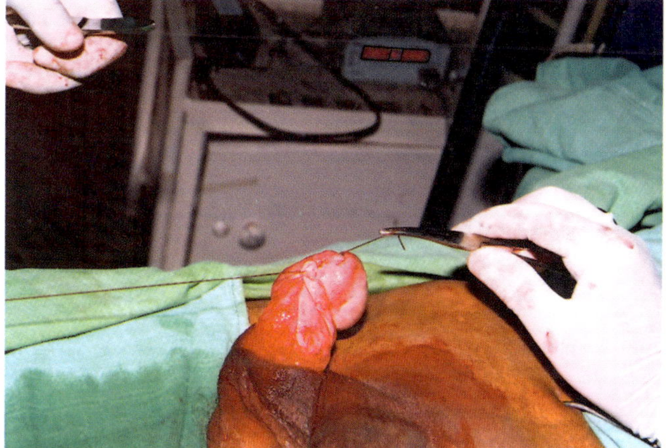

Fig. 90.4 Eversion of sac stitching of everted margins

Eversion of Sac (Fig. 90.4): Jaboulay's Operation

If the sac is large but thin walled, it is not excised but its free margins are united behind epididymis and cord with 0 running hemostatic sutures. Care should be taken to avoid strangulation of the cord by leaving an adequate gap between the tunical suture line and the cord.

Hydrocelectomy/Sac Excision

Excision of the sac may be performed in case of thick walled sacs and multiloculated hydrocele. Excise the sac leaving a reasonable margin to avoid injury to epididymis. The edges are then over sewned with continues 2/0 catgut sutures. This stops bleeding from the wound (Fig. 90.5).

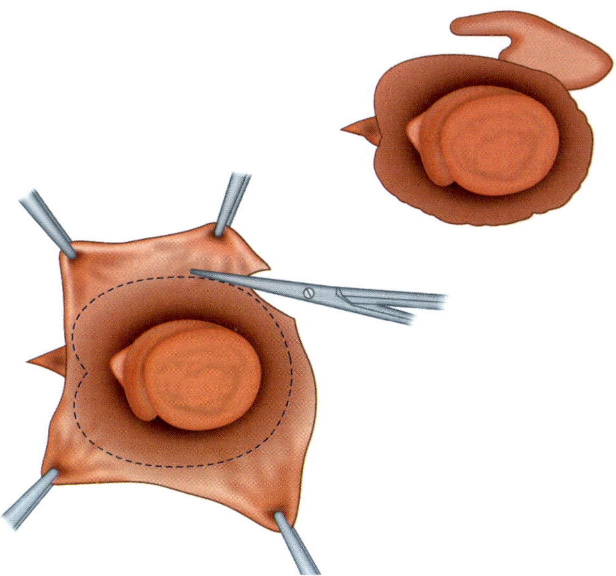

Fig. 90.5 Excision of sac

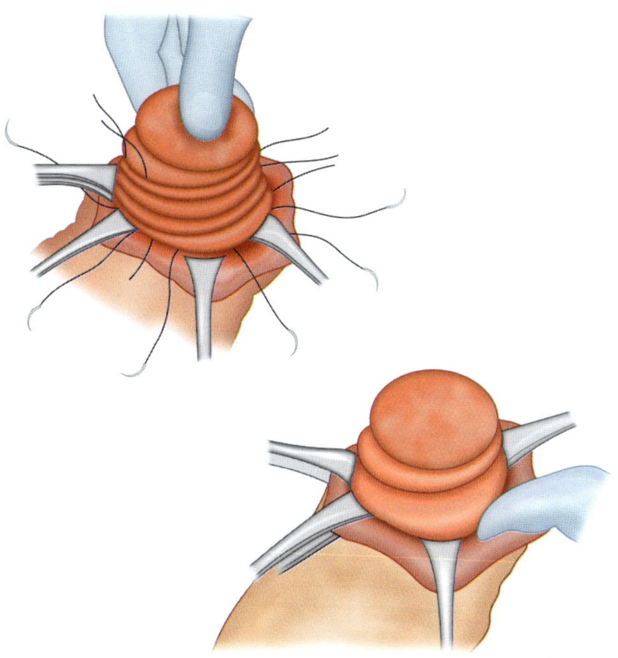

Fig. 90.6 Plication

Lord's Plication

In case of small thin walled tunica vaginalis sac the redundant tunica vaginalis may be plicated by five or six gathering stitches radiating outwards from its attachment to the testis towards its cut end (Fig. 90.6). This achieves the same effect as the Jaboulay procedure without risking vascular compromise of the cord. The advantage of the plication technique over excision technique is that they require less dissection and hence, less risk of hematoma.

Closure

- Check hemostasis
- A corrugated rubber drain may be inserted and brought through separate stab wound
- Dartos may be closed by interrupted absorbable suture
- Skin is closed by interrupted mattress suture using non-absorbable materials.

POSTOPERATIVE CARE

- Apply scrotal suspensory bandage to reduce edema and bleeding
- Administer antibiotics and analgesic
- Remove sutures after 7 days.

POSTOPERATIVE COMPLICATIONS

- *Hematoma:* A large hematoma indicates inadequatae hemostasis and may require re-exploration to evacuate blood clots and secure hemostasis
- Sepsis.

CHAPTER

91

Vasectomy

Dhiraj Choudhury

INDICATION

For male sterilization, vasectomy is the most popular operation.

PREOPERATIVE PREPARATION

Counseling and consent by husband and wife.

OPERATIVE PROCEDURE

Conventional Method/Scalpel

- *Position:* Supine
- *Anesthesia:* Usually local
- *Technique:* The area is prepared and draped. The vas is palpated through skin at the root of the scrotum and manipulated to superficial position and steadied between finger and thumb. It may be kept fixed by underpinning with a needle (Fig. 91.1) 1 or 2% Xylocaine (plain) is infiltrated into skin and around the cord.

Incision

A small vertical incision is made over the vas on scrotal surface.

Exposure

The incision is deepened through its coverings till the vas is exposed. The vas is picked up with Allis' forceps and delivered through the wound, after division of fascial coverings (Fig. 91.2). A vas ring can be inserted to hold the vas.

Vasectomy

A short segment 1–2 cm of the vas is divided between two pairs of artery forceps and the divided ends of the vas are

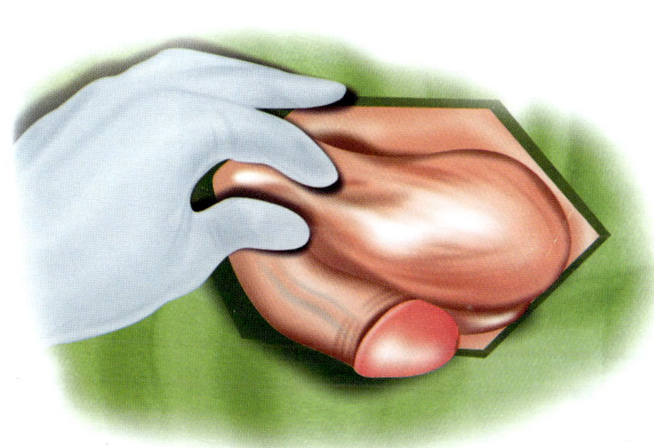

Fig. 91.1 Fixation of vas between finger and thumb

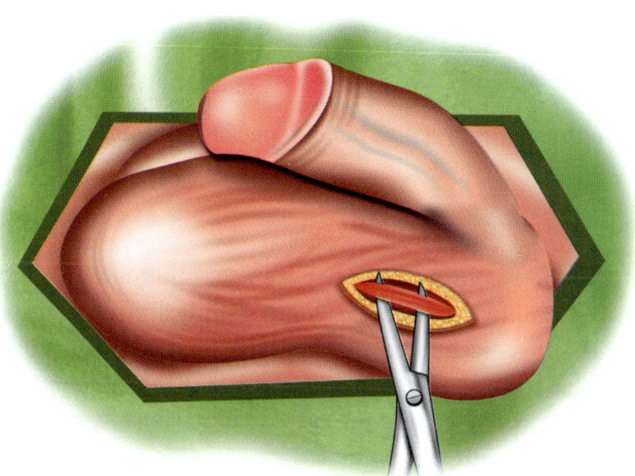

Fig. 91.2 Exposure of vas

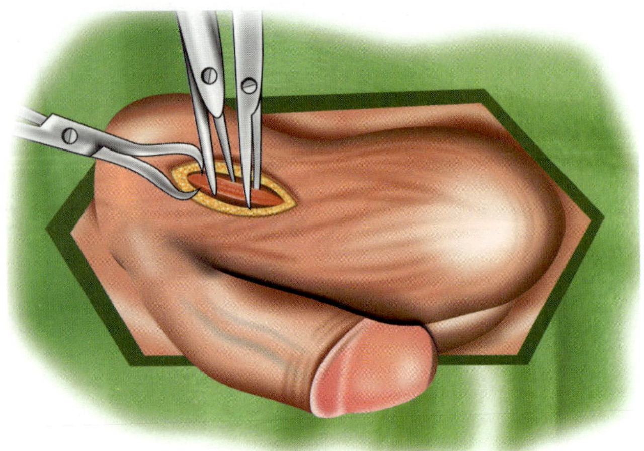

Fig. 91.3 Vasectomy

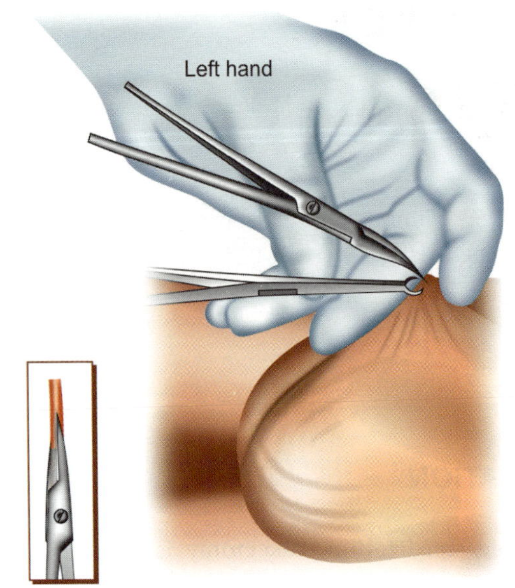

Fig. 91.4 Exposure of vas

ligated with silk or catgut (Fig. 91.3). Folding back the vas or fascial interposition may be used to prevent recanalization.

Closure

The wound is closed with absorbable suture.

No Scalpel Vasectomy

This was first performed in China in 1974.

Advantages

- Less invasive
- Causes fewer complications like hemorrhage, infection
- Better acceptance.

Disadvantage

Requires surgical skill to handle special instruments.

Steps

Hold the vas in position between the thumb and middle finger and place the index finger slightly above the thumb (three finger technique to isolate vas).

Raise the skin weal by injecting 1% lignocaine over the vas. The skin overlying the vas is held in ring forceps and is punctured with sharp pointed forceps (Fig. 91.4). The skin margins are then gently separated. The vas is picked up by one pointed blade of the forceps and lifted out of the wound releasing the ring forceps at the same time (Figs 91.5 and

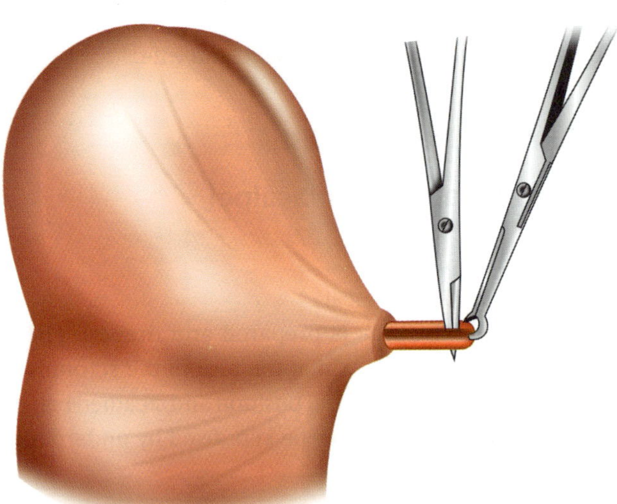

Fig. 91.5 Manipulation of vas

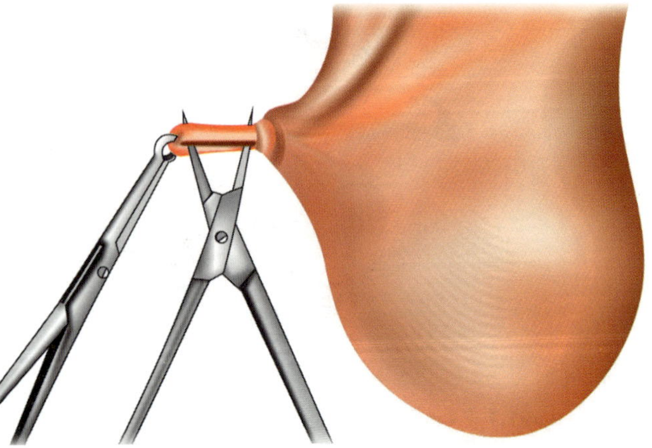

Fig. 91.6 Manipulation of segment of vas

91.6). The pulled vas is then ligated and divided. The ends are allowed to slip back into the scrotum. The other side is similarly operated. The wound is simply dressed.

POSTOPERATIVE CARE

- Patient is immediately discharged
- Analgesic is advised.

POSTOPERATIVE COMPLICATIONS

Short Term

- Hemorrhage, hematoma
- Sepsis
- Sperm granuloma.

Long Term

Less than 1% failure rate due to recanalization.

CHAPTER

92

Varicocelectomy

Dhiraj Choudhury

Varicocele, a varicose condition of the pampiniform plexus is mostly idiopathic in nature. Secondary varicocele may be found on the left side caused by renal vein obstruction by renal tumor (Fig. 92.1).

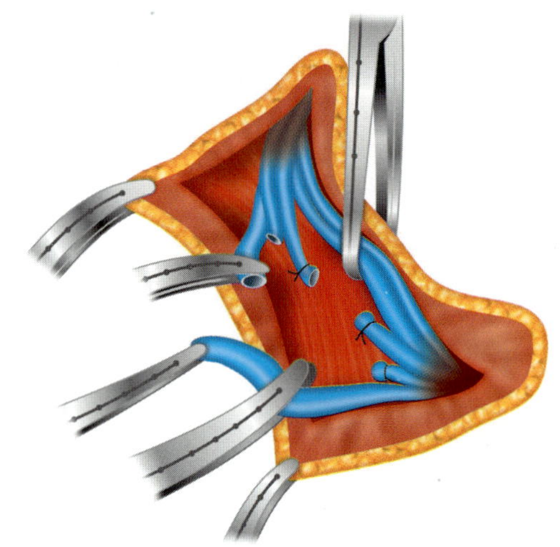

Fig. 92.1 Exposure and excision of pampiniform veins

INDICATIONS FOR INTERVENTION

- For treatment of male infertility.
- Symptomatic varicocele, should be judiciously selected for operation if symptoms are not relieved by reassurance, scrotal support and analgesic.

TYPES OF INTERVENTION

- Laparoscopic method
- Embolization
- Open method

Laparoscopic Method

- The simplest procedure is laparoscopic ligation of the testicular vein above the inguinal ligament where the pampiniform plexus has coalesced into one or two veins.
- The patient's bladder is emptied and he is positioned supine with a 20° left lateral tilt side. The surgeon stands at the right side of the patient. Three laparoscopic ports are inserted one 10 mm at umbilicus for laparoscope, a 10 mm port in midline half-way between pubis and umbilicus and one 5 mm at the left side of the rectus sheath lateral to umbilicus. Adhesion between the sigmoid colon and lateral pelvic wall are freed until the vas and testicular vessels are seen entering the deep inguinal ring. The testicular vessels are mobilized and veins clipped but artery left intact.

Embolization

- Embolization of testicular vein under radiographic control can be tried as an alternative method.

Open Method

- *Position:* Supine.
- *Anesthesia:* General or spinal.
- *Incision:* Inguinal approach is most popular. A 4" long incision is made above and parallel to medial part of the inguinal ligament.
- *Exposure:* The inguinal canal is opened by excising the external oblique aponeurosis. The spermatic cord is encircled and delivered to the wound. Deliver the testis out of the scrotum.
- *Technique:* The structures of the cord are dissected free. All the dilated tortuous internal spermatic veins are ligated and removed (Fig. 92.1).
  Check hemostasis and return the testis to scrotum.
- *Closure:* Close external oblique aponeurosis with continues 0 chromic catgut. The skin is closed with intermittent ethilon stitches.

POSTOPERATIVE CARE

- Analgesic
- Scrotal suspensory bandage.

POSTOPERATIVE COMPLICATIONS

- Hemorrhage
- Sepsis.

CHAPTER

93

Excision of Epididymal Cyst

Dhiraj Choudhury

Epididymal cysts are the most common intrascrotal cystic swellings and are benign.

INDICATIONS FOR OPERATION

The vast majority are asymptomatic. The indications for surgery may be pain or cosmesis.

STEPS

- The patient lies supine.
- The operation is done under general a spinal anesthesia.
- *Incision:* The skin is incised over the cyst parallel to skin vessels.
- The incision is deepened through the layer of the dartos.
- As the incision is extended between fascial layers, it is usually possible to manipulate the thin walled cyst. The layers of fascia should be gently pushed away, by fine sharp dissection.
- The dissection will leave the cyst attached at its base to the epididymis. The pedicle needs to be crossclamped and tied with absorbable ligature.
- *Closure:* The wound is closed in layers.

SECTION

17

Adrenals

CHAPTER

94

Surgery of Adrenals

Dhiraj Choudhury

ADRENALECTOMY

Indications

- Neoplasia
  - Adrenocortical adenoma
  - Adrenocortical carcinoma
  - Phaeochromocytoma (Medullary tumor)
  - Ganglioneuroma
  - Neuroblastoma
- Hyperplasia
- For management of endocrine dependent disease
  - Advance carcinoma of breast.

PREOPERATIVE PREPARATION

- In order to combat hormone insufficiency, adrenalectomy should be carried out under cortisone control, both pre- and postoperatively
- In case of pheochromocytoma, adequate control of blood pressure is necessary preoperatively, intraoperatively and postoperatively.

METHODS

- Laparoscopic adrenalectomy
- Retroperitoneoscopic adrenalectomy
- Laparoscopic or retroperitoneoscopic adrenalectomy has become the gold standard in the resection of adrenal tumors except for those with signs of malignancy.
- *Open adrenalectomy*: It should be considered if radiological signs, distant metastasis, large tumors (7.8–10 cm) or hormonal pattern suggest malignancy.
- *Laparoscopic adrenalectomy*: Transperitoneal approach requires creation of 4–5 ports on the side to be operated after pneumoperitoneum.
- *Right adrenalectomy*: After mobilization of right lobe of the liver, the adrenal vein is identified, divided and clipped. The dissection is then carried till complete or subtotal removal of the adrenal.
- *Left adrenalectomy*: The patient is positioned on his or her right side; mobilization of the spleen will result displacement of the tail of the pancreas medially. The left adrenal vein will be identified by putting incision on Gerotas fascia. The left adrenal vein is divided and clipped. This is followed by transection of left adrenal.
- *Retroperitoneal adrenalectomy*: The advantage of this approach is minimal dissection required. The first port is placed at the distal end of the 12th rib with patient in prone position. After digital dissection into retroperitoneum Gerotas fascia is displaced ventrally.

The right adrenal vein is covered by retrocaval posterior aspect of the adrenal gland. The left adrenal vein is usually located at the medial inferior pole of the adrenal gland.

OPEN ADRENALECTOMY

Posterolateral Approach

Position: The patient lies on one side with affected side uppermost.

Anesthesia: General with endotracheal intubation.

Right adrenalectomy: The right adrenal is exposed by right posterolateral approach as described for exposure of kidney. After mobilization of right lobe of liver the adrenal vein is identified running to right side of inferior vena cava. The vein is exposed by careful blunt dissection. The vein is ligated and divided. Adrenal artery is small and variable and coagulated. The fascial connection between adrenal and kidney is divided and the gland removed.

Left adrenalectomy: The left adrenal is exposed by left posterolateral approach. Mobilization of the spleen will displace the pancreas medially. The fascia of Gerota is incised to identify left adrenal vein which is ligated and divided at its point of entry into left renal vein. The artery is dealt with diathermy. The resection is completed by transection of the gland. For large suspected malignant tumor, thoracoabdominal approach should be considered.

Bilateral adrenalectomy: By anterior approach.

Anesthesia: General with endotracheal intubation.

Position: Dorsal position with thoracolumbar region slightly arched over the raised bridge.

Incision: A curved transverse incision convex upwards, 5 cm above the umbilicus.

The left adrenal is approached first by dividing the lienorenal ligament. The spleen is turned upwards and to right of the patient together with tail of the pancreas and splenic vessels. The left kidney and adrenal is now visible. The gland is recognized by its orange color. It is cleared after securing the vessels—particularly on the medial border. The gland is removed. The spleen and pancreas are replaced in their original position.

The right adrenal gland is searched in subhepatic pouch, in an area bounded by the lower border of the liver, right side of the vena cava and renal vessels. The liver is gently retracted upwards while the kidney is drawn downwards. The posterior peritoneum is incised around upper pole of the kidney. Elevation of peritoneal flap will display right adrenal which can be brought to view by a finger inserted above it. The gland is gently rotated so that vessels related to its medial surface particularly large but short vein which joined inferior vena cava, can be safely secured. The fascial connections are divided and the gland is removed.

SECTION

18

Vascular Surgery

CHAPTER

95

Exposure of Major Peripheral Arteries

Dhiraj Choudhury, Saugata Deb

INDICATIONS

Emergency

- Arterial injuries
- Acute arterial occlusion due to thromboembolism.

Elective

- Arteriography
- For preliminary ligation in case of radical cancer surgery
- Arterial bypass for chronic ischemia
- For regional perfusion
- A-V fistula.

COMMON CAROTID ARTERY

Indications

- Trauma
- Endarterectomy
- Carotid body tumor.

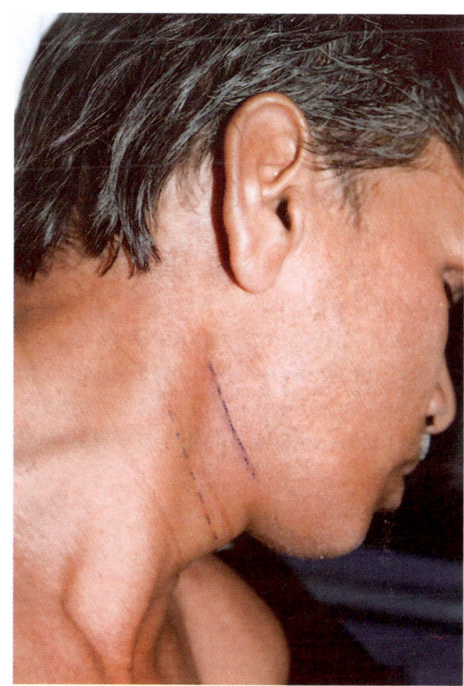

Fig. 95.1 Skin incisions for common carotid (lower) and external and internal carotid (upper)

Operative Procedure

- *Position:* The patient lies in supine position with neck slightly extended and head turned to opposite side.
- *Anesthesia:* Patient is given general anesthesia with endotracheal intubation.
- *Incision:* A transverse crease incision is made at the level of cricoid cartilage (Fig. 95.1).
- *Exposure:* The incision is deepened through subcutaneous tissue, platysma and deep fascia. The sternomastoid muscle is retracted laterally and omohyoid downwards to expose carotid sheath.
  The sheath is opened longitudinally to expose common carotid artery.

Closure

The skin is closed with interrupted sutures.

EXTERNAL AND INTERNAL CAROTID ARTERIES

Operative Procedure

- *Incision:* A crease incision is made below the angle of mandible (Fig. 95.1).
- *Exposure:* The incision is deepened through subcutaneous tissue and platysma. The deep fascia is divided to expose the sternomastoid muscle which is retracted posteriorly.

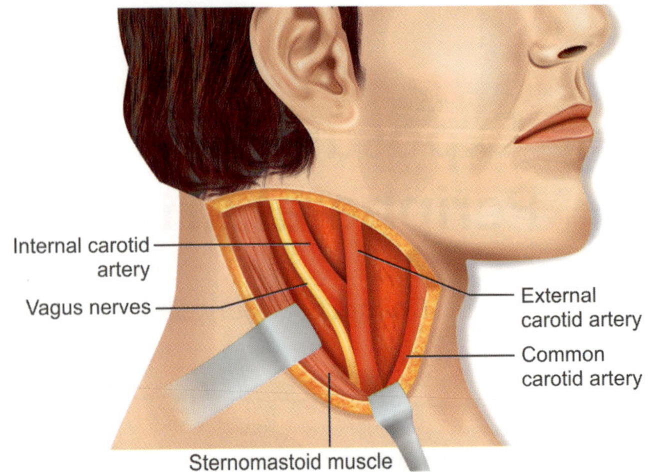

Fig. 95.2 Exposure of common carotid artery and its terminal branches

The common facial vein is divided and ligated at the upper end of the incision.

The carotid sheath is opened to expose external and internal carotid arteries (Fig. 95.2).

- *Identification:* The external carotid artery is identified by presence of branches in neck. The internal carotid artery lies initially posterolateral to external carotid and then deep to it. The hypoglossal nerve crossing these vessels should be protected.
- *Closure:* The skin can be closed with interrupted 2/0 ethilon sutures.

SUBCLAVIAN ARTERY

Indications

Trauma, aneurysm and atheromatous occlusions are main indications for exposure of subclavian artery.

Operative Procedure

- *Position:* The patient lies in supine position.
- *Anesthesia:* General anesthesia with endotracheal intubation is given.
- *Incision:* A transverse incision is made ½″ above and parallel to middle-third of clavicle.
- *Exposure:* The incision is deepened through subcutaneous tissue, platysma and deep fascia. The external jugular vein may require ligation. The second part of the sub-clavian artery is exposed by division of sternomastoid and scalenus anterior muscle (Fig. 95.3). The omohyoid muscle is retracted upwards to expose 3rd part of subclavian artery.

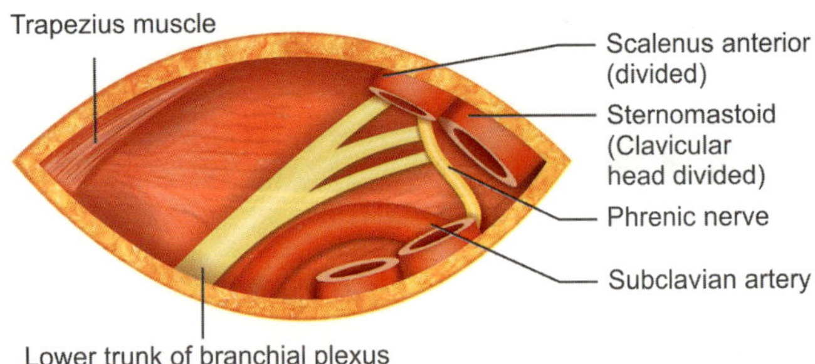

Fig. 95.3 Exposure of 2nd part of subclavian artery

The scalenus anterior muscle lies medially and upper and middle of brachial plexus laterally.

- *Closure:* The wound is closed in layers.

AXILLARY ARTERY

Indications

Embolectomy and operation for aneurysm are main indications of exposure of axillary artery.

Operative Procedure

- *Position:* The patient lies in supine position with arm at right angle on an arm-rest.
- *Anesthesia:* General anesthesia with endotracheal intubation is given.
- *Incision:* An incision is made along the line of (pulsatile) artery up to lower border of pectoralis major muscle.

  The groove between coracobrachialis and triceps is a guide to the artery.
- *Exposure:* The incision is deepened through subcutaneous tissue and deep fascia. The clavicular head of the pectoralis major muscle is retracted upwards and medially, to provide exposure of axillary artery which is sufficient for embolectomy. But for wider exposure, the sternocostal head of pectoralis major muscle and pectoralis minor muscle require division.
- *Closure:* Skin is closed with interrupted sutures with 2/0 ethilon.

BRACHIAL ARTERY

In Arm

Embolectomy, repair of injury and arteriography are main indications for exposure of brachial artery.

Operative Procedure

- *Position:* The patient lies in supine position with arm supported on arm rest.
- *Anesthesia:* General anesthesia with endotracheal intubation.
- *Incision:* An incision is made along the inner border of the biceps (line of artery) above the elbow.
- *Exposure:* The incision is deepened through subcutaneous tissue. The deep fascia is divided. The biceps muscle is retracted laterally and median nerve which crosses the artery superficially, is retracted laterally.

  The brachial artery with its two venae comitans is now exposed (Fig. 95.4).

Fig. 95.4 Exposure of brachial artery in arm

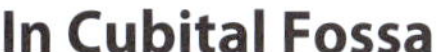

In Cubital Fossa

Trauma and embolism are main indications for exposure.

- *Incision:* A longitudinal incision is made in the middle of cubital fossa along medial side of biceps tendon. An S-shaped incision is considered better (Fig. 95.5).
- *Exposure:* The incision is deepened through subcutaneous tissue. The main cubital vein is ligated.

  The bicepital aponeurosis is divided when the median nerve is expected.

  The biceps tendon is retracted laterally and pronator teres medially to expose the brachial artery (Fig. 95.6).
- *Closure:* Skin is closed with interrupted ethilon sutures.

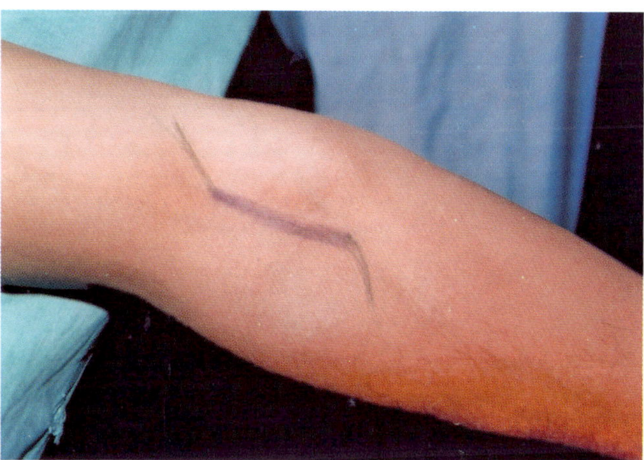

Fig. 95.5 Incision for brachial artery in cubital fossa

RADIAL ARTERY

Indication: The most common indication of exposure of radial artery at wrist is for creation of arteriovenous shunt for dialysis in renal failure.

Operative Procedure

- *Position:* The patient lies in supine position with arm fully supinated.
- *Anesthesia:* General anesthesia with endotracheal intubation is applied.
- *Incision:* A longitudinal or transverse incision, centered 3–4 cm above the radial styloid process is made (Fig. 95.7).
- *Exposure:* The incision is deepened through subcutaneous tissue and superficial fascia. The lower end of cephalic vein lies in superficial fascia at radial side of wrist.

  The radial artery lies at a deeper level between brachioradialis and flexer carpi radialis.

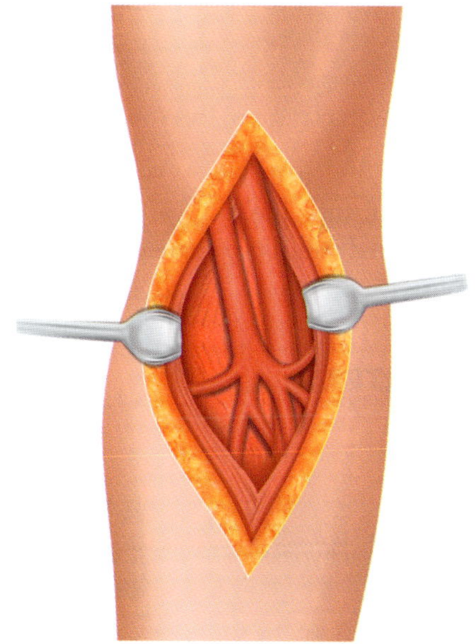

Fig. 95.6 Exposure of brachial artery in cubital fossa

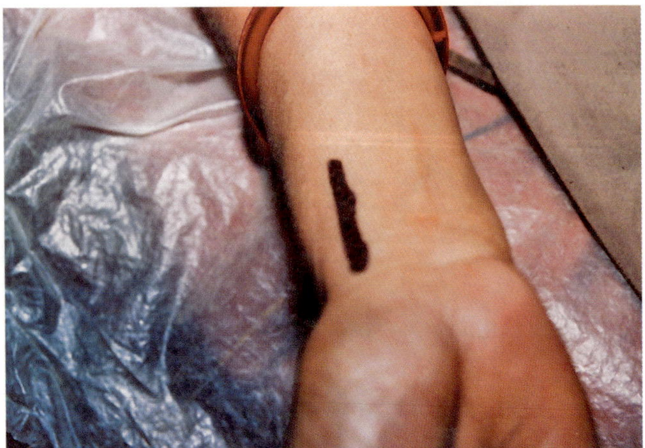

Fig. 95.7 Incision for radial artery

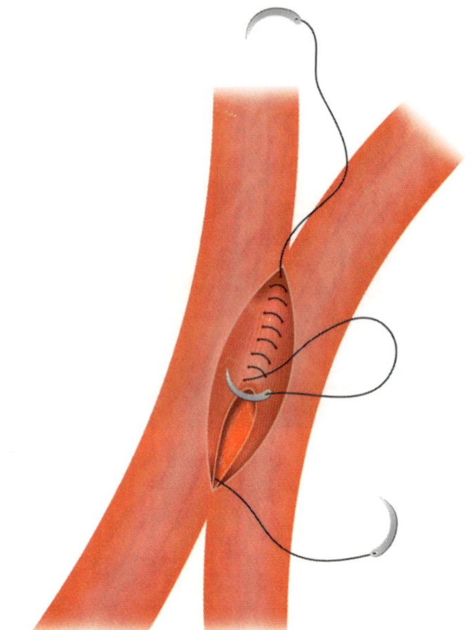

Fig. 95.8 AV fistula (Radial) artery and cephalic vein

- *Procedure:* AV fistula. The radial artery and cephalic vein can be mobilized and approximated to allow side-to-side anastomosis (Fig. 95.8).

FEMORAL ARTERY

Indications

- Embolectomy
- Femoro-popliteal bypass
- Repair of injury.

Operative Procedure

- *Position:* The patient lies in supine position.

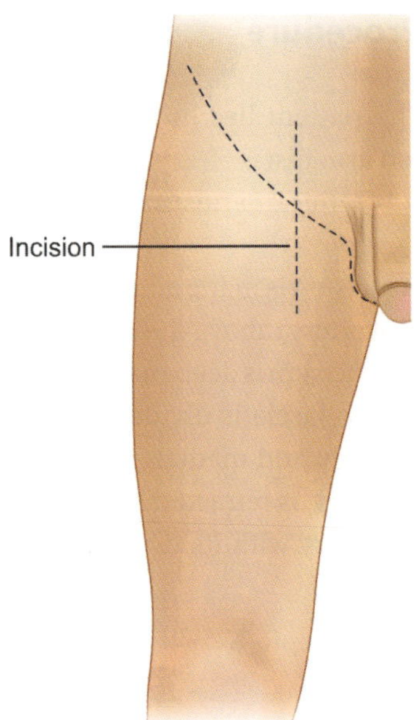

Fig. 95.9 Incision for femoral artery

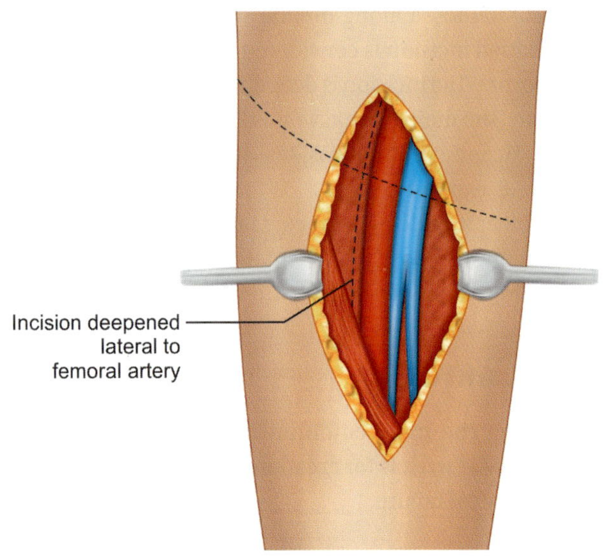

Fig. 95.10 Exposure of femoral artery

- *Anesthesia:* General anesthesia with endotracheal intubation.
- *Incision:* A vertical incision is made along a line running from mid-inguinal point to apex of femoral triangle (Fig. 95.9).
- *Exposure:* The incision is deepened through skin, subcutaneous tissue, superficial and deep fascia.
  The superficial external pundendal artery is ligated.
  The femoral sheath is opened to expose common femoral vessels. The femoral artery lies laterally to femoral vein and is dissected circumferentially (Fig. 95.10).
  The profunda femoris artery lies posterolaterally.

- *Closure:* The skin is closed with interrupted sutures. The incision and exposure made over CFA using a somewhat lateral approach to avoid the lymphatic pad.

In Hunter's Canal

- *Incision:* A longitudinal incision is made along the line of anterior border of the sartorius muscle.
- *Exposure:* The incision is deepened through subcutaneous tissue. The fascia covering the subsartorial canal is incised after retraction of sartorius muscle, to expose femoral artery and vein.
  The femoral vein lies lateral to femoral artery which is crossed by long saphenous vein.
- *Closure:* After completion of procedure, skin is closed with interrupted stitches.

POPLITEAL ARTERY

Indications

Exposure of popliteal artery may be required for:
- Trauma
- Bye-pass
- Aneurysm.

Operative Procedure

- *Position:* The patient is placed in prone position.
- *Anesthesia:* General anesthesia with endotracheal intubation.
- *Incision:* A vertical incision is made over popliteal fossa (Fig. 95.11).
- *Exposure:* The incision is deepened through subcutaneous tissue, superficial and deep fascia. The short saphenous vein may require ligation at its termination.
  Division of fascial roof exposes the medial and lateral popliteal nerves. The popliteal vessels are exposed following retraction of semimembranous and biceps above, and two heads of gastrocnemius below. The popliteal vein lies lateral to and superficial to artery and is retracted to expose popliteal artery (Fig. 95.12).
- *Closure:* Skin is closed with interrupted ethilon stitches.

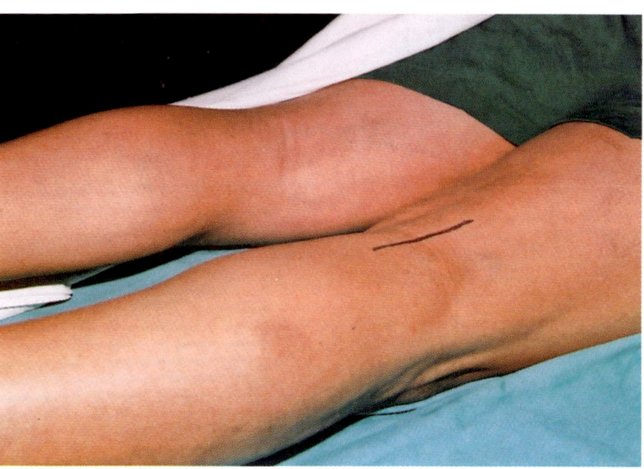

Fig. 95.11 Incision for popliteal artery

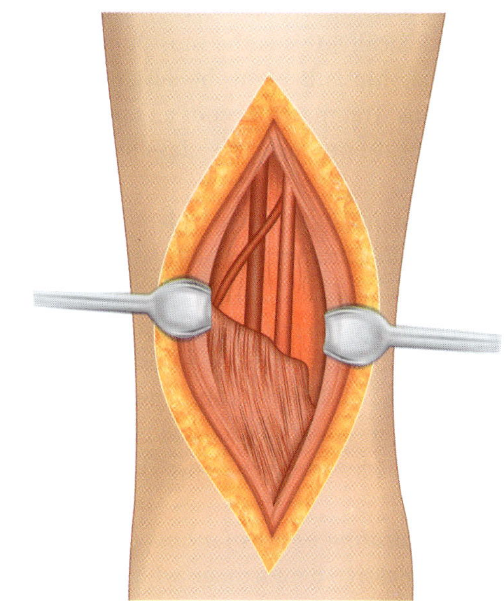

Fig. 95.12 Shows exposure of popliteal artery in popliteal fossa

CHAPTER

96

Vascular Trauma

Krishnendu Mukherjee

INTRODUCTION

This is a very complex topic, impossible to do justice in a short chapter. Paradoxically, this is the most important chapter since the readership is likely to be surgical trainees and younger surgeons. Trauma transcends all surgical specialties. Probably, the best approach is a classification based on clinical scenarios.

Isolated unilateral limb trauma with or without fractures, open or closed with 'hard' signs of vascular injury, e.g. absent distal pulses.

Same as above, as a part of polytrauma. Here, chest and significant abdominal injuries and some head injuries get higher priority, but the limb cannot wait too long either. Temporary vascular shunts should be considered here to 'buy' time. Even a Ryles tube may be used between a proximal and distal artery.

Solitary penetrating injury of a limb (including stab or gunshot) with massive hemorrhage with or without distal ischemia.

- Abdominal and thoracic injuries.
- Closed or penetrating neck injuries.
- Complex injuries, e.g. 'blasts', disasters, etc.

The first golden rule is to approach every patient along Advanced Trauma Life Support (ATLS) protocol. (The importance of ATLS cannot over-emphasized to all medical graduates). A MAP of 80–90 is generally adequate. Rapid infusion of fluids is not always required. The next question is how much to investigate?

Routine chest X-ray, a blood sample for Hb, grouping, glucose, urea-electrolytes and a urine sample for microscopy are essential. A cervical spine and pelvis X-ray and a screening abdominal ultrasound are also appropriate. Some situations do not need any investigation at all, except a blood sample for cross-match. A penetrating abdominal trauma with severe hypotension or a bullet injury of the groin with massive hemorrhage can and should proceed straight to theater.

Once an isolated limb injury is confirmed, vascular assessment follows the ALI protocol. Is the limb viable? Attempts to re-perfuse a non-viable limb are futile and may be fatal. (This underscores the need for the prevention of a missed diagnosis. All limb injuries *closed* or *open* must be clinically assessed for distal neurovascular signs. X-rays alone is not sufficient. A transient posterior dislocation of the knee which has spontaneously snapped back into position may have a normal X-ray. The popliteal artery may have sustained severe injury).

Once potential viability is established (preferably including hand-held Doppler assessment), no time should be lost before surgical exploration.

A preop CTA or MRA may be very helpful but is not mandatory. Conventional catheter-based DSA may be performed only in the absence of fractures if good endovascular expertise is available because treatment may be possible.

Time permitting, it is, however, more important to do an ultrasound mapping of the great saphenous vein (GSV). In lower limb injuries, the contralateral GSV is mapped.

The following principles are next followed at the operation:

Both the affected limb and the mapped leg must be prepped and draped, should a vein harvest be required.

Dislocations are reduced first before surgical exploration.

Fractures, however, are dealt with later.

Exceptions include supracondylar fracture of the humerus and rarely non-communited fractures of distal femur. Here, closed fracture reduction itself may make the pulse return.

If a normal pulse is palpable after reduction, exploration is not needed but a clinical reassessment must be made within 12 hours. On long-term follow-up these patients may rarely develop pseudoaneurysms or traumatic AVF.

In all other situations surgical exploration should commence at and proximal to the site of injury, area of bruising/swelling or an open wound. The target is to dissect a normal proximal artery (Fig. 96.1).

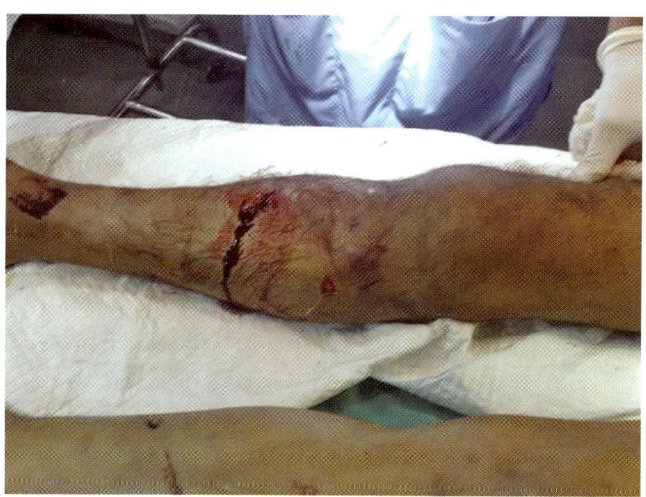

Fig. 96.1 Compound fracture from within—small punctured wound. Pulseless leg

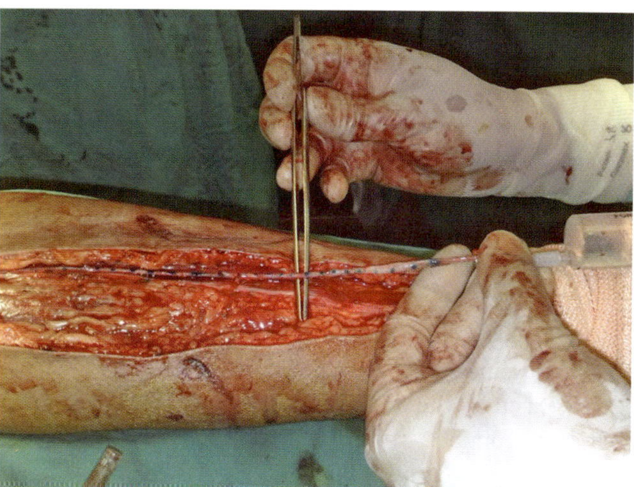

Fig. 96.3 Great saphenous vein (GSV) harvest. Gentle distension with heparinized saline

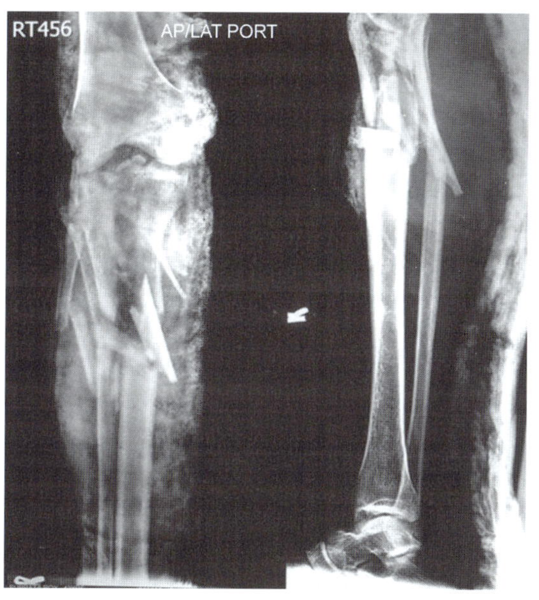

Fig. 96.2 X-ray of same patient. Severe communicated fracture of tibia and fibula with popliteal artery injury

If a preop angiogram has demonstrated a deep main artery is injured (Fig. 96.2) (e.g. distal popliteal artery in upper leg with comminuted fracture of proximal tibia), a plan of doing a femorodistal bypass may have already been made. Instead of going in the site of injury, the femoral artery in adductor canal and posterior tibial artery in lower third of leg may be exposed first.

After debridement and hemostasis of the injured area, fracture fixation is undertaken *before* the vascular reconstruction. Internal or external skeletal fixation is undertaken (depending on closed/open injury) while simultaneously the GSV harvest can be commenced in the unaffected leg by another team.

TECHNIQUE OF GREAT SAPHENOUS VEIN HARVEST (Fig. 96.3)

An incision is made above the medial malleolus and the GSV identified. The incision is extended upwards preferably by scissors few cms at a time while constantly keeping the vein in view. Perivenous dissection is commenced and the tributaries tied off and divided between fine silk ligatures. Clips may be faster but should be avoided on the vein side of the tributary if tunneling is considered a possibility. Before actually mobilizing the full vein off its bed, it is prudent to mark the anterior surface (12 'O' clock line) of the vein with dots of sterile gentian violet with a blunt nerve hook or fine tipped mosquito forceps (Methylene blue does not adhere to the adventitia). The extension of the incision follows the course of the vein.

It is important not to raise too much flaps to avoid seromas and the vein handled with extreme care. It is finally divided at the ankle level and a truncated 16 G Jelco cannula introduced and double tied over the vein with silk. 'Double-Distal' is a useful pneumonic. It is *this* side of the vein which will form the proximal arterial anastomosis. Gradual hydrostatic dilatation can then begin via the cannula with heparinized saline. The whole vein never distends uniformly, segments of spasm are invariable. Gentle digital pressure on the distended segments helps to propagate the dilatation. The hepsaline is flushed with intermittent "soft-push"; forceful overdistension must be avoided. Leaks visible must be repaired *in situ* with 7-0 or 8-0 polyprophylene or PTFE sutures. Once adequate length is achieved, the proximal end is tied with a single ligature or clipped and the vein divided. The Jelco is capped to retain hep-saline in the vein and the harvest is preserved in a small bowl of cold hepsaline admixed with patient's own blood. Near and above the knee, the GSV is surprisingly deep. The wound is closed and dressing applied. Closure of the harvest wound is best achieved by a direct running continuous subcuticular suture. Only a few interrupted absorbable sutures may be used in the subcutaneous level.

If the GSV is unavailable or unsuitable, the SSV or cephalic vein of the upper limb may be used, or two segments "spliced' together by anastomosing them on the bench.

By this time the fractures would have been fixed if two teams are working.

The 'run-in' and 'run-off' vessels are once again re-assessed. 5000 IU heparin is administered systemically and the artery cross-clamped the distal anastomosis is usually performed first because a gentle Fogartization is of the distal vessel and hep-saline irrigations are required. Some back-bleed should be present. Most surgeons will complete the distal anastomosis but not tie the anchoring knot to assess pulsatile flow across the anastomosis after the release of proximal clamps at the end of reconstruction and to "bleed out" air bubbles in the vein.

Before the proximal anastomosis (with the distal end of the vein!) two considerations are vitally important. Some bed or a new tunnel? And, what is the appropriate length? Usually a short bridge graft (Fig. 96.4) is required and it may lie in the same bed of the injured area. But if heavy contamination or devitalization is present or soft-tissue cover unlikely to be possible, then a new subcutaneous tunnel may be needed. In this case, possible future incision sites for orthopedic reconstruction or fasciotomy incision sites must be avoided. The vein elongates slightly when sustaining arterial flow. When crossing a joint, flexion and extension need to be taken into account. It should be tension free yet not too redundant.

The proximal anastomosis is next completed after cutting the vein to appropriate length. Both an end-to-end bridge graft or an end-to-side bypass graft are acceptable (Figs 96.5 to 96.7). The traumatized artery is usually in a bruised segment

Fig. 96.4 Reversed great saphenous vein bridge graft from popliteal to posterior tibial artery. Note the external skeletal fixator

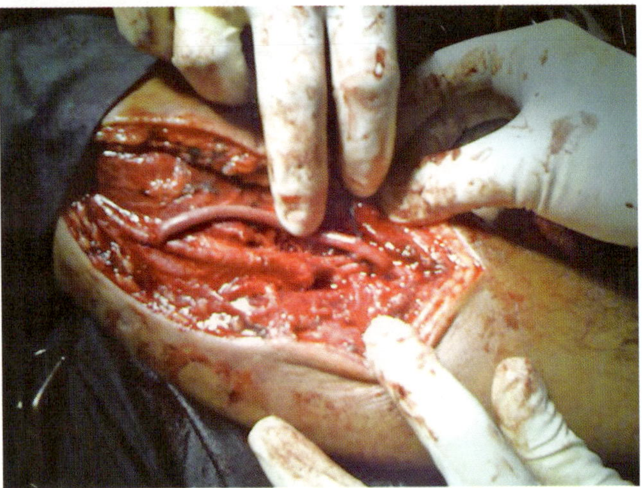

Fig. 96.5 Reversed great saphenous vein bypass graft. Note the traumatized neurovascular segment

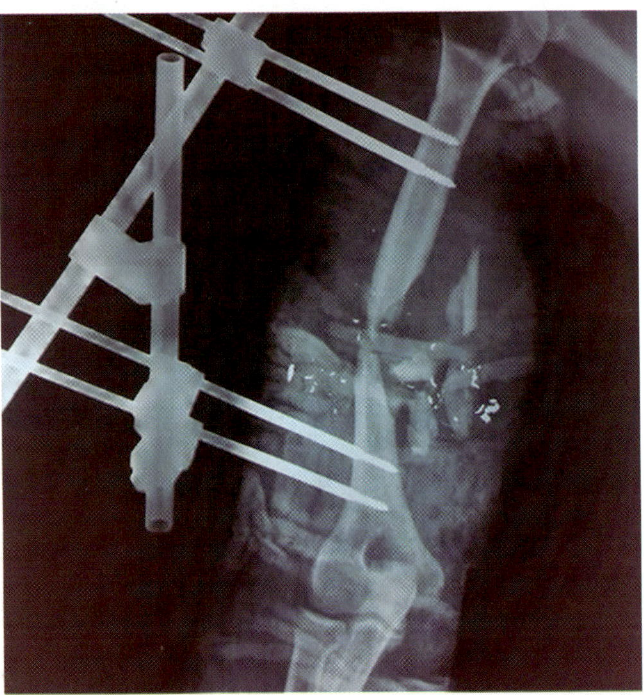

Fig. 96.6 Mid-brachial artery injury. Communicated fracture humerus. External skeletal fixation

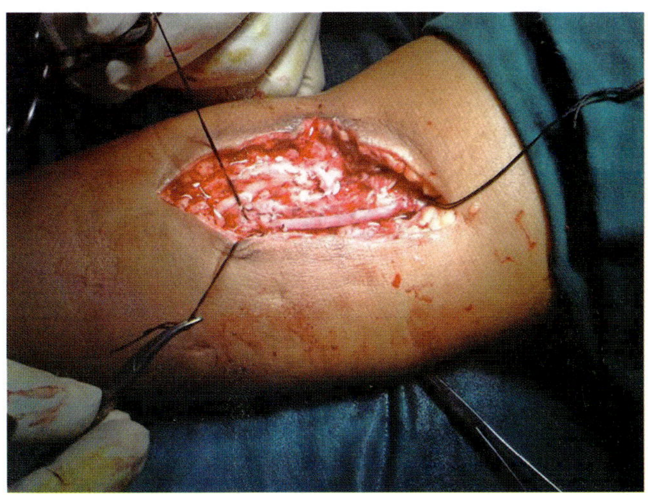

Fig. 96.7 Reversed great saphenous vein bridge graft repair of brachial artery

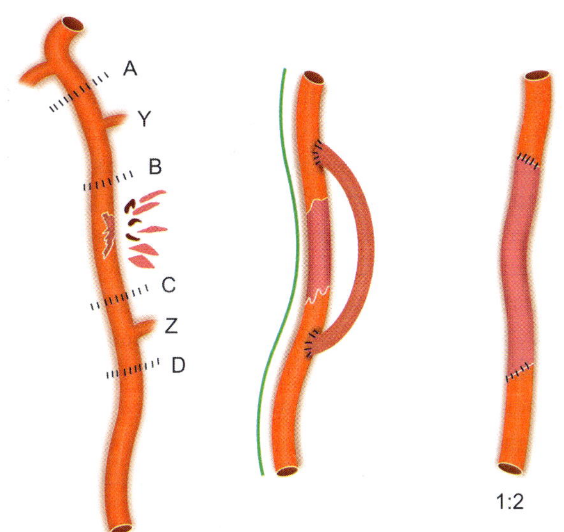

Fig. 96.8 Bypass graft and bridge graft. Proximal and distal controls. Note that B and C will be effective (i.e. just proximal to the site of interest). A and D will be ineffective because of branches Y and Z. A very proximal control may also help. Note the vein ends are fish-mouthed, i.e. an obliquity created

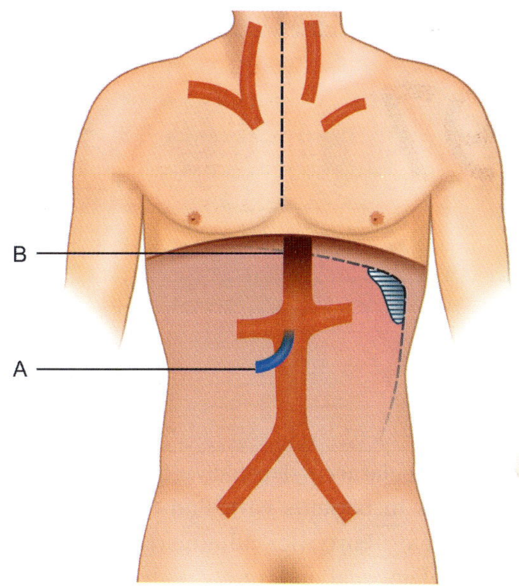

Fig. 96.9 Massive abdominal hemorrhage. At laparotomy, rapid supra-celiac (B) control of the abdominal aorta is usually effective. As soon as possible, the control can be shifted to infra-renal aorta (A)

of a neuro-vascular bundle with a thrombosed segment with intimal flap. Trying to resect this artery may damage the nerve. But hemostasis at this area must be rechecked before closure.

Suction drains may be safely placed in the area. Pedal pulses are not always immediately palpable despite a successful reconstruction. A 'shoot' angiogram in C-arm or Doppler assessments of distal signals should be performed on table.

Heparin should be continued (e.g. 5000 IU, SC 8 hourly for 2–3 days) and antiplatelets commenced as soon as possible.

In limb injuries, where severe hemorrhage is the initial problem, the wound is best managed with pack and pressure while rapid proximal control is obtained by surgical exposure of the appropriate vessel (e.g. External iliac artery for groin or mid-thigh injuries, CFA for lower thigh or upper leg injuries) (Figs 96.8 and 96.9).

CHAPTER

97

Vascular Access

Krishnendu Mukherjee

Long-term vascular access is usually required for maintenance hemodialysis in patients with End Stage Renal Disease (ESRD). Chemo-Ports (for administering chemotherapy drugs in malignancy) and, rarely, nutritional support, are other indications.

SHORT-TERM DIALYSIS CATHETERS

These are double lumen, non-cuffed central venous catheters (CVC). They are considerably bigger than CVC used for general intravenous access or CVP measurements, even the triple lumen catheters commonly used in hospitals. Dialysis catheters, therefore, are more prone to evoke inflammatory response within axial veins and cause stenosis (Fig. 97.1). Any central vein stenosis jeopardizes the future of surgically created vascular access in the ipsilateral limb. Subclavian veins are notorious for stenosis, hence CVC for dialysis should not be placed in subclavian veins.

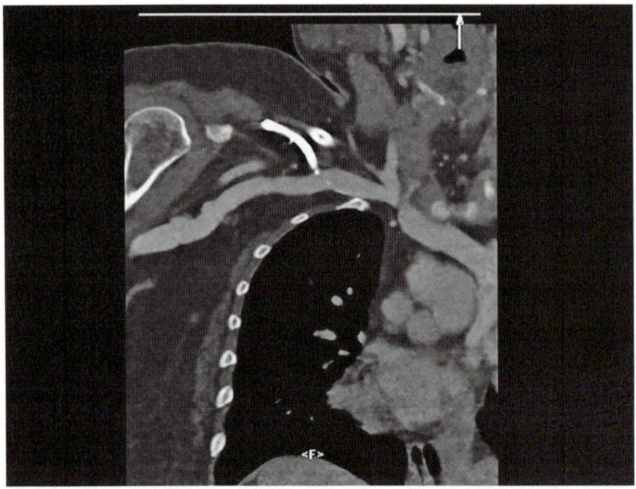

Fig. 97.1 A CT–venogram showing a stenosis at the beginning of right brachiocephalic vein. Dialysis catheters in central veins are notorious to cause this kind of stenosis

Right internal jugular (RIJ) vein is the preferred site followed by right external jugular vein followed by left internal jugular (LIJ) vein. Femoral veins can be used to access the IVC but are second line choice. They are easier to place but limit mobility and carry a higher infection rate.

LONG-TERM DIALYSIS CATHETERS

While short-term CVC may serve the purpose for 4–6 weeks, these CVC may be used for months to years. These are cuffed, tunneled double lumen catheters, commonly referred to as 'Permcaths'. Here too, the RIJ is the preferred site. Percutaneous placement is possible; the catheter in tunneled from an infraclavicular exit point (local anesthesia is required) with the cuff lying within the tunnel. The end of the CVC should be in the right atrium with arterial hole facing the mediastinum.

Operative technique for an RIJ dialysis CVC placement will be described in detail.

The procedure must be explained and the patient reassured.

- The patient is positioned supine with the neck slightly extended and turned to left. A small but comfortable cloth roll may be used between the scapulae. A slight 'head-down' position helps in distending the vein.
- Pulse oximetry and a cardiac monitor must be in place; this is not a minor procedure.
- Skin prep and drapes are placed; the operator follows strict aseptic principles.
- US-guided puncture and fluoroscopy is recommended but not always possible. For a Permcath placement, they are essential. Coagulation parameters are checked only if relevant history is present.
- The anatomical landmarks (Fig. 97.2) are palpated first; the carotid pulse is felt. The IJV lies lateral to the artery but rare anatomical variations may be present; a posterolateral location is the most common anomaly.

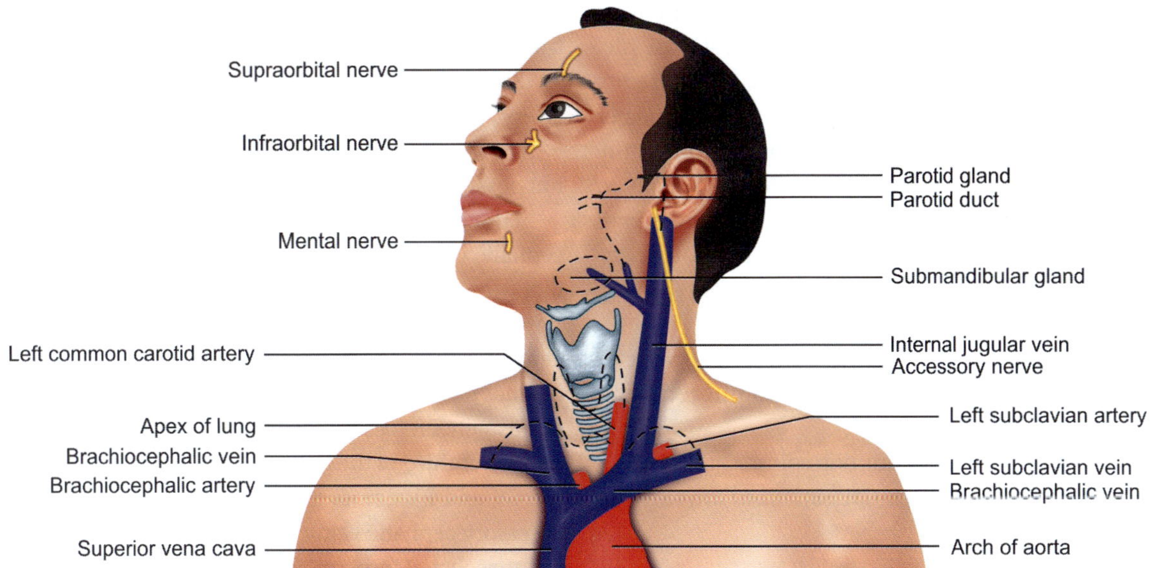

Fig. 97.2 Anatomy of central veins

Since the vein and the artery are enclosed in the same sheath, trying to displace the artery medially does not help; it renders the vein lumen rhomboid due to medial pull.

- Less experienced operators may choose to use a smaller needle to locate the vein first ('seeker needle'). Approaching the vein just medial to the medial border of sternocleidomastoid or at the apex of the triangle formed by the two heads of the muscle is appropriate.
- A 45 degree angle and direction towards the ipsilateral nipple usually helps. Free aspiration of venous blood confirms successful puncture. The 'seeker needle' is left *in situ* and the larger needle introduced.
- Accidental arterial puncture must be detected at this phase. ESRD patients often have higher venous pressure due to fluid overload. But the brisk spurt of carotid artery and the color of the blood should alert the operator.
- Holding the needle securely in left hand, the right-handed operator starts to push in the guidewire (GW) after removing the syringe (Some sets have novel side entry or "through-the-syringe" ports).
- The GW should pass freely without resistance. A few ectopic beats on the monitor are common and denote entry into right heart.
- Local anesthesia is instilled at the puncture site and a small stab incision made, only the skin needs to be incised.
- CVC for dialysis are bigger; hence gradually increasing size of dilators are used. Hence, it is essential to detect inadvertent arterial entry before the bigger dilators are used.
- Once the appropriate dilator is in place, the CVC is handled, preferably with fresh gloves and passed over the GW after removing the dilator.
- It is vitally important to grip the end of the GW first before introducing the dilators and finally the CVC. GW embolism is a serious complication. Therefore, the GW has to be gradually pulled out till it exits from the back of the dilator and CVC.
- Free aspirations of blood from both lumens are confirmed and both are flushed by hep-saline.
- More local anesthetic is instilled, suture fixation completed and an antibiotic ointment (preferably mupirocin) is used before applying a small but secure sterile dressing. Large dressings 'hide' hematomas!
- A chest X-ray is immediately asked for.

The X-ray is reviewed as soon as possible for correct placement (the tip of the CVC should be in SVC) and presence of any pneumothorax/hemothorax is excluded.

If an accidental arterial puncture has occurred, another attempt at venepuncture should not be made before 5-10 mins of pressure.

If 2 or 3 attempts fail to locate the vein, it is best to abandon the procedure and await US-guided puncture. If emergency dialysis is required; an alternative site should be tried.

A femoral CVC will be easier.

COMPLICATIONS OF CENTRAL VENOUS CATHETERS

- *Neck hematoma:* A hematoma following a dialysis CVC placement is never a minor affair. The patient should be set up, the hematoma marked, transferred to intensive care, coagulation parameters sent for and, if possible, a CT scan arranged. If there is any degree of respiratory distress or stridor, the patient should be taken to theater immediately. It is futile to attempt intubation in the intensive care unit or the ward. The attempt is likely to fail. Intubation should be performed in the theater with standby fiberoptic bronchoscope and tracheostomy sets. The hematoma should be surgically explored but the CVC can be usually preserved.

- *Catheter malfunction:* Kinks, fibrin-sheaths, pericatheter thrombus are more commonly encountered with permcaths.
- *Infections* remain the most common complication.
- *Pneumothorax, hemothorax, GW embolism* are rare but serious complications.

SURGICAL ACCESS

The superficial veins are easy-to-cannulate, specially in the upper limbs. However, the flow is inadequate to sustain hemodialysis. A vein, however, can be "arterialized" by anastomosing it to an artery.

The arterial flow increases further because the cardiac output increases in response to the fall in peripheral resistance. Over a period of weeks, the fistulated vein "matures" with high flow and slightly thickened walls to be able to withstand repeated needle trauma for dialysis. The classical Appel - Cimino - Brescia fistula was created near the wrist by anastomosing the cephalic vein to the radial artery. There is adequate international consensus in this arena today.

The nondominant forearm is preferred and a native AV fistula (AVF) placed as distally as possible in the forearm is the first procedure of choice.

If this is not possible or has failed, a similar AVF should be tried in the other forearm.

Subsequent choice is a native AVF based on the brachial artery.

Prosthetic grafts should be used only when native AVF is not possible or has failed.

Though highly variable, most persons have a lateral cephalic vein (CV) (Fig. 97.3) and a medial basilic vein (BV) in the forearm. The CV courses from the anatomical snuff box upwards laterally into the arm and ends in the subclavian vein. It remains subcutaneous in most of its course till it reaches the deltopectoral groove. The BV courses up medially but usually pierces the deep fascia at the junction of middle and lower third of the arm. The median cubital vein connects the CV and BV across the antecubital fossa, often, a medial accessory cephalic vein courses from lateral to medial in the flexor aspect of forearm and drains in the BV at elbow. When placing an intravenous cannula in a patient with CKD, these veins are best avoided in the nondominant hand.

A wrist or distal forearm radiocephalic AVF is the preferred access. A brachiocephalic (Fig. 97.4) AVF is also commonly performed. Brachiobasilic AVF has the disadvantage of shorter needling space from where the BV enters the deep fascia in the lower arm, it may be 'superficialized' to aid needling or alternatively the whole BV may be mobilized and re-routed through a new subcutaneous tunnel in the anterior arm to anastomosed end-to-side to the brachial artery (basilic vein transposition).

When 'native' options are exhausted, prosthetic grafts are used. Standard wall ePTFE grafts (e.g. GOREFEX) are suitable; however, trilaminar ePTFE grafts (e.g. Flixene, ATRIUM) (Fig. 97.5) appears to be superior. These are often implanted as a "U" loop configuration (Fig. 97.6) in the forearm between

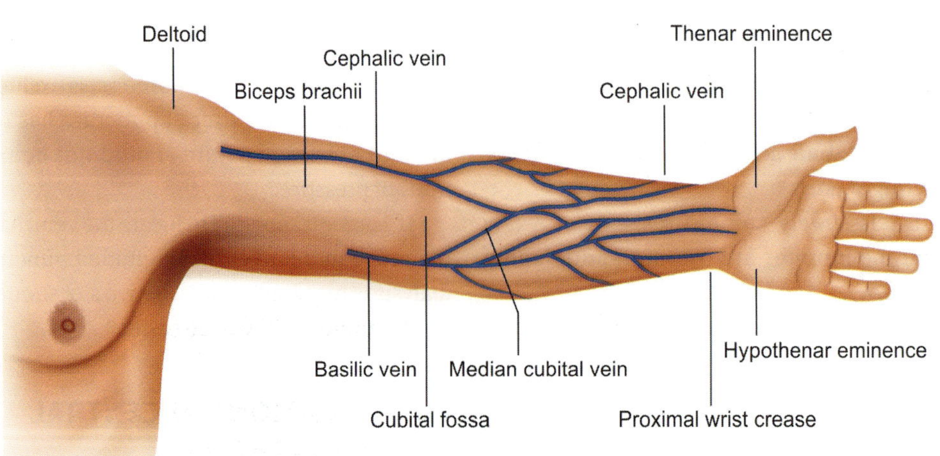

Fig. 97.3 Anatomy of superficial veins of upper extremity. Note the basilic vein passes under the deep fascia in lower arm

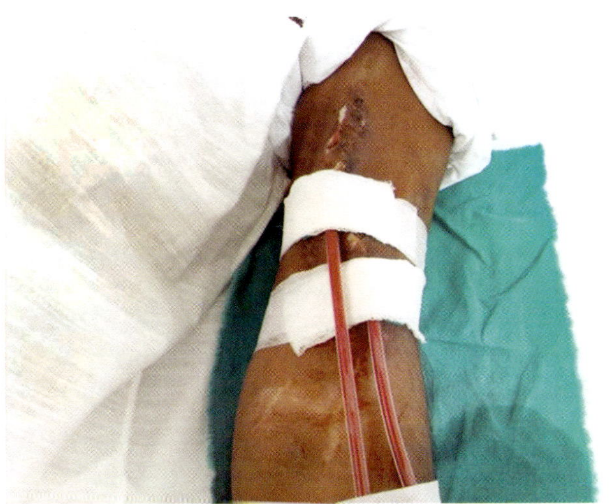

Fig. 97.4 A brachiocephalic AV fistula in arm is being used for dialysis. Note the two needles and tubes; the arterial tube is below, the venous (rectum) line is above, i.e. more proximal

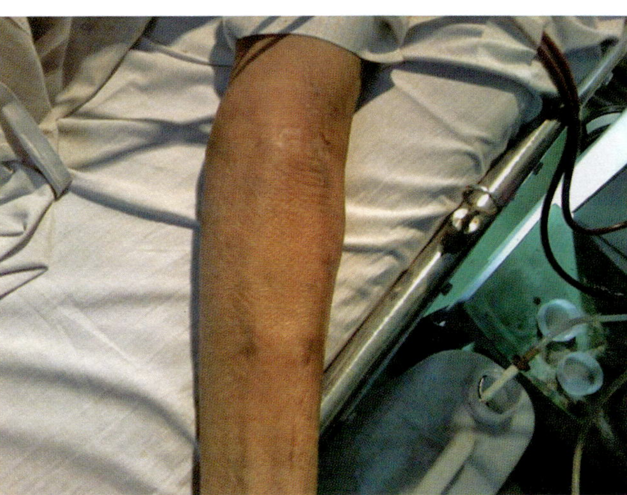

Fig. 97.6 A forearm U-loop graft. Though common in the West, this configuration has poorer outcome in South Asia

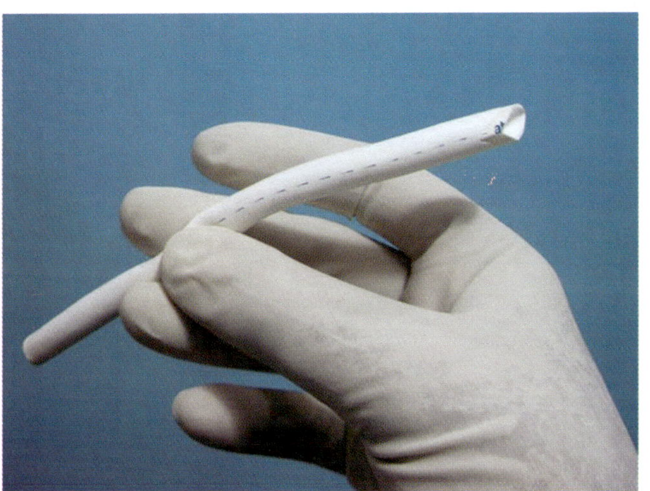

Fig. 97.5 A 6 mm ePTFE vascular graft

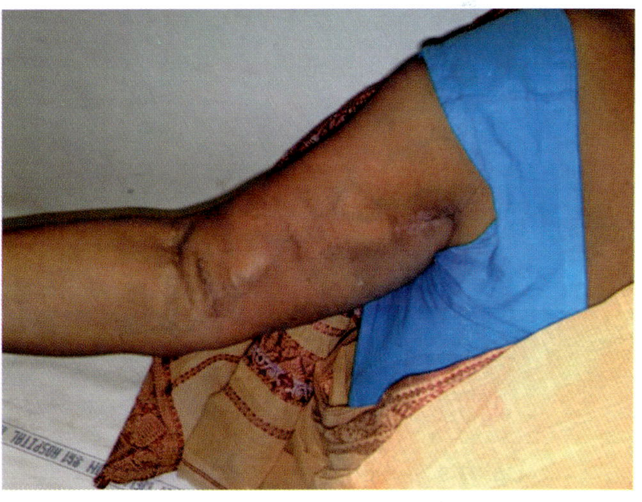

Fig. 97.7 An arm graft, brachial artery to axillary vein

the brachial artery and any of the superficial or deep veins in the antecubital fossa.

The most common cause of late failures of AV grafts is obstruction at the venous end from intimal hyperplasia due to turbulence. In South Asian population, probably due to narrower caliber of outflow veins, loop grafts work poorly. A straight or gently curved configuration of an arm graft from the brachial artery to the bigger axillary vein gives the most optimum results (Fig. 97.7).

Complex access procedures are required in some patients e.g. axillo-axillary (Necklace) grafts (Fig. 97.8) saphenous or femoral vein translocations, femorosaphenous grafts, etc.

COMPLICATIONS OF SURGICAL VASCULAR ACCESS

Reactionary and secondary hemorrhage, pseudoaneurysms, thrombosis and steal syndrome (Fig. 97.9) are important complication. Rupture of pseudoaneurysms and mycotic (infected) (Fig. 97.9) aneurysms can lead to catastrophic hemorrhage. High output cardiac failure and ischemic neuropathies are rare complications (Figs 97.10 and 97.11).

Noncaucasian race, female sex (increased subcutaneous fat), diabetes, increasing age, multiple forearm infusions, multiple CVC insertions contribute to access failure and complications.

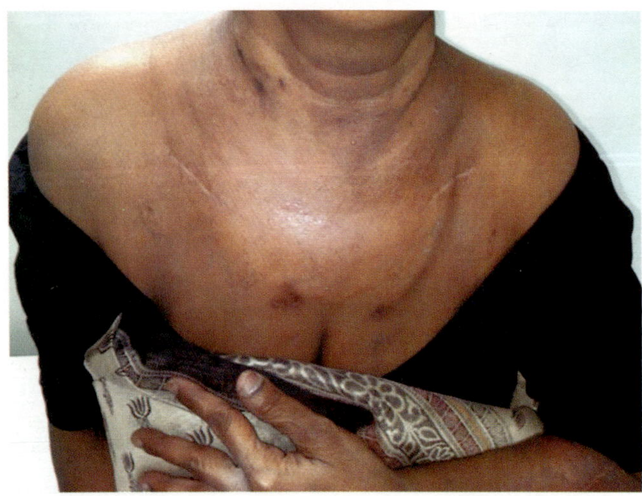

Fig. 97.8 A "necklace" graft. A graft is tunnelled ante-sternal between first part of axillary artery to third part of axillary vein

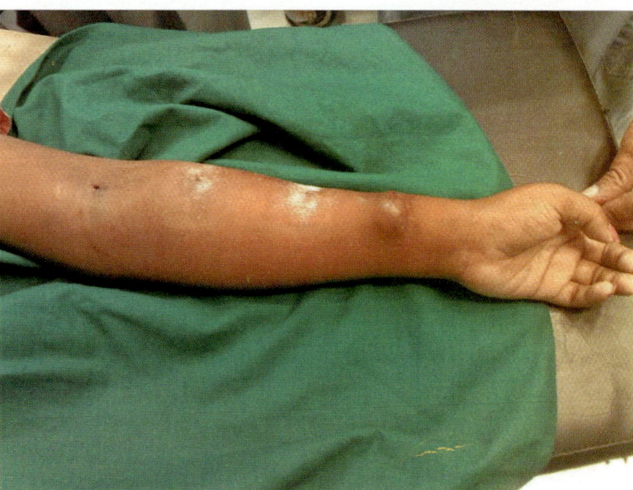

Fig. 97.10 Anastomotic aneurysm of a radiocephalic AVF

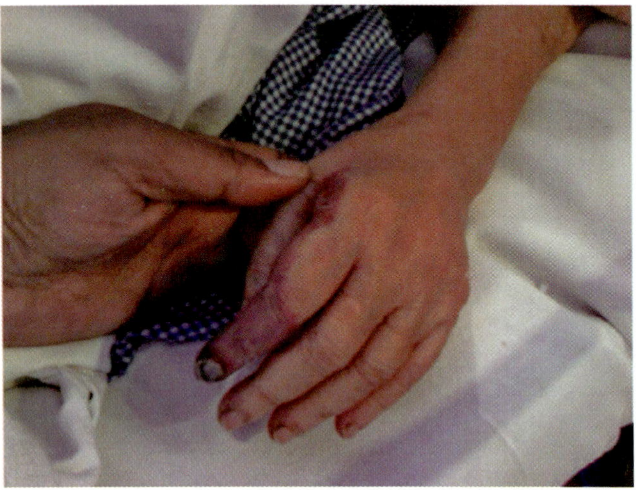

Fig. 97.9 Severe "steal syndrome" caused by a high-flow brachial artery based AVF

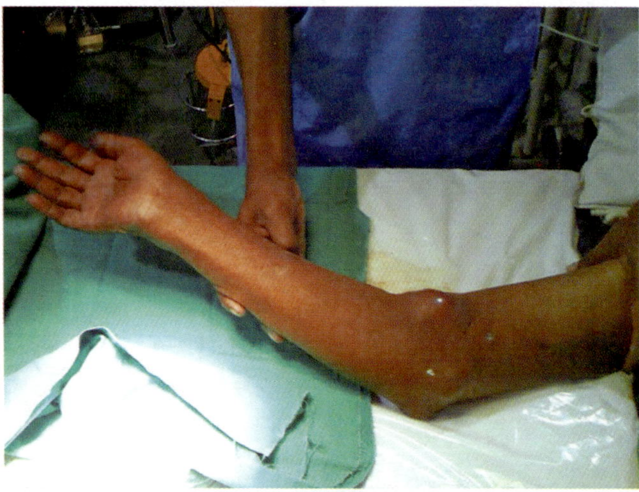

Fig. 97.11 A mycotic (infected) aneurysm of a brachial AVF. Note the medial blister and 'steel' causing color change of index finger

OPERATIVE TECHNIQUE: THE RADIOCEPHALIC ARTERIOVENOUS FISTULA

Adequate preoperative assessment is vital. Clinical examination with a tourniquet is often enough but needs patience. The quality, course and tributaries of the vein and both radial and ulnar pulses are felt.

Allen's test may not always be appropriate in dark races. When pulses are doubtful or course of a segment of the vein is doubtful, a hand-held Doppler is useful. However, Duplex imaging should be employed if clinical assessment remains borderline.

- The procedure is performed under local anesthesia, infiltration needs to be subcutaneous and away from the vein with a tiny (e.g. 26 G) needle.
- Usual aseptic precautions and drapes are applied. The patient is lightly sedated and remains supine with the arm abducted in an operating side-table or table extension.
- A longitudinal incision is made and deepened to subcutaneous fascial level. Dissection in this plane exposes the vein; the deep fascia need not be reached at this point. A cutaneous branch of the radial nerve is encountered and preserved. The vein is carefully mobilized and tributaries ligated. The vein-side of even

the small tributaries must be ligated, not cauterized because arterial flow is soon expected. The vein should not be stripped of the adventitia except for few mm near the anastomosis. The distal part is ligated and the vein divided.

- Gradual and gentle hydrostatic dilatation is performed with heparinized saline. Some surgeons gently pass 2 mm or 3 mm vessel dilators or baby Ryles tube.
- Once the vein appears suitable, the artery is exposed and dissected. Bipolar diathermy of tiny branches avoids spasm; however, should spasm occur, a spray of papaverine hydrochloride is effective. Non-atheromatous 'young' arteries are more prone to spasm.
- An arteriotomy is next made between bulldog clamps taking care not to injure the posterior wall. Lifting up the anterior wall with a small curved needle may help. Iris scissors or small Potts scissors are used to extend the arteriotomy to a 10–12 mm size. Both clamps are released sequentially to test the antegrade and retrograde arterial flow. The vein is now prepared with fish-mouthing or a linear cut-back to create a 'Cobrahood'. An end-to-side anastomosis is created by parachute or anchor technique usually employing 7-0 or 8-0 prolene, magnification loupes are strongly recommended. Retrograde flow from the vein may obscure view during the anastomosis, digital pressure on the skin or a soft venous clamp may be needed.
- Hemostasis is usually achieved spontaneously after the release of clamps within one or two minutes provided the technique was correct. The lie of the vein is reviewed to check for kinks or rotations.

This mobilized portion of the vein which 'swings' to the artery has received new attention in recent years.

The most common site of stenosis in an AVF is juxta-anastomotic, where the vein makes a bend from its original bed. Turbulence is believed to be the cause. Hence the 'swing vein' must lie as straight as possible or in a smooth curve. Thrill should be palpable instantaneously.

The wound is closed after checking hemostasis and a stethoscope is used to listen to the bruit. If this is absent, the area should be repainted and re-explored immediately.

Being a common procedure with very low risk profile for the patient for major complications or mortality, trainees may find this a good opportunity to develop basic skills. However, a failed primary access may cause enormous morbidity to the patient. Hence adequate senior supervision should be always present.

CHAPTER

98

Acute Lower Limb Ischemia

Krishnendu Mukherjee

This is one of the most common clinical scenarios presenting to the vascular surgeon.

Acute limb ischemia (ALI) is a surgical emergency usually affecting the lower limbs. Sudden onset pain and paresis/paresthesia is the classical symptom at presentation but pain is not invariable. Sudden onset monoparesis with numbness alone may be the initial symptom. Whenever a patient presents with a symptomatic limb, with or without a history of trauma, distal vascular assessment should be routinely performed. If you examine the distal pulse in every case, you will not miss a limb ischemia.

The most common cause is an acute arterial thrombosis in a previously diseased atherosclerotic artery. Embolism from a proximal source of thrombus is the less frequent cause (Table 98.1).

Causes of acute limb ischemia (in the absence of trauma)

Thrombotic: Acute or chronic event in an atherosclerotic individual; usually males, >50 years, other risk factors (diabetes, hypertension, smoking, etc.) and h/o claudication may be present.

Acute event in existing vasculitic syndromes (e.g. with SLE, TA) (usually females, may be younger).

Table 98.1 Examination of lower limb ischemia

Femoral pulse	*Area of prep and drape*
Ipsilateral present	Full groin to foot, may require popliteal artery exploration. Great saphenous vein should be assessed preoperatively.
Ipsilateral absent, contralateral present	Both groins and lower abdomen; may need a femoro-femoral crossover bypass graft.
Both absent	Both groins and whole abdomen up to cheek and neck; likely to be far more serious; Aorto-iliac disease or saddle embolus. May require aorto-bifemoral or axillo-bifemoral bypass.

Embolic: Mural thrombus; recent MI, atrial thrombus, presence of AF, etc. (Proximal source of embolus must be evident to be able to diagnose embolism).

Rarer causes include external compression, vasoconstrictor drugs, hypercoagulable states.

It is vital to appreciate that ALI is a clinical diagnosis. Investigations are needed to help plan the management but the most important evaluation remains clinical with a handheld Doppler (HHD) (Fig. 98.1). Ankle-Brachial Pressure Index (ABPI or ABI) is reliable objective marker which can directly translate to decision making. ABI is not infallible, especially in diabetics with calcified arteries. Nevertheless, it remains an important criteria. An ABI of <0.35 or a 50 mm of Hg arterial pressure at posterior tibial or dorsal pedis artery generally denotes critical limb ischemia.

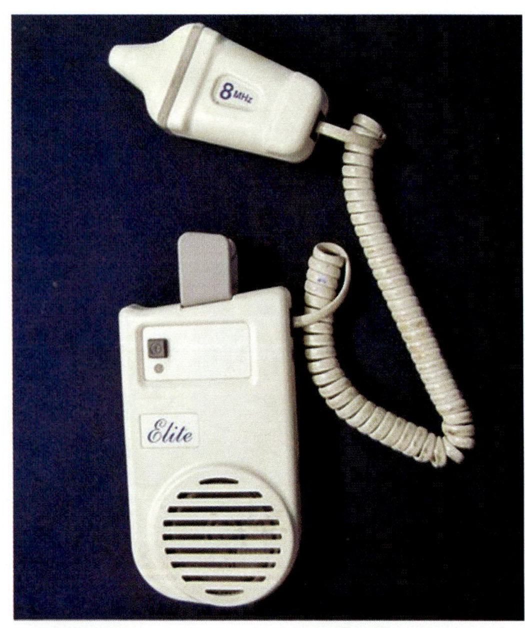

Fig. 98.1 A handheld Doppler (HHD)

ASSESSMENT AND DECISION MAKING

There is adequate consensus on the following classification:
Grade 1: Limb is viable. There is no motor or sensory loss, both arterial and venous signals are present in HHD.
Grade 2a: Limb is threatened. There is sensory loss with minimal or no color change, i.e. there is blanching. There is no motor loss. Arterial signals are dampened or absent. ABI, if measurable, is critical.

Grade 1 is suitable for endovascular therapy. Grade 2a is suitable for either endovascular or surgical intervention. There is time for more elaborated investigation, e.g. CT or MR angiogram provided hours are not wasted.
Grade 2b: Limb is severely threatened but may be salvageable.

There is some motor loss and sensory loss. Discoloration is mostly blanching. No arterial signals but venous signals present in HHD.

There is no time for endovascular approach. Unless easily available, there is no time for higher investigations. Should proceed straight to surgery.
Grade III: Unsalvageable.

Complete sensory motor loss with tense compartment. Fixed discoloration (staining) present. There are no venous signals.

Counsel appropriately and plan for an urgent primary amputation. This algorithm may not be required in all cases; e.g. A young female with known rheumatic heart disease presents with ALI. Ipsilateral femoral pulse is present. The limb is viable. One may proceed straight for an embolectomy (Table 98.1).

Initial Management (Parallel with Assessment and Definitive Decision-making)

- Heparin 5000–10000 IU I/V bolus, 1000 IU/hr infusion
- Oxygen and hydration (crystalloids only)
- Analgesia
- Antibiotics
- Prophylaxis for GI bleed and constipation
- Basic investigations. [Hb, Grouping, TC-DC, Random glucose, urea, creatinine, Na^+, K^+, APTT, CXR, ECG, echocardiogram. USG screening of abdomen and marking of both great saphenous veins (GSV) in both lower limbs].
- Clean the groins and the limbs with soap and water.
- Keep the limb at 0 degree. Do not elevate or depress.
- Catheterize (Usually required).
- If endovascular option is pursued, do not wait for CT or MR angiogram (CTA/MRA). If surgical option is pursued, provided inordinate delay is not expected, a CTA/MRA will be helpful.

Alert theaters about the use of C-arm for on-table angiogram and availability of contrast agents.

ENDOVASCULAR APPROACH

The target area is approached usually by ipsilateral or contralateral femoral arterial access. The initial arteriogram should always include proximal shoot films to visualize the aortoiliac segment. This assessment is extremely important because should the thrombolytic fail, surgical options will be dictated by the anatomy of 'run-in' and 'run-offs'.

Catheter-directed thrombolysis starts by infusion of rTPA 15 mg or streptokinase 1,00,000 IU or urokinase. Heparin is also infused along the arterial sheath and systemic heparin adjusted accordingly. APTT is checked every 6–8 hrs. Re-assessment is made over a 12–24 hr period by taking the patient back to cathlab for contrast imaging. Several mechanical thrombectomy and atherectomy devices and aspiration thombectomy catheters are available and are often used in conjunction with thrombolysis. RCTs have shown, specially in category I patients, thrombolysis is as effective as surgery.

Subsequent discovery of a stenotic lesion may be amenable to angioplasty.

Complications

- Hemorrhage
- CVA
- Distal embolization
- Hemorrhage from puncture site (may require aprotinin, plasma, protamine). APTT should be monitored every 6–8 hrs.

Contraindications to Thrombolysis

- Pregnancy
- Polytrauma
- H/o CVA, any neurosurgical procedure or GI bleed within 2 months
- Any other major surgery within 2 weeks.

(Depending on risk assessment for surgical approach in individual cases, contraindication may become relative rather than absolute).

SURGICAL APPROACH

It is essential to remember that what appears to be a femoral bifurcation embolism, may not turn out to be a simple femoral embolectomy. The possible requirement of autogenous veins as bypass conduits, different range of prosthetic grafts, on-table angiogram, blood transfusions, and abdominal exploration—all possibility should be considered during preoperative planning.

The femoral pulse is a reasonably good guide.

If possible, both legs and feet should be in transparent bags with ultrasound gel on feet (Figs 98.2 to 98.4).

Femoral Embolectomy

In an emergency, longitudinal or curvilinear incisions across the groin are preferred. If local anesthesia is being used, an anesthetist must be present for monitored anesthetic care. The wound is deepened in the same plane till the sheath of femoral vessels is reached. Common femoral artery is dissected longitudinally. A sudden change in size (tapering) denotes the origin of profounda femoris (deep femoral artery, DFA). A medial and lateral circumflex artery will be encountered if CFA is dissected more proximally. This may require division of the inguinal ligament which should be repaired later.

All arterial branches are preserved, if possible; held in slings and controlled by bulldogs. An arteriotomy (slightly oblique is preferred to longitudinal in South Asian patients) is

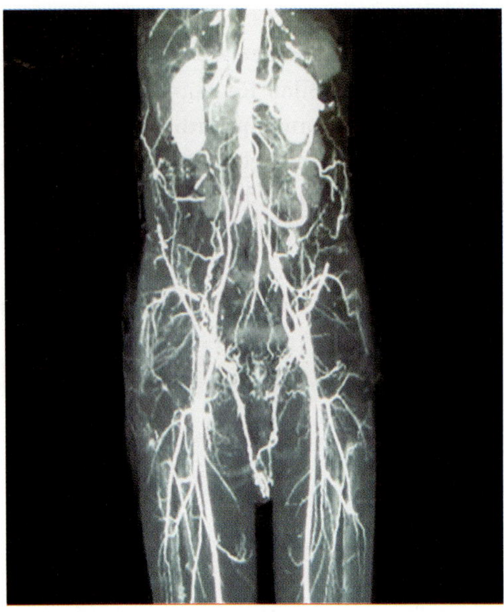

Fig. 98.2A Bilateral acute limb ischemia CT angiogram reveals aorta-iliac occlusion. Extensive collaterals denote chronic disease

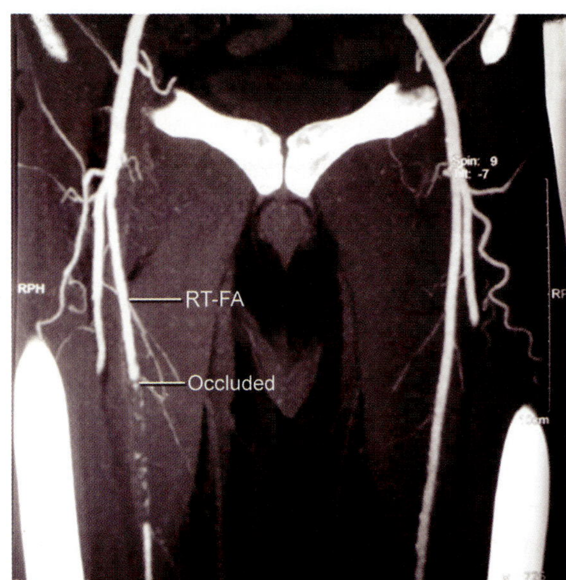

Fig. 98.2B Acute limb ischemia, there was h/o claudication, CT angiogram – SFA obstruction. Note cork-screw collaterlas' chronic disease. A femoral embolectomy will fail here

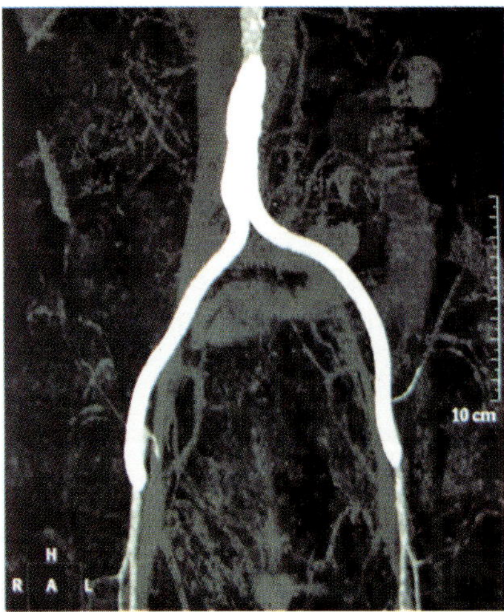

Fig. 98.3 Treated by urgent aorta-bifemoral bypass

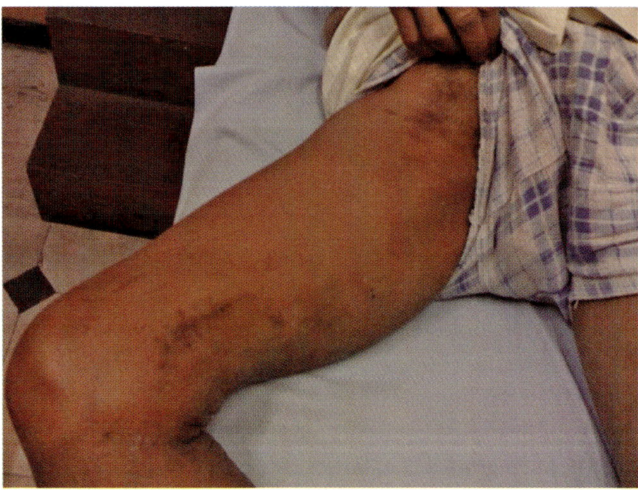

Fig. 98.4 Emergency direct femoro-popliteal bypass. A prosthetic graft (Heparin-bonded PTEE) was used

made. Release of proximal clamp tests the 'run-in' flow. If this is normal, a Fogarty catheter, usually 5F/6F is passed down the SFA and DFA.

The Fogarty balloon should be de-aerated on the trolley and accurate measurements of volume of heparinized saline needed for optimal inflation noted. During pull-back gradual distension is increased. Clots retrieved are usually sent for both histopathology and microbiology. This is repeated till optimal back-bleed is seen but back-bleed should not alone be taken as an adequate endpoint of the procedure. Return of pedal pulses is a satisfactory endpoint but is often not present. An HHD assessment is more important. A normal triphasic signal on PTA and DPA is adequate. Whenever in doubt, an angiogram should be obtained but interpreting an on-table C-arm arteriogram is not always easy. The limb should be externally rotated and repeat shots taken. Contrast leak from the arteriotomy can be controlled by a Zavid clamp or even a lightly applied Babcock forceps.

CHAPTER

99

Treatment of Varicose Veins

Dhiraj Choudhury, Saugata Deb, Krishnendu Mukherjee

TREATMENT OPTIONS FOR VARICOSE VEINS

Conservative Method

It includes reduction of obesity, avoidance of prolonged standing and use of elastic stocking.

Indications

- Mild symptoms
- Varicosity during pregnancy
- Patient unfit for surgery.

Injection Method

Fegan's sclerotherapy

Indications

- Small varicose veins below knee
- Recurrent varicosity after operation.

Operative Methods

Indications

- Varicosity with incompetent saphenofemoral or saphenopopliteal junction
- Severe symptoms
- Venous ulcer (complicated).

Types of Operations

- *Trendelenburg's operation:* High ligation of sapheno-femoral junction
- Long saphenous strip
- High ligation of saphenopopliteal junction with or without stripping
- Avulsion of varicosity/multiple phlebectomy
- Subfascial ligation.

TRENDELENBURG'S OPERATION: JUXTA-FEMORAL FLUSH LIGATION

- *Preoperative step:* The long saphenous vein and the prominent incompetent perforators are marked with a marker.
- *Position:* The patient lies supine with legs slightly abducted and head-down position to avoid embolism.
- *Anesthesia:* General or spinal anesthesia may be given.
- Incision: An oblique incision is made below and parallel to inguinal ligament in groin, over saphenofemoral junction (1" below and lateral to pubic tubercle (Fig. 99.1).
- *Exposure:* The incision is deepened through subcutaneous tissue to expose the long saphenous vein under the deep fascia. Trace the tributaries of the long saphenous vein namely superficial epigastric, superficial external pudendal and superficial circumflex iliac veins entering the proximal part of the long saphenous vein and divide them between ligatures (Fig. 99.2).

The long saphenous vein is carefully dissected up to its junction with femoral vein. Display the femoral vein about 1 cm above and below the junction.

HIGH LIGATION OF THE LONG SAPHENOUS VEIN

Ligate the long saphenous vein at its junction with femoral vein with silk (double ligature is preferred) and divide it. Hold the lower end of the vein temporarily occluded with a hemostats if stripping of the vein has been decided (Figs 99.3A and B).

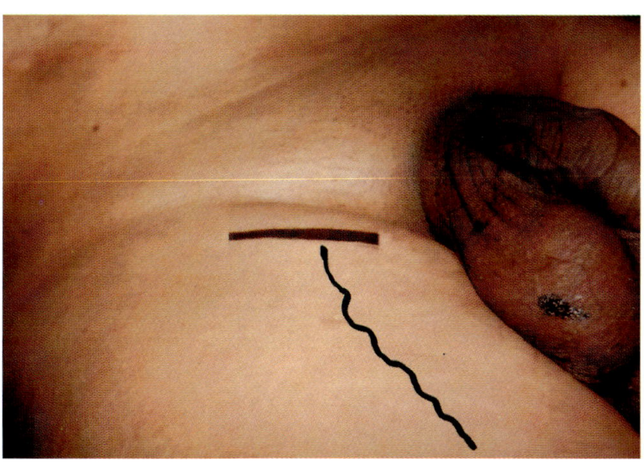

Fig. 99.1 Skin incision for Trendelenburg's operation

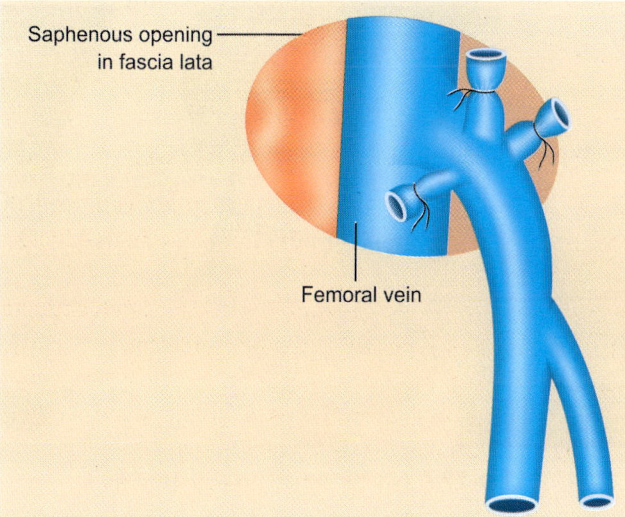

Fig. 99.2 Ligation of tributaries of long saphenous vein (schematic diagram)

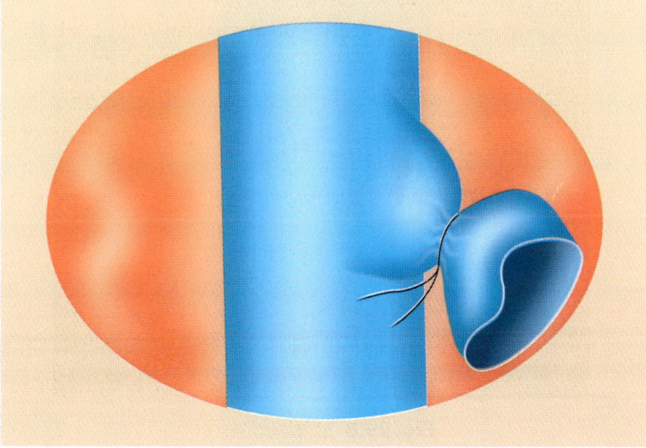

Fig. 99.3A High ligation of long saphenous vein (schematic diagram)

STRIPPING OF LONG SAPHENOUS VEIN

Long saphenous vein is traditionally stripped from the groin to the ankle. But the incidence of saphenous nerve injury when stripped below knee is unacceptably high. Moreover, it has been found that stripping below the knee is not essential for the treatment of long saphenous vein varicosity. Therefore, nowadays stripping is done from the groin to below knee only. The remaining portion may be avulsed with multiple small incisions.

Steps

The stripping of the long saphenous vein can be done with Myer's stripper which consists of a coiled spring with a wire core, 35 inch long with an acorn-shaped head fitted to one end and olivary tip at the other end (Fig. 99.4).

Following high ligation and division of the long saphenous vein in the groin, the stripper is inserted through the distal end of the vein (Fig. 99.5) and gently manipulated down the vein until it reaches below the knee. Apply an acorn head of adequate size (8 mm) at the top end of the stripper in the groin (Fig. 99.6).

Make an oblique incision below the knee over the tip of the stripper. Dissect the vein carefully and apply two ligatures. Tie the distal ligature. Make a small incision (venotomy) on the vein through which the tip of the stripper can be delivered and fitted with T-shaped handle (Fig. 99.7). Withdraw the stripper until it is arrested up by the acorn head at the groin. A ligature is tied around the vein containing the long saphenous vein is stripped from groin to knee with steady downward traction on the handle. The stripped vein will be found telescoped against the acorn head (Fig. 99.8).

If stripping of the whole length of the saphenous vein is decided, the lower end of the long saphenous vein is exposed by a small transverse incision over the medial malleolus. The vein is dissected taking care of the saphenous nerve. Pass two ligatures around the vein and tie the distal ligature (Fig. 99.9).

The tip of the stripper can be brought out by an incision on the anterior wall of the vein above the distal ligature and fitted with a T-shaped handle. The stripping is then performed by downward traction on the handle. The process can be done in a reverse way by inserting the stripper at the level of the medial malleolus, and passing it in proximal way. It is less likely to be obstructed by valves.

Problem

The stripping of the whole length of the long saphenous vein may not be completed in this simple manner in all cases.

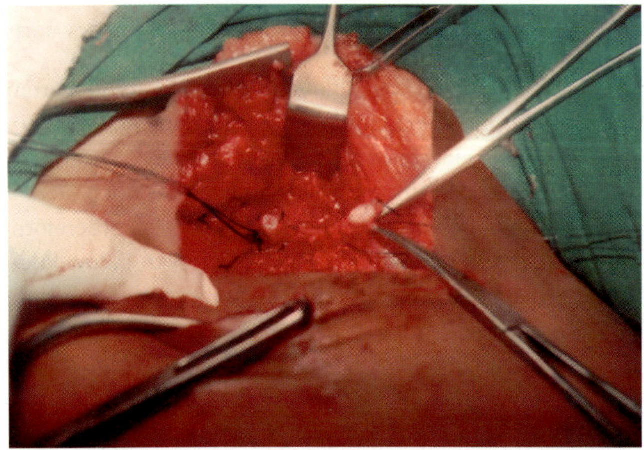
Fig. 99.3B High ligation of long saphenous vein

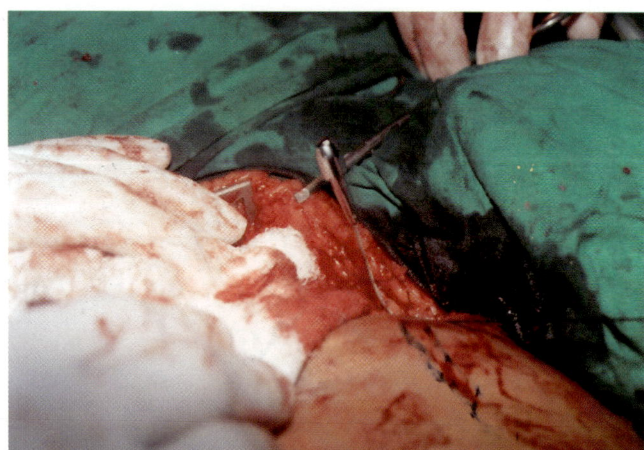
Fig. 99.6 Application of a corn head

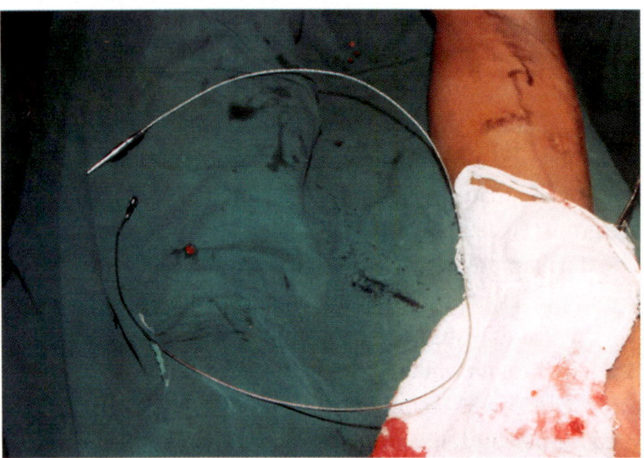
Fig. 99.4 Myer's stripper

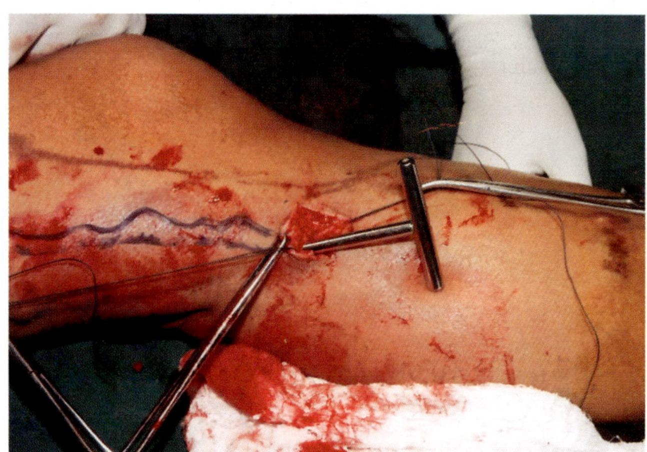
Fig. 99.7 Application of T-shaped handle

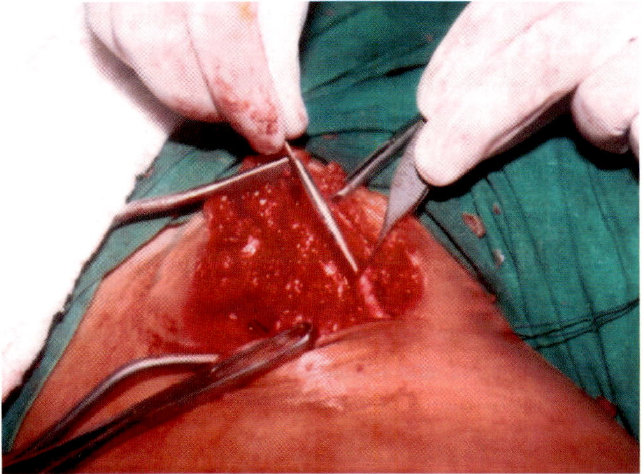
Fig. 99.5 Introduction of stripper

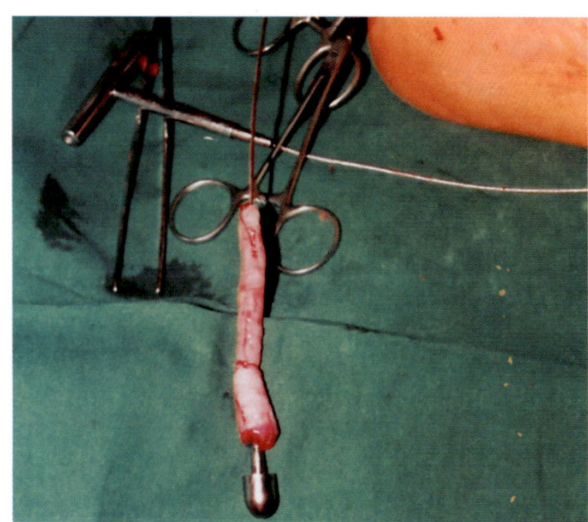
Fig. 99.8 Stripped vein

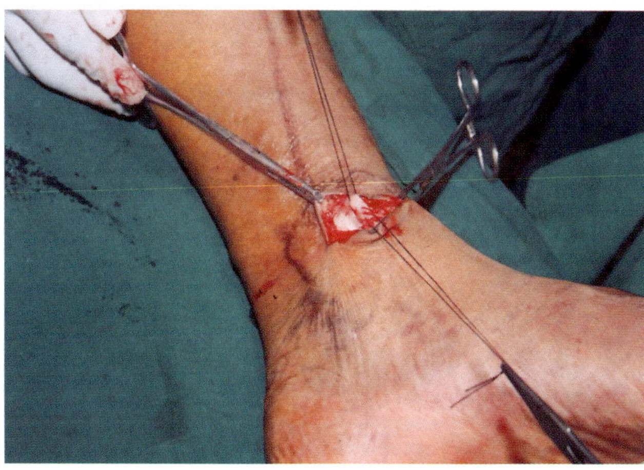

Fig. 99.9 Exposure to long saphenous vein over medial malleolus

Frequently the stripper is arrested at the level of the knee, when it is necessary to cut down upon the tip of the instrument and manipulate under direct vision. Sometimes, it may be necessary to strip the segment of the vein already traversed. The remaining vein may be stripped after re-insertion of the stripper.

Closure

The deep fascia is closed by interrupted 2/0 chromic catgut or vicryl. The skin is closed with subcuticular suture or interrupted 3/0 ethilon suture.

Compression Bandage

Bleeding from the stripper track can be minimized by raising the limb above and application of elastic crape bandage from below upwards.

SAPHENO-POPLITEAL LIGATION AND STRIPPING

Preoperative step: It is preferable to have the junction of short saphenous vein and popliteal vein marked with a marker by Doppler assessment.

Indication

Short saphenous vein varicosity with saphenopopliteal incompetence.

Operative Procedure

- *Position:* The patient lies prone on the table with knee flexed
- *Anesthesia:* General endotracheal or spinal
- *Incision:* A transverse incision is made on the lower part of the popliteal fossa
- *Exposure:* The incision is deepened through subcutaneous tissue to expose the short saphenous vein. It is often accompanied by sural nerve
- *Flush ligation:* The short saphenous vein is identified, ligated and divided at the level where it pierces the deep fascia to join popliteal vein
- *Stripping:* The stripper is introduced into the short saphenous vein in a downward direction and its exit is made by a short incision just below the lateral malleolus. The short saphenous vein is ligated and divided above the ligature. An acorn head is attached to upper end and handle at lower end. The vein is now stripped in downward direction.
- *Closure:* Close the wounds with interrupted ethilon sutures.

AVULSIONS OR MULTIPLE PHLEBECTOMY

Indication

Presence of varices not in close proximity to saphenous veins.

Operative Procedure

A very small incision is made over the vein in marked places. The vein is grasped with the mosquito forceps or special vein hook and a loop of the vein is drawn out. Divide the loops between the forceps and ligate the cut ends. Repeat the process in different places already marked (Figs 99.10A to C).

- *Closure:* Each wound is closed with fine sutures or steristrip.

SUBFASCIAL LIGATION (COCKET AND DODD'S)

This can be done by conventional method or endoscopically, for incompetent perforator causing venous ulcers.

Operative Procedure

- *Position:* Supine with legs partially above.
- *Anesthesia:* General endotracheal or spinal.
- *Incision:* A long vertical incision is made 2 cm behind the medial margin of tibia in the lower half of leg.
- *Exposure:* The incision is deepened to expose the deep fascia. The deep fascia is divided.
- *Subfascial ligation:* The perforators can be seen passing through holes in the deep fascia. They are ligated and divided.

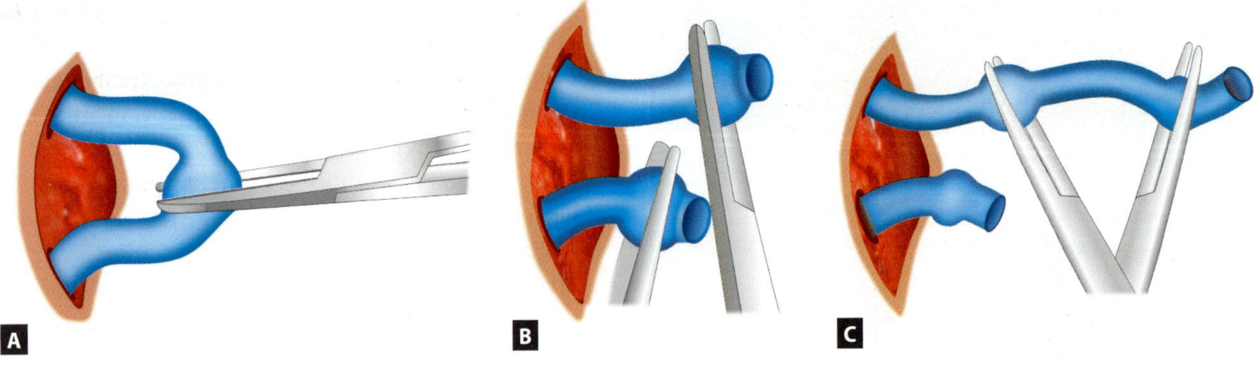

Figs 99.10A to C Phlebectomy

- *Closure:* The deep fascia is not closed. The skin is closed with interrupted stitches
- *Postoperative:* The leg is bandaged with elastic crepe bandage.

Postoperative Care

- Raise foot-end of the bed
- Immobilize the patient as soon as fully recovered from anesthesia
- Keep elastic crepe bandage
- Remove stitches after 6–7 days.

POSTOPERATIVE COMPLICATIONS

- Hemorrhage
- Sepsis
- Lymphatic edema.

ENDOVASCULAR OPTIONS

Catheter and guidewire based interventions for varicose veins is a relatively recent phenomenon and commenced with the use of radiofrequency waves for ablation of refluxing great saphenous vein. Subsequently, in 2002, laser was approved for endovenous use. Over the years, further improvements in technology have established endovenous thermal ablation techniques as the procedure of choice for most patients with varicose veins.

Our understanding of the anatomy and international consensus on the taxonomy of the venous system of lower limbs have also evolved with times. Superficial veins, embryologically, develop with the superficial nerves as opposed to the deep venous system which develops with the arteries. The great saphenous vein (GSV, previously referred to as long saphenous vein) and the short saphenous vein drain usually constant territories; however, have considerable anatomical variations at their termination. The anatomy of these variations are now well documented. The posterior and anterior accessory veins (PAGSV, AAGSV), the thigh circumflex veins and vein of Giacomini are also well understood. The word "Communicating" vein is used to denote intravenous tributaries within the superficial system while "Perforators" are veins between the deep and superficial territories. Eponymous description of perforators (e.g. Boyd, Dodd, Cockett, etc.) are largely replaced by landmarks of anatomy and measurement (by ultrasound), e.g. Adductor canal, paratibial, posterior tibial, etc.

Every patient is clinically assessed using the CEAP classification system. C (Clinical) ranges from 1–6, (e.g. C1 is telangiectasia, C2 is varicosity, C5 is healed ulcer, C6 is active ulcer etc.), E (Etiologic) e.g. primary or secondary, A (Anatomical) and P (Pathophysiologic), i.e. refluxive or obstructive. A detailed Duplex Doppler Scan is next performed before planning treatment.

Endovascular/Venous Laser Ablation

- The procedure can be performed under LA with sedation, GA or regional anesthesia.
- The varicose veins are marked preoperatively with an indelible marker (Figs 99.11A to C).
- Position of the patient is usually supine except when operating on the short saphenous system where the prone position is preferred. The operating table must be able to tilt seamlessly. Head-up and head-down positions may be required several times.
- Usual asceptic precautions are followed and the "treatment limb" is prepped and draped up to the groin and lower abdomen. EVL may be combined with ambulatory phlebectomies and rarely, conversion to conventional surgery may be needed.

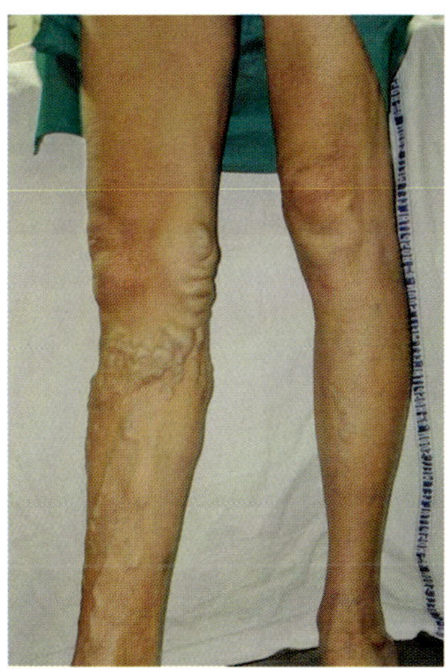

Fig. 99.11A Varicose veins

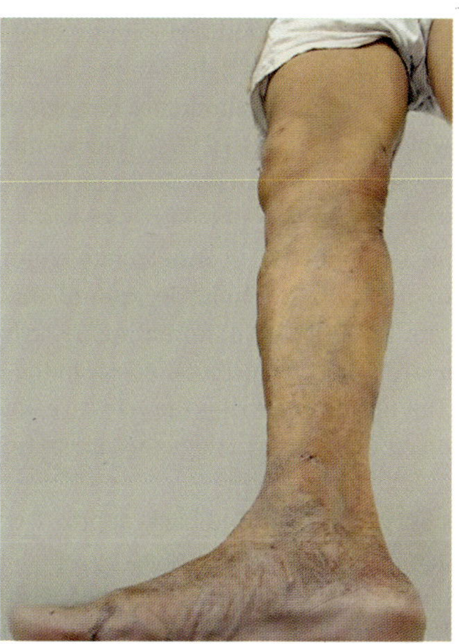

Fig. 99.11C 3 weeks later endovascular/venous laser ablation (EVLA) is now the gold standard treatment option for varicose vein

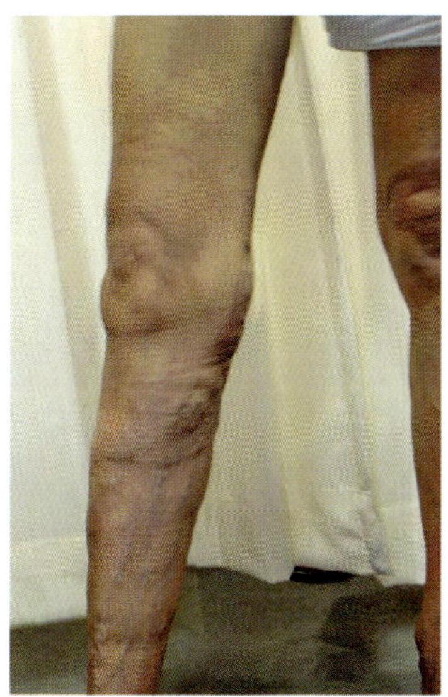

Fig. 99.11B 24 hours post-endovascular/venous laser ablation (EVLA)

- The procedure starts with a quick ultrasound evaluation by the surgeon, referred to as "reading the veins". A good quality Duplex ultrasound is essential for the operation. The probe is taken along with copious ultrasound gel within a sterile laparoscope camera cover.
- A head up position is used to scan the veins. Percutaneous access is gained under ultrasound control, usually by a 16G needle. At times, by locating the access point, a 1 cm incision may be made and tiny retractors used to locate the point.
- All subsequent manipulations will be through this access site. If tortuosity or other problems in negotiating guidewires (GW) create technical difficulties, new segmental accesses may have to be created in more proximal sites. GW technology has also evolved considerably and several wires are available to the operator. Movement and locations of GW are guided as per the ultrasound image, e.g. the Sapheno-Femoral Junction (SFJ) is identified by the "Rabbits' ear" sign or "Mickey-Mouse" sign and exact GW positioning is performed.
- The GW entry point is dilated by the tip of a mosquito forceps and a 4 Fr sheath is negotiated through the veins.
- When satisfactory sheath placement is achieved, the GW is removed and the laser wire placed.
- Though Nd-YAG laser has been used for treating telangiectasias, diode lasers are most commonly used for venous work. The wavelength (WL) selected is important. Lower WL, 940 nm, 980 nm and 1040 nm are hemoglobin specific (HSLW). 1340 nm, 1470 nm are water specific (WSLW). WSLW offers advantages. The laser is absorbed by the water in the endothelium. This causes lesser pain and bruising but ablation rates are similar. The laser generator has specific settings to select the Wattage, pulse-times, frequency and fire sequences. The surgeon has to select the settings depending on the patients' requirement. Generally, one Joule of energy is delivered by one Watt (1J = 1W); the total energy required for ablation will depend on what segment and veins are being treated.

- The laser fiber is synchronized to emit a light (Aiming-beam) near the tip, this light can be visualized by the surgical team as it transilluminates through the skin and differs when it is at subfascial level. If accidently traversing a deeper vein, e.g. in muscles, the beam disappears from view.
- The table is tilted back to anti-Trendelenburg position to allow the veins to collapse around the fiber and tumescent fluid (ice-cold normal saline, xylocaine and sodi-bicarb) is injected percutaneously in the perivenous space. This tumescence helps the veins to collapse further and protects the skin and cutaneous nerves from the heat scatter.
- The fiber is gradually pulled back, approx 1 cm at a time after each "fire" which is operated by a pedal switch by the surgeon. Gentle pressure is applied with a swab on the fire zone to further compress the veins. It also gives a "feedback" to the surgeon's tactile sensation by a "popcorn-burst" feeling. This feel and the visualization of the aiming beam is very important throughout the pull-back time.
- A pressure dressing is applied in the limb at the end of the procedure. Patient may be allowed out of bed after 12–24 hours but home-rest should be advised for one week with minor analgesics.

Complications

- Inadvertent deep vein fire leading to DVT is the most dangerous complication. Accurate use of Duplex Ultrasound on-table and visualizing the nature of aiming beam at all points are, therefore, crucial.
- Skin burns, wire perforations, nerve and arterial injury are recognized complications but are rare.
- Variable degrees of bruising and minor hypoesthesia in lower leg are common but are self-limiting.

SECTION 19

Miscellaneous

CHAPTER 100

Sympathectomy

Dhiraj Choudhury, Saugata Deb

CERVICODORSAL SYMPATHECTOMY

In this operation, the sympathetic trunk from the lower/half of the stellate ganglion to just below third thoracic ganglion is removed.

Indications

- Excessive sweating of upper limb (hyperhidrosis)—good result
- Raynaud's disease—the effect is often short lived
- Intractable pain in upper limb
- Buerger's disease involving upper limb
- Repair of subclavian aneurysm.

Preoperative Preparations

- Mark the side
- Counseling about the risk of Horner's syndrome.

Approaches

- **Anterior supraclavicular approach**
  Advantages:
  - Less postoperative pain
  - Rapid convalescence
  - Both sides can be done at one sitting

  Disadvantage
  - Dissection is relatively difficult
- **Axillary approach**
  Advantages:
  - Gives easy and direct approach to upper thoracic ganglia but not to stellate ganglia
- **Transthoracic approach:** For endoscopic thoracic sympathectomy (see page 417) this is the route of choice. At present endoscopic-thoracic sympathectomy is considered the best option if the surgeon is experienced.

Anterior Supraclavicular Approach

- *Position:* The patient lies in the supine position with sandbag under shoulders, with neck extended and head turned away.
- *Anesthesia:* General anesthesia with endotracheal intubation
- *Incision*: A transverse 3 inches long incision is made 1 cm above and parallel to medial half of the clavicle (Fig. 100.1)
- *Exposure:* Deepen the incision through platysma and deep cervical fascia. Dissect, divide and ligate the external jugular vein.

Next, divide the clavicular head of sternomastoid to expose the scalenus anterior muscle and phrenic nerve (Figs 100.2A and B).

Protect the phrenic nerve. Mobilize the scalenus anterior muscle down to the first rib and divide it at its insertion. The second part of the subclavian artery is now exposed.

The subclavian artery which in now exposed, is gently mobilized and retracted downwards. Be careful about

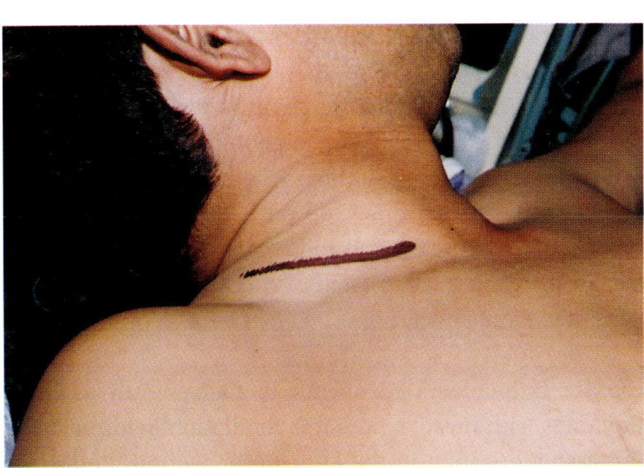

Fig. 100.1 Skin incision for anterior supraclavicular approach

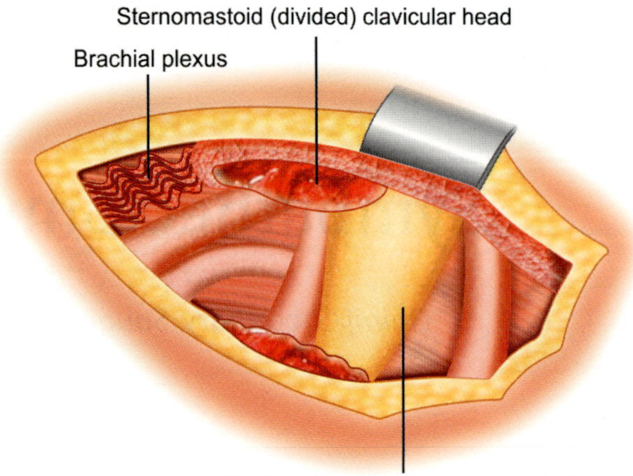

Fig. 100.2A Exposure of scalenus anterior after division of sternomastoid (clavicular head)

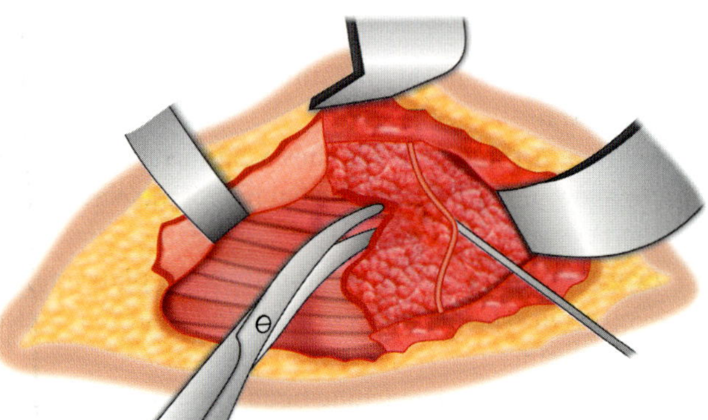

Fig. 100.2B Division of scalenus anterior muscle with retraction of phrenic nerve

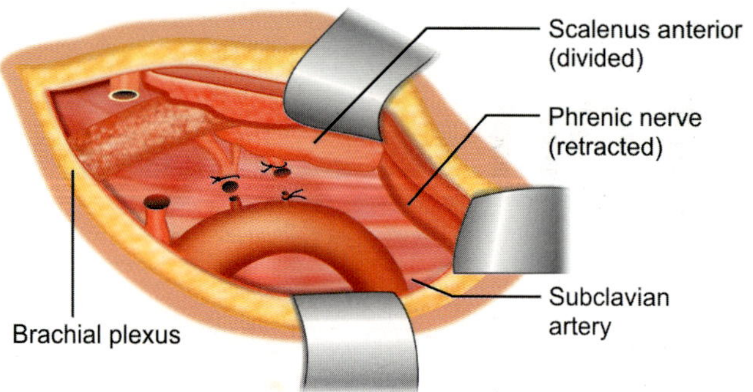

Fig. 100.3A Exposure of subclavian artery

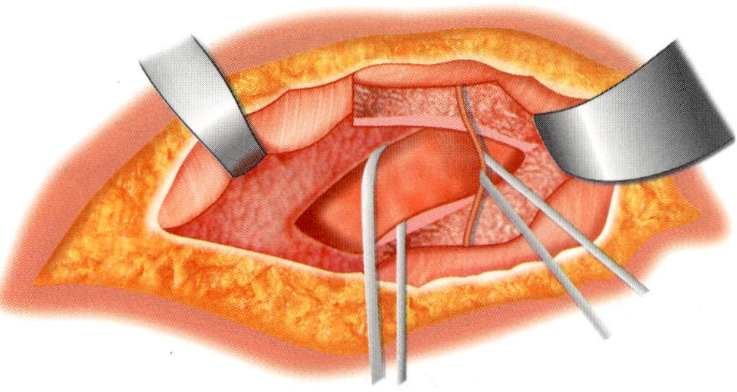

Fig. 100.3B Subclavian artery mobilized and pulled below

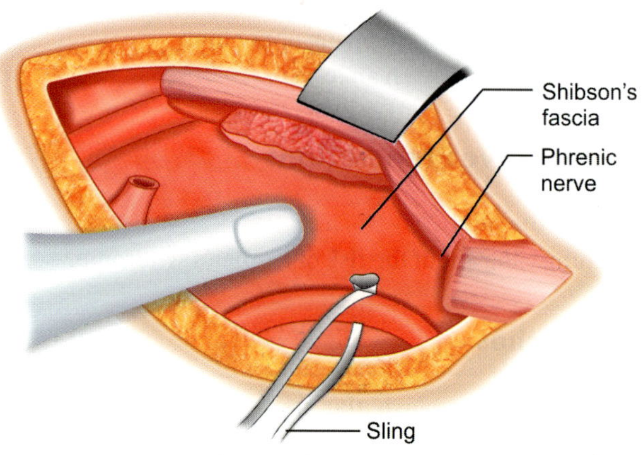

Fig. 100.4 Exposure of shibson's fascia

brachial plexus posteriorly. The thyrocervical artery is seen and ligated with silk. A tape is passed around subclavian artery to act as a sling for retraction (Figs 100.3A and B).

Identify the inner border of the first rib and detach the suprapleural membrane by swab, dissection and push the pleura downwards. Expose the neck of first three ribs (Fig. 100.4).

Technique: The sympathetic chain is identified crossing the neck of the ribs-stellate ganglion on the first rib. The sympathetic chain is divided below the third thoracic ganglion. The upper segment is drawn upwards and laterally and rami passing to and from the 2nd and 3rd ganglia are divided. The stellate ganglion is left to avoid Horner's syndrome. Send the specimen for histology (Figs 100.5A and B).

Closure: If the pleura are opened in inadvertently re-inflate the lungs with positive pressure ventilation before closing. Put a suction drain in the floor of the wound. Repair the sternomastoid muscle with catgut. Close the wound in layers.

Postoperative care

- Analgesic should be advised
- Systemic antibiotic.

Postoperative complications

- Horner's syndrome if stellate ganglion are damaged
- Pneumothorax due to damage to apical pleura
- Damage to phrenic nerve causing paralysis of hemidiaphragm
- Damage to thoracic duct.

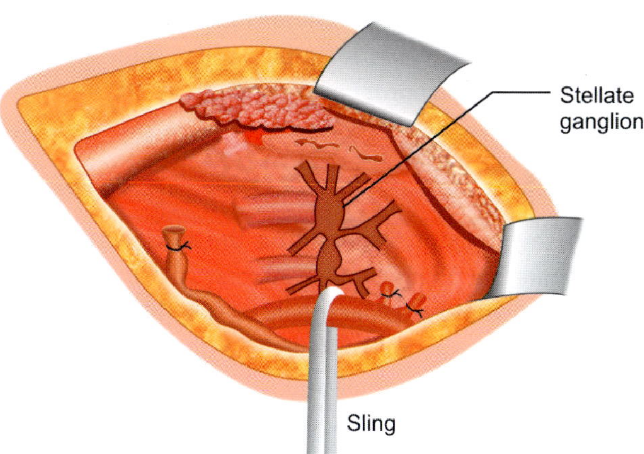

Fig. 100.5A Exposure of cervicodorsal sympathetic chain

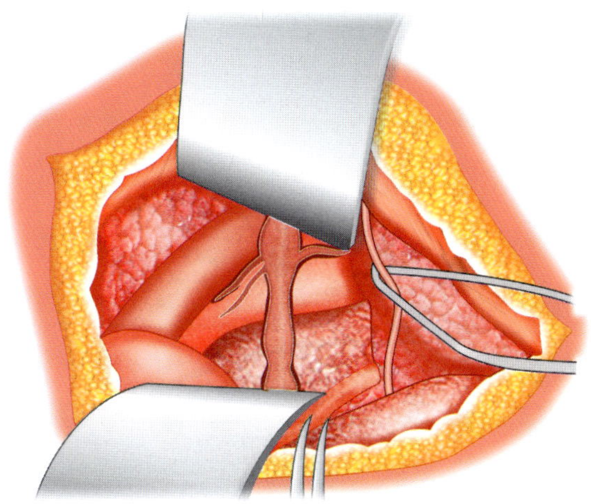

Fig. 100.5B Sympathetic chain displayed (stellate ganglion)

Axillary Approach

- *The incision:* A 4 inches long incision is made in the medial wall of the axilla along the line of 2nd intercostal space
- *Exposure:* The incision is deepened through the fibers of serratus anterior muscle until the space is reached, taking care of nerve to serratus anterior posteriorly.

The pleural cavity is entered by dividing the intercostals muscles. The intercostal space is enlarged by a rib spreader.

The lung is pushed downwards by gentle gauze dissection.

Technique

The sympathetic chain can be seen through parietal pleura. Identify the various ganglia—the stellate over neck of the first rib.

The overlying pleura is now incised exposing the sympathetic chain, which is divided below the 3rd thoracic ganglion.

The divided chain is now turned upwards and rami communicantes are divided above the 2nd ganglion and removed. Hemostasis is secured.

Closure

The wound is closed with an intercostal drain.

TRANSTHORACIC APPROACH ENDOSCOPIC

Preoperative Preparation

- A chest X-ray should be done
- *Position:* Supine with both arms abducted to 60°
- *Anesthesia:* General endotracheal preferably with double tubes.

Procedure

Once the particular lung has been deflated, insert a Veress needle through 5 cm incision in the third intercostal space and establish pneumothorax. Slowly introduce 1 liter of CO_2 into the pleural space. Insert a 5 mm thoracoscope through a cannula introduced through the same incision. Advance the thoracoscope under vision until ribs are identified. Identify the sympathetic ganglia and chain over the neck of the ribs. Through a separate stab wound in the 5th intercostal space in anterior axillary line. Insert a pair of endoscopic shears via an insulated cannula. Dissect carefully the second thoracic ganglia over the second rib and divide under direct vision. Now cut the chain as it crosses the third rib and remove the nerve. Hold the thoracoscope ready while the lung is re-inflated and then remove it. Close the skin wounds.

LUMBAR SYMPATHECTOMY

This is a paraganglionic sympathectomy because fibers supplying the vessels of the lower limb have their cell stations in the sacral ganglia which are not disturbed.

Indications

- Buerger's disease—lower limb. Sympathectomy has no place in the treatment of intermittent claudication. Patient having rest pain, pregangrene or dry gangrene may show transient improvement with sympathectomy
- Hyperhydrosis of the lower limb
- Causalgia of the lower limb
- Traumatic arterial spasm

- Acrocyanosis frigida.
  Both sides can be done in one sitting. But during bilateral operation first lumbar ganglion one side should be preserved to avoid sterility due to paralysis of ejaculatory mechanism.

Preoperative Preparations

Test vibration sensation in feet in diabetic patient to exclude neuropathy.

Extraperitoneal Approach

- *Position:* The patient lies in a supine position with a sandbag beneath the flank on the side of operation to give 20° tilt
- *Anesthesia:* General anesthesia with endotracheal intubation is used
- *Incision:* A transverse or oblique incision is made starting midway between anterior superior iliac spine and costal margin to lateral border of the rectus (Fig. 100.6).

Exposure

Deepen the incision by dividing the muscles (external oblique, internal oblique and transversus abdominis) in the same line to expose extraperitoneal fat (Fig. 100.7).

The peritoneum is displaced medially and forwards off the posterior abdominal wall, raising ureter and genital vessels with it. Retract the peritoneum with a large Deaver retractor (Fig. 100.8). The sympathetic chain is identified lying in the groove between vertebral bodies and psoas muscle. It is felt like a cord. The following structures can be mistaken for lumbar sympathetic trunk genitofemoral nerve lymphatic chain, and tendon strip of psoas muscle (Fig. 100.9).

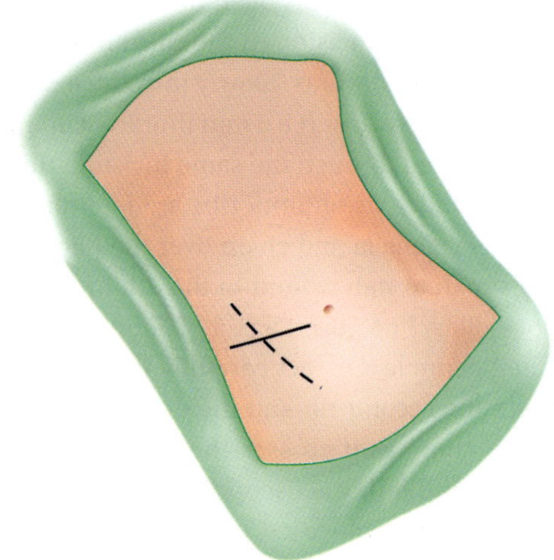

Fig. 100.6 Skin incisions for lumbar sympathectomy

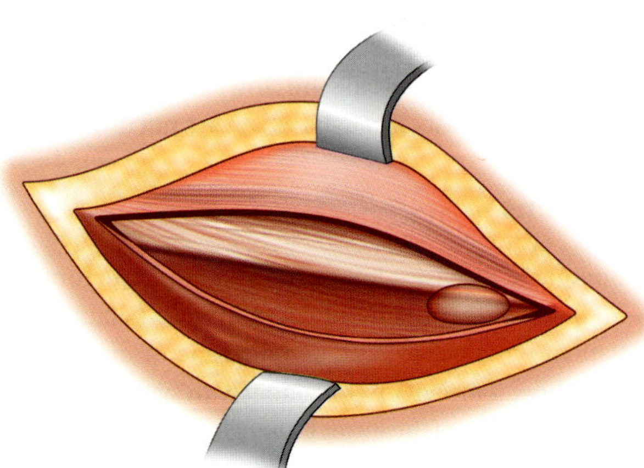

Fig. 100.7 Division of muscles

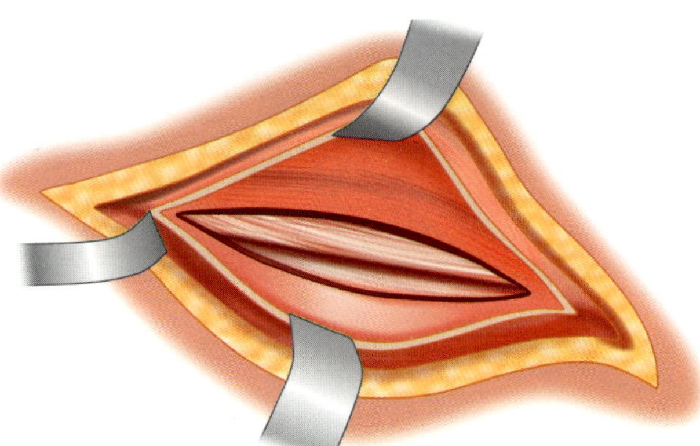

Fig. 100.8 Exposure of extraperitoneal space

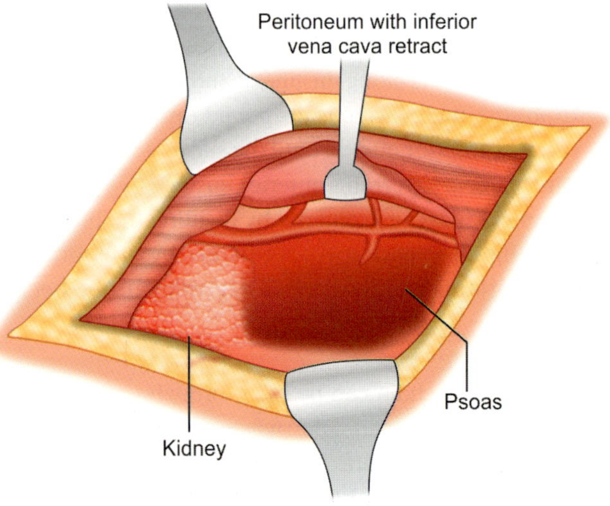

Fig. 100.9 Exposure of (R) sympathetic trunk

On the right side is behind inferior vena cava and on the left side it is overlapped by aorta. The lumbar veins crossing the sympathetic chain are ligated and divided. Bleeding from accidental injury should be initially treated by pressure packing and then definitive step (Figs 100.10 and 100.11).

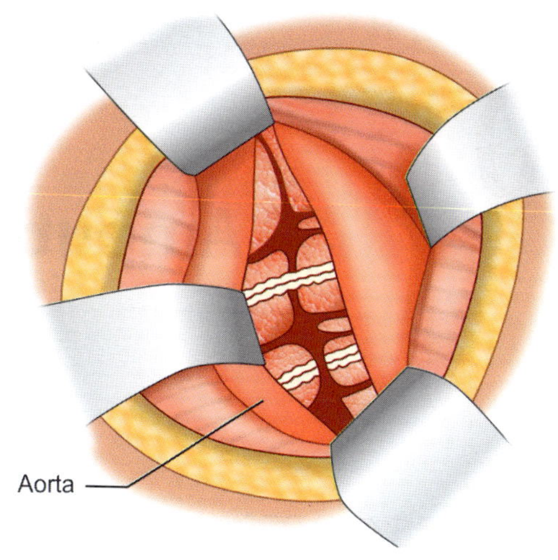

Fig. 100.10 Exposure of (L) lumbar sympathetic chain

Technique

The sympathetic chain is picked up with forceps and dissected upwards and downwards.

The first right lumbar ganglia lies behind duodenum and 4th behind common iliac vessels. The second lumbar ganglion is large.

The L2, L3, L4 ganglia with their white and grey rami are excised and held with a long curved forceps and removed. Send the tissue for histological confirmation.

Closure

The wound is closed in layers—muscles with interrupted catgut stitches and skin with interrupted ethilon/silk stitches.

Postoperative Care

- Intravenous fluid for 24–48 hours
- Nasogastric suction particularly in bilateral cases, to prevent ileus.

Postoperative Complications

- Retroperitoneal hematoma
- Paralytic ileus
- Postsympathectomy neuralgia in the distribution of genitofemoral nerve
- Bilateral removal of 1st lumbar ganglia will impair ejaculation.

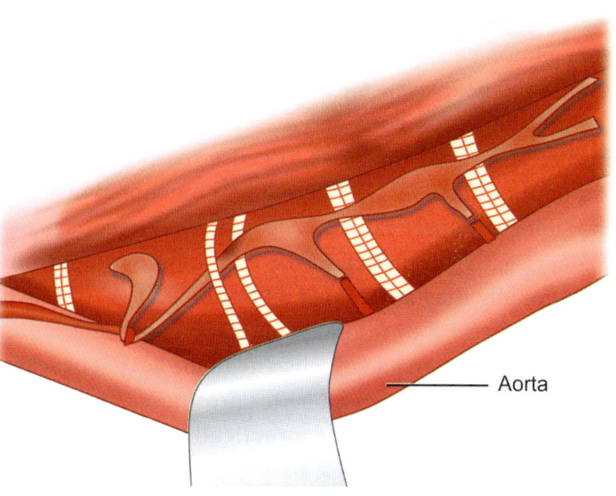

Fig. 100.11 Exposure of (L) lumbar sympathetic chain

CHAPTER

101

Amputations and Disarticulations

Subhayan Bera

INTRODUCTION AND DEFINITION

The word amputation has been derived from the Latin word amputare, which means to cut off, or to prune. It means the removal of a limb or other appendage or outgrowth of the body. Generally, it is used to describe the operation, by which a distal part of lower or upper limb is removed.

Amputation is one of the oldest surgical procedures, known to medial science. Leprosy, ergotism and punishment were major causes in the past. Dysvascular conditions, trauma and neoplasma are common causes nowadays.

Amputation is considered to be an irreversible and mutilating procedure, so as to cause the permanent loss of a limb or part of it with permanent functional disability. Psychological upset can also accompany. Surgeons usually take a negative approach to the operation of amputation. Traditionally they are trained and oriented towards saving limbs and lives. They resort to amputation only after months of pain, debilitation and expanse. With the advent of science and technology, better and better prostheses are available nowadays. These provide practically good functional recovery. It is considered only when other and better alternative methods are not available.

Amputation can be life-saving in certain situations. Satisfactory amputation stump with a well-designed prosthesis may provide good and satisfying functional recovery. This result is dependent on age, general medial condition, pathological condition and motivation of the patient. The profession of the patient is also important. In upper extremity amputations, recognition of dominant had or side is to be kept in mind.

Fairly clear distinction exists between indications of upper limb and lower limb amputations. In lower limb amputations, stability and strength helping in good quality ambulation is important. In upper limb useful function is more important to stability. Deformed or short arm with useful function may be preferable to prosthesis. Prior discussion to explain the cause and level of amputation increases acceptance of the procedure by the patient and relatives.

Amputation of toe, finger or part of them is generally considered as minor amputations as functional debility is minimum in most of the cases. Whereas amputation through leg, thigh, forearm or arm are considered as major amputations as functional debility arising afterwards is considerable.

On many situations, independent clinical opinion from a clinician, not involved in the direct management of the patient, is sought, regarding the necessity and justification of amputation. Opinions from other speciality like physical medicine, vascular surgeons, and plastic surgeons with special expertise in microvascular surgery may be necessary.

In selected cases in investigation with plain X-ray to see bone involvement is required. Arterial tree can be studied with Doppler study, contrast angiogram, DSA or MRI angiogram. CT scan, oximetry, plethysmography, may be selectively needed to assess the need for amputation. The status of skin circulation may be assessed by clearance of radioxenon, quantification of skin fluorescein delivery by fiberoptic fluorometry, transcutaneous PO_2 or oxymetry, thermography.

Amputation of part of lower limb is the most common type of amputation. Most of the techniques described are largely suitable for this type of amputation.

DISARTICULATION

Disarticulation is the special name given to an amputation, where the procedure is done through a joint. Here bone is not divided but nonbony structures of joint are divided so that the joint opens up. Skin, muscles, tendons, vessels, nerves and other structures are divided following the rules of amputation, specific to that part of the limb.

Indications

Dead, damaged, dangerous and deformed limbs (4Ds) are four basic groups of indications for amputations. However, with advent of modern science and technology indications are ever-changing. Lower limb amputation is much more common than upper limb amputations. The *vascular disease and infection due to diabetes constitute indications in nearly 80% of cases.* Of these about 20% will have diabetes. In about 10% cases, the limb loss is due to injury. A brief account of the indications follows. Absolute indications are to save life. Relative indications are to relieve pain or restoration of health and functions.

Vascular diseases with arterial insufficiency or ischemia of acute or chronic variety are the most common cause of lower limb amputation in the western world. These include Buerger's disease, atherosclerosis, diabetes, thromboembolic disease, arteriovenous fistula and peripheral aneurysm. Failure or inappropriate candidate for revascularization procedure is also indications.

Venous disease with ulceration is an uncommon indication.

Acute *infection* like diabetic cellulitis with toxemia or gas gangrene may require amputation some times. Other fulminating infection may cause extensive irreversible damage. Chronic infection of bone and joints like osteomyelitis and septic arthritis, fungal infections, extensive tissue necrosis, leprosy may lead to amputation procedures.

Gangrene is an almost absolute indication for amputation. The extent of gangrene is important to select the level. In dry gangrene due to vascular insufficiency amputation can wait until the demarcation has appeared. In wet or moist gangrene urgent amputation is often required.

Wounds and injuries to a limb may necessitate amputation. Limb may not be salvageable due to severe injury with massive loss of soft tissues and vascular injury, combined soft tissue and bone injury or irreversible damage with traumatic amputation or avulsion. Attempt to save mangled limb also has dangers.

Thermal injury (burn) and cold injury (frostbite) may lead to amputation.

Amputation may be necessary to treat *malignant tumors* or *large benign tumors* of the extremities. Some of these are large carcinoma infiltrated to bone, osteosarcoma, osteoclastoma. Ewing's sarcoma, Kaposi's sarcoma, Marjolin's ulcer, malignant melanoma, secondary deposits.

Severe *deformity* needing amputation may be congenital or acquired. This is mostly applicable in lower limb deformities. Cerebral palsy, myelomeningocele, infantile paralysis, painful paralyzed limb are some causes.

Paralytic limbs in acute anterior poliomyelitis, neurological deficit after injury or disease are rare indications.

Congenital limb abnormalities with absent limb or part of limb may be an uncommon indication for amputation. Polydactylism or supernumerary digit may need amputation. Carefully planned amputation is done for prosthetic fitting.

Complications or failure of *prosthetic surgery* is a relatively new indication.

Principles

General Considerations

According to the clinical situation, the amputation can be of emergency, urgent or elective type. In these cases, minor variation or adjustment in techniques may be required for the same amputation. Primary objectives are to be achieved and time available for amputation is to be considered in conducting an amputation procedure. Occasional necessity for revision procedure is to be kept in mind as well. This needs to be informed to patients and relatives. Motivation of the patient and usability for the stump are important considerations.

An Ideal Amputation Stump

An ideal amputation stump should fulfill the criteria as follows. Truly speaking an ideal stump hardly ever exists, as it has some theoretical concepts incorporated in its description.

Ideally amputation should be through the site of election. The shape should be conical without any projecting bony spur or any redundant muscle mass. It should be firm. It should heal by primary intention, without leaving any adherent, thin or folded scar in the skin. It should be bob-tender. The scar should be away from prosthesis contact or pressure bearing area, preferably in transverse disposition. The joint above the amputation should have good power and range of mobility.

Optimum Levels of Lengths of Amputation

If the clinical situation allows, functions desired should be considered in planning the length of stump. This is markedly different in upper and lower limbs. Longer stump is preferable up to a certain point. It must be kept in mind that, long stump can be revised but too short stump is not repairable. Certain optimum levels are given in Table 101.1. These should be accepted with some flexibility. Availability of type of prosthesis is also important in planning the length of the stump.

Tabel 101.1 Optimum levels of lengths of amputation

Leg	14 cm of tibia, minimum length is 8 cm
Thigh	25–30 cm from tip of greater trochanter
Forearm	20 cm from the tip of olecranon, minimum length is 8 cm
Arm	20 cm from acromion, above this as much as possible

Basic Methods

Surgical technique can vary according to need or necessity of the procedure. Clinical situation can affect the method as well. In extreme cases, initial emergency or urgent procedure is primarily aimed at lifesaving measures with provision of revision or definitive later on.

Principles of techniques fall in one of the three classes of amputation methods.

The standard or conventional methods use different types of flaps with bases near the site of amputation.

Osteomyoplastic amputations and myodesis are relatively newer concepts. These provide improved functions. Slightly longer muscles and osteo-periosteal flaps are sutured over bone end to plug the marrow and cover bone end in osteomyoplastic technique. In myodesis cut ends of muscles are sutured to bone end through drill holes.

The third technique is open or provisional guillotine method. This is the oldest method. It can be used for release of a caught limb in an accident or to amputate grossly infected limb, causing toxemia in a severely ill person.

The basis methods of initiation and planning of amputations, assure a sound skin cover with an almost ideal stump. Different methods are briefly described below.

Flap method: This method is used most commonly. Usually one or two semicircular flaps are created to cover the stump. Length of the single flap or combined length both flaps should be one and half times the diameter of the limb at the site of amputation. For proper healing good vascularity of the flap or flaps is ensured. Proximal part of flap should contain adequate muscles which are cut obliquely to make thinner towards the end, where it contains skin and deep fascia. In initial planning length of flaps should be kept longer rather than shorter. The longer flaps can be trimmed easily if the necessity arises.

Oval or elliptical method: This technique forms a side scar. Skin and soft tissues are divided in elliptical or oval shape. Proximal site and side of amputation are marked first. Lower end of incision on the opposite side is marked then. Bone is divided at the level of proximal part of incision. Soft tissues are divided obliquely.

Circular method: The determination of level of bone division is decided first. Skin, muscle and other soft tissues are divided below equal to the diameter of the limb at that level. It can be used where the limb is almost cylindrical like arm. It creates a terminal scar.

Racquet incision: A circular or elliptical incision is made. A straight incision is carried proximally from this to expose the site of bony division. This method is useful in proximal disarticulation of fingers and toes.

Fish-mouth incision: Two almost equal elliptical anterior and posterior flaps are joined laterally on both sides. Elevating these flaps exposes the site of bony section. This method is used in fingers and toes.

Equal lateral and medial flap method: This technique is adopted in amputation through proximal part of fingers.

Guillotine method: This is the oldest and primitive method of amputation. Usually all tissues including are divided at the same level. The wound is left open and allowed to granulate. This is useful when amputation has to be performed at the spot for trapped limp in an accident. As the results are unsatisfactory revised corrective amputation is often necessary.

General Steps and Basic Techniques

General, spinal-epidural or regional anesthesia is adequate. Forefinger and toe amputations local anesthesia without adrenaline may be adequate. Controlled hypotensive anesthesia may be useful in proximal amputation to be reducing bleeding.

Proper positioning of the patient and limb is required. Most of the amputation sites necessitate access to the limb from all sides.

The amputation site and side should be marked beforehand including in emergency procedures with special reference to the site of election. At operation, marking of the incision site or flaps is important. Initial planning should include liberal sizes of flaps to avoid tension during closure. Blood supply to flaps needs special attention. Anatomical blood vessels are carefully identified to avoid bleeding or to assess the degree of ischemia. During muscle division, degree of bleeding is noted. Myodesis or myoplasty gives better mobility and strength to the stump. Division of bone should be smooth without sharp corners or projections. Too much subperiosteal dissection might create sequestrum, which may be ring shaped. Placement of scar should be well planned, preferably on a side. Avoidance of tension during skin closure is extremely important. Techniques or number of stitches of skin should not cause ischemia of the skin.

Toothed forceps are better avoided particularly in ischemic disease. Hemostasis should be adequate to avoid hematoma formation at amputation site. Nerve division should be well above so that it does not adhere to scar. Neither it should form neroma. Immobilization of proximal joint may be necessary.

In vascular disease tourniquet is avoided. Stump revision may be necessary in some cases. It sepsis wound may have to left open to allow secondary healing.

Special retractors and amputation knife are useful adjuncts. Overall dissection should be very clean with minimum crushed or devitalized tissue.

Whenever possible veins and arteries are ligated separately, to avoid arteriovenous fistula formation. Drain is used almost always.

Choice of Levels in Different Diseases

In vascular disease of lower limb, in about 2/3rd cases, below-knee (BK) amputation is possible. Metabolic expenditure of walking is 20% greater in BK amputation and 100% greater in above-knee (AK) amputation, when compared to normality. Ghormley described the below knee amputation with long posterior flap in 1947. Higher level of amputation can be avoided by preceding reconstructive vascular surgery or endovascular revascularization, in selected cases.

In diabetic gangrene without frequent involvement of large vessels, relatively conservative amputation is attempted.

In benign tumors local ablation, but in malignant tumors more radical approach is necessary.

In children, maximum possible length is preserved. As amputation might affect the major growing epiphysis, proportionate amputations are not advisable in children. Disarticulation through knee or ankle is useful considerations. Bony overgrowth necessitates the need for revision surgery.

Primary or secondary skin grafting or skin flap repair is to be kept in mind in trauma with skin loss or developing injury, to preserve the length of stump.

In sensory neuropathy with foot ulcer or bone involvement, conservative approach is taken. In sepsis, level of amputation is decided by the extent of gangrene, which might need secondary procedures.

AMPUTATION OF LOWER LIMB

Amputation and Disarticulation of the Toes

Amputation of toes can be partial or complete. If the clinical condition allows, functionally useful stump of toe should be kept. Partial amputation preserves part or whole of phalanges.

Partial amputation is preferred to disarticulation. A vascular cartilage at the joint might interfere with healing. Whenever possible tendon insertions are preserved. This also acts as spreader and prevents some deformities of toes. Preservation of base of proximal phalanx preserves metatarsal arch. A long plantar flap is created for partial amputation, so that scar will on the dorsal side away from pressure.

Complete amputation or disarticulation of a toe is done through racket shaped incision, with the straight part extending proximally up to neck of metatarsal. Skin is closed with nonabsorbable interrupted stitches.

Amputation in the Foot

Though amputation through the foot disrupts arch and affect walking to some extent, a shoe-filler prosthesis gives a good functional result. The common indications are trauma, diabetes and vascular disease. This can be done as transmetatarsal, tarsometartarsal (Lisfranc's) or midtarsal (Chopart's) amputations.

Whenever possible along volar flap is constructed. Interrupted skin stitches are kept for nearly two weeks. In diabetic gangrene, ray amputation, in which individual ray consisting of toe with its metatarsal can be excised. This heals up by secondary intention.

Amputation at the Ankle Joint

Amputation through ankle is rarely performed now a days, limb filters do not prefer this. Though this is end bearing, may develop painful stump ulcers.

The amputations through ankle are Syme's amputation, modified Syme's amputation and Pirogoff's amputation.

James Syme, Scottish surgeon, described his method in 1842. The incision starts below the tip of lateral malleolus and is carried to a point 2 cm below medial malleolus with a backward inclination. The two ends are then joined across the front by shortest possible line. All structures are divided down to bones. Dividing the anterior capsule the ankle joint is opened and after this lateral ligaments are cut. The ankle joint is dislocated gradually posterior ligaments, detachment of tendocalcaneous and dissection of calcaneous from heel flap are done. Preservation and protection of blood supply of heel flap is of utmost important. Parts of malleoli are removed from immediately above ankle joint. Wound is closed over drain with few interrupted stitches.

Modified Syme's amputation involves elliptical incision and division of the tibia and fibula slightly higher. In Pirogoff's modification, posterior part of calcaneum is retained in heel flap to get a longer stump.

Amputation Through Leg

Below Knee Amputation

This amputation is possibly the most common major amputation, done often. In about 80% of patients with ischemic gangrene, amputation at this level can be done successfully. Whenever possible amputation is done through middle third of leg. The ideal tibial stump length should be 14 cm but not less than 8 cm. Much work has been done on this amputation, including properly fitting prosthesis for rehabilitation. Many techniques have been described. All techniques take advantage of the fact that due to the presence of the large muscle mass posteriorly, posterior flap is relatively vascular and large posterior flap can be used to cover the end of the stump.

Applied Anatomy

Of the two bones, the major weight bearing bone is tibia, and somewhat posterolateral to this is fibula. Both are anchored by tough interosseous membrane in their deeper margins. Septae from other margins from both bones diverge to be attached to deep fascia to form four anatomical compartments, which contains muscles.

The anterior or extensor compartment in the upper part contains tibialis anterior, extensor hallucis longus and extensor digitorum longus. The lateral or peroneal compartments contain peroneus longus and brevis. The posterior or flexor compartment has two subdivisions, superficial and deep. The superficial muscles are gastrocnemius and immediately deep to its soleus. The deep muscles are flexor digitorum longus. Flexor hallucis longus and tibialis posterior.

The anterior tibial artery and nerve (deep peroneal nerve) lie on the anterior surface of interosseous membrane. The posterior artery or nerve lie in between the superficial and deep muscles of calf. The peroneal artery lies on the back of interosseous membrane close to fibula and superficial peroneal nerve lie deeply near fibula between the peroneal muscles. The long saphenous vein ascends up on the medial side and short saphenous vein on the posterior surface of leg.

Surgical Technique

The technique described by Ghormly in 1947 and popularized by EM Burgess (1981), uses a long posterior flap with calf muscles to cover the transected bones. In vascular disease tourniquet is not used (Fig. 101.1). The proposed level of bone section is marked with a marker pen. The short anterior flap is marked transversely about 1 cm distally (Fig. 101.2). The long posterior flap, almost one half-times the diameter of the leg is marked out from the ends of transverse anterior flap (Fig. 101.3).

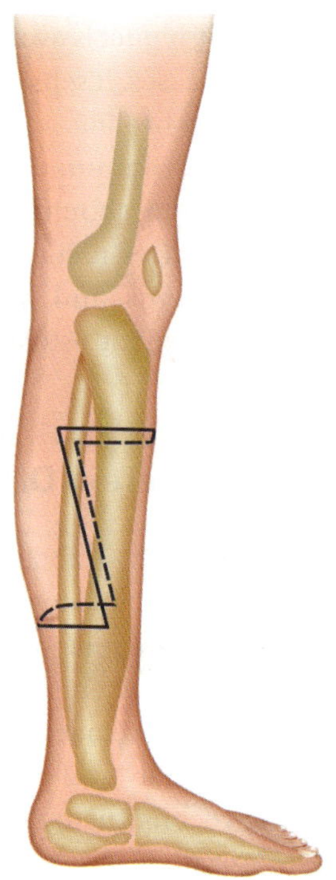

Fig. 101.1 Incision for below-knee amputation

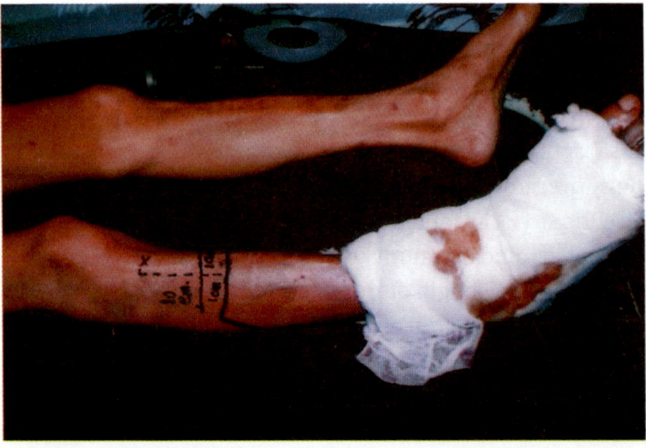

Fig. 101.2 Skin incision (anteriorly)

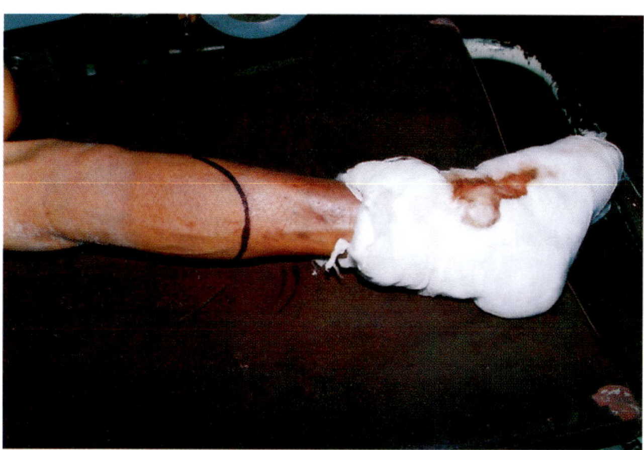

Fig. 101.3 Skin incision posteriorly

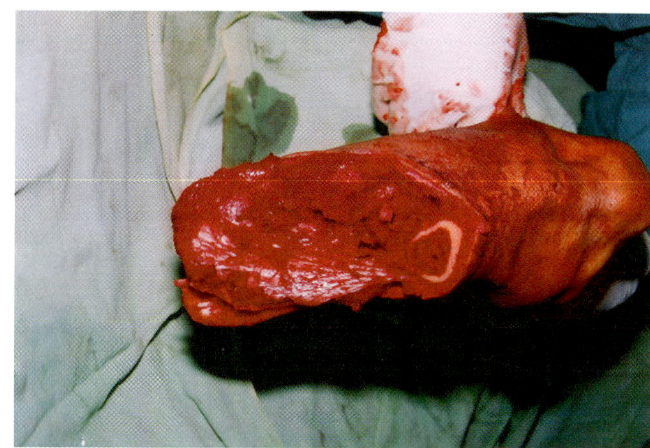

Fig. 101.4 Muscles of posterior flap

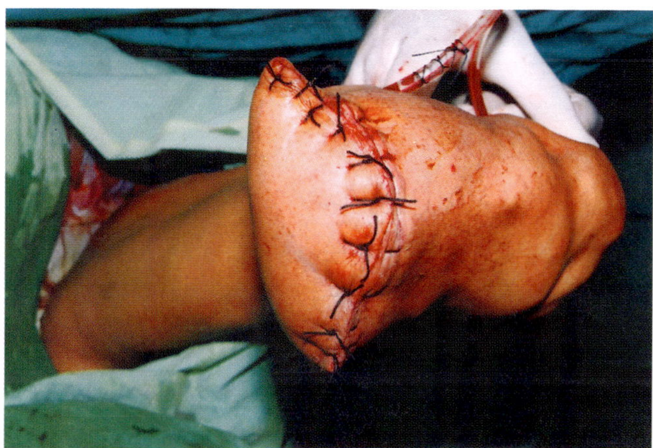

Fig. 101.5 Skin closure with suction drain

The anterior incision is deepened to divide the deep fascia and muscles. The anterior tibial vessels are ligated and divided. Periosteum from the exposed tibia is elevated for about 1 cm. A triangular piece of tibia is removed to avoid sharp anterior bony projection and tibia is divided with Gigli or power-saw.

Muscles are elevated from the fibula and interoseous membrane and fibula is divided 1 cm higher than tibia.

The posterior incision is deepened to expose muscles. The lower ends of the divided bones are retracted. Calf muscles are divided obliquely to the line of skin incision gradually. In the process, posterior tibial nerve and vessels are secured. Drain is usually used (Fig. 101.4).

Too bulky posterior flap due to muscles is to be avoided. Bone ends are rounded. Hemostasis is achieved. Deep fascia is closed with synthetic absorbable sutures. The skin is closed with nonabsorbable material in interrupted fashion with section drain (Fig. 101.5).

In skew-flap technique of below knee amputation, equal anteromedial and posterolateral flaps are raised and the suture line runs obliquely.

Postoperatively plaster of Paris cast may be used to avoid gradual flexion deformity. Drain can be taken out after 3 days and stitches are removed after 10 days.

Farabeuf's amputation through upper third of leg, the old site of election is obsolete now.

Amputation Through Knee Joint

In disarticulation through knee joint, unequal anterior and posterior or equal lateral and medial flaps may be used. This is not very popular. It leaves a large bulbous stump. It is difficult to level the knee center in prosthesis.

Supracondylar (Gritti-Stokes) amputation leaves a longer stump than above knee amputation. However, it is difficult to fit an internal knee mechanism in prosthesis. A long anterior flap with patella is constructed. Knee joint is dislocated by dividing ligamentum patellae. Femoral condyles and articular surface of patella are removed. Patella is then anchored to femoral end with wire.

Amputation Through Thigh

Amputation through thigh can be through lower, middle or upper third. Amputation in the lower thigh is called above-knee (AK) amputation.

Above-knee Amputation

Amputation through the lower third is called above-knee amputation some time. Ideally 25–30 cm of femur from tip

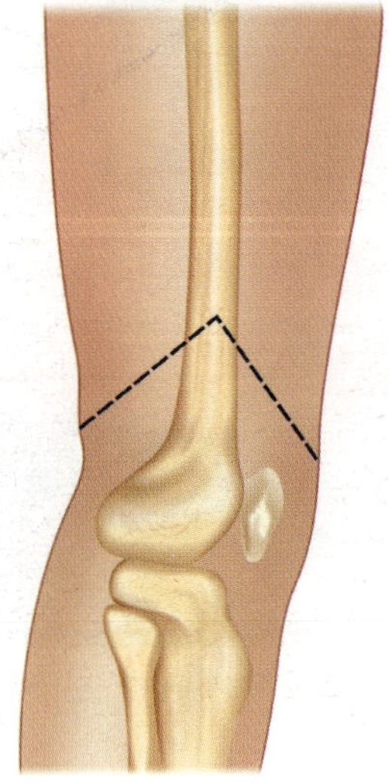

Fig. 101.6 Skin incision making equal flaps

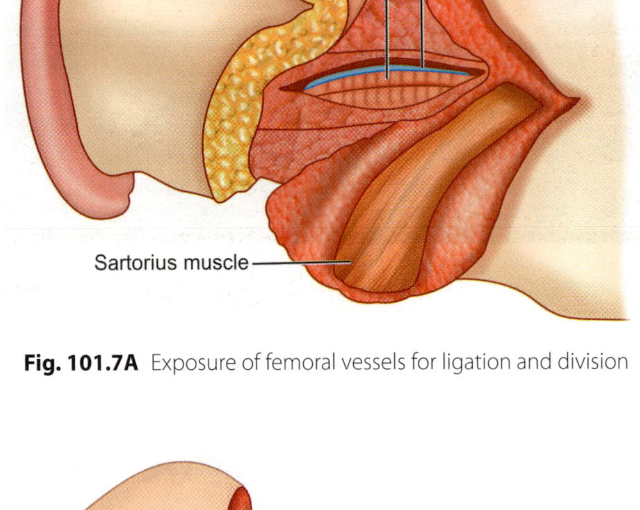

Fig. 101.7A Exposure of femoral vessels for ligation and division

of greater trochanter or 70% of the length of femur should be kept, which is about 8–10 cm from knee joint. This is done in trauma or when below-knee amputation is not possible. Prosthesis lies in total contact. Some weight is taken by ischial tuberosity. Strong muscles with femur acting as lever move the prosthetic limb.

Mark out equal anterolateral and posteromedial flaps by adequate skin incision (Fig. 101.6). The skin flaps are reflected proximally and muscles are divided. The sartorius and quadriceps are divided. The femoral vessels are identified beneath sartorius and doubly ligated with Silk (Fig. 101.7A). Medially the adducer muscles are divided. The posterior muscles are divided in same plane as anterior group. The sciatic nerve is dealt with in usual manner. The femur is divided with saw (Fig. 101.7B). The anterior and posterior group of muscles are sutured together (Fig. 101.7C). Flaps are stitched over a drain (Fig. 101.8).

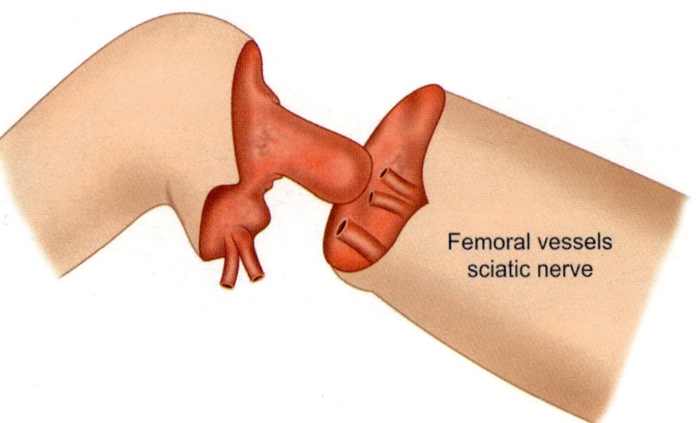

Fig. 101.7B Site of division of femur

Amputation (Disarticulation) at the Hip

This is required for trauma or tumors of thigh. Either single posterior flap method, which is better for prosthesis or anterior racquet method with handle at the line of femoral vessels can be used. In both methods, femoral vessels are carefully secured initially. Femoral nerves are divided. Anterior muscles are divided and hip joint is opened from the front. Adductors, gluteus and hamstrings are divided leaving some part. Obturator and gluteal vessels and sciatic nerve are dealt with gradually. The skin is closed over drain with interrupted sutures.

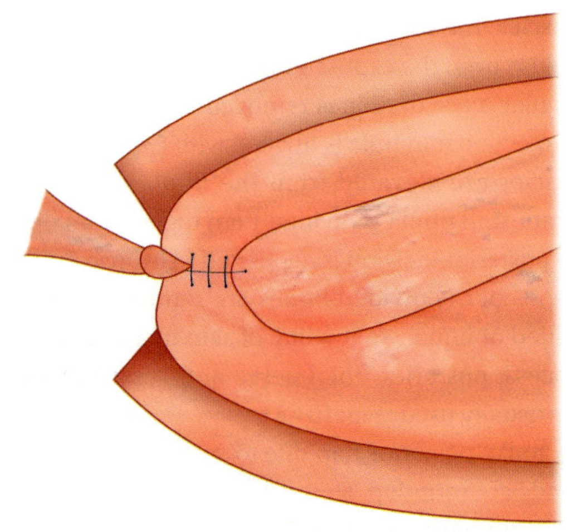

Fig. 101.7C Closure of muscles

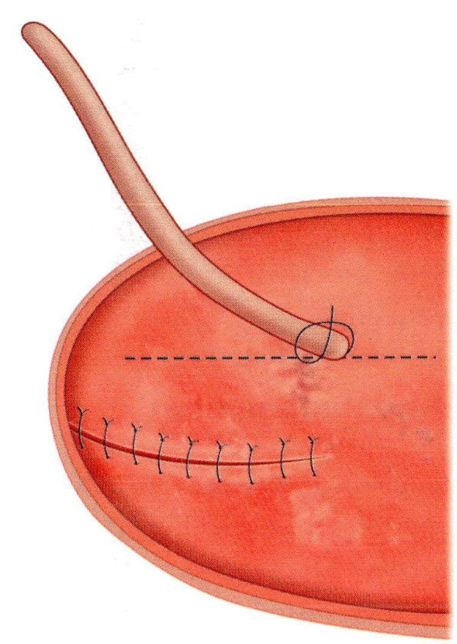

Fig. 101.8 Closure of skin with suction drain

Interinnomino–abdominal Amputation (Hind-Quarter)

This is performed for malignant growth of pelvic bones or upper thigh and trauma. It is relatively rarely practiced now a days. An elliptical incision is employed. The innominate bone with attached lower limb is removed. Important considerations are muscles attached to the pelvic bone, large vessels and nerves. Vascularity of posterior gluteal flap can ensured by preserving superior gluteal vessels.

AMPUTATION OF UPPER LIMB

Amputation in the Fingers and Hand

The most common indication for amputation through fingers or hand is injury. Other causes include infection, vascular diseases or tumors. The basic principles are to conserver as much as possible. Amputation through phalanx is preferable to disarticulation. This preserves attachment of flexor and extensor attachments. In addition to mobility of joints, dominant hand function and profession are also important considerations. Local flaps are preferred to split skin graft.

Amputation of terminal phalanx is started with a transverse incision at the dorsum 5–6 mm distal to amputation level and then creation of a long rectangular palmar flap. Once the bone is divided, palmar flap is folded upwards to stitch to dorsal skin with few-interrupted monofilament no absorbable stitches.

Amputation through middle and proximal phalanx is done by long or sole longer palmar flap. Digital vessels need to be secured. Middle phalanx should be preserved as much as possible. If half or more cannot be preserved in case of index or little finger, they should be shortened through metacarpal head obliquely.

To preserve palmar ligament of metacarpal arch and interossei muscles, amputation of middle and ring fingers are best done through the base of proximal phalanx with the creation of two lateral flaps. The digital vessels are ligated. The skin flaps falling together are closed with few interrupted stitches.

Disarticulation of metacarpophalangeal joint is done by racquet shaped incision over metacarpal neck. The flexor and extensor tendons, digital arteries, palmar ligament, collateral ligament and interosseous tendons need to be dealt with. In case of index or 5th finger, oblique excision of heads can be done, without disturbing metacarpal arch.

As much as possible, the thumb should be preserved. Even reconstruction, re-implantation or grafting procedures should be considered as thumb function is preeminent. Removal of bone is kept to minimum and flaps are made from available skin.

In case of hand as much as possible should be preserved. No formal amputation is necessary. Even if the fingers or metacarpals are lost, palm of hand can be useful for opposition. In manual workers, metacarpal heads give a broad palm and grip.

Disarticulation at the Wrist Joint

This is rarely practiced. Amputation through lower part of forearm is preferred as pronation or supination cannot be transmitted to artificial limb.

Amputation through the Forearm

The site of election is 16–20 cm from the tip of olecranon, the minimum length is 8 cm, when it is done in upper forearm it is called below-elbow amputation. Circular incision or equal dorsal and volar flaps are used in distal forearm. In proximal procedures flaps can be constructed.

Krukenberg Amputation

In bilateral loss of arms, this method can be done at one side. Separation of radius and ulna distally provides crude grasp and pincer function.

Disarticulation at the Elbow Joint

It is not done commonly. It leaves a bulbous or club-shaped end. Depending on the local condition, flap, racquet, oval or circular method can be applied. Along with muscles, tendons and capsule of joint, brachial artery and median, ulnar and radial nerves need to be dealt with.

Amputation through Arm

20 cm stump from tip of acromion is the optimum length. At this level, it is called above-elbow amputation. Above this level much as possible should be kept. Flap, curcular or elliptical method can be employed. Principal structures encountered are muscles (biceps, brachialis, coracobrachialis, triceps), vessels (cephalic vein, brachial artery) and nerves (median, ulnar, radial and musculocutaneous). Bone is divided with power or Gigli saw. This amputation and amputation through upper arm preserve shoulder contour.

Amputation at the Shoulder (Disarticulation)

Spence described the method in 1856. The handle or racquet incision starting near coracoids process passes downwards along arm and encircles arm at the level of axillary fold. The dissection starts at the handle. Which is continued distally. Abduction and rotation facilitate dissection. Anterosuperior capsule is divided first. Early dealing with brachial vessels and nerves is helpful.

Interscapulo-thoracic Amputation (Fore-Quarter)

The indication of this mutilating operation is malignancy. This can be done, preferably by classic anterior approach advocated by Berger (1887) or by posterior approach of Littlewood. This operation removes upper limb with scapula and lateral two-thirds of clavicle. Anterior horizontal part of incision is placed just above the medial two-thirds of clavicle. At the lateral end, anterior limb of incision passes obliquely downwards over clavicle, coracoids process, middle of axillary fold to the inferior angle of scapula. Posterior limb is created by continuing the above incision upwards across the scapula and supraclavicular fossa to meet the bifurcation. At the outset, anterior dissection is done to divide the clavicle and control of axillary-subclavian vessels and brachial plexus. Pectorals are then divided. Posterior dissection is then carried up to the medial border of scapula. Division of attached muscles of scapula to trunk (trapezius, latissimus dorsi, levator scapulae, serratus anterior) complete the major part of operation.

Preoperative Preparation

In trauma patient, correction of hypovolemia with fluid and electrolytes and blood is necessary. In proximal amputations blood transfusion may be needed, as bleeding can be more than expected. Appropriate prophylaxis for tetanus or gas gangrene is to be kept in mind. Associated injuries will need appropriate care. Diabetes control is extremely important. Prophylactic antibiotics and analgesia will be chosen on the basis of clinical circumstances. In vascular disease, cardiac status should be assessed. Antiplatelet or thrombolytic therapy needs attention.

Postoperative Management

Most of the preoperative measures are to be continued in the postoperative period. As the healing progresses and gradual recovery takes place, supportive and treatment measures need to be modified or reduced accordingly. Analgesia is of prime importance in this phase, initially intravenous or intramuscular and later on orally. Rest and immobilization of proximal joint during the period of initial healing can be helpful in some case. Psychotherapy can be a useful adjunct. In early postoperative period, back care should be directed to prevent formation of bed store.

Wound inspection starts at about third day and continues at regular intervals. Through in most cases drain can be removed on third postoperative day, it may need to stay longer in some. In infective cases, early removal of few stitches may be necessary to drain local collection.

In lower limb with normal blood supply stitches are removed in 12–14 days. In arterial disease, stitches may have to be left up to 3 weeks.

Early physiotherapy and exercises of the limb may be started, once the pain settles and acute complications are unlikely to arise, usually by the end of a week. Walking with aids and assistance, gradual weight bearing, trial prosthesis and consideration of rehabilitation will come into play gradually. Pneumatic postamputation mobility (PAM) can be applied after a week. Here pneumatic bag is inflated to act as socket. Gradually less emphasis is put on bandaging.

Complications

A brief account of possible complications, related to amputation, is listed below.

Reactionary hemorrhage—in the immediate postoperative period.

Hematoma formation—due to improper hemostasis or inadequate drain.

Secondary infection—antibiotics, avoidance of hematoma formation and ischemia, adequate drainage—can reduce this.

Secondary hemorrhage—due to infection.

Ischemic flap necrosis—due to suturing under tension, wrong level selection or improper assessment of flap vascularity.

Delayed healing—may be due to infection, diabetes, malnutrition, uremia.

Pain—due to operation or primary disease. Low dose, less potent or less frequent analgesic medicines.

Causalgia—due to sympathetic nerve growth.

Phantom limb and phantom pain—due to persistence of image of limb in sensory cortex.

Osteomyelitis—due to spread of infection to bone.

Spurs and Osteophytes—careful division of bone is necessary

Scar-adherent or uncomfortable, ulceration of the stump—due to infection and ischemia

Thickened lymph edematous skin, eczema, fungal infection—due to poor ventilation and hygiene.

Sebaceous cyst, implantation dermoid—due to pressure

Stump neuroma—failure to divide nerve high enough

Adventitious bursa—due to poor fitting socket

Jactitation and tremor—intermittent spasms due to imbalance between synergists and antagonists.

Aneurysms and arteriovenous fistula—fare complication due to improper dealing with blood vessels.

Fixed flexion deformity and stiffness—due to inadequate pain relief, failure to provide cast support or inadequate physiotherapy

Muscle herniation—due to gap in deep fascia or slipping from bone end

Nonunion—in Gritti-Stokes, between patella and femur

Psychological depression—due to loss of functional part or even job

Failure to use prosthesis—due to lack of physical, mental capability and determination.

Rehabilitation and Prostheses

Early physiotherapy is almost an essential step in the proper rehabilitation of an amputee in both lower and upper limb amputations. Measurement and assessment of stump by a prosthetist should start in the early postoperative period.

In lower limb amputee, early use of wheelchair should be taught. Walking with stick, crutches, walking frame or between parallel bars is useful to gain confidence.

If the healing is good, in trauma patients with normal vascularity, partial weight hearing can be allowed by the end of second week, which can be increased progressively. In vascular disease, it should be started later. The use of early walking aids, like modified pylons rocker, foot and knee hinge with side lock has also been recommended.

In the early weeks after amputation, the stump is bulky due edema. This undergoes gradual shrinkage, which can be enhanced by pneumatic prosthesis. The stump can take up to 3 months for maturation. During this time elastic net sock can before useful than bandaging. As a preparatory measure, it is better to provide simple removable temporary prosthesis initially. Definitive permanent prosthesis, which may expensive, is provided later.

In lower limb, BK amputation, it can be advantageous, if a temporary prosthesis with well-fitted total-contact socket and an endoskeletal pylon, having adjustment facility and an attached solid ankle cushion heel (SACH) foot is advised. The socket can be changed to align the prosthesis according to the need and gait pattern, total contact patellar tendon bearing plastic socket with attached SACH foot is used often. The artificial limb is suspended by circumferential strap at supracondylar level. Light-weight carbon fiber modular prostheses are now available.

In above knee amputee, prosthetic knee can be used. The limb is suspended by waist belt or by suction socket with negative pressure.

Older classification of end bearing or side bearing prosthesis are not followed rigidly as our understandings are much more clear and technology is more advanced.

In upper extremity amputations, early prosthesis helps to maintain cortical representation, which may be lost early otherwise. Therapy in arm training school is essential, for it needs much longer rehabilitation. Movement can be initiated from scapular or shoulder muscles. Expensive myoelectric prostheses with electrical signals from stump muscles are also available. Biomechanical principles are applied here.

As certain degree of functional loss is inevitable in amputation, change of profession is to be considered in many cases.

Prosthesis

Prosthesis is used to replace a missing limb or its part, in an attempt to restore and provide function. Ideal prosthesis should be similar to the missing part.

Prosthesis has five basic components. These are socket, body, harness or suspension system, control system and terminal device. In upper extremity, in terminal device might be purely cosmetic without control mechanism, body powered hooks or externally powered hooks, prosthesis may be exoskeletal with a tube like outer shell or endoskeletal with inner central road like structure.

Prognosis

Half the patients undergoing BK amputation can use artificial usefully.

The operative mortality for isolated tumor, trauma or infection is about 3%. In atherosclerosis, this increases by two-fold to 6%. The mortality increases with more proximal amputations. The causes of death are cardiac in half and lung in quarter of cases.

In BK amputation for vascular diseases 70–80% heal by primary union. In vascular disease, about 1/3rd will die in 2 years and 2/3rd will die in five years. In vascular disease one in 10 will need amputation of the other limb in every year or so.

In malignancy grade and stage of the primary disease with spread, affect prognosis significantly. In other case, primary disease affects the overall prognosis and survival.

CONCLUSION

Amputation is a mutilating operation with loss of a limb or part of it. If primary disease can be recognized early, its treatment can reduce the need for amputation. Modern life style increases the incidence of high blood pressure, diabetes and hyperlipidemia, which are responsible for many vascular diseases. Lifestyle modification may reduce this type of disease-related amputations.

In accident victims, early and expert treatments with reconstructive, microvascular or reimplantation surgery may salvage limbs in some.

Even when the amputation inevitable modern occupational and physical medicine helps in rehabilitation phychological counseling, prosthesis replacements or even occupational change helps the amputee considerably.

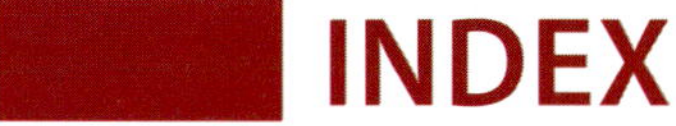

INDEX

Page numbers followed by *f* refer to figure and *t* refer to table.

G

H

U

V

W

X